T0382646

Fetal Medicine

Advanced Skills Series

Fetal Medicine

Edited by

Bidyut Kumar, MD FRCOG

Consultant Obstetrician and Gynaecologist, Wrexham Maelor Hospital, Betsi Cadwaladr University Health Board, Wrexham, North Wales, Honorary Lecturer, Cardiff University, and Honorary Senior Lecturer, School of Healthcare Studies, Bangor University, Gwynedd, Wales, UK

Zarko Alfirevic, MD FRCOG

Professor of Fetal and Maternal Medicine and Head of Department of Women's and Children's Health at the University of Liverpool and Honorary Consultant Obstetrician at Liverpool Women's Hospital, UK

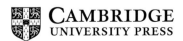

CAMBRIDGE
UNIVERSITY PRESS

CAMBRIDGE
UNIVERSITY PRESS

University Printing House, Cambridge CB2 8BS, United Kingdom

Cambridge University Press is part of the University of Cambridge.

It furthers the University's mission by disseminating knowledge in the pursuit of education, learning and research at the highest international levels of excellence.

www.cambridge.org
Information on this title: www.cambridge.org/9781107064348

© Cambridge University Press 2016

First published 2016

Printed in the United Kingdom by Clays, St Ives plc

A catalogue record for this publication is available from the British Library

Library of Congress Cataloguing in Publication data
Names: Kumar, Bidyut, editor. | Alfirevic, Zarko, editor.
Title: Fetal medicine / edited by Bidyut Kumar, Zarko Alfirevic. Other titles: Fetal medicine (Kumar) |
Advanced skills series. Description: Cambridge; New York : Cambridge University Press, 2016. |
Series: Advanced skills series | Includes bibliographical references and index.
Identifiers: LCCN 2015046515 | ISBN 9781107064348 (hardback) Subjects: |
MESH: Fetal Diseases–diagnosis | Fetal Monitoring | Fetus–physiology | Abortion, Induced |
Pregnancy, Multiple Classification: LCC RG627 | NLM WQ 211 | DDC 618.3/2–dc23
LC record available at http://lccn.loc.gov/2015046515

ISBN 978-1-107-06434-8 Hardback

Additional resources for this publication at www.cambridge.org/9781107064348

....

Contents

Contents

List of contributors

Umber Agarwal MRCOG
Department of Fetal and Maternal Medicine,
Liverpool Women's Hospital, Liverpool, UK

Zarko Alfirevic MD FRCOG
Centre for Women's Health Research and
University of Liverpool Department of Obstetrics
and Gynaecology, Liverpool Women's Hospital,
Liverpool, UK

R. Bryan Beattie MD FRCOG
Department of Fetal Medicine, University Hospital
Wales, Cardiff, UK

Amarnath Bhide MD FRCOG
Fetal Medicine Unit, Blackshaw Road, London, UK

Leanne Bricker FRCOG
Fetal Medicine Unit, Corniche Hospital, Abu
Dhabi, UAE

Lyn S. Chitty PhD MRCOG
Genetics and Genomic Medicine, UCL Institute of
Child Health; Great Ormond Street Hospital for
Children NHS Foundation Trust, and Fetal Medicine
Unit, University College London Hospitals NHS
Foundation Trust, London, UK

Thomas R. Everett BSc MB BS MD
Fetal Medicine Unit, University College London
Hospitals NHS Foundation Trust, London, UK

Alan Fryer MD FRCP FRCPCH
Department of Clinical Genetics, Liverpool Women's
NHS Foundation Trust, Liverpool, UK

Manish Gupta BSc MRCP MRCOG
Department of Obstetrics and Gynaecology, Whipps
Cross University Hospital, London, UK

Mark D. Kilby DSc MD FRCOG FRCPI
Department of Fetal Medicine, Birmingham
Women's Hospital, Birmingham, UK and the Centre
for Women's and Children's Health, University of
Birmingham, Birmingham, UK

Bidyut Kumar MD FRCOG
Department of Obstetrics and
Gynaecology, Wrexham Maelor Hospital,
Wrexham, UK

Geeta Kumar MD FRCOG
Department of Obstetrics and
Gynaecology, Wrexham Maelor Hospital,
Wrexham, UK

R. Katie Morris PhD MRCOG
Birmingham Centre for Women and Children's
Health, University of Birmingham, Birmingham
Women's Hospital, Birmingham, UK

Kristina Naidoo BMedSci MRCOG
St Mary's Hospital, Manchester, UK

Manju Nair MD MRCOG
Department of Obstetrics and Gynaecology, Royal
Gwent Hospital, Newport, UK

Kate Navaratnam MRCOG
Centre for Women's Health Research and
University of Liverpool Department of Obstetrics
and Gynaecology, Liverpool Women's Hospital,
Liverpool, UK

Ezechi Cally Nwosu FRCOG
Department of Obstetrics and Gynaecology, St
Helens and Knowsley Teaching Hospital NHS Trust,
Prescot, UK

Gianluigi Pilu MD
Department of Obstetrics and Gynaecology,
University of Bologna, Italy

Ashis Sau MD FRCOG
Department of Obstetrics and Gynaecology,
University Hospital Lewisham, London, UK

Neil J. Sebire MD DRCOG FRCPath
Department of Histopathology, Great Ormond Street
Hospital, London, UK

Andrew Sharp BSc PhD MRCOG
Centre for Women's Health Research, Liverpool
Women's Hospital, Liverpool, UK

Ai-Wei Tang MRCOG
Department of Fetal Medicine, Liverpool Women's
NHS Foundation Trust, Liverpool, UK

Fred Usakov MD
Fetal Medicine Unit, University College London
Hospitals NHS Foundation Trust, London, UK

Orhan Uzun MR FRCP
Division of Paediatric Cardiology, University Hospital
Wales, Cardiff, UK

Preface

The practice of fetal medicine has seen many significant advances over the last decade or so. Those that come to mind are the introduction of non-invasive screening for Down syndrome, the ability to diagnose and appropriately counsel more complex fetal abnormalities, better understanding of the role of fetal Doppler studies in the areas of growth restriction and red cell allo-immunisation and the rapidly expanding indications for fetoscopic and open fetal therapy.

To appropriately train the future generation of fetal medicine specialists, the Royal College of Obstetricians and Gynaecologists (RCOG) has prescribed a curriculum for subspecialty training for those super specialists who will be based in tertiary referral centres, acting as the hubs in the so-called 'hub and spoke' model of clinical network system of healthcare service provision. In any such system a vital role is played by the specialists that form the spokes of this system. Most of them will be based in district hospitals; they will carry out the job of a general obstetrician and gynaecologist but harbour and maintain a special interest in the discipline of fetal medicine.

The RCOG's advanced training skills module (ATSM) in fetal medicine aims to educate and train such specialists. When we planned to write this book, our intention was to create a one-stop source of knowledge for the ATSM in fetal medicine. We enlisted the authorship of renowned experts and wanted to contain the depth and breadth of their knowledge, expecting them to focus on the ATSM syllabus. However, as readers will testify, on many occasions we were unsuccessful in curbing their enthusiasm and desire to share their vast knowledge and clinical experience. We do hope that the end result, although aimed primarily at those who wish to complete the ATSM in fetal medicine, will also serve as a ready source of knowledge in the day-to-day work of many fully trained practitioners who have a special interest in this area.

This book draws on knowledge acquired from our many successes, but also provides lessons from those clinical episodes that did not go according to plan. If this book helps readers to avoid those clinical errors which we have made, then our effort as editors will have been worthwhile.

We thank all the authors for their dedication in writing their chapters and going through the laborious process of both responding to our editorial queries and proofreading their own work. We acknowledge the tireless help and effective support of the staff at John Spalding Library, Wrexham Maelor Hospital, in their timely assistance with online searches and provision of copies of required published material.

Before we conclude, we must thank our patients, who have been the biggest source of education and learning, and without whom this book would be both impossible to compile and rendered purposeless.

Bidyut Kumar
Zarko Alfirevic
January 2016

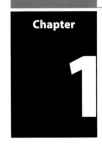

Chapter

1

Genetics of fetal anomalies

Alan Fryer

The counseling of families with known or possible genetic disorders is discussed in Chapter 2. In this chapter, two important preliminary questions are addressed:

- what types of genetic disorders are there and how do they arise?
- what methods are available for diagnosing them?

Types and classification of genetic disorders

The unit of inheritance is the gene and there are an estimated 21,000 protein-encoding genes in the human genome. These genes are arranged on 23 pairs of chromosomes (22 autosomes and one pair of sex chromosomes) in the nucleus of the cell. In addition, there are 37 genes in each of the thousands of mitochondria in each cell. These genes are arranged in a circular structure and their products all have a function within mitochondria in oxidative phosphorylation. The replication of mitochondrial genes is controlled by the products of nuclear genes.

Whilst each somatic cell contains the same genes, within each tissue some genes will be expressed and others will be silenced. The control of gene expression is a complex process and errors in this process can result in cellular malfunction. Alterations in gene expression may be caused by various factors that are not yet fully understood but are not (in many situations) due to alterations in the structure of the genes themselves, and hence are termed "epigenetic" changes.

Disorders due to alterations (mutations) in chromosomes and genes can thus be classified as follows.

Constitutional chromosome disorders

Numerical abnormalities

In these cases, instead of 46 chromosomes per cell, the actual number of chromosomes may be reduced or increased in number. This numerical imbalance may be present in all cells examined or just in a proportion ("mosaicism"). Where mosaicism is present, the percentage of abnormal cells may vary from tissue to tissue.

Structural abnormalities

In this situation, there may be the correct number of chromosomes, but one or more chromosomes may be structurally abnormal and have segments deleted or duplicated, or there may be complex inter- or intrachromosomal rearrangements, such as translocations, inversions, insertions, etc. These complex rearrangements may lead to the disruption of the function of genes and hence be "unbalanced," or alternatively they may not alter function and be "balanced" rearrangements.

Single-gene disorders

Mutations in individual genes within the nucleus (which may lead to loss or gain of function) can be of sufficient effect as to result in phenotypes that follow Mendelian patterns of inheritance. Mendelian disorders may be classified by their pattern of inheritance:

- Autosomal dominant conditions, e.g. Huntington's disease (HD), neurofibromatosis types 1 and 2, tuberous sclerosis, adult polycystic kidney disease, etc.
- Autosomal recessive conditions, e.g. cystic fibrosis (CF), hemoglobinopathies, spinal muscular atrophy, congenital adrenal hyperplasia, etc.

Fetal Medicine, ed. Bidyut Kumar and Zarko Alfirevic. Published by Cambridge University Press. © Cambridge University Press 2016.

- X-linked disorders (usually X-linked recessive), e.g. Duchenne muscular dystrophy (DMD), hemophilia A and B, Fragile X syndrome, etc.

Some disorders may follow more than one pattern of inheritance. For example, there are autosomal dominant, autosomal recessive and X-linked forms of retinitis pigmentosa, the most common inherited form of visual impairment. There are also a few examples of disorders that in some families result from mutations in two separate genes ("digenic inheritance"); examples include some cases of Bardet–Biedl syndrome and retinitis pigmentosa. In these cases of digenic inheritance, it is likely that the genes involved encode proteins that act in the same cellular pathway. Counseling families with nuclear gene disorders is discussed in detail in Chapter 2.

In addition to the nuclear genes, there are 37 mitochondrial genes. Mitochondrial DNA (mtDNA) gene mutations, such as those that account for Leber's optic neuropathy and some mitochondrial myopathy syndromes e.g. mitochondrial disease-encephalopathy (MELAS), lactic acidosis and stroke-like episodes, myoclonic epilepsy-ragged red fibres (MERRF) and neurogenic weakness, ataxia, retinitis pigmentosa (NARP), do not follow Mendelian patterns as mitochondria are exclusively inherited via the oocyte. Therefore, a woman who carries a mitochondrial gene mutation will theoretically transmit that mutation to all of her offspring, whereas a man carrying a mitochondrial gene mutation will not transmit the disorder to any of his offspring. It must also be noted that each human cell contains thousands of copies of mtDNA. A mutation may be present in only some of the mitochondrial genomes. This situation is termed "heteroplasmy." If the mutation is present in all of the mitochondrial genomes in the cell, then there is "homoplasmy." Prenatal genetic testing and interpretation of test results for mtDNA disorders are difficult because of mtDNA heteroplasmy. The percentage level of mutant mtDNA in a chorionic villus sampling (CVS) biopsy may not reflect the percentage level of mutant mtDNA in other fetal tissues, and the percentage level may change during development and throughout life; therefore, for most heteroplasmic mtDNA mutations, prenatal diagnosis is not recommended. However, the mutations m.8993T>G and m.8993T>C (typically but not always associated with a NARP phenotype) show a more even tissue distribution and successful prenatal diagnosis has been achieved. In the situation of homoplasmy, the mutation will be transmitted to all offspring.

In addition to mtDNA point mutations, mtDNA deletions and duplications occur, which usually arise de novo. The risk of transmission of an mtDNA deletion from an affected woman is low and estimated at 4%[1].

Multifactorial disease

Many conditions, including many congenital abnormalities, are more common among family members but the pattern in families does not follow Mendelian inheritance. The familial pattern is due to the combined effect of a number of gene variants interacting with each other and with the environment. The number of predisposing gene alterations may be few (oligogenic) or many (polygenic) and risk of occurrence of a disease cannot be calculated accurately from simple principles and as such, recurrence risk counseling is based on empiric data.

Somatic genetic diseases

Many disorders (such as all cancers) are due to mutations or an accumulation of mutations in somatic cells. In this situation, gonadal cells are not involved and the disorders are not heritable.

Epigenetic disorders

Epigenetic factors are noninherited changes in the DNA (e.g., methylation of certain DNA bases) or in the folding or position of the chromatin within the nucleus, which do not affect the sequence of bases in a gene but influence its expression (i.e., whether it is switched on or off). A small percentage of genes (probably less than 1%) are only expressed on either the paternally derived or the maternally derived chromosome – these are said to carry a paternal or maternal "imprint." In Prader–Willi syndrome (PWS), for example, the genes responsible on chromosome 15 are only expressed on their paternal copies (the copies on the chromosome inherited from the child's mother are "switched off"). If a mutation (usually a deletion) affects the paternally derived genes, then no copies of these genes will be expressed and an abnormal phenotype results. This same result can occur if the child has two maternal copies of chromosome 15 and no paternal copy (a situation known as "maternal uniparental disomy"). For the large majority of the genome, uniparental disomy (two copies present) of paternal or maternal chromosomes or chromosome regions has no phenotypic effect, but if the chromosome region contains "imprinted" genes, a phenotype may result. Other well-known imprinting disorders are Angelman syndrome and Beckwith–Wiedemann syndrome (BWS). In the above example of PWS, the phenotype results from silencing of genes that should be expressed. In other disorders, the phenotype may result from expression of genes that are normally silenced. Altered methylation of DNA underpins many of these conditions. In BWS, the cause of the loss or gain of methylation is usually unknown but not heritable.

Structure of the genome

Chromosome structure

Genetic material consists of DNA that is packaged into 46 chromosomes in humans. This packaging is achieved by complexing the DNA with DNA-binding proteins called histones. This complex of DNA and histones is termed "chromatin." For each autosome, there is disomy in each DNA-containing cell apart from the gametes, which should contain one copy of each autosome and one sex chromosome. Normally in each somatic cell, one copy of each autosomal gene has come from the father ("paternal allele") and one from the mother ("maternal allele"), with the term "allele" simply meaning an alternative form of the same gene. There are about 21,000 protein-encoding genes located on these 46 chromosomes. Other genes encode various RNA species, and mutations in these genes can cause genetic disease, but for the purposes of this chapter we shall only consider the protein-encoding genes.

DNA is a double-stranded molecule made of four nucleotides or bases: adenine (a purine base that pairs with thymine on the opposite strand), thymine (a pyrimidine base that pairs with adenine), guanine (a purine base that pairs with cytosine) and cytosine (a pyrimidine base that pairs with guanine), which are usually referred to by their initial letters – A, T, G and C. These bases are bonded to each other in each DNA strand by strong phosphodiester bonds, whereas the bonds that hold together the double helix are hydrogen bonds, which are weak electrostatic bonds.

Gene structure and function

Figure 1.1 illustrates three important processes in molecular biology, i.e., DNA *replication*, *transcription* of the DNA code into RNA and the *translation* of the RNA code into a polypeptide/protein molecule. When cells divide, the DNA has to replicate itself (a process requiring substrate and DNA polymerases), and this

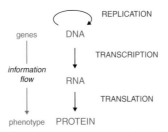

Figure 1.1 The classical paradigm of Mendelian genetics – genes encode proteins.

TRANSLATION and the GENETIC CODE

The genetic code is a TRIPLET CODE

Groups of 3 bases (TRIPLETS or "codons") specify one amino acid, e.g.

DNA	RNA	protein
ATG	AUG	methionine M
AAA	AAA	lysine K
TCC	UCC	serine S
CAG	CAG	glutamine Q

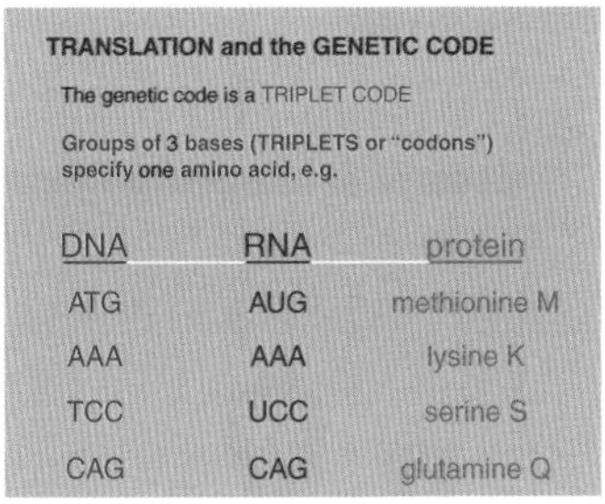

Figure 1.2 Translation and the genetic code: The diagram shows four codons with their DNA and RNA sequences and the amino acid that they encode; each amino acid is represented by a letter. The genetic code is "degenerate" with, on average, each amino acid specified by about three different codons.

process results in copy errors or mutations. We shall return to this later in the chapter. One of the two DNA strands (the template strand) serves as a template for RNA synthesis; the RNA strand produced (requiring an RNA polymerase enzyme) is complementary to the template strand and has the same base sequence (except that uracil replaces thymine) as the opposite, nontemplate strand.

With regard to protein synthesis, the genetic code is a triplet code: many triplets (or groups of three bases or "codons") encode amino acids (examples given in Figure 1.2) but one triplet (AUG) is a start codon and there are three stop codons (UAA, UAG and UGA).

The sequence of bases in the DNA strands does not form one continuous "read-out." The sections of the gene that will encode the protein molecule reside within "exons" and the intervening DNA segments are termed "introns." During transcription, all the exons and introns are transcribed, but then the RNA molecule is modified so that the intron sequences are "spliced out" and the molecule has other modifications made to it (a methyl cap – a methylated guanosine molecule – on the 5' end and poly-A tail on 3' end) before a mature messenger RNA (mRNA) molecule is produced as illustrated in Figure 1.3.

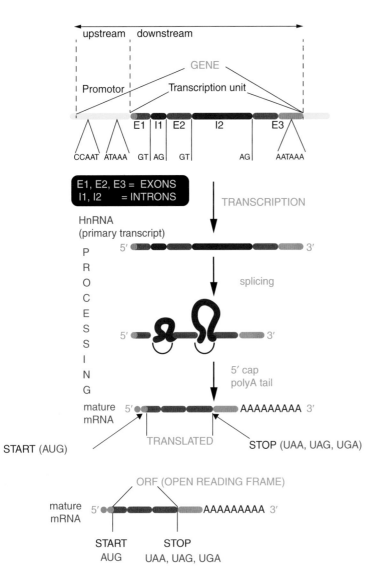

Figure 1.3 (a) The stylized gene template strand has three exons (E1, 2 and 3) and two introns (I1 and I2). Exon 1 contains the 5′ untranslated region (UTR) and exon 3 contains the 3′ UTR. Transcription produces an RNA molecule that is then modified to produce mRNA.
(b) A mature mRNA molecule. The open reading frame lies between the start and stop codons. Exon sequences also contain the 5′ and 3′ UTRs.

Translation takes place on the ribosomes in the cytoplasm, with transfer RNA acting as an adaptor between each amino acid and its codon.

Genome organization

Only approximately 1% of our DNA is comprised of protein-encoding exons (some exons/parts of exons encode untranslated regions). However, we now recognize that an additional (approximate) 15% of the human genome is functional, i.e., controls the expression of protein-encoding genes in different cells and at different developmental stages. These regulatory elements include promoters, enhancers, insulators and silencers etc., which provide exquisite control of gene expression. A pseudogene is a DNA sequence that is very similar to that of a functional gene but is itself nonfunctional. Long interspersed nuclear elements are a class of repetitive DNA sequences, and long terminal repeats are low copy number repeats. Figure 1.4 summarizes the complexity of the genome.

As is clear from Figure 1.4, there is an abundance of repetitive DNA within the genome. Throughout the genome, large deletions or duplications often seem to result from nonhomologous recombination between direct repeat sequences (unequal exchange between repeats on homologous chromosomes or sister chromatids), as illustrated in Figure 1.5.

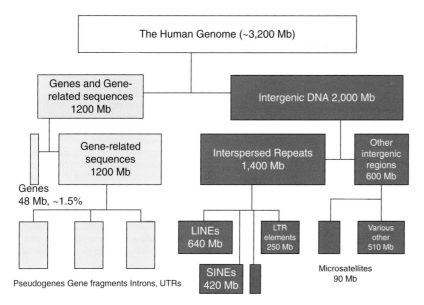

Figure 1.4 The structure of the genome.

The exon sequences or "exome" (labeled "genes" in the diagram) account for only 1.5% of the total cellular DNA. Over 80% of the genes in the exome currently have no known role in disease. LINEs, long interspersed nuclear element; LTR, long terminal repeats; SINEs, short interspersed nuclear element; UTRs, untranslated regions.

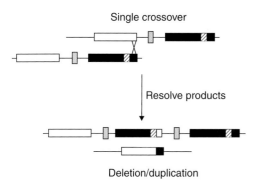

Figure 1.5 Misalignment and recombination between homologous chromosomes leading to deletion/duplication. The white and black boxes have very similar sequences and there is a gene in between (grey box). If the white and black boxes mispair at meiosis so that the white box pairs with the black box and a recombination (crossover) event occurs as shown, the resultant chromosome will contain either a deletion of the gene sequence (no grey box) or a duplication (two grey boxes).

Figure reproduced from Blanco P, Shlumukova M, Sargent CA, Jobling MA, Affara N, Hurles ME. *J Med Genet* 2000; 37: 752–8. With kind permission of BMJ Publishing.

Types of mutation

Large-scale rearrangements

- Deletions and duplications
- Inversions and insertions

For some disorders, these types of mutations are common mutational mechanisms. Deletions and duplications may involve part of, or the whole of, a gene. For

example, in DMD and Becker muscular dystrophy, approximately 66% of cases are due to deletions of one or more exons of the dystrophin gene and in type 1 spinal muscular atrophy, 95% of cases have a homozygous deletion of the *SMN1* gene. Large deletions of several genes are often mediated by repeated sequences and result in several well-known microdeletion syndromes, e.g. DiGeorge syndrome (22q11 deletion) and Williams' syndrome. One of the best-known duplication syndromes is hereditary motor and sensory neuropathy type 1A, which is due to a duplication of the *PMP22* gene on chromosome 17. One of the best examples of an inversion mutation is in hemophilia A, where 50% of severe cases are due to an intron 22 inversion (Figure 1.6).

Point mutations

- Base substitutions
- Small insertions /deletions

These point mutations can result in a variety of possible consequences, as illustrated in Figure 1.7. A nonsense mutation results in the generation of a stop codon, which would terminate protein translation. In the example in Figure 1.7, the conversion of C to T results in production of TGA that is transcribed into UGA in mRNA, which encodes a stop codon. Such mutations are therefore usually pathogenic. Similarly, the frameshift mutation illustrated by the deletion of one cytosine residue results in the production of a downstream stop codon (UAA). Mutations in splice sites can

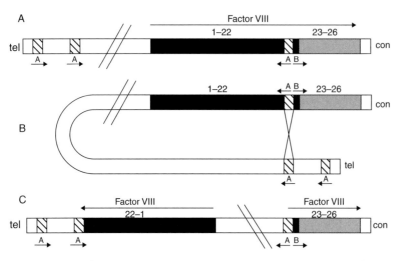

Figure 1.6 Intron 22 inversion in the factor VIII gene as a major cause of severe hemophilia A.

(a) The factor VIII gene is represented as a black box (exons and introns 1–22) and a grey box (exons and introns 23–26). A repetitive sequence "A" (hatched box) in intron 22 of the factor VIII gene is present in two additional copies 360 kb and 435 kb "upstream" of the gene. The arrows represent the relative orientations of the three copies of "A."
(b) During male meiosis, this part of the X chromosome has no pairing partner and the repetitive sequences "A" may pair, forming a loop. The repetitive segments are orientated in the same direction. A crossover can occur as indicated.
(c) A crossover has occurred. This causes an inversion of the black box segment (exons 1–22) and totally disrupts the gene structure.

Figure reproduced from Purandare SM, Patel PI. Recombination hot spots and human disease. *Genome Res* 1997; 7: 773–86. With kind permission of CSH Press.

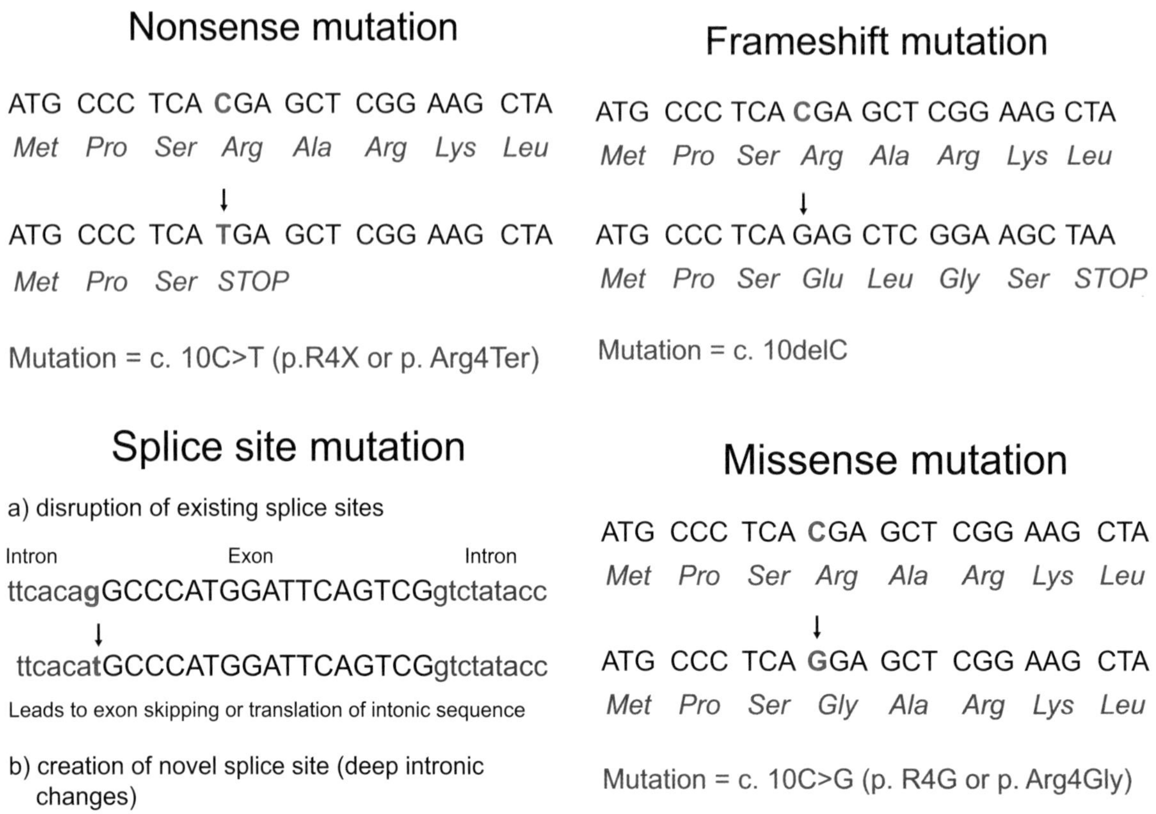

Nonsense mutation

ATG CCC TCA **C**GA GCT CGG AAG CTA
Met   Pro   Ser   Arg   Ala   Arg   Lys   Leu

↓

ATG CCC TCA **T**GA GCT CGG AAG CTA

Met   Pro   Ser   STOP

Mutation = c. 10C>T (p.R4X or p. Arg4Ter)

Frameshift mutation

ATG CCC TCA **C**GA GCT CGG AAG CTA
Met   Pro   Ser   Arg   Ala   Arg   Lys   Leu

↓

ATG CCC TCA GAG CTC GGA AGC TAA

Met   Pro   Ser   Glu   Leu   Gly   Ser   STOP

Mutation = c. 10delC

Splice site mutation

a) disruption of existing splice sites

Intron   Exon   Intron
ttcaca**g**GCCCATGGATTCAGTCGgtctatacc

↓

ttcaca**t**GCCCATGGATTCAGTCGgtctatacc

Leads to exon skipping or translation of intronic sequence

b) creation of novel splice site (deep intronic changes)

Missense mutation

ATG CCC TCA **C**GA GCT CGG AAG CTA
Met   Pro   Ser   Arg   Ala   Arg   Lys   Leu

↓

ATG CCC TCA **G**GA GCT CGG AAG CTA

Met   Pro   Ser   Gly   Ala   Arg   Lys   Leu

Mutation = c. 10C>G (p. R4G or p. Arg4Gly)

Figure 1.7 Some types of point mutation.

cDNA is the DNA sequence complementary to the mRNA sequence. Thus, c.10C>G means that at the 10th nucleotide in the cDNA sequence, cytosine has been replaced by guanine. c, complementary; del, deletion.

result in failure to splice out the intron sequences or failure to splice in the next exon. Missense mutations that result in a change of amino acid (e.g., in Figure 1.7, arginine is converted to glycine) are the most difficult to interpret in terms of determining pathogenicity. Interpretation may involve a variety of steps including searching databases to see if the mutation has been reported previously in patient cohorts (in which case it may be pathogenic) or in the general population (in which case it may be a benign variant or "polymorphism"), and asking whether it changes the nature of the amino acid (e.g., polar to nonpolar), if it potentially affects splicing, if it is in an evolutionarily conserved region of the gene (in which case it may be affecting a region of great functional significance), if it affects a region of known functional significance, if mutations have been reported in the same codon, and whether it segregates with the disease in the family (if there are other affected family members available for testing).

Expanding trinucleotide repeats

This is an important mutational mechanism that is illustrated in Figure 1.8, along with a number of disorders where this is the sole or main mutational mechanism.

Organization of genetic services

In the UK, genetic services are currently organized in regions serving populations of between 2 and 5 million. The clinical genetic service is staffed by consultants in clinical genetics and genetic counselors. There is usually an allied genetic laboratory that provides chromosome and gene analysis using a variety of techniques. There are close links between the genetic laboratories in each region and biochemical genetics and specialist hematology laboratories for the prenatal diagnosis of inborn errors of metabolism and hematologic disorders. Samples that are sent to the laboratory for prenatal testing include amniotic fluid, chorionic villus samples, fetal blood and increasingly maternal blood (noninvasive prenatal testing (NIPT)).

Detecting chromosome abnormalities: methods

Karyotyping

Karyotyping involves assessing the chromosomes using a light microscope and requires dividing cells, so the tissue has to be cultured to stimulate cell division (mitosis); the cell cycle is arrested at metaphase, cells harvested, slides made and stained, and then analysed. The cells to be examined can be obtained from amniocentesis, CVS or fetal blood sampling. Long-term culturing takes 7–10 days and in the UK, professional best practice guidelines indicate that a prenatal report should be issued within 14 days in 95% of cases.

Culture failure is rare and if it occurs it is usually if the sample is small or heavily blood-stained or contaminated. Best practice guidelines indicate that a report should be issued successfully in 99% of amniocentesis and chorionic villus samples. Some authors have suggested that failure of amniotic fluid cell growth may be related to fetal aneuploidy, but this has not been observed by others.

With an amniocentesis, cytogenetic results are highly reliable – sources of error could be maternal contamination or failure to detect fetal mosaicism. The risk of a false-negative result for a chromosome abnormality due to maternal cell contamination has been estimated at between 1 in 4,000 and 1 in 8,000. When mosaicism is detected, the laboratory has to decide whether the mosaicism is likely to be "true" or whether it may have arisen during the culturing process in the laboratory ("pseudomosaicism"). Diagnostic and counseling issues arise when true mosaicism is detected (0.3% of amniocenteses), particularly when it involves rare trisomies.

Expanding trinucleotide repeats

Normal (polymorphic)

⬛ = Trinucleotide repeat e.g CAG

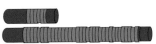

Affected (expanded into affected range)

Expanding trinucleotide repeats

- CAG = HD / SCA's / SBMA
    (Affected range 40–120 repeats)
- CTG = Myotonic dystrophy
    (Affected range 50–3000 repeats)
- CGG = Fragile X (Frax A)
    (Affected range 200–3000 repeats)
- GAA = Friedreich Ataxia
    (Affected range 100–2000 repeats)

Figure 1.8 Trinucleotide repeat expansion mutations. The left upper diagram shows two alleles, one with eight CAG repeats and another with nine repeats. The left lower diagram shows an expansion in one allele to 36 repeats. The right-hand list contains important disorders for which trinucleotide repeat expansions are the sole or main mutational mechanism. HD, Huntington's disease; SBMA, spinobulbar muscular atrophy; SCA, spinocerebellar ataxia.

With CVS, chorionic villi can be examined directly or after short-term culture (when the source of cells is trophoblast) or after long-term culture (when it is the mesenchymal core of the villus that is the source of cells). Analysis of direct CVS cultures has largely been replaced by quantitative fluorescent polymerase chain reaction (QF-PCR) or fluorescent in situ hybridization (FISH) for rapid identification of the common aneuploidies. With CVS, false-negative results are very rare following long-term culture. There is, however, the potential for false positives or diagnostic difficulty due to "confined placental mosaicism" (CPM), i.e. the abnormal cell line is present in the placenta but not in the fetus. The incidence of true mosaicism identified in chorionic villus tissue is about 2.1%, with 1.9% being CPM and 0.2% being true fetal mosaicism. If mosaicism is detected a follow-up amniocentesis is usually recommended. If the amniocentesis suggests that there was CPM, one may still need to consider the possibility of an abnormal phenotype in the fetus due to trisomy rescue, resulting in uniparental disomy if the chromosome involved contains an imprinted gene (e.g., chromosomes 7, 14 or 15).

The resolution of chromosome analysis by karyotyping is in the region of 5–10 megabases (Mb) on a postnatal blood sample, but at amniocentesis or CVS the resolution tends to be in the region of 10–20 Mb, and is therefore only sufficient to exclude aneuploidy and large structural rearrangements.

Fluorescent in situ hybridization

FISH can be performed on cultured or uncultured cells. Unlike karyotyping, this is a targeted approach to identifying specific chromosome abnormalities using fluorescently labelled DNA probes (single-stranded DNA sequences that will hybridize to complementary sequences in the target region). It can be used for rapid aneuploidy screening, detecting specific deletions or additional material (e.g., 22q11 deletion in a fetus with a congenital heart defect detected on a scan or the presence of an additional 12p isochromosome seen in Pallister–Killian syndrome in the fetus with a diaphragmatic hernia) or detecting specific balanced and unbalanced familial translocations. The recommended reporting time for a rapid result on uncultured cells is 3 working days – occasionally cultured cells are required, but this can only be determined on a case-by-case basis. FISH can also be used to confirm and/or characterize a possible karyotype anomaly, and can help give positional information when an imbalance has been identified by microarray.

Quantitative fluorescent polymerase chain reaction (PCR-based copy number analysis)

QF-PCR analyses DNA sequences along chromosomes 21, 13, 18 and the sex chromosomes that are specific for those chromosomes in DNA extracted from CVS or amniotic cells. It is a test designed for the rapid detection of trisomies of these chromosomes. The target turnaround time is 3 working days but in most cases a result is achieved within 24 h. Abnormal results are confirmed by karyotyping and/or FISH. In the case of Down's syndrome (DS), karyotyping is essential to exclude a translocation form of DS, such as a Robertsonian translocation. QF-PCR may not detect mosaicism or structural rearrangements of the chromosomes.

Microarray-comparative genome hybridization

Microarray-comparative genome hybridization (microarray-CGH) is a hybridization method whereby single-stranded DNA in the patient sample is compared with a reference DNA sample when hybridized to complementary sequences that are spotted on to a slide. It is a method that has a huge capacity for miniaturization and automation. The surfaces used are microscope slides or nitrocellulose coated glass surfaces onto which individual oligonucleotides are spotted in individual locations. Thus the "array" of thousands of oligonucleotides fixed to the slide becomes the set of probes to which the patient's DNA is added after being labeled with a fluorophore (usually Cy3 (green) and Cy5 (red)). Two DNA samples – one from the patient and one control sample (made from mixing DNA from several individuals) – are "denatured" (made single-stranded), and each is labeled with a different fluorophore and then hybridized together onto the "microarray" (the slide onto which the oligonucleotides are spotted) (Figure 1.9). Following hybridization, bound label is detected using a high-resolution laser scanner; the signal intensity obtained is analyzed with digital imaging software.

Possible results include:

- No copy number imbalance detected – a normal report with a standard rider is issued.
- Copy number variant (CNV) detected that is a known benign polymorphism – a normal report is issued.
- Known pathogenic CNV detected.
- Pathogenic CNV that has been found to be more prevalent in cohorts of patients with learning

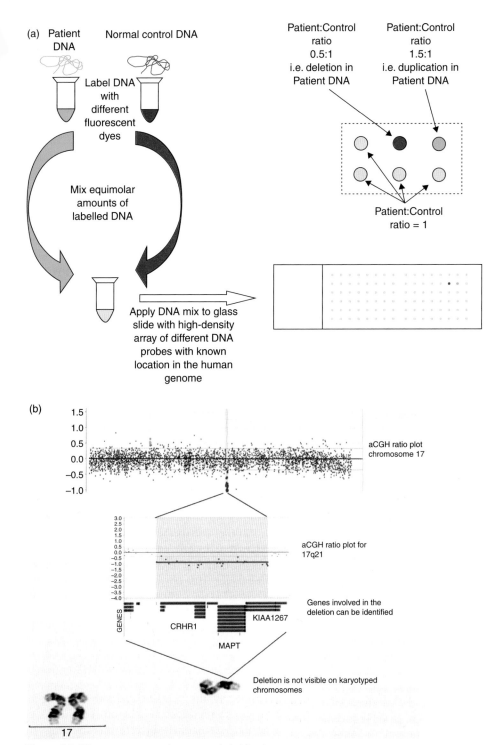

Figure 1.9 Microarray-comparative genome hybridization:

(a) The diagram illustrates the patient sample labeled with green dye being mixed with the control (reference sample) labeled red. The mixture is then hybridized to the array onto which is spotted thousands of unique oligonucleotides. The green- and red-labeled DNA should hybridize equally to complementary sequences on the array; a deletion in the patient DNA will result in more red than green hybridizing (resulting in an orange colour) and a duplication in the patient sample results in excess green.

(b) The diagram illustrates the result when an array has been exposed to a high-resolution laser scanner and the signal intensity obtained analyzed with digital imaging software. The computer analysis shows a deviation from a linear output with an excess of red indicating a deletion; in this example a very small deletion at 17q21.31 that would not be visible down a microscope. The array result also gives information about the genes that are in the deleted region.

Reproduced from Sharkey FH, Maher E, Fitzpatrick DR. *Arch Dis Child* 2005; 90: 1264–9 and Tadros S, Morrogh D, Scott RH. *Arch Dids Child Educ Prac Ed* 2013; 98: 134–5. With kind permission of BMJ Publishing.

disability or neurodevelopmental problems but may be carried by apparently neurologically normal individuals ("neurosusceptibility loci"). These CNVs thus show reduced penetrance – penetrance being the probability that a person carrying this variant will manifest an abnormal phenotype. Some of these neurosusceptibility CNVs can also be associated with birth defects.

- Copy number imbalance detected but is neither a known pathogenic CNV nor a known benign polymorphism. The imbalance is validated using another method, e.g. FISH. If confirmed, parental bloods are requested. If imbalance is de novo, it may be reported as likely to be pathogenic depending on the gene content. If it is found to be familial, it is reported as "significance uncertain."

Where a variant of uncertain significance (VOUS) is found, several factors are considered as well as whether it is familial or de novo. Databases of CNVs known to occur in healthy individuals and in known patient cohorts are consulted. Other considerations are: does the variant overlap a "known syndrome"?; does it contain morbid genes?; and is it a gene-rich or a gene-poor area?

The advantage of microarray-CGH is primarily that it is more sensitive and accurate than conventional karyotyping, i.e., there is a higher abnormality detection rate (DR) and it can reveal specific genes that have been deleted or duplicated. It can also detect mosaicism down to a level of around 20%. The typical arrays currently used in postnatal analysis have an average resolution of 60 kb with increased clustering of probes in known microdeletion/duplication regions. A wider range of array designs and formats are now available and higher resolution arrays that detect deletions and duplications, even down to the single exon level, are becoming increasingly used in a clinical setting.

The possible disadvantages are that arrays will not detect balanced rearrangements and that they will detect variants of uncertain significance or reduced penetrance, and may detect (very rarely) an "unexpected" finding of clinical significance unrelated to the reason for the test (e.g., deletion of a breast cancer gene). Best practice guidelines suggest a target reporting time of 28 calendar days or 56 days where parental follow-up is required for postnatal samples.

Microarray-CGH has revolutionized the postnatal detection of chromosome abnormalities and is being introduced into prenatal testing. There is a significant body of literature that shows that the use of arrays when applied to fetuses with a major structural ultrasound abnormality results in an increased diagnostic yield of 4–6% pathogenic CNVs in the presence of a normal karyotype[2]. Following the results of the National Institute of Health study in the USA[3], the American College of Obstetricians and Gynecologists issued a recommendation that "in patients with a fetus with one or more major structural abnormalities identified on ultrasonographic examination, and who are undergoing invasive prenatal diagnosis, chromosomal microarray replaces the need for karyotyping"[4]. In the UK, there is also support for the use of prenatal arrays (after the common trisomies have been excluded by QF-PCR) in the context of:

- one or more structural anomalies identified on an ultrasound scan
- isolated nuchal translucency ≥3.5 mm when crown–rump length measures from 45 mm to 84 mm (at approximately 11 weeks 0 days to 13 weeks 6 days
- fetuses with a sex chromosome aneuploidy that is unlikely to explain the ultrasound anomaly (e.g., XXX, XXY and XYY).

Most laboratories introducing prenatal arrays are using the same array platform (with the same sensitivity) that they currently have in place for postnatal arrays. It has been recommended that any variant that will potentially inform the management of the pregnancy *or* of the family, in the clinical context in which the array was done *or* in the future should be reported, regardless of size of imbalance. This obviously includes pathogenic variants related to the indication for the array but can also include:

- high-penetrance neurosusceptibility loci that are associated with a risk of a severe phenotype to enable discussion about the overall likely phenotype of the child
- neurosusceptibility loci associated with an increased incidence of anomalies detectable on a scan, as reporting these may help direct further scanning
- unsolicited pathogenic findings fulfilling the above criteria, such as deletion of a known cancer predisposition gene, e.g., BRCA1 or a female fetus carrying a deletion in the dystrophin gene (responsible for the X-linked condition DMD).

It has been recommended that incidental findings that should not be reported include any finding that is not linked to potential phenotypes for the future child in question or has no clinically actionable consequence for that child or family in the future, e.g., VOUS that cannot be linked to a potential phenotype on the basis of genes involved, low-penetrance neurosusceptibility loci and unsolicited pathogenic variants for which there is no available intervention.

Given the complexity of the potential findings, careful counseling of the patient is required prior to undertaking prenatal microarray-CGH analysis, and often afterwards, as some findings may be pathogenic but with very variable phenotypes, which may include normality.

Detecting chromosome abnormalities: protocols

Given the variety of techniques available, what protocols are practiced? Laboratories will usually offer a rapid test (QF-PCR or FISH on uncultured cells in most cases) followed by karyotyping. As stated above, microarray is replacing karyotyping in the investigation of the fetus with ultrasound scan abnormalities. The developments in NIPT are likely to result in radical changes to these protocols of care.

Detecting single-gene disorders

This can be achieved in a variety of ways.

- Look for phenotypic effect, e.g., ultrasound scanning in skeletal dysplasias or other dysmorphic syndromes.
- Testing the presence or activity of the gene product. Biochemical testing is frequently employed where the fetus is at risk of inheriting an inborn error of metabolism. For this author, if a gene mutation or mutations is known in the family then using DNA methods may be preferable as he has come across (very rarely) false-negative enzyme testing on CVS.
- DNA testing. Nowadays, most DNA-based antenatal testing for single-gene disorders involves direct testing for a specific gene mutation (or mutations in the case of an autosomal recessive disorder where the affected child is a compound heterozygote). In the past, when the gene mutation was often unknown, antenatal diagnosis could be offered by tracking the gene that carried the mutation with nearby DNA polymorphisms ("linkage approach"). Such linkage approaches are rarely required these days but are occasionally requested; for example, in so-called "prenatal

exclusion testing" in HD – this will be described in some detail later in this chapter.

Testing for a single gene disorder in antenatal practice usually requires knowledge of the mutation within the family. Many genetic disorders display "locus heterogeneity" whereby there could be several possible genes responsible and one requires knowledge of which gene is responsible in the individual presenting family. For example, tuberous sclerosis can be caused by a mutation in the *TSC1* gene (located on chromosome 9 at 9q34) or in the *TSC2* gene (located on chromosome 16 at 16p13); in any one family the mutation could be in *TSC1* or *TSC2*, and it is essential to find the mutation in an affected family member before an invasive prenatal test can be offered.

Even if there is no locus heterogeneity, there will frequently be "allelic heterogeneity"; the type and site of the mutation within any one gene may vary enormously between affected individuals in different families, even if there are "hot spots" for mutations in some genes. It is important to emphasize here that usually one needs to know the family mutation before antenatal testing can be offered.

"Blind testing" in prenatal genetics can only be considered when a genetic disorder is always or usually due to one specific mutation or type of mutation or where most cases are due to one of a "set" of mutations that can be readily tested in a single assay. Such situations may include:

- disorders where the large majority of cases are due to large gene rearrangements, including whole exon deletions, e.g. DMD
- disorders where all cases are due to a small number of specific mutations (e.g., achondroplasia or sickle cell disease) or where most cases are due to one of a series of mutations that can all be screened in a single test (e.g., CF)
- disorders where all cases are due to the same mechanism of trinucleotide repeat expansion (e.g., HD, myotonic dystrophy, Fragile X syndrome).

In most of the above situations, if the affected family member (or members) was a relative of one of the couple, then testing would be offered to the "at-risk" parent rather than testing the fetus, and only if the "at-risk" parent was a mutation carrier would fetal testing be considered. For example, a pregnant woman may report that she had a maternal uncle who died some years previously from "muscular dystrophy," presumed DMD. It is not possible to confirm the diagnosis in the maternal uncle as no DNA was stored from him whilst he was alive. The woman and her family may be counseled cautiously that *if* the diagnosis was DMD, then as 60–70% of the mutations in the dystrophin gene (the gene responsible for DMD) are large deletions, her DNA could be screened for large dystrophin deletions; if these are not present, her risk of being a carrier is significantly reduced (but not eliminated). If of course she is shown to carry a dystrophin deletion, then she is a carrier and the risk to a male fetus would be 50%. Fetal testing could then be offered and a male fetus tested for the specific deletion identified in the woman. If the woman is not a carrier on "blind testing", then an offer could be made to test her mother (if available) in the same manner. If the woman's mother is found to carry a dystrophin deletion that is not carried by the woman herself, then the fetus is not at any increased risk of DMD and the couple can be reassured. Similar principles apply to the other situations listed above. For example, if a woman has a family history of a male relative with Fragile X syndrome she can be directly tested for her carrier status by measuring the size of the CCG repeat in the first exon of both copies of her FRAXA gene (*FMR1*). If both copies fall within the normal range she can be reassured. Such counseling, however, will always have the caveat that the diagnosis of Fragile X syndrome is correct in the male relative – this should be confirmed if possible as he may have another X-linked mental retardation syndrome, or indeed a syndrome that follows an entirely different inheritance pattern.

Blind testing in the fetus can be performed in the achondroplasia group of skeletal dysplasias. If limb shortening is detected on antenatal scanning (and neither parent has a skeletal dysplasia) and the appearance suggests achondroplasia or thanatophoric dysplasia, genetic testing may confirm or refute the suggested diagnosis. These conditions are usually due to new autosomal dominant gene mutations in the *FGFR3* gene. Achondroplasia is caused (in 99% of cases) by one of two mutations at the same base, i.e. c.1138G>A or c.1138G>C, and in thanatophoric dysplasia (TD), two common mutations (p.Arg248Cys and p.Tyr373Cys) account for 60–80% of TD type I, and p.Lys650Glu has been identified in all cases of TD type II.

What if the mutation(s) in the family is/are unknown and one is dealing with a condition where blind testing in the parent or fetus is not possible, and yet the pregnancy could be or is at high risk? It is important to establish if the affected family member is available and would be willing to consent to providing a sample for DNA analysis. If the affected family member is deceased (or the affected individual was a fetus in a previous pregnancy) it is important to try and establish if any DNA is available for analysis and to obtain consent from an appropriate person to access the sample. Guidance on the issues relating to consent and confidentiality have been reported[5].

To find an unknown mutation in a family will depend on a number of factors – notably what condition one is dealing with. For a disorder with marked locus heterogeneity, this may not be realistic in the short window of early pregnancy. If it is conceivable that one might be able to find a mutation if DNA is available from the affected family member, most laboratories are capable of screening an average-sized gene in 1–2 weeks, though it would take longer to screen a large gene or multiple genes.

Finding mutations usually involves gene sequencing. The standard method used is Sanger sequencing, which was first introduced in the mid 1970s and became automated in the 1990s. New strands of DNA are synthesized with fluorescently labeled bases, and the order of the bases is "read" as the fragments are separated by size using capillary electrophoresis.

Sanger sequencing will detect the presence of the sequence, but not how many copies of the sequence are present. In autosomal conditions, Sanger sequencing often has to be supplemented by a quantitative method to detect whole or partial gene deletions or duplications. The most common method employed for this quantitative analysis is the "multiplex ligation probe assay" (MLPA), which is briefly discussed below.

Once a mutation is identified, a rapid method for direct detection of the relevant mutation(s) can be developed. This will involve using PCR to amplify just the relevant DNA sequence from the sample obtained from the parent (if carrier testing) or fetus (if CVS tissue) for direct mutation analysis. The analyses

Table 1.1 Analysis performed on amplified DNA

Sequencing methodologies	Fragment analysis
Sanger sequencing	Dosage analysis: multiplex ligation probe assay (MLPA)
Pyrosequencing	Microsatellite typing
Next-generation sequencing (NGS)	Detecting trinucleotide repeat expansions
	Detecting altered DNA methylation

DNA amplification-PCR

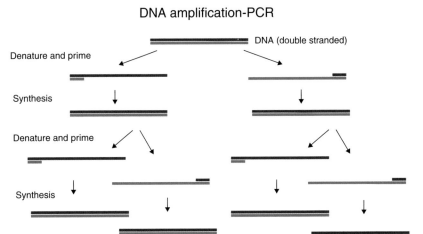

Figure 1.10 Polymerase chain reaction (PCR). The double-stranded DNA is "denatured" (made single-stranded) by heating up the reaction mixture. DNA replication occurs in the presence of substrate, heat-resistant DNA polymerase and primers for the 5′ and 3′ ends of the DNA segment to be amplified. From two strands, two new strands are synthesized making four copies in all. The DNA synthesis is stopped by cooling when the strands will anneal together. The cycle then begins again resulting in the production of eight copies of the target sequence.

undertaken can be subdivided into either sequencing or fragment analysis (Table 1).

For PCR, it is necessary to know the normal sequence of the section of the gene that it is to be amplified. Primers are constructed – often 20–30 nucleotides long – to bind to the DNA flanking this section. Heat-stable DNA polymerase (e.g., Taq polymerase) is added and deoxynucleotide triphosphates dATP, dCTP, dGTP and dTTP are present as substrate. After about 30 cycles (3–5 min per cycle) the PCR products include the starter sequence and about 100,000 copies of target sequence (Figure 1.10).

The amplified target DNA segment can then be sequenced by Sanger sequencing to look for the presence or absence of the mutation. In most situations, the assay is designed to detect the specific mutation or mutations within a family. In some disorders, where one is seeking to detect the same mutation in every patient, pyrosequencing is very effective. This method does not require electrophoresis but can only analyze very short sequences (10–20 bases), and hence has a limited role in prenatal diagnosis. Detailed descriptions of these sequencing technologies are beyond the scope of this chapter.

Next-generation sequencing (NGS). The problem of finding mutations in multiple genes, and even whole exomes or genomes, is being approached by new sequencing technologies. There are a number of different NGS platforms but, in essence, all of them result in the sequencing of millions of small fragments of DNA in parallel (hence the other name of "massive parallel sequencing"). The capacity of an NGS platform is many orders of magnitude greater than Sanger sequencing by

capillary electrophoresis – in fact it is now possible to sequence a whole human genome in a single test. In whole-genome sequencing, each of the three billion bases is sequenced multiple times. Genomic DNA (gDNA) is first fragmented into a library of small segments that can be uniformly and accurately sequenced in millions of parallel reactions. The newly identified strings of bases, called *reads*, are then reassembled using bioinformatics software using a known reference genome as a scaffold (a process called *alignment*). Multiplexing enables large sample numbers to be simultaneously sequenced during a single experiment. To accomplish this, individual "barcode" sequences are added to each sample so they can be differentiated during the data analysis. The term "coverage" generally refers to the number of sequencing reads for any given base within the sample DNA. This is usually averaged across a gene or across multiple genes. Coverage is variable across the genome – the more GC-rich the sequence the lower the number of reads achieved.

An alternative to whole-genome sequencing is to sequence only the coding regions of known genes (the exome) or part of the exome or a panel of selected genes. In order to achieve this, a "target capture" step is introduced at the start of the process to select out from the gDNA only those genes or regions of genes to be sequenced.

In a whole-genome or whole-exome sequencing run, it is currently not possible to accurately read every single base of every gene. If coverage of certain exons is poor, the gaps may have to be covered by Sanger sequencing. Additionally, at the present time, if a possible mutation is identified by NGS technologies, confirmation by Sanger sequencing is recommended.

Detection of CAG repeat expansion in HD

Figure 1.11 Detection of CAG repeat expansion in Huntington's disease (HD).

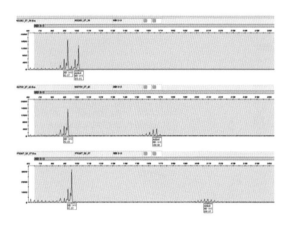

Normal 17, 20 repeats

Affected 17, 42 repeats

Affected 18, 57 repeats

The role for NGS in prenatal testing is developing. At present, it is primarily offered commercially for the detection of aneuploidy by NIPT. If cell-free fetal DNA (cffDNA) is sequenced in this way and the sequence reads assigned to each chromosome are then counted, whether a chromosome is over- or underrepresented can be calculated. This can be achieved by a whole-genome sequencing approach or by a targeted approach for sequences on selected chromosomes, and is currently being offered on a commercial basis for the detection of trisomies 21, 18 and 13, with quoted DRs of around 99.9% for trisomy 21 but lower rates of around 97% for trisomy 18 and 87% for trisomy 13 (largely reflecting the higher GC content of chromosomes 13 and 18). As NGS power increases and data accrue these DRs will be revised upwards. Some companies are now also able to offer testing for defined chromosomeal microdeletions.

Fragment analysis uses the same automated capillary electrophoresis as sequencing but the order of the bases is not "read." Instead the fluorescently labeled amplified DNA sequences are simply separated by size (smaller fragments run faster). This is illustrated in the diagnosis of the trinucleotide repeat disorder HD (Figure 1.11) where the peaks represent the allele sizes in samples from three individuals – one unaffected patient with 17 and 20 repeats and two affected patients with 42 and 57 repeat expansions, respectively.

Fragment analysis as described above is not feasible for very large expansions, such as can be seen in Fragile X syndrome and myotonic dystrophy. In these situations, one may require an old technique called Southern blot analysis to size the expansion.

As indicated above, fragment analysis can also be used to type microsatellite repeats in linkage testing (discussed below) and to detect DNA methylation alterations. In this latter case, the DNA has to be pretreated with sodium bisulfite, which converts cytosine to thymine in unmethylated DNA and so produces a new sequence. The PCR reaction is then designed using primers that are specific for either modified or unmodified cytosines in the primer-binding site. The outcome of the PCR test will thus result in either the presence or absence of a product.

Fragment analysis can not only determine the size of a DNA fragment, but it can also be used to determine the relative amount of a given DNA fragment compared with others generated in the same PCR based test, i.e. it is able to detect a deletion or duplication of a defined fragment of DNA. This requires multiple PCR products to be generated in a single reaction. The presence of large numbers of different primers can cause problems if one is trying to quantify the amount of DNA present as the efficiency of different primer pairs is not equal. MLPA is a method by which large numbers of specific sequences are able to be amplified simultaneously with only *one* set of PCR primers. This method is thus used for the detection of deletions and duplications not detectable by Sanger sequencing.

Testing using linked polymorphisms including exclusion testing

As discussed above, occasionally prenatal testing can be performed by "gene tracking" in those situations where the gene's chromosomal location is known. Indeed this form of prenatal haplotyping rather than direct mutation testing forms the basis of preimplantation genetic diagnosis (PGD) in some PGD centers. In order to perform this testing, polymorphisms in or close to the gene (in close "linkage") have to be identified. DNA polymorphisms are variations within the DNA sequence at a given location – a segment of DNA or a gene sequence is said to be polymorphic if it has two or more alleles with an allele frequency of at least 1%. There are a variety of polymorphisms that can be utilized. In the past, restriction fragment length polymorphisms (RFLPs) were used – these rely on variations in gene sequence that create or abolish a "restriction enzyme site," which are short sequences that are recognized and cut by specific enzymes. There are approximately 10^5 RFLPs in the genome, but they are only two-allele systems (site present/site absent). RFLPs became replaced in clinical usage by variable number of tandem repeat polymorphisms (VNTRs), particularly "microsatellite" VNTRs, which are multiple allele systems, and there are approximately 10^5 of these in the genome. A "microsatellite" consists of a small number of nucleotides (usually 2–6) tandemly repeated, e.g. CACACA or (CA)n. Another important type of polymorphism is the single nucleotide polymorphism – these are very numerous ($n \sim 10^7$) and can be typed on a massive scale, but like RFLPs, are only two-allele systems. RFLPs and VNTRs are illustrated below.

One particular application of the use of polymorphisms is in "prenatal exclusion" testing in HD. HD

is an autosomal dominant condition with an onset usually in mid-adult life. Although genetic testing for this condition is, in most cases, technically straightforward (as the condition is due to a CAG expansion in the first exon of the Huntingtin gene on chromosome 4), many young adults at risk choose not to have a presymptomatic (predictive) test for themselves as they prefer not to know whether they will develop this devastating neurodegenerative disorder, preferring to remain at 50% risk. Nevertheless, they may not want to risk transmitting the disorder to a child and request exclusion testing. In this form of testing, polymorphic markers are identified that can be tracked through the family so that two scenarios may occur, illustrated in Figure 1.12.

(1) The fetus inherits a copy of chromosome 4 that has come from the affected grandparent – the risk to the fetus rises to 50% and termination of pregnancy is offered.
(2) The fetus inherits a chromosome 4 from the unaffected grandparent – the risk to the fetus becomes negligible.

A microsatellite polymorphism is identified close to the HD gene. There are three alleles or alternative forms of the gene in this family (A, B and C) and the "at-risk" parent types AB. His affected father types BB and so he has inherited allele B from his father – it is allele B that carries with it the 50% risk. He has inherited allele A from his unaffected mother. His wife types

Figure 1.12

(a) RFLPs – a 2-allele system – as shown below:

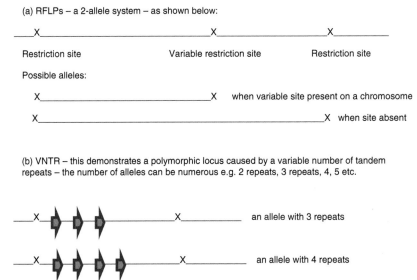

(b) VNTR – this demonstrates a polymorphic locus caused by a variable number of tandem repeats – the number of alleles can be numerous e.g. 2 repeats, 3 repeats, 4, 5 etc.

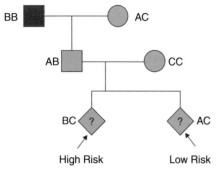

Figure 1.13 Chromosome 4.

CC and will therefore pass allele C to the fetus. If he passes allele B, the risk to the fetus rises to approximately 50%, and if he passes allele A the risk falls to a very low level.

This testing requires the couple to terminate a pregnancy at 50% risk. In practice, a few couples when put in this situation have opted not to terminate and others have opted for predictive testing, which would result in either both the at-risk parent and the fetus being shown to be unaffected or alternatively the "double whammy" of both parent and fetus being shown to be mutation carriers.

Why is the result quoted "high risk" or "low risk"? This is because homologous chromosomes pair and recombine during meiosis (as shown in Figure 1.5). If a recombination occurs between the locus of the polymorphic marker and the locus of the gene mutation, then an incorrect prediction will be made. The closer the marker to the site of the gene mutation, the lower would be the risk of an incorrect prediction. The availability of flanking markers further promotes accuracy of prediction.

NIPT using cffDNA: current usage and future applications

cffDNA was first identified in maternal plasma in 1997 and is present in greater concentration than fetal cells. It can be detected in the maternal circulation as early as 32 days and accounts for between 4–10% of circulating cell-free DNA during pregnancy. The cell-free fraction of maternal blood is isolated and the DNA extracted, and can be studied using quantitative and qualitative analysis. It is rapidly cleared, with a half-life of 16–30 min (longer if woman has pre-eclampsia), and is virtually undetectable within hours of delivery. The levels alter depending on the wellbeing of the syncitiotrophoblast, i.e., a placental effect. The presence of cffDNA allows the possibility of NIPT and uses include:

- Rhesus typing
- sexing of the fetus – useful in X-linked disorders and those conditions where fetal sex influences management, e.g., congenital adrenal hyperplasia. The test involves detection of male-specific sequences. Detection of such sequences indicates a male fetus and failure to detect such sequences indicates a female fetus
- diagnosis of autosomal dominant disorders where father carries the mutation
- exclusion of autosomal recessive disease by exclusion of the paternal mutation (where it differs from the maternal mutation)
- diagnosis of conditions with specific de novo mutations, e.g., achondroplasia, Apert syndrome
- detection of fetal aneuploidy – using next-generation sequencing technology.

NIPT is usually performed after 7–8 weeks of pregnancy. Most experience in the UK within the National Health Service has been for Rhesus testing and for fetal sexing. In the UK, the Bristol Institute for Transfusion Sciences (BITS) and International Blood Group Reference Laboratories (IBGRL) perform 400 cffDNA Rhesus blood group tests per year, and these are currently only being performed in high-risk pregnancies, i.e., in women who already have antibodies[6]. They have found that if performed after 11 weeks there is 99% sensitivity, and after 24 weeks 100% sensitivity. Fetal sexing has so far been the second most common indication – it has usually been performed at around 8–9 weeks' gestation, and an audit of two UK laboratories over a 3-year period (2006–2009) recorded 672 pregnancies tested and NIPT was highly accurate after 7 weeks' gestation (99.5%)[7]. This author's only experience of a false prediction probably resulted from a pregnancy that was initially a twin pregnancy. Parents should be advised of the small risk of discordant results and the possible need for repeat testing to resolve inconclusive results.

The use of next-generation sequencing technology or of digital PCR technology makes a broader range of diagnostic applications possible. NIPT for the detection of aneuploidies is now widely available through commercial providers. A small number of false positives have been identified (presumably mainly due to confined placental mosaicism, though occasionally and theoretically from other mechanisms, such as maternal mosaicism, demised twin and maternal malignancy). These findings mean that NIPT must still be regarded as a screening test pending confirmatory invasive testing. Additionally, this same technology is now being used in the detection of microdeletion syndromes (e.g., 22q11 deletions) and even for familial single-gene disorders where the mother is a carrier (e.g., detection of relative haplotype dosage allowing diagnosis of X-linked disorders, such as DMD).

Example scenarios

(1) Laura, a young white British woman, presents in her first pregnancy. Her partner has a daughter with CF from a previous relationship. Laura does not have any details about what genetic testing has been performed in her partner and the affected child. Her partner is in the Army and is currently serving overseas. She is counseled that CF is an autosomal recessive disorder and (assuming paternity) her partner will be a carrier. Her child is only at risk of having CF if she is also a carrier – it is explained that 1 in 20 to 1 in 25 people are carriers (she has no family history of CF herself). It is explained that she can be tested for the 50 most common CF mutations that occur in the local population using a commercial kit – if she is found to be a carrier, then the risk to the pregnancy rises to 1 in 4, and if she is not a carrier of any of these mutations the risk will fall to about 1 in 400. (The 50 mutations include DF508, which accounts for approximately 70% of the mutations in northern European populations. The next most common mutations G542X, G551D, W1282X and N1303K each account for only 1–2% of known mutations[8]). She opts for carrier testing and does not carry any of the mutations in the assay. She is happy with the low risk and no further testing is performed.

(2) Agnes and her husband have moved to the UK from Poland and Agnes presents in her first pregnancy. She reports that her father back in Warsaw has severe hemophilia. She wants testing in the pregnancy and would request termination of an affected male fetus. It is explained that, assuming paternity, she will be an obligate carrier of this X-linked recessive condition and that the gene mutation would need to be known in order to offer DNA-based diagnosis via a CVS at 11 weeks' gestation. She offers to contact her father to try to get confirmation of the diagnosis (i.e., if it is hemophilia, and if so, if

it is hemophilia A or B). Assuming the likeliest scenario that her father has hemophilia A, she is tested for mutations in the factor VIII gene – initially for the common intron 22 inversion mutation that accounts for approximately 50% of severe hemophilia A. In the meantime she is offered fetal sexing via NIPT, which shows she is carrying a male fetus. Results come back within 2 weeks revealing that she is a carrier of the factor VIII intron 22 inversion. She is offered a CVS, which shows an affected male fetus and she requests termination of pregnancy.

(3) Lucy is 22 years of age and her brother has DMD. She is in her first pregnancy and knows that she is a carrier as she was tested when she was 16 years old. She is aware that she can be offered prenatal diagnosis. The local clinical genetics service confirms that she has been tested and that the family mutation is a deletion of exon 45 of the dystrophin gene. She is counseled that there is a 50% chance that any son will be affected. She decides not to have fetal sexing by NIPT as she says that she wants a CVS for a definitive test and would request this even if NIPT suggested that she was carrying a girl. It is explained that usual practice is to sex the fetus on the CVS tissue initially and not to perform carrier testing if the fetus is shown to be female (once maternal contamination has been excluded). It is explained that the service tries to avoid inadvertent carrier testing and tends to only perform this in X-linked disorders if there is a medical reason for doing so (e.g., if a girl would be tested anyway during childhood for health reasons). She is happy with this management plan and undergoes a CVS, which shows a female fetus. The pregnancy continued uneventfully.

References

1. Chinnery PF, Di Mauro S, Shanske S, et al. Risk of developing a mitochondrial DNA deletion disorder. *Lancet* 2004; 364: 592–6.

2. Callaway JL, Shaffer LG, Chitty LS, et al. The clinical utility of microarray technologies applied to prenatal cytogenetics in the presence of a normal conventional karyotype: a review of the literature. *Prenal Diagn* 2013; 33: 1119–23.

3. Wapner RJ, Martin CL, Levy B, et al. Chromosomal microarray versus karyotyping for prenatal diagnosis. *N Engl J Med* 2012; 367: 2175–84.

4. Committee opinion no. 581: the use of chromosomal microarray analysis in prenatal diagnosis. American College of Obstetricians and Gynecologists Committee on Genetics. *Obstet Gynecol* 2013; 122: 1374–7.

5. Royal College of Physicians, Royal College of Pathologists and British Society for Human Genetics. Consent and confidentiality in clinical genetic practice: guidance on genetic testing and sharing genetic information, 2nd edn. Report of the Joint Committee on Medical Genetics. London: RCP, RCPath, 2011. www.bsgm.org.uk (accessed January 30, 2014).

6. Finning K, Martin P, Summers J, et al. Effect of high throughput RHD typing of fetal DNA in maternal plasma on use of anti-RhD immunoglobulin in RhD negative pregnant women: prospective feasibility study. *BMJ* 2008; 336: 816–8.

7. Hill M, Finning K, Martin P, et al. Non-invasive prenatal determination of fetal sex: translating research into clinical practice. *Clin Genet* 2011; 80(1): 68–75.

8. Firth H, Hurst J. *Oxford Desk Reference – Clinical Genetics*. Oxford, UK: Oxford University Press, 2005.

Bibliography

Strachan T, Read A. *Human Molecular Genetics* 4th edn. Garland Science, Taylor & Francis Group, LLC, 2011.

Gardner RJM, Sutherland GR, Shaffer LG. *Chromosome Abnormalities and Genetic Counselling*, 4th edn. Oxford, UK: Oxford University Press, 2012.

Acknowledgments

I would like to thank Mr Roger Mountford, Miss Una Maye, and Mrs Magda Ainscough of the Cheshire and Merseyside Genetics Laboratory for helpful discussion.

Chapter

2

Antenatal counseling

Bidyut Kumar and Alan Fryer

It is essential that good communication exists between the obstetric team and the regional clinical genetics service in order to optimize the care of families where there are known genetic disorders or where definite or possible genetic disorders come to light during the pregnancy. There are two main situations where communication should take place:

(1) the unexpected finding of either structural abnormalities (usually multiple) on antenatal ultrasound scans or of a chromosomal anomaly following invasive testing by amniocentesis or chorionic villus sampling (CVS)

(2) a history is obtained in the antenatal clinic of a known genetic disorder in the couple's families – sometimes there is more than one genetic disorder uncovered on history taking.

A full discussion of the links and communications between clinical genetics departments and maternity units is given in the report of a prenatal genetics group of the Clinical Genetics Society[1]. The aim of these communications is to enable accurate diagnosis (if possible) of any genetic disorder, and to provide appropriate information to the couple and their family about the prognosis (if known), recurrence risks and what choices may be available to them.

The basic principle of genetic counseling is to seek to be nondirective. The aim is to provide accurate facts about the diagnosis, prognosis, risks and options available. The presentation of these facts should be empathic and tailored to the individual or couple's knowledge, emotional state, religious, ethnic and cultural views. Continued support should be offered and this may involve other health professionals. It should be emphasized that the decision to continue or discontinue a pregnancy belongs to the couple themselves. The counselor helps the patient reach decisions that the patient thinks are correct. Prevention

of handicap is an important but secondary aim, and the improvement of the human gene pool (eugenics) is not an aim, even if it were possible. Very occasionally, a couple may request termination of pregnancy (TOP) for a condition that may be considered "mild" or "treatable" by the counselor. In such circumstances, access to an alternative opinion should be provided.

Genetic assessment involves taking a full medical history and family history, usually constructing at least a three-generation pedigree, and may involve physical examination of the pregnant woman, her partner or other family members (depending on which member is affected), and performing appropriate investigations. Following this, the counselor may be able to assess the risk to the pregnancy and the likely severity of the disorder in any affected child.

The indications for antenatal genetic counseling, some of which are discussed below, are as follows:

- advanced maternal age
- positive maternal serum screen test result (see separate chapter)
- previous pregnancy with fetal aneuploidy
- patient or family member with a known genetic disorder
- detection of unexpected chromosome abnormality
- family history of congenital anomaly or mental retardation
- ultrasound detected fetal abnormality
- recurrent pregnancy loss or stillbirth (outside the scope of this book)
- carrier screening based on ethnicity
- consanguinity
- maternal disease
- maternal teratogen exposure (see separate chapter)
- parental concern.

Fetal Medicine, ed. Bidyut Kumar and Zarko Alfirevic. Published by Cambridge University Press. © Cambridge University Press 2016.

Advanced maternal age

Advanced maternal age is associated with an increased risk of chromosomal trisomy in the fetus. Table 2.1 shows the approximate incidence of trisomy at different reproductive stages and demonstrates that the large majority of trisomic conceptions miscarry. The different birth incidence of the common trisomies (Tables 2.2 and 2.3) partially reflects this – some trisomies are less lethal in utero. Not all chromosomes are equally likely to result in a clinically recognized trisomy – chromosomes 16, 21 and 22 together account for 50% of all trisomies in clinically recognized pregnancies.

Trisomic conceptions result from meiotic nondisjunction (Figure 2.1). Nondisjunction could arise from failure of separation of the homologues at meiosis I or failure of chromatid separation at meiosis II. Alternatively, there is evidence that failure of pairing of homologues (and chiasma formation) or distal positioning of chiasmata predispose to aneuploidy. In this alternative hypothesis, the unpaired chromosomes may undergo "pre-division," whereby the chromatids separate during meiosis I rather than meiosis II and may then randomly segregate, creating in some cases disomic gametes. Not all chromosomes are equally susceptible to meiotic nondisjunction. A study in sperm by Spriggs et al. found that the mean frequencies of disomy for chromosome 21 and the sex chromosomes were significantly higher than for the other autosomes[2].

The effect of advanced maternal age has been considered to operate predominantly at meiosis I. It may result in a disorganized spindle that results in irregular segregation of the homologous chromosomes or the ability of a compromised exchange (due to altered chiasma events) to ensure proper segregation.

Autosomal aneuploidy overwhelmingly has its origin in oogenesis (mainly meiosis I, though in some cases, e.g., trisomy 18, meiosis II may be a major site). Male gametogenesis has a major role, however, in sex chromosome aneuploidy – in 47XXY, 50% of cases arise from paternal errors and 45X is mostly due to the absence of the paternal sex chromosome.

In Down's syndrome (DS), 90–95% of all cases have free trisomy 21 (i.e., the additional chromosome 21 lies unattached to any other chromosome and the cells have 47 chromosomes), and in about 95% of these cases the extra chromosome is of maternal origin; among maternal meiotic errors about 75% are due to meiosis I nondisjunction and 25% have a meiosis II origin.

Table 2.1 Clinically recognized trisomies

Reproductive stage	Approximate incidence of trisomy (%)
Liveborns	0.3
Stillbirths	4.0
Spontaneous abortions	35
All clinically recognized pregnancies	5
Pre-implantation embryos	20
Fertilised oocytes	20–25

Table 2.2 Age-related incidence of liveborn trisomy 21[3]

Maternal age (years)	Liveborn incidence of trisomy 21
15–19	1/1560
25	1/1350
28	1/1110
30	1/890
32	1/660
35	1/355
38	1/170
40	1/97
43	1/31
45	1/23

Table 2.3 Age-related incidence of liveborn babies with trisomy 18 and 13[4]

Maternal age (years)	Liveborn incidence trisomy 18[a]	Liveborn incidence trisomy 13[a]
20	1 in 10,000	1 in 14,000
30	1 in 7,000	1 in 11,000
35	1 in 3,600	1 in 5,300
38	1 in 1,500	1 in 2,400
40	1 in 700	1 in 1,400

[a] Approximate values adapted from reference 4.

The MI reductional division   The MII equatorial division

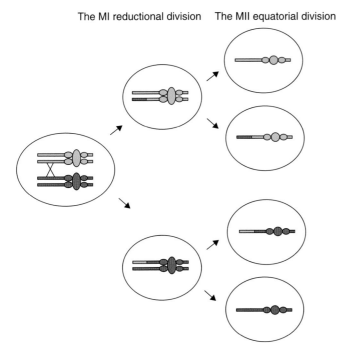

Figure 2.1 Meiosis. At the outset, each chromosome replicates itself forming sister chromatids. The homologous chromosomes pair and non-sister chromatids exchange material (this is a crossover or recombination event and the point at which exchange takes place is called a chiasma). At meiosis I (MI), the homologous chromosomes separate. At meiosis II (MII), equatorial division occurs so that each gamete contains only one copy of each chromosome.

Previous pregnancy with fetal aneuploidy

Here we consider the situation of a couple with normal (or presumably normal) chromosomes who have had a child or fetus with aneuploidy. It is not usually necessary to analyze the parental chromosomes of a child with free trisomy 21 – it is, however, essential to do so in the case of a baby with a translocation form of DS (parental Robertsonian translocations are discussed later in this chapter).

Risk of recurrence for any chromosomal abnormality in a liveborn infant after the birth of a child with free trisomy 21 is increased by about 1% above the population age-related risk. The risk is probably 0.5–1% for trisomy 21 and 0.5% for other chromosomal abnormalities[4,5]. For trisomy 13 or 18, the risk of recurrence for the same trisomy or for another viable trisomy is also increased, though numbers are small[6]. For sex chromosome aneuploidy, there is no firm evidence that a recurrence risk above age-specific figures exists[7].

Women with a previous history of aneuploidy should be offered a diagnostic test during the antenatal period, though this offer could be considered discretionary in the case of sex chromosome aneuploidy. For those with a previous history of a fetus with DS, the couple should have the option of choosing between first-trimester combined DS screening test or a diagnostic test involving CVS or amniocentesis. Prenatal noninvasive testing on free fetal DNA in maternal blood may also be considered.

Patient or family member with a known genetic disorder

A genetic counselor can offer such couples information about the chance of passing on the disorder in question and the availability and accuracy of antenatal testing for the specific disorder. This process might involve assessment of the parents or the fetus or both.

If one of the parents is reported to be affected by, or a carrier of, a genetic condition, the diagnosis may need confirmation by review of medical records, clinical assessment and laboratory tests. The risk to the fetus will depend on the pattern of inheritance. If there is a history of a genetic disorder in a relative of one of the parents, it may be necessary to perform an assessment of the parents, and then offer assessment of the fetus if the risk is deemed to be high and testing is available.

Assessment of the parents could involve clinical assessment and/or laboratory tests. In terms of clinical assessment, an example would be if Mr A, the father of the fetus, has a relative with neurofibromatosis type 1 (NF1). Clinical examination of Mr A may be sufficient to determine if the fetus is at risk of having NF1. Similarly, laboratory testing may be performed on the mother or on her partner (or both) if concern is raised about a known or possible genetic disorder in one or other family. Common examples are family histories of DS and cystic fibrosis (CF). If a woman reports a history of DS in her partner's nephew, it may be possible, with appropriate consent, to access the records of the DS child to see if the child has trisomy 21 (in which case the recurrence risk is not increased above population level) or a translocation (in which case there could be a higher risk). Alternatively, if this information is not readily available, it may be reasonable to simply check her partner's chromosomes by karyotyping to confirm or refute that he is a carrier of a balanced translocation. Similarly, if a woman reports that she has a sibling with CF, it may be possible to assess her carrier status if the mutations are known in her sibling. Alternatively, it would be reasonable to simply assess her partner's carrier status as the risk will be very low if he is not a carrier of the common CF mutations (see Example 1 in Chapter 1).

Assessment of the fetus may be offered where there is a known genetic disorder in the family and the fetus is at high risk. The indication for testing in this latter scenario may be because the parents would request TOP if the fetus was shown to be affected, but sometimes it may be to plan the method of delivery (e.g., third-trimester amniocentesis in hemophilia), place of delivery (in hospital with neonatal intensive care facilities if the child is predicted to be at risk of congenital myotonic dystrophy) or to stop or continue treatment (e.g., fetus at risk of congenital adrenal hyperplasia where the mother is treated with dexamethasone to reduce the likelihood of an affected female fetus being virilized).

Let us consider the risks relating to both chromosomal and single-gene disorders.

Chromosomal disorders

The most commonly encountered problem is where one of the parents is known to carry a balanced rearrangement though occasionally a parent carries an unbalanced one. In these situations, the consequences to the fetus depend on the nature of the rearrangement. It is beyond the scope of this book to consider the counseling of the myriad of possible rearrangements – suffice

to say that the advice of a clinical geneticist should be sought on each occasion. The most common rearrangements are briefly considered below.

Balanced translocations

Robertsonian translocations involve the acrocentric chromosomes 13, 14, 15, 21 and 22. The majority are nonhomologous (i.e., 13:14, 14:21, etc.) but rarely one sees homologous translocations (e.g., 21:21). The risk of a liveborn child with an unbalanced karyotype depends on which chromosomes are involved. The highest risk relates to those translocations involving chromosome 21 (e.g., 14:21, 13:21; 15:21; 21:22), where the likelihood of a liveborn child with DS being born to a female carrier is usually quoted at 10%. Prenatal diagnosis should be offered. The risk to a male carrier is much less (usually quoted as 1–2%), but still at a level where prenatal diagnosis should be offered. The risk of having a liveborn child with DS to a 21:21 carrier is 100%.

Segregation of chromosomes in this situation is shown in Figure 2.2.

There is an additional concern in carriers of translocations involving chromosomes that carry imprinted genes (see Chapter 1), such as 13:14, 13:15 and 14:15. There is the very small but theoretical risk of a zygote having an unbalanced karyotype followed by trisomy rescue resulting in uniparental disomy (UPD). For example, in the case of a 13:15 translocation, if an egg containing both the 13:15 translocation chromosome and the free copy of chromosome 15 is fertilized, the zygote will contain the translocation chromosome, the maternal free copy of chromosome 15 and a paternal free copy. If "trisomy rescue" occurs and the paternal chromosome 15 is lost, the fetus will be disomic but have two maternal copies of chromosome 15. Maternal UPD for chromosome 15 results in Prader–Willi syndrome. Abnormal phenotypes are also associated with paternal UPD for chromosome 15 (Angelman syndrome) and for paternal and maternal UPD 14. Prenatal testing for these rare conditions is usually offered.

Reciprocal translocations occur when two chromosomes exchange segments. Segregation of the chromosomes at meiosis carries a risk of the gamete having an unbalanced karyotype with a deletion of one chromosome segment and a duplication of the other. The risk of a liveborn child with an unbalanced karyotype depends on a number of factors that need to be considered by the genetic counselor – namely, which

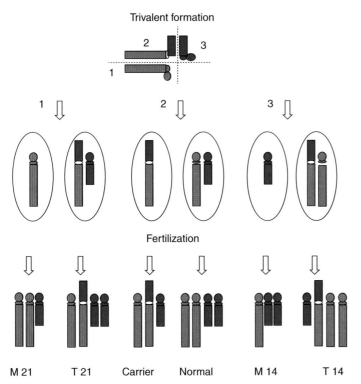

Trivalent formation

Fertilization

M 21   T 21   Carrier   Normal   M 14   T 14

Figure 2.2 Segregation of chromosomes at meiosis in Robertsonian translocations. Meiosis in a 14:21 translocation. Here, instead of two homologous chromosomes pairing, the three chromosomes (the free copies of 14 and 21, and the translocation chromosome) form a trivalent arrangement. As the three chromosomes segregate, the six possible gametes are shown, and following fertilization, possible viable outcomes include normal, carrier and trisomy 21. Trisomy 14 may be viable if trisomy rescue occurs. M, monosomy; T, trisomy.

chromosomes are involved, the size of the segments (i.e., degree of monosomy and trisomy) and possible modes of segregation at meiosis (Figure 2.3). The other factor to be considered is the mode of ascertainment in the family – if the family was ascertained through the birth of a child with an unbalanced karyotype, the risk is significant. If, however, the ascertainment was via recurrent miscarriage, the risk may be low.

A female carrier of an X-autosome translocation is a special case – if she is fertile, counseling needs to consider the potential outcomes if she were to have a female fetus with the balanced translocation (probably phenotypically normal if the parent is phenotypically normal), a male fetus who carries the balanced translocation and a female fetus with an unbalanced translocation.

Inversions

Inversions occur whereby a segment of a chromosome has flipped upside down and been reinserted into the chromosome. They are divided into those that are pericentric and those that are paracentric. Pericentric inversions occur when the breakpoints are on either side of the centromere; in paracentric inversions the breakpoints are both on the same side of the centromere. The

risk of a liveborn child with an unbalanced karyotype in carriers of pericentric inversions depends on which chromosome is involved and the length of the inverted segment. Paracentric inversions tend to be innocuous.

Supernumerary marker chromosomes (SMCs)

A phenotypically normal parent may carry an SMC – sometimes this is a fragment of chromosome material that does not contain any genes but sometimes the SMC does contain significant genetic material but is only present in a proportion of cells (i.e., the parent is mosaic). Counseling should consider the risk if the fetus was nonmosaic.

Single-gene disorders

Gregor Johann Mendel (1822–1884) described a pattern of inheritance that applies to disorders caused by a defect in a single gene (unifactorial inheritance). Genes are inherited in pairs, one of each pair inherited from each parent. An allele is one of a pair of genes that can act in a dominant or recessive manner. Segregation of alleles occurs at meiosis so that each gamete receives only one allele. Alleles at different loci in a chromosome segregate independently.

(a)

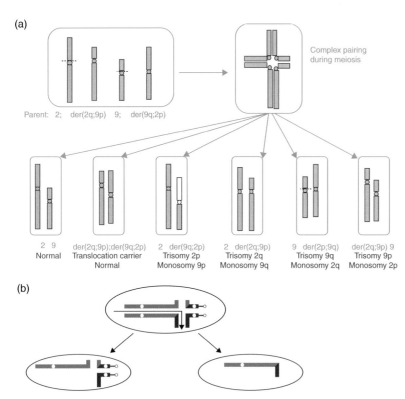

Parent: 2; der(2q;9p) 9; der(9q;2p)

Complex pairing
during meiosis

2 9	der(2q;9p);der(9q;2p)	2 der(9q;2p)	2 der(2q;9p)	9 der(2p;9q)	der(2q;9p) 9
Normal	Translocation carrier Normal	Trisomy 2p Monosomy 9p	Trisomy 2q Monosomy 9q	Trisomy 9q Monosomy 2q	Trisomy 9p Monosomy 2p

(b)

Figure 2.3 Segregation of chromosomes at meiosis in reciprocal translocations:

(a) Reciprocal translocation with 2:2 segregation at meiosis. An illustration of a reciprocal translocation between chromosomes 2q and 9p. A quadrivalent forms at meiosis as homologous segments pair with each other. The diagram shows six possible segregants when there is 2:2 segregation. Four of these segregants are unbalanced.

(b) Reciprocal translocation with 3:1 segregation at meiosis. 3:1 segregation may be favored if one of the derivative chromosomes following the translocation is small. This can occasionally result in a liveborn child with an unbalanced karyotype. The most common example is the 11q23:22q11, which, following 3:1 segregation, can result in a fetus who is effectively trisomic for part of chromosome 22 and part of chromosome 11. In this diagram, chromosome 11 is blue and chromosome 22 is red – one product of cell division contains one copy of chromosome 11, one copy of chromosome 22 plus the additional chromosome – as a result, the gamete would thus have additional 11q and 22q material.

Table 2.4 shows the typical features of single-gene disorders.

Autosomal dominant

Disorders that follow this pattern of inheritance can create significant dilemmas. Usually, the advice of a clinical geneticist should be sought. The basic principles are listed in Table 2.4. The caveats associated with autosomal dominant conditions are listed below.

- **Age-dependent penetrance**. The term penetrance is the probability that a person inheriting the mutation will manifest evidence of it. Some mutations are fully penetrant (penetrance = 1) but the penetrance can be age-dependent. Some disorders do not manifest until adult life, sometimes late adult-life (e.g., Huntington's disease), and if a gene carrier dies before they would have manifested the condition, there can be the appearance of a "skipped generation."
- **Reduced penetrance**. Some autosomal dominant disorders regularly show reduced penetrance, and it can be very difficult to reassure family members

who have no clinical signs of the disorder. Gene testing is invaluable in these situations.

- **Variable expression**. Even if a disorder is fully penetrant, the expression within and between families may be extremely variable, and accurately predicting the outcome in a fetus who inherits the mutation is usually impossible. There are many disorders where mildly affected parents have had more severely affected children, and vice-versa.
- **New mutations**. In many severe disorders, the majority (if not all) cases represent new mutations and the parents are unaffected. Some disorders with a high mutation rate show a paternal age effect. This is striking in achondroplasia and Apert syndrome, where the incidence of new mutations rises sharply with increasing paternal age. This has been shown to be due to the nature of the mutation giving a selective advantage to spermatogonia that carry the mutation.
- **Germ-line (gonadal) mosaicism**. If a person carries the mutation in only some of his or her cells (i.e., mosaicism) it is likely that the manifestations will be milder and may not be recognizable. In some

Table 2.4 Mendelian disorders

	Autosomal dominant	Autosomal recessive	X-linked recessive	X-linked dominant
Some common disorders	Achondroplasia Acute intermittent porphyria Familial adenomatous polyposis Familial breast cancer (BRCA1,2) Familial hypercholesterolemia Huntington's disease. Myotonic dystrophy Neurofibromatosis type 1 and 2 Osteogenesis imperfecta Tuberous sclerosis	Congenital adrenal hyperplasia Cystic fibrosis Friedreich's ataxia Galactosaemia Hemochromatosis Homocystinuria Phenylketonuria Sickle cell disease Tay–Sach's disease Thalassaemia	Duchenne muscular dystrophy Becker muscular dystrophy Color blindness Fragile-X syndrome G-6-P-D deficiency Hemophilia A, B Ocular albinism Retinitis pigmentosa (some) Hunter syndrome Complete androgen insensitivity syndrome	Vitamin D-resistant rickets Incontinentia pigmenti Rett syndrome
Typical pattern of inheritance	Both sexes equally affected. Transmitted by both sexes. An affected person is usually a heterozygote for the mutation (i.e., has a mutation in one copy of the gene and the other copy of the gene is normal "wild-type"). Homozygotes are rare and may be lethal in some disorders. Every time that person has a child there is a 50:50 (1 in 2) chance of the gene being transmitted and as the disorder is dominant, one would expect any child inheriting the mutation to manifest the disorder. Hence, successive generations are affected. Male-to-male transmission occurs.	Both sexes equally affected. Both parents are unaffected carriers. Unaffected siblings have a 2 in 3 chance of being carriers. In some cases increased incidence of parental consanguinity.	Males affected almost exclusively. Transmitted by carrier females. Every time a carrier female has a child there are four possible outcomes: an affected male; an unaffected male; a carrier female (who will usually be clinically unaffected like her mother); and a non-carrier female. Male-to-male transmission does not occur. Daughters of affected males are carriers. Sons of affected males are always unaffected.	Affects both hemizygous males and heterozygous females. Females may be less severely affected than males. Females transmit to half their sons and half their daughters. Males transmit to all daughters and none of their sons. No male-to-male transmission.

disorders, such as neurofibromatosis type 2, a high proportion of new cases have been shown to be mosaic for the mutation. If a person carries the mutation in mosaic form in somatic and gonadal cells (gonosomal mosaic) or just in the gonadal cells (gonadal mosaic), they will be at risk of transmitting the disorder to a child. If, therefore, a child has an autosomal dominant disorder and the parents appear unaffected, one should still consider the possibility that one or other parent may be a gonosomal or gonadal mosaic. This has been identified several times in some disorders (e.g., tuberous sclerosis) but very infrequently in others (e.g., neurofibromatosis type 1). In tuberous sclerosis, for example, even if one can show that neither parent of an affected child carries the affected child's mutation, a small recurrence risk of 2–3% is usually quoted, and some families in this situation will request prenatal testing in a future pregnancy.

- **Parent-of-origin effects/"anticipation."** For some autosomal dominant disorders, the sex of the affected parent influences the phenotype in the child. This is specifically an issue for the trinucleotide repeat disorders myotonic dystrophy and Huntington's disease. Congenital myotonic dystrophy nearly always follows maternal rather than paternal transmission of the mutation, and juvenile Huntington's disease follows paternal rather than maternal transmission.

- **Parent-of-origin effects/"imprinting."** As discussed in Chapter 1, a small proportion of the genes in the human genome exhibit epigenetic silencing (imprinting). An important example is the gene UBE3A, implicated in Angelman syndrome on 15q11. This gene is silenced on the paternal chromosome. If a man transmits a mutation in UBE3A, his child will be unaffected as the paternal copy would have been silenced anyway. If the child inheriting the mutation is a daughter, then she would be at 50% risk of having an affected child when she becomes a parent, as there is a 50% chance that she will transmit the mutation-carrying copy of chromosome 15 that has come from her father. As this will now be a maternal copy, the child will be affected.

Autosomal recessive disorders

In many ways, these present fewer counseling issues. If a child has an autosomal recessive disorder, he or she will have inherited a mutation in the same gene from both parents. Both parents are heterozygotes. This may be exactly the same mutation (e.g., both parents may carry the DF508 mutation in the CF gene) and the child is said to be a homozygote for the mutation, or the parents may carry different mutations in the same gene (e.g., one parent carries DF508 and the other carries G551D in the CF gene) and the child is said to be a compound heterozygote. In general, when counseling, one tends to ignore the small possibility that one of the mutations is a new (de novo) event. Where the mutations are known and the parents have been tested, there have been very few reports of new mutations being identified – more often, the failure to find the mutation in a parent suggests an alternative explanation such as

nonpaternity. If a couple have an affected child, one usually counsels a 1 in 4 recurrence risk for each future pregnancy. If a couple asks about the potential severity in a future affected child, penetrance tends to be complete and the degree of variability is generally less than in autosomal dominant disorders.

If one of the parents has an autosomal recessive disorder (e.g., oculocutaneous albinism), the risk to their child is low as their partner would have to be a carrier in order for them to have an affected child. If the disorder is rare and their partner is not a relative, it would be unlikely that the partner would be a carrier.

If a disorder is rare, the risk of recurrence in the wider family is low unless there is consanguinity. Approximate risks can be calculated if the heterozygote frequency in the population is known. In the case of CF, approximately 1 in 20 northern European white Caucasians are carriers. If a healthy person has a sibling with CF, that person has a 2 in 3 chance of being a carrier. Assuming their partner has no family history of CF and is not a blood relative, then this partner's carrier risk is 1 in 20. The risk of this couple having a child with CF can be calculated as $2/3 \times 1/20 \times 1/4 = 1$ in 120.

Issues arise in counseling when consideration has to be given to consanguinity and the fact that the heterozygote frequency may vary with geographical or ethnic group. These issues are discussed further below.

X-linked disorders

Most such disorders are recessive and a female carrying a mutation in one copy of an X-linked gene will have (almost always) a normal copy on her other X-chromosome and be unaffected. A male, however, who inherits an X-linked mutation will be expected to manifest the disorder. If a woman presents with a family history of an X-linked disorder, advice should be sought from a clinical geneticist. Testing the daughter of an affected male for a mutation is virtually a paternity test, and if undertaken, should be preceded by careful counseling.

As with autosomal dominant inheritance, one has to consider the possibility of a new mutation when a male has an X-linked disorder and there are no other affected family members. Similarly, if a woman has two affected sons and there is no other family history, then one has the following possibilities to consider:

- she is a carrier and her mother is also a carrier
- she is a carrier but the mutation arose in her mother's egg or father's sperm
- she is a gonadal mosaic.

Mutation analysis to detect carriers is extremely important in X-linked disorders, particularly those severe disorders where many women will request prenatal diagnosis. Duchenne muscular dystrophy (DMD) creates a particular issue as the incidence of germline mosaicism is high (18%), and so, even if a woman who has had a son with DMD does not carry the mutation in her blood cells, it would be routine to offer prenatal testing for the mutation in a future pregnancy and offer mutation-based carrier testing to any daughter when that daughter reaches an appropriate age[9].

Some X-linked disorders are dominant or semi-dominant, and in these cases a significant proportion of female carriers will have clinical signs and symptoms. An example occurs with the Fragile X mental retardation syndrome. It is often a difficult counseling situation when a woman is a carrier of a Fragile X pre-mutation. Fragile X mental retardation syndrome is a trinucleotide repeat expansion disorder (see Chapter 1). Carriers with an expansion of 50–200 CGG repeats usually have normal learning ability ("pre-mutation carriers"). These expansions are unstable, and when transmitted to a fetus, may expand into the "full mutation" range (>200 repeats). Learning disability is inevitable in a male who inherits a full mutation. Approximately 50% of females who inherit a full mutation also have learning disability. Some couples would request TOP if a female full mutation carrier is identified, especially if they have experience of a severely affected female in their family.

There are some X-linked dominant disorders where almost all the affected patients are female (e.g., Rett syndrome). This is because these conditions demonstrate male lethality. On the other hand, there are some rare X-linked dominant disorders where the clinical phenotype tends to be more severe in the female than the male (e.g., craniofrontonasal dysplasia).

The process of X-inactivation can also influence the phenotype in a female. Where there is more than one X chromosome in a cell, it is usual for all except one of the X chromosomes to be inactivated. Not all parts of the additional X chromosomes are inactivated – some sections remain active, including the pseudoautosomal region on the short arm of the X chromosome (Xp). The process of X-inactivation is random, and one would expect in 50% of a female's cells that her paternally derived X would be inactivated and in the other 50% it will be her maternally derived X. By chance, this percentage may be skewed so that a woman who carries a mutation in one of her X-linked genes may manifest the disorder if an excessive percentage of her "normal" X chromosomes have been inactivated (or vice-versa, she may be protected from an X-linked dominant mutation if the mutation-carrying chromosome has been preferentially inactivated by chance).

Y-linked disorders

The major genes on the Y chromosome relate to testis determination and spermatogenesis, and mutations in these genes affect reproductive medicine and gynecology practice rather than obstetrics, and will not be considered further in this chapter.

Mitochondrial DNA disorders

The inheritance of mitochondrial DNA disorders is discussed in Chapter 1.

Chromosome abnormalities detected unexpectedly at prenatal diagnosis

This may arise if karyotyping is performed and a numerical or structural chromosome abnormality is found that is probably coincidental to the reason for performing the test. An example is where a karyotype is performed because of abnormal scan findings and the fetus is found to have sex chromosome aneuploidy (e.g. 47,XXY, 47,XXX, 47,XYY or a mosaic pattern such as 45,X/46,XY, 45,X/46,XX etc.), a SMC or an apparently balanced translocation or inversion. The situation can similarly arise if a microarray is performed, as this might detect sex chromosome aneuploidy even if it will not detect a balanced rearrangement. The main features of some of these coincidental but possibly significant findings are listed in Table 2.5.

Pretest counseling should include the possibility of detecting a coincidental but clinically significant abnormality. Advice should be sought from a clinical geneticist if such an abnormality is found. In the case of finding an apparently balanced translocation or inversion or an SMC, the laboratory will usually recommend performing karyotyping on the parents to see if the rearrangement has arisen de novo or whether it has been inherited. Transmission from a phenotypically normal parent predicts a low risk of abnormality in the fetus or subsequent child. Care should be taken with SMCs if a parent is found to be mosaic. Microarray or fluorescent in situ hybridization

Table 2.5 Main clinical features in some chromosome disorders that are commonly identified as coincidental findings

Karyotype abnormality	Some of the main clinical findings
47,XXY Klinefelter syndrome	Tall stature, azoospermia, hypergonadotrophic hypogonadism, modest reduction in IQ of 10–15 points (i.e., most have IQ within normal range), 50% require speech therapy, tendency to passive, unassertive behavior. Occasional other issues e.g., gynecomastia.
47,XXX	Tall stature, modest reduction in IQ of 10–15 points (so most have IQ within normal range), 50% require speech therapy. May be a slightly increased risk of premature ovarian failure. Most are fertile and have chromosomally normal babies.
47,XYY	Tall stature, modest reduction in IQ of 10–15 points (i.e., most have IQ within normal range), 50% require speech therapy. Behavioral problems are more common than in the general population, particularly amongst those with some learning problems; no association with criminality per se. Most are fertile and have chromosomally normal children.
45,X Turner syndrome	If liveborn, short stature, gonadal dysgenesis, IQ usually normal. Cardiovascular malformations, particularly coarctation and ventricular septal defect in 15–50%. Renal anomalies, especially horseshoe kidney in one-third. Some phenotypic changes in 50% cases – neck webbing, cubitus valgus, wide-spaced nipples, etc.
45,X/47,XXX	This depends on the proportion of 45,X cells to 47,XXX, which may vary from tissue to tissue.
45,X/46,XY	Most have normal male external genitalia.
Idic 15	If this is found and it does not contain any material from the Prader–Willi/Angelman region, it will be associated with a normal outcome providing uniparental disomy 15 is excluded.

analysis may be undertaken to see if the SMC contains any significant genes.

If a balanced Robertsonian translocation (whether inherited or de novo) is found, and the chromosomes involved contain imprinted genes, testing for UPD should be offered.

De novo rearrangements will occasionally be unbalanced and microarray analysis is often undertaken to check for submicroscopic imbalances. If no imbalance is detected on array, further consideration still needs to be given as to whether the breakpoints could disrupt a gene that could be directly causing the scan findings (or even "unmasking a recessive," whereby the chromosome breakpoint disrupts a gene and unfortunately the same gene on the homologous chromosome carries a mutation – the result being that the function of both copies of the gene is impaired). Counseling in this situation can be very difficult and one is often left with a degree of uncertainty. The problems related to microarray analysis in general are discussed in Chapter 1.

Family history of congenital anomaly or mental retardation

Genetic disease, chromosomal abnormalities and in-utero exposure are amongst the causative factors that can lead to mental retardation and congenital

anomaly. Some common conditions follow a multifactorial inheritance pattern, which means that both genetic and environmental factors contribute to their development. Meticulous history taking can help differentiate between isolated conditions and problems that occur as part of a larger constellation of findings.

Examples of typical clinical cases are as follows.

(1) If one parent or a previous child was born with a congenital abnormality, such as a congenital heart defect or a facial cleft, personal and family history may help identify a specific genetic or environmental cause. If no specific cause is identified, empiric figures are often available to help assess the risk to the fetus (Table 2.6).

(2) If a healthy couple has already had a child with congenital abnormalities or learning disability, the recurrence risk depends on whether a diagnosis has been reached in the affected child. If the diagnosis is unknown, an empiric recurrence risk of about 5% may be quoted, although there are some situations where one feels concerned that the condition resembles some disorders that follow autosomal recessive inheritance and the risk of recurrence may be 25%. If the offspring is deceased (or was a fetus that miscarried or the pregnancy was terminated for fetal anomalies), consideration should be given to performing a karyotype in the

Table 2.6 Recurrence risks to siblings and offspring risks with nonsyndromic defect and no other family history[10]

Congenital abnormality in parent or sibling	Recurrence risk to sibling	Offspring risk to child	Comment
Cleft lip +/- cleft palate	2–6%	4%	Varies with severity of cleft.
Isolated cleft palate	2–3%	4%	—
Congenital heart disease	1–3% for most defects – may be higher for some e.g. isomerism sequence.	2–7%	In general the risks to offspring are greater to affected mothers than affected fathers. With left sided obstructive defects assessment of first degree relatives is indicated.
Neural tube defect	2–5%	4%	Risk depends on population incidence – figures given are without folate supplementation.
Bilateral Renal agenesis	3–8%	NA	Risk higher if parent has renal anomaly e.g. unilateral renal agenesis.

Adapted from reference 10. Comments may apply where there is a range of risk. NA, not applicable.

parents in case that offspring had an unbalanced chromosome translocation transmitted by a parent with balanced translocation. This is particularly the case if chromosome analysis had not been performed on the fetus or was unsuccessful. This may also be worth considering if a fetal karyotype was achieved but the quality of the chromosome banding was low – if fetal DNA is available, microarray analysis on fetal DNA can be performed; if fetal DNA is not available, parental karyotyping should be considered.

(3) One of the couple (with a previous partner) has had a child with one or more congenital abnormalities or learning disability. If the diagnosis is unknown, particular consideration should be given as to whether one could be dealing with a "high-risk" scenario, such as an unbalanced chromosome translocation in the child (and the parent being a balanced translocation carrier) or an X-linked recessive disorder (if the affected child is a male child of the female partner).

(4) One of the couple has a relative (or relatives) with congenital abnormalities (single or multiple) or learning disability. Again, one needs to consider whether one might be dealing with a potential high-risk situation, such as a chromosome rearrangement or an X-linked recessive disorder as in (3). Often pedigree analysis can provide

reassurance about the risk of an X-linked disorder occurring in the couple's offspring.

Ultrasound-detected fetal abnormality

Fetal anomalies can be detected quite unexpectedly both in the first trimester during a first-trimester pregnancy dating scan or during a routine anomaly scan at 18 to 21 weeks' gestation. Some ultrasound markers (e.g., increased nuchal translucency, echogenic fetal bowel and choroid plexus cyst) can be associated with an underlying genetic and chromosomal disorder. In other cases, actual anomalies are detected, but it may be unclear if they are associated with an underlying genetic or chromosomal disorder. Family history, and drug and disease history, might allow for better assessment of genetic risk. Genetic counselors can help patients by explaining the significance of ultrasound findings and the availability of further testing through CVS, amniocentesis or fetal echocardiogram. The interpretation of the results from these tests may need input from a geneticist to help couples make decisions about the management of their pregnancy.

Examples of cases encountered in clinical practice are as follows.

(1) A 28-year-old primigravida, at her routine 20-week scan, was found to have a fetus with a short barrel-shaped chest, hyperextended spine,

short ribs, partial agenesis of cerebellar vermis, unilateral talipes, hyperechogenic bowel, absence of stomach bubble and significantly shortened long bones. The patient opted for TOP. Fetal karyotype was found to be normal. Postmortem examination including radiology suggested a diagnosis of Jeune asphyxiating thoracic dystrophy (JATD). She was reviewed by a geneticist and informed that JATD is inherited in a recessive manner and there would be a 1 in 4 chance that any future pregnancy might be affected with the same disorder. Prenatal diagnostic DNA testing is only available for this disorder if the causative mutations are identified but DNA was banked from the fetal tissue in case analysis became necessary in the future.

(2) A 38-year-old third gravid patient, at her routine 20-week scan was found to have a fetus with exomphalos containing bowel and bladder, lumbosacral spina bifida with a myelomeningocele at L5–S1 level. She was seen by a multidisciplinary team (MDT), including a pediatric neurosurgeon, and counseled in detail. The likely diagnosis was omphalocele-extrophy-imperforate anus-spinal defect (OEIS) complex. Fetal karyotype was normal. Following prolonged consideration and discussion with the MDT, the couple opted for TOP.

(3) During a dating ultrasound scan, the fetus of a 40-year-old third gravid was found to have abnormal appearance of her lower limbs. CVS produced a normal karyotype. At 18 weeks, the fetus was found to have very short and deformed long bones, an abnormally shaped thorax and abnormal fetal face. The patient opted for a TOP. Postmortem examination suggested a diagnosis of osteogenesis imperfecta II. A geneticist reviewed the patient. The majority of such fetuses inherit this condition as a de novo mutation in the genes. The recurrence risk was said to be higher than the background population risk because of the possibility of germ line mosaicism or a rare autosomal recessive form of lethal osteogenesis imperfecta.

Carrier screening based on ethnicity

Some genetic disorders are more likely to occur among people who trace their ancestry to a particular geographic area. People within an ethnic group may share disease-causing mutations inherited by descent. Examples of genetic conditions that are more common in particular ethnic groups are sickle cell anemia, which is more common in people of African, African-American or Mediterranean heritage, and Tay–Sachs disease, which is more likely to occur among people of Ashkenazi (eastern and central European) Jewish or French Canadian ancestry. It is important to note, however, that these disorders can occur in any ethnic group.

One in five people of Ashkenazi descent are carriers of at least one of the main Jewish genetic disorders. Tests can be offered for Tay–Sachs (frequency, 1 in 30), Canavan (1 in 40), Niemann–Pick type A, familial dysautonomia, Fanconi anemia type C, glycogen storage disease type 1a, Bloom syndrome, mucolipidosis type IV as well as CF. In the UK, screening for Tay–Sachs disease in the Ashkenazi Jewish population has National Screening Committee approval, and carrier testing is funded by the National Health Service. Screening tests for the other disorders can be arranged privately.

CF has a carrier frequency of 1 in 25 amongst Caucasians, and is known to be more frequently associated with the finding of fetal echogenic bowel on ultrasound scan in the second trimester.

Consanguinity

There is an increased risk of an autosomal recessive disorder in the offspring of a consanguineous partnership. It is likely that in any unselected population, everyone carries at least one harmful autosomal recessive gene. In marriages between first cousins, the chance of an offspring inheriting the same recessive gene from both parents that originated from one of the common grandparents is 1 in 64. Polygenic conditions are also more common in this situation. A recent study from Bradford, UK calculated that consanguinity accounted for almost one-third of congenital anomalies in babies of Pakistani origin[11].

If a couple are blood relatives (e.g., first cousins), the risk to a child of a serious genetic disorder depends on whether there is further consanguinity in the family. In a first-cousin relationship with no previous consanguinity, there is an empiric risk of 4.0–4.5% for serious congenital and genetic disorders diagnosed by 1 year of age, rising to 8% to include conditions diagnosed later in childhood. For second cousins or first cousins once removed, the risk of serious disorders diagnosed by 1 year of age is 3.0–3.5%. If the couple come from an inbred family the risk is higher.

Every case will need to be dealt with individually, but in general, detailed fetal anomaly scanning is offered to all. Specific screening tests can be offered to the couple depending on their ethnic origin:

- northern European – CF
- Mediterranean – hemoglobinopathy and CF
- Ashkenazi Jewish – Tay–Sachs and CF (and possibly other conditions)
- African–American, Afrocaribean, African – hemoglobinopathy and CF
- Indian/South-East Asian – hemoglobinopathy and CF.

Maternal diseases

Some maternal diseases may act as a teratogen that can adversely affect a developing fetus. Examples of such diseases are thyroid dysfunction, phenylketonuria, insulin-dependent diabetes mellitus, seizure disorder and lupus. In such cases, it may remain unclear whether the maternal pathology itself or the medication used to treat the disorder is implicated in the risk. Therefore, in this regard, a genetic counselor will work with the physician to inform and discuss about the potential risks and benefits of medications, and to determine the best course of action for the patient.

References

1. Clinical Genetics Society. Clinical Genetics and Antenatal/Fetal Medicine: Liaison and Training. A report of the Clinical Genetics Society Prenatal Genetics Group, February 2008. www.clingensoc.org (accessed January 30, 2014).

2. Spriggs EL, Rademaker AW, Martin RH. Aneuploidy in human sperm: the use of multicolor FISH to test various theories of nondisjunction. *Am J Hum Genet* 1996; 58(2): 356–62.

3. Hecht CA, Hook EB. The imprecision in rates of Down syndrome by 1-year maternal age intervals: a critical analysis of rates used in biochemical screening. *Prenat Diagn* 1994; 14: 729.

4. Gardner RJM, Sutherland GR, Shaffer LG. *Chromosome abnormalities and Genetic Counselling*, 4th edn. Oxford University Press, 2012; 408.

5. Kingston HM. Common chromosomal disorders, In: *ABC of Clinical Genetics*, 3rd edn. BMJ Books, 2003; 19.

6. Evans MI, Johnson MP, Yaron Y, Drugan A. Epidemiology of aneuploidy. In: *Prenatal Diagnosis*. McGraw-Hill, 2006; 22.

7. Gardner RJM, Sutherland GR, Shaffer LG. *Chromosome Abnormalities and Genetic Counselling*, 4th edn. Oxford University Press, 2012; 290.

8. Gardner RJM, Sutherland GR, Shaffer LG. *Chromosome Abnormalities and Genetic Counselling*, 4th edn. Oxford University Press, 2012; 293.

9. British Society for Human Genetics. Report on the genetic testing of children 2010. www.bsgm.org (accessed January 31, 2014).

10. Firth HV, Hurst JA. *Oxford Desk Reference Clinical Genetics*. Oxford University Press, 2005.

11. Sheriden E, Wright J, Small N et al. Risk factors for congenital anomaly in a multiethnic birth cohort: an analysis of the Born in Bradford study. *Lancet* 2013; 382(9901): 1350–9.

Bibliography

1. Gardner RJM, Sutherland GR, Shaffer LG. *Chromosome Abnormalities and Genetic Counselling*, 4th edn. Oxford University Press, 2012.

2. Firth HV, Hurst JA. *Oxford Desk Reference Clinical Genetics*. Oxford University Press, 2005.

2. Harper PS. *Practical Genetic Counselling*, 7th edn. Edward Arnold (Publishers) Ltd., 2010.

3. Kingston HM. *ABC of Clinical Genetics*, 3rd edn. BMJ Books, 2003.

Chapter

3

Antenatal screening for fetal anomalies

Manju Nair and Bidyut Kumar

Obstetricians have an ethical and legal duty to inform women about reasonably available tests capable of providing useful information about the presence of fetal disease and malformation. Such information upholds the autonomy of pregnant women and their partners, and supports them in decisions about whether to continue a current gestation based on facts about fetal health, presence or absence of anomalies and the implications of anomalies for the future of the child and family.

Screening is the process of surveying a population, using a specific marker or markers and defined screening cut-off levels, to identify the individuals in the population at higher risk for a particular disorder. Screening is applicable to a population; diagnosis is applied at the individual patient level.

Criteria for implementing screening tests

The criteria for screening mentioned in the classic World Health Organization report by Wilson and Jungner are worth quoting here[1]. These criteria are accepted as the "gold standard" for assessment and decision making about a screening policy.

(1) The condition sought should be an important health problem.

(2) There should be an accepted treatment for patients with recognized disease.

(3) Facilities for diagnosis and treatment should be available.

(4) There should be a recognizable latent or early symptomatic stage.

(5) There should be a suitable test or examination.

(6) The test should be acceptable to the population.

(7) The natural history of the condition, including development from latent to declared disease, should be adequately understood.

(8) There should be an agreed policy on whom to treat as patients.

(9) The cost of case-finding (including diagnosis and treatment of patients diagnosed) should be economically balanced in relation to possible expenditure on medical care as a whole.

(10) Case-finding should be a continuing process and not a "once and for all" project.

Pretest counseling

It is essential that prior to implementing any screening test, the parents be provided with appropriate information. The DISCERN methodology defines a set of criteria by which the quality of genetic screening information can be judged[2]. The interested reader may wish to discover that pretest counseling should include information on sensitivity (detection rate (DR)) and false-positive rate (FPR) of the screening test, alternative options if the result is 'screen positive' and information that a screening test may lead to risky invasive diagnostic tests for confirmation of diagnosis. Even if termination of pregnancy is not considered, some parents may like to have all the information to be better prepared for the birth and care of an affected infant. The care provider should allow the couple unbiased information and sufficient time to make an informed choice.

Fetal Medicine, ed. Bidyut Kumar and Zarko Alfirevic. Published by Cambridge University Press. © Cambridge University Press 2016.

Principles of screening tests

The four measures that are used to evaluate screening tests are:

(1) percentage of the total number of diseased or affected people identified by a test (sensitivity)
(2) proportion of all those who did not have the disease and tested negative (specificity) (also expressed as a percentage)
(3) positive predictive value (PPV) is the percentage of all those who tested positive and actually had the disease
(4) negative predictive value (NPV) of a test is the percentage of actual negative (absence of disease) amongst those who had a negative screening test result.

The first two measures are of epidemiologic importance, whereas PPV and NPV are perhaps of more interest to the clinician, because it is only after a "positive" screening result that the patient becomes interested.

To further explain these measures, refer to the illustration below.

	Disease positive	Disease negative
Test positive	X	Y
Test negative	M	N

Sensitivity = X/X+M; specificity = N/Y+N.

PPV= X/X+Y; NPV= N/ M+N.

FPR = Y/ X+Y.

Generally speaking, sensitivity and specificity do not vary as a function of prevalence of the disorder, but PPV and NPV do. In a population with low risk of the disorder (or low prevalence of the disorder), the proportion of positives that will be false positive will be much higher than in a population in which the prevalence is very high. In the latter case, the vast majority of positives will, in fact, be true positives.

As screening performance improves, the FPR decreases and the sensitivity or DR increases. A risk cut-off might be determined based upon the desired DR, FPR or both. A risk cut-off is expressed as the risk or likelihood of the condition being present in the fetus at term or at the time of the screening test.

In the UK, antenatal screening is routinely offered for the following conditions:

- fetal anomaly (ultrasound screening between 18 weeks 0 days and 20 weeks 6 days)
- Down's syndrome (DS; combined test in the first trimester and quadruple test in the second trimester)
- hematologic conditions (screening for hemoglobinopathy)
- infections (asymptomatic bacteruria, human immunodeficiency virus, hepatitis B, syphilis and rubella).

Screening for neural tube defects

Alpha-fetoprotein (AFP) is a glycoprotein produced by the yolk sac and the liver during fetal development. Beginning at the end of first trimester, fetal serum AFP levels decline steadily. In pregnant women, fetal AFP levels can be monitored in urine. AFP is cleared strongly from the kidneys allowing AFP to tend to mirror fetal serum levels. In contrast, maternal serum AFP levels are much lower but continue to rise until about week 32. This is thought to be because the mother is not utilizing the AFP, and therefore clears it from her system without issue. The exact role and function of AFP in humans remains unclear.

AFP is excreted by fetal kidneys and is then passed with fetal urine into the amniotic fluid. Peak concentrations of amniotic fluid AFP is reached at around 12 weeks' gestation. Falsely elevated levels of maternal AFP can be present when amniotic fluid is contaminated with fetal blood. AFP reaches maternal circulation by transplacental diffusion and by transamniotic diffusion. Excess AFP in amniotic fluid due to fetal disorders diffuses across the amnion. The restrictive amniotic membrane, in combination with a relatively high transplacental diffusion of normal background AFP, makes measurement of maternal serum AFP (MSAFP) less sensitive.

A screening strategy used to detect open neural tube defects (NTDs) involves converting MSAFP levels to multiples of the median (MoM) value for gestational age, and then classifying 2% of all screened pregnancies as having an elevated result (2.5 MoM or higher).

A case control study involving 219,000 consecutive pregnancies between 1995 and 2002, compared the ability of routine ultrasound and MSAFP levels to detect NTDs. Of 189 identified fetuses with NTDs, 102 were screened with MSAFP and 25% of these were screened as negative. Of the 186 NTDs identified prenatally, 62% were initially detected by routine second-trimester ultrasound, 37% detected by targeted ultrasound prompted by high MSAFP levels, and the remaining 1% were diagnosed by pathology examination after miscarriage[3]. There was another study in the early 1990s investigating the value of MSAFP in screening for NTDs, which produced sensitivity of about 86% and specificity of 98%, positive (LR+) and negative (LR−) likelihood ratios of 35.16 and 0.15, respectively[4].

The current recommended practice in the UK is that when routine ultrasound screening is performed to detect NTDs, screening with the use of MSAFP is not required.

Screening for Down's syndrome

Maternal age

The origin of the most common type of DS is associated with a free extra chromosome 21 (trisomy 21 or T21) and differs from the more rare types that are dependent on extra chromosome 21 material caused by a structural chromosome rearrangement. In particular, it is exclusively this common type that is associated with an increase dependent on maternal age, a rise which is especially dramatic at later reproductive ages from maternal age of around 35 years onwards. Prevalence of DS at birth increases from about 1 in 1500 at age 20 years to about 1 in 900 at age 30 years and 1 in 350 at the age of 35 years. Thereafter, a more rapid rise of risk is seen, reaching about 1 in 85 at age 40 years and 1 in 35 at the age of 45 years.

Historically, the term advanced maternal age denotes a woman 35 years of age or older (at the time of delivery), and reflects the age at which the risk of giving birth to a living child with any chromosomal abnormality (1/204) roughly equals the risk of a fetus dying from complications of genetic amniocentesis (approximately 1/200).

Gestational age also influences the risk for a woman to have a pregnancy affected by DS because a greater proportion of pregnancies with DS fetus are spontaneously miscarried than pregnancies with normal fetus. Thus, the risk will be higher for any given maternal age, the earlier in pregnancy a screening test is performed. Furthermore, the risk of miscarriage varies according to the woman's age, being lower in the younger age group.

In recent decades, there has been an important upward shift in maternal age at delivery, and this has substantially influenced both the DR and FPR at the age cut-off of 35 years. For example, in 1980, women at or above the age of 35 years accounted for 5% of all pregnancies and all of these women were assumed to be "screen positive." The FPR in this age group was thus about 5%. The DR for DS in this age group was about 25%. In 1990, the FPR increased to 9% and the DR to 42%, and in year 2000 these rates were 13% and 54%, respectively.

Development of more modern screening tests, as described below, makes it possible to achieve much higher DR and lower FPR. Therefore, screening by maternal age is no longer recommended as a DS screening strategy.

Tests used for Down's syndrome screening

Screening for DS takes place during either the first or second trimester by either ultrasound or maternal serum biochemistry, or a combination of both. Measurements of the biochemical markers are converted into MoM for gestational age, and adjusted for maternal weight and ethnicity.

Screening tests, which have been implemented or tried, include the following. Those appearing in italics are no longer undertaken in common clinical practice.

- 11–14 weeks
  - nuchal translucency (NT)
  - combined test: NT + human chorionic gonadotropin (hCG) + pregnancy-associated plasma protein A (PAPP-A)

- 15–20 weeks
  - *double test (hCG + unconjugated estriol (uE3))*
  - *triple test (hCG, uE3, AFP)*
  - quadruple test (hCG, uE3, AFP, inhibin A)

- *11–14 weeks and then at 15–20 weeks*
  - *total integrated test (combined test at 11–14 weeks, followed by AFP, uE3 and inhibin A at 15–20 weeks)*
  - *serum integrated test (PAPP-A and hCG at 11–14 weeks, followed by AFP, uE3 and inhibin A at 15–20 weeks).*

First-trimester screening (11–14 weeks)

Nuchal translucency

Of all the markers, increased NT has the most significant association with aneuploidy. The definition of raised

NT varies in different studies with values expressed in millimetre (mm) or centiles (greater than 3 mm or greater than the 95th or 99th centile). Measurements of NT greater than 99th centile (3.5 mm) in the first trimester are strongly associated with chromosomal abnormalities, major cardiac defects and other abnormalities[5]. The risk of an abnormality is directly proportional to the value of NT. A study by Kagan et al., which included 11,315 pregnancies, showed that the incidence of aneuploidy was directly proportional to the value of NT and noted the incidence to be 7% (at NT of 3.4 mm), 20% (at 3.5–4.4 mm), 50% (at 5.5–6.4 mm) and 75% when NT ≥8.5 mm[6].

- **Aneuploidy.** Several studies have been conducted to assess the performance of NT as a screening tool. One of the pioneering studies was by Snijders et al. in 1998 (96,127 patients from 22 centers at 10–14 weeks of gestation). They found that a risk assessment based on the measurement of NT and maternal age had a DR of 82% for trisomy 21 at a FPR of 8% and a DR of 77% at a FPR of 5%[7]. The SURUSS trial of 47,053 pregnancies from 25 maternity units (24 in the UK and one in Austria) noted a DR of 63% for a 5% FPR[8]. The FASTER trial (33,557 patients) noted a DR of 70% at 11 weeks and 64% at 13 weeks with a 5% FPR[9].
- **Cardiac defects.** Compared to the general population, there is an increased risk for congenital heart defects in fetuses with increased NT. The risk of congenital heart defects varies between 2% (when NT values at 95th centile) to 5% (for NT value at 99th centile, 3.5 mm). Septal defects are the most commonly noted abnormality[10].
- **Other congenital abnormalities.** In fetuses with increased NT and normal karyotype, other abnormalities have been noted, such as skeletal dysplasia, diaphragmatic hernia, abdominal wall defects, body stalk anomaly and genetic syndromes. Noonan syndrome is currently the only molecular genetic condition that has been shown to have a clear association with raised NT.
- **Miscarriage or fetal demise.** An increased risk has been noted in fetuses with increased NT and the risk is directly proportional to the measurement of NT, with an increased incidence in cases of hydrops. It can vary from 1.6% in pregnancies with NT between 95–99th percentile to about 20% for NTs measuring greater than 6.5 mm[11].

- **Association with maternal infection.** This is mostly in cases of persistent second- or third-trimester nuchal edema and hydrops. Parvovirus B19 is the only specific pathogen that has been shown to have a direct association with increased NT due to the effect of fetal anemia or fetal myocardial infarction.
- **Normal outcome.** The chance of delivering a baby with no abnormality was 70% for values of NT measurement between 3.5–4.4 mm, 50% for NT of 4.5–5.4 mm, 30% for NT of 5.5–6.4 mm and 15% for values >6 mm[12].
- **Further investigations.** In cases of enlarged NT >3.5 mm, a diagnostic test for fetal karyotyping should be considered. In addition, fetal echocardiography either in early or mid second trimester, along with a detailed fetal anatomical survey, should be carried out.

Various theories have been proposed to explain the mechanism of development of increased NT. The mechanism for increased NT is thought to differ based on the associated abnormality. One of the proposed theories in trisomy 21 is the abnormal collagen with more accumulation of fluid. In fetuses with cardiac anomaly, many theories have been proposed, including endothelial dysfunction, venous congestion of the head or neck, fetal anemia and cardiac dysfunction[12].

The ideal gestation to measure the NT is between 11 and 13 weeks 6 days of gestation or crown–rump length measurement of 45–84 mm. This time period has the additional advantage of assessment of the fetal anatomy in line with the normal embryologic development. After 14 weeks, the fetal position may not be favorable and an increased NT might resolve.

For details of the technique of NT measurement, readers are referred to the chapter on ultrasound assessment of fetal anatomy.

Compared to the serum screening modalities, screening involving NT measurement has the advantage of being less affected or unaffected by smoking, ethnicity or parity. It is also useful in multiple pregnancies. However, it has the limitation of being operator and gestational age dependent. Hence, it requires quality control and audit of clinical practice.

Cystic hygroma

Cystic hygroma is a congenital malformation of the lymphatic system in which obstruction between the lymphatic and venous pathways leads to accumulation of lymph in the jugular lymphatic sacs. It can be septated or nonseptated. Septated cystic hygroma has a 50% chance of being associated with aneuploidy. It may be difficult to differentiate a cystic hygroma from a simple increased NT, but a few differentiating points would be a generalized edema and multiple septations in cystic hygroma compared with more localization in NT. The evaluation would be the same in both cases but counseling with regards to the risk differs. Compared to increased NT, cystic hygroma has a higher risk of aneuploidy (fivefold), cardiac anomalies (12-fold) and fetal demise (sixfold)[13]. The other causes of cystic swelling in the nuchal region, such as posterior encephalocele, cervical meningocele and cystic teratoma, should be excluded. Due to the strong association with aneuploidy, it is reasonable to directly offer invasive testing in the case of prenatal diagnosis of cystic hygroma. The outcome depends on the presence of associated abnormalities and the size of the cystic hygroma.

Fetal nasal bone

The nasal bone can be normally visualized as a thin echogenic line within the bridge of the fetal nose. Absence of the nasal bone or nasal bone hypoplasia (measurements below 3.5 mm or 2.5th percentile) is considered to have a strong association with trisomy 21. Different methods have been used to define nasal bone hypoplasia, for example, measurement of less than 2.5 mm or less than the 2.5th percentile.

A meta-analysis by Moreno-Cid et al. analysed 21 studies relevant to fetal nasal bone and risk for DS[14]. They estimated a LR+ of 40.08 and a 95% confidence interval (CI) of 18.10–88.76, with an absent nasal bone and a NPV of 0.71 (95% CI, 0.64–0.79). The LR+ for hypoplastic nasal bone was 15.15 (95% CI, 8.15–28.16) with a NPV of 0.47 (95% CI, 0.34–0.64). They found that there was no significant difference between the different methods of defining nasal bone hypoplasia, and screening performance was found to be better with nasal bone measurements expressed as MoM or percentiles rather than as a ratio of biparietal diameter and nasal bone length, as noted in some other studies.

Addition of this marker to the combined screening test has been shown to increase the DR to about 97% for a FPR of 5%, or a DR of 95% for a FPR of 2%[15].

Tricuspid regurgitation

Several studies have reported an increased DR of aneuploidies using tricuspid regurgitation (TR) as an additional screening tool. A study by Kagan et al. estimated that if tricuspid flow measurement is added to a screening policy based on maternal age, fetal NT, fetal heart rate, serum-free n chorionic beta-hCG and PAPP-A, the DR of trisomy 21 would be 96%, and the DR of trisomy 18, trisomy 13 and Turner syndrome would be 92%, 100% and 100%, respectively, at FPR of 3%[15].

Technique for measurement. The pulsed Doppler gate should be placed across the tricuspid valve in the four-chamber view of the heart with the angle of insonation <20°. Diagnosis of TR is made when the regurgitant jet is at least 80 cm/s and extends to more than half of systole.

Ductus venosus Doppler

Several studies have reported reversed a-wave in the ductus venosus Doppler in DS (59–93%). However, it could be present in 3–21% of normal fetuses. There can be difficulties in obtaining the measurement in the first trimester due to the small size of this vessel. FPVs with absence of the flow due to sampling of the inferior vena cava blood flow and false-negative readings can be obtained with presence of a-wave due to sampling of the umbilical vein. Hence, it should be performed only by trained operators and may be used as an adjunct to modify the priori risk[16].

The combined screening test

The combined test includes assessment of the NT, serum beta-hCG and PAPP-A levels. This test is done between 11 and 13 weeks 6 days.

The FASTER trial demonstrated that adding the serum markers to measurement of NT increases the DR of DS from 70–87% with a 5% FPR[9]. The other finding of this trial was that at a gestation of 11 weeks, the combined test performed better with a DR of 87% compared with that at 12 weeks (DR of 85%) and 13 weeks (DR of 82%). This is because the NT and PAPP-A tests perform better at 11 weeks compared with 13 weeks. Some of the other studies, such as the Biochemistry, Ultrasound and Nuchal Translucency (BUN) study with 8,216 patients showed a DR of 79% at a FPR of 5%[17].

Apart from the advantage of increased DR, the combined screening test has the added benefit of earlier results and opportunity for diagnostic testing by chorion villus sampling (CVS) at an earlier gestation compared to amniocentesis. If required, women have the option of earlier termination of pregnancy, which is relatively safer.

One of the main factors affecting the success of the first-trimester screening, is the accuracy of estimation of the NT and ensuring that women have access to this service in the narrow window period of 10–13 weeks 6 days. For a positive screening test result, there is the need for provision of early invasive testing by CVS, which is a more skilled procedure and carries a slightly increased miscarriage rate when compared to amniocentesis.

Second-trimester serum screening

In the UK, it is common practice to offer the quadruple test (AFP, hCG, uE3, inhibin A) to those women for whom the combined test could not be carried out for whatever reason. Other tests of historical interest are the triple test (AFP, hCG, uE3) and double test (AFP, hCG). These are offered between 15 weeks 0 days and 20 weeks 0 days.

Estimates from the SURUSS and FASTER trials show a DR of 81% for a FPR of 5%. The evidence from the SURUSS trial does not support the double test (DR 60%, FPR 5%), triple test (DR 70%, FPR 5%) or NT measurements on their own because of their increased FPR without increasing the DR, thereby increasing the rate of unwarranted invasive diagnostic tests[8,9].

In the UK, the current national screening policy recommends a screening test with a DR of >90% for a screen positive rate (SPR) of <2% for the combined test, and a DR of >75% for a SPR of <3% for those undergoing quadruple screening[18]. The threshold for risk assessment is 1 in 150 for the above two tests.

Rationale for selection of the serum analyates

The serum levels of each analyate are different at each period of gestation. The values are expressed as MoM after population-based medians are established, thereby eliminating the effect of gestational age on the result. This enables us to compare an individual woman's risk to that of the entire population.

Human chorionic gonadotropin

hCG is a complex glycoprotein produced exclusively by the syncytiotrophoblast. It increases rapidly in the first 8 weeks of gestation, reaches a peak by 10 weeks and declines steadily until 20 weeks when it plateaus. Free beta-hCG has slightly increased sensitivity in detecting trisomy 21 when compared with total hCG[19,20].

Alpha-fetoprotein

In the early second trimester, AFP increases by 15–20% per week. It is a major protein in the fetus and is synthesized in the yolk sac, gastrointestinal tract and liver of the fetus. Antibodies against AFP do not have significant cross-reactivity, which has enabled the development of a variety of antibody based assays for reliably measuring AFP in amniotic fluid and maternal serum.

Unconjugated estriol

uE3 is produced by the placenta from precursors provided by the fetal adrenal glands and the liver. In the early second trimester, estriol level increases by 20–25% per week.

Pregnancy associated plasma protein-A

PAPP-A is a high molecular weight zinc containing metalloprotein, produced by the trophoblast. PAPP-A levels increase by 30–50% per week between 10 and 13 weeks of gestation. In addition to being a marker of chromosomal aneuploidy, it is an indicator of early pregnancy failure and placental insufficiency.

Inhibin A

Inhibin A is a glycoprotein synthesized by the gonads, corpus luteum, decidua and placenta. The levels increase in the first trimester until 10 weeks and then remain stable until 25 weeks of gestation. Thereafter, it increases to reach a peak by term.

If the individual performance of each marker is compared, hCG and inhibin A perform the best, followed by uE3 and AFP.

Affected pregnancies

Compared to unaffected pregnancies, in affected pregnancies with T21, the levels of second-trimester AFP and uE3 are, on average, 0.70–0.75 MoM and levels of beta-hCG and inhibin A are about 2.0 MoM. First-trimester PAPP-A levels are approximately 0.4 MoM and free beta-hCG is about 1.8 MoM. PAPP-A levels are 2 to 2.5 times lower in DS. This difference is significant in the first trimester, but it loses the significant difference between affected and unaffected pregnancy around 14 weeks.

The exact mechanism for these changes is not clearly understood. It has been hypothesized that it could be due to poorly functioning fetal tissue with compensatory placental hyperfunction as reflected by an increase in the placental secretory products, such as hCG and inhibin, and a decrease in the fetal secretory products, such as AFP and estriol[19].

In trisomy 18, the serum-free beta-hCG, estriol and PAPP-A levels are much lower. In trisomy 13, the first-trimester analyte pattern is similar to that of trisomy 18, but more variable. It is characterized by low to very low PAPP-A (median 0.36 MoM) and free beta-hCG (median 0.41 MoM)[21].

Factors affecting the screening results

- Maternal weight has an inverse relation with the levels of all four markers, possibly due to increased dilution.
- Ethnicity
- Concentrations of maternal serum AFP, PAPP-A, total hCG, and free beta-hCG are increased and inhibin A levels are decreased in African–American compared with Caucasian women.
- Smoking
- AFP and inhibin A levels are higher and uE3, beta-hCG and PAPP-A levels are lower in smokers than in nonsmokers.
- Diabetes mellitus
- Maternal serum levels of AFP and uE3 are noted to be decreased in women with diabetes.
- In-vitro fertilization: maternal serum beta-hCG and inhibin A levels tend to be increased and uE3 levels decreased as a consequence of the hormonal treatment to stimulate the ovaries for in-vitro fertilization.
- Multiple pregnancy
- It is difficult to interpret the serum screening levels in multiple pregnancies.
- Selection of risk cut-off. Each patient is given a numerical risk based on age and screening test results. For a given test, as the risk cut-off becomes higher, fewer women are screen positive and fewer affected pregnancies will be identified. If less stringent risk cut-offs are chosen, a greater number of affected pregnancies will be identified, but there will be more false-positive tests and more invasive testing.

Role of the midtrimester scan in screening for aneuploidy

Many fetuses with chromosomal abnormality are found to have unusual findings on ultrasound examination or clear, well-defined abnormalities. Some of the unusual findings are not significant anomalies on their own, but have a known association with aneuploidy. These unusual sonographic findings could also be a normal variant and could disappear at a later gestation. Various terms have been used for these unusual findings, such as "soft markers." "Genetic sonogram" refers to a combination of using second-trimester ultrasound markers and serum markers to estimate a risk for aneuploidy, but is not in common use. Various studies have reported the association between abnormal ultrasound findings and trisomy 21, with DR ranging between 53.1% and 92.8%[22].

Sonographic signs associated with trisomy 21, 18 and 13

Trisomy 21

Major defects include cardiovascular defects (atrioventricular septal defect (AVSD), tetralogy of Fallot), duodenal atresia, cystic hygroma and hydrops.

Other abnormal findings might include increased nuchal fold thickness, mild ventriculomegaly, renal pelvicalyceal dilatation, echogenic bowel, echogenic cardiac focus, short femur/humerus, clinodactyly, sandal sign, widened iliac angle, growth restriction, hypoplastic nasal bones and brachycephaly[13].

Trisomy 18

Major defects include cardiac defects (double outlet right ventricle, ventricular septal defect (VSD), AVSD), meningiomyelocele, agenesis of corpus callosum, omphalocele, diaphragmatic hernia, clubbed or rocker bottom feet, orofaial cleft, cystic hygroma and hydrops.

Other markers include increased nuchal fold, mild ventriculomegaly, short femur/humerus, enlarged cisterna magna, echogenic bowel, choroid plexus cysts, micrognathia, strawberry-shaped skull, clenched or overlapping fingers, single umbilical artery and growth restriction.

Trisomy 13

Major defects include holoprosencephaly, orofacial clefting, cyclopia, proboscis, omphalocele, cardiac defects (VSD, hypoplastic left heart), polydactyly, rocker bottom feet, echogenic kidneys, cystic hygroma and hydrops.

Other abnormal findings include increased nuchal fold, mild ventriculomegaly, echogenic bowel, echogenic cardiac focus, short femur or humerus, overlapping fingers, single umbilical artery and growth restriction.

Interpretation of results and calculation of risk

Renal pyelectasis

Results of a meta-analysis of 10 observational studies of 2,148 cases has shown that isolated fetal pyelectasis in the second-trimester ultrasound is associated with a pooled LR+ of 2.78 (95% CI, 1.75–4.43) and LR– of 0.99 (95% CI, 0.98–1.00)[23]. The cut-off used in most of the studies in the meta-analysis was 4 mm.

Echogenic bowel

Echogenic bowel refers to increased echogenicity of the bowel, which is similar to or greater than the surrounding bone. Whilst making the diagnosis, it is important to have the lowest gain setting of the machine. A higher transducer frequency (8 MHz) can give a false-positive diagnosis.

It can be a normal finding in the third trimester due to the presence of meconium in the bowel. The detection of echogenic bowel is of significance in the second trimester. The possible causes of increased echogenicity are swallowing of blood by the fetus due to the presence of blood or blood components in the amniotic cavity due to placental bleeding. The other causes are CF (due to the increased viscosity of the meconium), fetal aneuploidy (possibly due to reduced bowel motility), congenital infection (mainly cytomegalovirus) and gastrointestinal obstruction.

A French multicenter study investigated and followed up 682 cases of echogenic bowel and noted multiple malformations in 6.9% of the cases, significant chromosomal anomaly in 3.5%, CF in 3% and viral infection in 2.8% of the cases[24]. Another study of 289 cases showed a prevalence of CF (7.6%), digestive malformations (7.0%) chromosomal abnormalities (3.7%) and materno-fetal infections (3.7%)[25].

Once the diagnosis is confirmed, parents should be offered CF carrier screening, maternal serologic testing for cytomegalovirus (CMV) and toxoplasmosis, and testing for fetal chromosomal abnormalities. A complete structural survey is required to exclude any other malformations, particularly bowel obstruction. Due to the associated risk of growth restriction, as noted in some studies, serial growth monitoring should be offered.

It is not uncommon for the echogenicity to resolve after a few weeks and also not to to have a definitive diagnosis. Long-term follow-up of these babies has not shown any abnormalities[26].

Short femur and humerus

A meta-analysis of second-trimester markers has shown that a short femur length (FL) has a LR+ of 3.72 (95% CI, 2.79–4.97) and a LR– of 0.80 (95% CI, 0.73–0.88) in detecting a fetus with trisomy 21. Short humerus length (HL) is associated with a LR+ of 4.81 (95% CI, 3.49–6.62) and a LR– of 0.74 (95% CI, 0.63–0.88)[27,29]. A short humerus has a better predictive value in detecting trisomy 21 compared to a short femur. Various criteria have been used for diagnosing a short femur/humerus, including a ratio of observed to expected HL/FL ratio less than 0.9. The expected value is calculated by the following formula:

Humerus: $-7.9404 + 0.8492 \times$ biparietal diameter (BPD)

Femur: $-9.645 + 0.9338 \times$ BPD.

Most recent studies, however, use the criteria of less than the 10th centile, 5th centile or 3rd centile for gestational age, with specificity increasing with lower threshold. It is also associated with other other causes like skeletal dysplasia, genetic syndromes and early signs of small-for-gestational-age fetus.

Echogenic cardiac foci

Echogenic cardiac foci are visualized as bright foci in either or both ventricles. It has been estimated that the probability of DS (assuming LR+ of 6.2) after an intracardiac echogenic foci has been detected would be 0.44% in a population with prevalence of 1 : 1,400, 0.62% with prevalence of 1 : 1,000 and 1.03% with prevalence of 1 : 600. The probability of a case of DS being detected was equal to the probability of an unnecessary miscarriage caused by amniocentesis when the background prevalence of DS was 1 : 770[29].

Cardiac anomalies

Several studies have reported abnormal cardiac findings to be associated with trisomy 21. These include VSD, endocardial cushion defect, right-to-left disproportion, outflow tract abnormalities, pericardial effusion and TR.

DR exceeding 90% have been noted if a fetal echocardiogram is performed along with a routine ultrasound examination[22]. However, this requires trained operators who can perform fetal echocardiography.

Calculation of risk based on second-trimester sonography

A meta-analysis of 56 studies involving 1,930 babies with DS and 130,365 unaffected fetuses has shown the following performance status for some of the ultrasound findings associated with aneuploidy[28].

Each ultrasound finding stated below is followed by its associated sensitivity, specificity, LR+ and LR− ratios.

- Thickened nuchal fold: sensitivity of 0.04 (95% CI, 0.02–0.10), specificity of 0.99 (95% CI, 0.99–0.99), LR+ of 17 (95% CI, 8–38), LR− of 0.97 (95% CI, 0.94–1.00).
- Choroid plexus cyst: sensitivity of 0.01 (95% CI, 0–0.03), specificity of 0.99 (95% CI, 0.97–1.00), LR+ of 1.00 (95% CI, 0.12–9.4), LR− of 1.00 (95% CI, 0.97–1.00).
- Femur length: sensitivity of 0.16 (95% CI, 0.05–0.40), specificity of 0.96 (95% CI, 0.94–0.98), LR+ of 2.7 (95% CI, 1.2–6.0), LR− of 0.87 (95% CI, 0.75–1.00).
- Humerus length: sensitivity of 0.09 (95% CI, 0–0.60), specificity of 0.97 (95% CI, 0.91–0.99), LR+ of 7.5 (95% CI, 4.7–12,) LR− of 0.87 (95% CI, 0.67–1.1).
- Echogenic bowel: sensitivity of 0.04 (95% CI, 0.01–0.24), specificity of 0.99 (95% CI, 0.97–1.00), LR+ of 6.1 (95% CI, 3.0–12.6), LR− of 1.00 (95% CI, 0.98–1.00).
- Echogenic intracardiac focus: sensitivity of 0.11 (95% CI, 0.06–0.18), specificity of 0.96 (95% CI, 0.94–0.97), LR+ of 2.8 (95% CI, 1.5–5.5,) LR− of 0.95 (95% CI, 0.89–1.00).
- Renal pyelectasis: sensitivity of 0.02 (95% CI, 0.01–0.06), specificity of 0.99 (95% CI, 0.98–1.00), LR+ of 1.9 (95% CI, 0.7–5.1), LR− of 1.00 (95% CI, 1.00–1.00).

A meta-analysis by Agathokleous et al. showed the following overall likelihood ratio for an isolated marker (derived by multiplying LR+ for the given marker by LR− of each of all other markers, except for short humerus, aberrant right subclavian artery and nasal bone)[29].

- Nuchal fold: 3.79
- Short humerus: 0.78
- Short femur: 0.61
- Mild hydronephrosis: 1.08
- Echogenic cardiac foci: 0.95
- Echogenic bowel: 1.65

- Aberrant right subclavian artery: 6.58
- Ventriculomegaly: 3.81
- Absent/hypoplastic nasal bone: 5.3

They calculated that in the absence of all markers, the risk for trisomy 21 would be reduced by 7.7-fold.

Various techniques have been described to modify the prior risk using the findings in the second-trimester scan. The incidence of each marker in aneuplodic fetus when divided by the incidence in normal pregnancy will give a likelihood ratio. The combined likelihood ratio of all the markers when adjusted with the background risk of maternal age can give the overall risk. The pre-test odds, derived from maternal age, second-trimester serum biochemical testing or first-trimester combined testing, is multiplied by the LR+ of each marker found to be present and the LR− of each marker looked for but not found[30].

Limitations of genetic sonogram

The value of these findings depends on the accuracy of detection and reliability with which it can be reproduced, for example, the diagnosis of echogenic bowel and the importance of accurate measurements of nuchal fold thickness or of the lateral ventricles. Secondly, some of these studies lack standardization of criteria for diagnosis of an abnormality. For likelihood ratios with a high confidence interval, one has to be cautious in giving an exact estimate of the risk.

Sonographic features, as mentioned above, may not be of practical value in detection of chromosomal abnormalities in a low-risk population. They should not be used as a primary screening tool as their use in this manner increases the FPR without increasing DR.

Current recommendations

Due to the above limitations sonographic markers should only be used as an adjunct to the other screening protocols. If it is used as a primary screening tool, it increases the FPR without increasing the DR.

The fetal anomaly screening program in the UK advises that the term "soft marker" should not be used[31]. Choroid plexus cyst(s), dilated cisterna magna, echogenic foci in the heart and two-vessel cord can be normal variants. Women who have a low risk through first- or second-trimester screening, or who have declined screening for DS, should not be referred for further assessment of chromosomal abnormality if the above features are detected at the second-trimester anomaly scan.

The American College of Obstetricians and Gynecologists recommends that it should be limited to centers with expertise in ultrasound and/or those centers engaged in clinical research to develop a standardized approach[32].

The genetic sonogram is valuable in the following situations:

- women who present at a later stage after the time period for second-trimester serum screening tests
- recalculation of the risk for those women who have been given a high risk of DS based on the serum markers but do not desire invasive testing.

Noninvasive prenatal testing

The main drive for the development of noninvasive prenatal testing (NIPT) in screening for aneuploidy is to reduce the number of invasive procedures. The initial research on NIPT focused on detecting intact fetal cells in maternal circulation using standard detection techniques, but this was not satisfactory for aneuploidy detection. Currently, NIPT has evolved to detect cell-free fetal DNA (cffDNA) in maternal blood, which contribute to 3–13% of the total circulating DNA, are placental in origin and are derived from apoptotic trophoblasts. The presence of cffDNA is not affected by maternal age, previous blood transfusions or fetal sex, but is increased in aneuploidy. They are undetectable in the maternal circulation after delivery, hence there is no cross-interaction from previous fetus/placenta.

Studies report a sensitivity of >99% for trisomy 21, and 100% and 91.7% for trisomy 18 and 13, respectively[32]. Hence, the overall number of invasive procedures will be reduced.

Other advantages of NIPT include fetal rhesus D genotyping and fetal noninvasive sexing from cfDNA for X-linked conditions.

Techniques for cffDNA detection

Various techniques have developed over the years to improve the detection of fetal DNA. These include parallel genomic sequencing, multiplex ligation dependent probe amplification (MLPA), quantitative fluorescence polymerase chain reaction (QF-PCR) and other variants of PCR. MLPA is a PCR-based technique that utilizes the amplification and quantification of the probes instead of nucleic acids. MLPA is a PCR-based technology that discriminates between copy numbers of specific sequences of DNA. In QF-PCR, repeats on

chromosomes 13, 18, 21, X and Y are identified using fluorescently labeled primers and PCR.

These techniques appear suitable for prenatal diagnosis in women undergoing invasive testing for aneuploidies alone. For women with risk factors such as structural malformations on ultrasound or a family history of chromosomal translocations, a full cytogenetic karyotype analysis is required[34].

Limitations

cffDNA only represents a fraction of the total DNA, which makes it difficult to distinguish fetal loci from maternal loci for point mutations. False-negative results are thus possible. False-positive results can occur due to mosaicism. The information is restricted to the specific chromosome, hence in the case of a positive result, confirmation by invasive testing is required. Ethical issues surrounding sex selection is another issue in certain countries.

Cost of the testing can be a limiting factor in adopting NIPT as a universal screening policy. One way of eliminating the cost factor is to use it in a selective population. For further details on NIPT the reader is referred to the chapter on genetics.

Cystic fibrosis

Cystic fibrosis (CF) is a multisystem disease involving the respiratory system, gastrointestinal system, sweat glands and the reproductive system in the males. It is the most common recessive disorder in the Caucasian population of northern European origin (prevalence of 1 in 2,500 to 3,300 live births). The diagnostic criteria for CF includes: presence of a typical clinical feature (respiratory, gastrointestinal or genitourinary); history of CF in sibling; positive newborn screening test in addition to abnormal sweat chloride concentration; two CF mutations; and abnormal nasal potential difference.

Genetics. CF is caused by mutations in a single large gene on chromosome 7 that encodes the CF transmembrane conductance regulator protein. This protein regulates the activity of the sodium and chloride channels of the epithelial surface of the respiratory, gastrointestinal and genitourinary system and the sweat glands. Hence, a dysfunction of this protein causes low water content in the secretions from this epithelium, causing them to be viscous.

Prenatal screening. Screening should be offered to women who have a strong family history of CF or

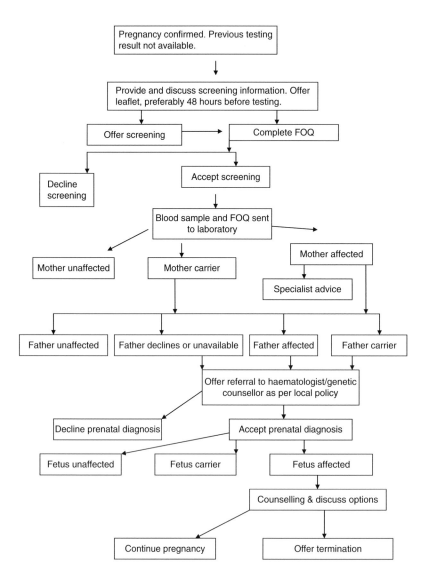

Figure 3.1 The step-wise process of screening for genetic disorder.

a finding of echogenic bowel in the second-trimester ultrasound scan.

Pretest counseling. As for every screening test, appropriate counseling is essential, particularly in this condition due to the complex genetics.

There are around 700 gene mutations described, which are divided into five different classes. The most common mutation is the delta F508, which is found in approximately 70% of Caucasian patients, while the most common mutation in individuals of Ashkenazi Jewish heritage is W1282X. The phenotypic expression of the disease varies according to the type of the mutation. For example, the above common mutations cause the classical multisystem affection of CF, whereas the

other rarer mutations may be associated with only an isolated feature of the disease affecting only one system (the R117H mutation is associated with congenital absence of the vas deferens).

The other aspect to be discussed is that a complex relationship exists between the genotype and the phenotype due to the presence of gene modifiers for CF mutations other than ΔF508 or W1282X (which are associated with classic CF). There is no simple, predictable relationship between genotype and phenotype.

If both partners carry a CF mutation, there is a 1 in 4 chance that their child will be affected. The severity of clinical disease in offspring varies as a function of the specific genetic mutations present.

A negative screening test means only that the individual does not carry any of the CF mutations in the screening battery; a negative result thus reduces the likelihood but does not completely exclude the possibility that the individual is a CF carrier.

It is also important to discuss further management in the case of a positive diagnosis. The prognosis of these children is improving gradually over the last few years, with an expected survival of up to 30–40 years as a minimum. With appropriate medical and psychologic support, these children cope very well and have an independent adult life[37].

Due to the above reasons, if the parental CF screen is positive, the individual should receive genetic counseling.

Screening for hemoglobinopathies

Hemoglobinopathy is a group of hemoglobin (Hb) disorders, which are inherited as an autosomal recessive trait. They mainly affect individuals whose origins can be traced to Asia, Africa, the Caribbean, the Middle East and the Mediterranean region, but

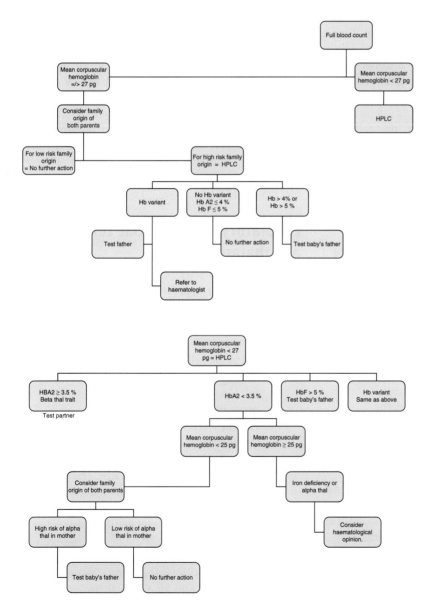

Figure 3.2 Algorithm for screening for haemoglobinopathy in low prevalence areas.

FBC: full blood count;
MCH: mean corpuscular hemoglobin.

because of the effects of migration and subsequent marriage and integration, can affect any ethnic group. The two most common types of hemoglobinopathies in the UK are the Hb variants (such as sickle-cell disorders), which are associated with the production of abnormal forms of Hb, and the thalassemias, in which there is an abnormality in the amount of Hb produced.

Normal adult Hb has four globin chains each associated with one hem moiety. Two of these globin chains are alpha and the other two may be beta (Hb-A, which forms 96% of adult Hb), delta (HbA2, 3.5% of adult Hb) or gamma (Hb-F, <1% of adult Hb). In the fetal life, all the Hb is of Hb-F type, which is gradually replaced by adult Hb after birth.

Many of the hemoglobinopathies are of no clinical significance, whereas others are associated with severe morbidity and mortality. Sickle-cell disorders often result in severe life-threatening clinical symptoms, and those with beta-thalassemia major require regular blood transfusions to maintain life.

Thalassemias are commonly of the following types: alpha-thalassemia and beta-thalassemia.

Alpha-thalassemia

Mutations in one or two of alpha genes, the condition called thalassemia trait.

If three abnormal alpha genes are inherited, the condition is called HbH disease. In the above two conditions, there are varying degrees of mild anemia with microcytic hypochromic red cell indices, such as reduced mean corpuscular volume (MCV) and mean corpuscular Hb (MCH).

If a fetus inherits no functioning alpha genes, no alpha globin is produced and the condition is called alpha-thalassemia major, which is incompatible with life.

Beta-thalassemia

When one mutant beta gene is inherited, the condition is called beta-thalassaemia minor (a carrier state). HbA2 levels are >3.5% of adult Hb. The affected person is not diseased but may pass on the abnormal gene.

When no normal beta gene is inherited, the condition is called beta-thalassaemia major. The affected person has severe disease and when untreated, can result in death of children in the first few years of life.

The National Health Service sickle-cell disease (SCD) and thalassemia screening programme was set up in 2001 by the UK National Screening Committee to implement a coordinated service for antenatal and neonatal hemoglobinopathy screening. Screening for SCD and thalassemia should be offered to all women, ideally by 10 weeks of gestation, in order to identify pregnant women at risk of carrying an affected fetus. Such women should then be offered counseling to facilitate informed decision making about prenatal diagnosis, and options about any subsequent action by the end of 12 weeks of gestation.

The type of screening depends on the prevalence of the disease, and can be carried out either in primary or secondary care. The aim is to offer universal screening in areas of high prevalence (fetal affection >1.5 per 10,000 pregnancies) and selective screening in areas of low prevalence (fetal affection ≤1.5 per 10,000 pregnancies).

Where prevalence of SCD is high, universal laboratory screening should be offered to all pregnant women to identify carriers of SCD and/or thalassemia. In low-prevalence areas, laboratory testing should be offered for relevant variants based on an assessment of risk determined by a questionnaire given to women about their family origin (Family Origin Questionnaire; available at: www.gov.uk/government/uploads/system/uploads/attachment_data/file/398766/FOQ_version_3_Feb_2014.pdf).

Laboratory tests for sickle cell disease and thalassemia

There are several tests that may be used in laboratory screening for thalassemia or SCD, and an explanation of those most commonly used in the UK are given below.

(1) Full blood count:

    (a) red blood cell (RBC) indices: a series of tests on RBCs (performed as part of the full blood count, which is offered to all pregnant women)

    (b) Hb: the level of Hb in the blood; this is low in anemia owing to iron deficiency or hemoglobinopathy

    (c) MCV: average volume of a RBC (measured as one of the RBC indices on the full blood count); this is low in thalassemia

    (d) MCH: average Hb level per RBC; this is low in thalassemia.

MCV does not appear useful for screening for beta-thalassemia, but may be more useful where there is a high prevalence of alpha-thalassemia. There is a good amount of evidence of fair quality that screening for beta-thalassemia by MCH has high sensitivity (100%) but low specificity (31%) with a cut-off of 27 pg.

Screening using RBC indices may be cost-effective for beta-thalassemia, even in areas of low prevalence.

(2) Additional tests:
   (a) ferritin test: this is a test performed on blood, which is low if the anemia is due to iron deficiency
   (b) electrophoresis: a non-automated test, which separates the Hb types present in a sample of blood
   (c) high-performance liquid chromatography (HPLC): an automated test, which separates the Hb types present in a sample of blood
   (d) sickle cell solubility test: a test that can be used to confirm the presence of sickle Hb in the blood.

The screening process involves testing a woman for carrier status early in pregnancy, and then testing her partner if she is proven to be a carrier. If both parents are confirmed as carriers, DNA analysis may be undertaken to confirm this. The unborn baby is tested using amniocentesis or CVS. The aim of antenatal testing for Hb disorders is to inform parents and to provide them with the option of pregnancy termination at an early stage of pregnancy if their child has a serious Hb disorder (See Figure 3.2).

Screening for infections

The following infection screen is routinely offered to all pregnant women in the UK:

asymptomatic bacteriuria (ASB)
rubella
hepatitis B
human immunodeficiency virus (HIV) infection
syphilis.

Asymptomatic bacteriuria

ASB is defined as persistent bacterial colonization of the urinary tract in the absence of symptoms. In the UK, it occurs in 2–5% of pregnant women. Compared with pregnant women without bacteriuria, pregnant women with untreated ASB have a higher risk of prterm birth and pyelonephritis. The increased risk among pregnant women with ASB ranges from 1.8% to 28%[28] for pyelonephritis and from 2.1% to 12.8%[40] for preterm birth.

Midstream urine (MSU) culture has been used as the "gold standard" for diagnosis of ASB. Disadvantages of this method are the delay of about 24 h in obtaining the result and the relatively higher cost compared with a reagent strip test (£0.14 versus culture at £1.40) [28]. The advantage of culturing MSU is in being able to identify the causative organism and determine antibiotic sensitivity. A number of other tests have been evaluated and none have been found suitable for diagnosis of ASB.

Studies have demonstrated that, compared to no treatment or placebo, antibiotic treatment for ASB reduced persistent bacteriuria during pregnancy, reduced risk of low-birthweight babies and reduced the risk of development of pyelonephritis[36], but a difference in preterm birth was not shown to be identifiable[37].

On current evidence, all women should be offered routine screening for asymptomatic bacteriuria by MSU culture early in pregnancy.

Rubella

Rubella infection is characterized by a febrile rash but may be asymptomatic in 20–50% of cases. Rubella screening does not attempt to identify current affected pregnancies because there is no treatment to prevent or reduce mother-to-child transmission of rubella for the current pregnancy. The aim of screening is to detect susceptibility during pregnancy so that postpartum vaccination may protect future pregnancies against rubella infection, prevent vertical transmission and reduce the risk of stillbirth and miscarriage due to rubella infection.

The UK National Screening Committee has recommended 10 IU as the lower cut-off level, which confers protection against infection[28]. To avoid misinterpretation, results of rubella screening should be reported as rubella antibody "detected" or "not detected," and not as "immune" or "susceptible." If rubella antibody is not detected, vaccination after pregnancy should be advised. Vaccination during pregnancy is contraindicated because of the possible teratogenic effect of the vaccine. However, an evaluation of surveillance data from the USA and some European countries of 680 live births from susceptible women who were inadvertently vaccinated during or within 3 months of pregnancy, none of the neonates were born with congenital rubella syndrome[28].

Rubella susceptibility screening should be offered to all pregnant women early in pregnancy.

Table 3.1 Interpretation of hepatitis B serologic test results

Tests	Results	Interpretation
HBsAg	Negative	Susceptible
Anti-HBc	Negative	
Anti-HBs	Negative	
HBsAg	Negative	Immune due to natural infection
Anti-HBc	Positive	
Anti-HBs	Positive	
HBsAg	Negative	Immune due to hepatitis B vaccination
Anti-HBc	Negative	
Anti-HBs	Positive	
HBsAg	Positive	Acutely infected
Anti-HBc	Positive	
IgM anti-HBc	Positive	
Anti-HBs	Negative	
HBsAg	Positive	Chronically infected
Anti-HBc	Positive	
IgM anti-HBc	Negative	
Anti-HBs	Negative	
HBsAg	Negative	Interpretation unclear; four possibilities:
Anti-HBc	Positive	1. Resolved infection (most common)
Anti-HBs	Negative	2. False-positive anti-HBc, thus susceptible
		3. "Low level" chronic infection
		4. Resolving acute infection

Anti-HBc, hepatitis B core antibody; anti-HBs, hepatitis B surface antibody; HBsAg, hepatitis B surface antigen; IgM, immunoglobulin M; IgM anti-HBc, IgM antibody to hepatitis B core antigen.

Hepatitis B

Hepatitis B is caused by infection with the hepatitis B virus (HBV). The incubation period from the time of exposure to onset of symptoms is 6 weeks to 6 months. HBV is found in the highest concentrations in blood and in lower concentrations in other body fluids (e.g., semen, vaginal secretions and wound exudates). HBV infection can be self-limited or chronic.

In adults, only approximately half of newly acquired HBV infections are symptomatic, and approximately 1% of reported cases result in acute liver failure and

death. Risk for chronic infection is inversely related to age at infection: approximately 90% of infected infants and 30% of infected children aged <5 years become chronically infected, compared with 2–6% of adults. Among persons with chronic HBV infection, the risk for premature death from cirrhosis or hepatocellular carcinoma is 15–25%. HBV is efficiently transmitted by percutaneous or mucous membrane exposure to infectious blood or body fluids that contain blood. The primary risk factors that have been associated with infection are: unprotected sex with an infected partner; birth to an infected mother; unprotected sex with more than one partner; men who have sex with other men; history of other sexually transmitted diseases (STDs); and illegal injection drug use.

Hepatitis B serologic testing involves measurement of several hepatitis B virus (HBV)-specific antigens and antibodies. Different serologic "markers" or combinations of markers are used to identify different phases of HBV infection, and to determine whether a patient has acute or chronic HBV infection, is immune to HBV as a result of prior infection or vaccination, or is susceptible to infection.

Interpretation of hepatitis B serologic test results are given in Table 3.1.

Hepatitis B surface antigen (HBsAg). A protein on the surface of HBV; it can be detected in high levels in serum during acute or chronic HBV infection. The presence of HBsAg indicates that the person is infectious. The body normally produces antibodies to HBsAg as part of the normal immune response to infection. HBsAg is the antigen used to make hepatitis B vaccine.

Hepatitis B surface antibody (anti-HBs). The presence of anti-HBs is generally interpreted as indicating recovery and immunity from HBV infection. Anti-HBs also develop in a person who has been successfully vaccinated against hepatitis B.

Total hepatitis B core antibody (anti-HBc). Appears at the onset of symptoms in acute hepatitis B and persists for life. The presence of anti-HBc indicates previous or ongoing infection with HBV in an undefined time frame.

Immunoglobulin M (IgM) antibody to hepatitis B core antigen (IgM anti-HBc). Positivity indicates recent infection with HBV (<6 months). Its presence indicates acute infection.

Hepatitis B e-antigen. This is a protein that is made by the virus. If this test is positive, it indicates that there is a lot of virus in the blood, which means that the virus can be more easily spread to others.

Hepatitis B e-antibody. Often as the virus stops replicating in the body, and the e-antigen disappears from the blood, the e-antibody appears. This can happen spontaneously or after treatment.

In the UK, prevalence of HBsAg in pregnant women has been found to range from 0.5–1%. Asian women appear to have a higher prevalence rate. About 85% of babies born to mothers positive for hepatitis B e-antigen will become HbsAg carriers and subsequently become chronic carriers, compared with 31% of babies who are born to mothers who are e-antigen negative. In England and Wales, about 21% of HBV infections in children below the age of 15 years are as a result of mother-to-child transmission. Mother-to-child transmission of HBV is approximately 95% preventable through administration of vaccine and immunoglobulin to the baby at birth. Therefore, serologic screening for HBV should be offered to all pregnant women.

Screening HBV infection consists of three stages:

(1) screening for HBsAg

(2) confirmatory test on a fresh blood sample for those who are positive for HBsAg

(3) where infection is confirmed, testing for hepatitis B e-markers in order to determine whether the baby will need immunoglobulin in addition to vaccine.

Human immunodeficiency virus

About 0.2% (2 of every 1,000) of pregnant women are HIV positive. Infection with HIV begins with an asymptomatic stage with gradual compromise of immune function eventually leading to acquired immunodeficiency syndrome (AIDS). The time between HIV infection and development of AIDS ranges from a few months to as long as 17 years in untreated patients. In the UK, prevalence in London is much higher than the rest of the country. If untreated, about one out of every three mothers will pass the virus to their baby before it is born. This is because the virus can cross to the baby from the mother's bloodstream through the placenta as early as a woman's 8th week of pregnancy. In addition, an HIV-positive mother can pass the virus to her baby at the time of the baby's birth, when there is an exchange of body fluids. It may not make a difference whether a woman delivers a baby vaginally, or by cesarean section, since in many cases the fetus may

have already been infected with HIV before its birth. Mother-to-child transmission is reduced to 8% with antiretroviral therapy with zidovudine. Combination antiretroviral treatment along with cesarean section and avoidance of breastfeeding can further reduce the risk of transmission to 1%[38].

The most common method to diagnose HIV infection is with a test for antibodies against HIV-1 and HIV-2. HIV antibody is detectable in at least 95% of patients within 3 months of infection. Early HIV diagnosis improves outcomes for the mother, and can reduce the rate of disease progression. Currently available HIV tests are more than 99% sensitive and specific for the detection of HIV antibodies. Available tests for HIV diagnosis in pregnant women include the enzyme immunoassay (EIA) and Western blot protocol, which is at least 99% and 99.99% sensitive and specific, and the "two-ELISA approach" protocol[6]. In both protocols, an EIA is initially used and if the results are unreactive, a negative report may be generated. If the reaction is positive, further testing with different assays is necessary. If both confirmatory tests are nonreactive then a negative report may be issued. If the confirmatory tests are reactive, one more test with a new specimen should be obtained in order to make sure that there were no procedural errors.

Pregnant women should be offered screening for HIV infection early in antenatal care because appropriate antenatal interventions can reduce mother-to-child transmission of HIV infection. A system of clear referral paths should be established in each unit or department so that pregnant women who are diagnosed with an HIV infection are managed and treated by the appropriate specialist teams.

Syphilis

Women who are pregnant can become infected with the same STDs as women who are not pregnant. Pregnancy does not provide women or their babies any additional protection against STDs. Many STDs are "silent," or have no symptoms, so women may not know they are infected.

Syphilis is an infectious disease caused by *Treponema pallidum* subspecies *pallidum*. This spirochete bacterium is usually transmitted through sexual contact and from an infected mother to fetus during pregnancy or at birth. Passing syphilis to a developing fetus can lead to serious problems, such as premature births, stillbirths and in some cases death, shortly after

Table 3.2 Classification of syphilis

Time after exposure	Classification
Early (infectious) syphilis	
9–90 days	Primary
6 weeks to 6 months (4–8 weeks after primary lesion)	Secondary
≤2 years	(Early) latent
Late (noninfectious) syphilis	
>2 years	(Late) latent
3–20 years	Tertiary
	Gummatous
	Cardiovascular
	Neurosyphilis
Congenital syphilis	
<2 years since birth (includes stillbirth)	Early congenital syphilis
≥2 years	Late congenital syphilis

birth. Untreated infants that survive tend to develop problems in multiple organs, including the brain, eyes, ears, heart, skin, teeth and bones. Screening for syphilis should be performed in all pregnant women during their first prenatal medical visit and repeated in the third trimester if the patient is considered to be at high risk. The classification of syphilis is shown in Table 3.2.

Syphilis is most infectious to other adults through sexual contact during primary and secondary syphilis, but transmission has also been recorded during early latent syphilis. Mother-to-child transmission can occur throughout early syphilis in the mother, which is also called *congenitally transmissible syphilis*. Transmission has been reported from mothers with late latent syphilis.

Syphilis tests detect antibodies to the bacterium that causes syphilis (*T. pallidum*) in blood, body fluid or tissue. The tests are used to screen for or to confirm a syphilis infection. The most commonly used method to screen for or diagnose syphilis is serology. Serologic tests include treponemal and nontreponemal tests. Nontreponemal tests, e.g., rapid plasma reagin (RPR) or venereal disease research laboratory test (VDRL), detect antibodies present from 4 to 8 weeks after infection. These tests can be quantified by serial serum dilution and changes in titers can help indicate successful treatment.

An important principle of syphilis serology is the detection of treponemal antibody by a screening test,

followed by confirmation of a reactive screening test result by further testing. The confirmatory test, or tests, should ideally have equivalent sensitivity and greater specificity than the screening test, and be independent methodologically so as to reduce the chance of coincident false-positive reactions. A second specimen should be tested to confirm the results obtained from the first specimen and to ensure that the patient details on the specimen were correct. A quantitative nontreponemal test and/or detection of specific treponemal IgM may be useful for assessment of the stage of infection and to monitor the effect of treatment. Serology cannot distinguish between the different treponematoses (syphilis, yaws, pinta and bejel).

Tests used to screen for syphilis

Venereal disease research laboratory test. The VDRL test checks for an antibody that can be produced in people who have syphilis. This antibody is not produced as a reaction to the syphilis bacteria specifically, so this test is sometimes not accurate. The test may be done on a sample of blood or spinal fluid. It is not very useful for detecting syphilis in very early or advanced stages.

Rapid plasma reagin test. The RPR test also detects syphilis antibodies.

Enzyme immunoassay test. This is a newer blood test that checks for antibodies to the bacteria that cause syphilis. A positive EIA test should be confirmed with either the VDRL or RPR tests.

Tests used to diagnose syphilis

Fluorescent treponemal antibody absorption (FTA-ABS) test. The FTA-ABS test checks for antibodies to the bacteria that cause syphilis and can be used to detect syphilis except during the first 3–4 weeks after exposure to syphilis bacteria. The test can be done on a sample of blood or spinal fluid.

***T. pallidum* particle agglutination assay (TPPA).** The TPPA test is used to confirm a syphilis infection after another method tests positive for the syphilis bacteria. The test detects antibodies to the bacteria that cause syphilis. It is not performed on spinal fluid.

Darkfield microscopy. This test uses a special microscope to examine a sample of fluid or tissue from an open sore (chancre) for the syphilis bacteria. It is used mainly to diagnose syphilis in an early stage.

Microhemagglutination assay for *T. pallidum* antibodies (MHA-TP). The MHA-TP is used to confirm a syphilis infection after another method tests positive for the syphilis bacteria.

Treponemal tests (e.g., FTA-ABS, MHA-TP and TPPA) are reactive slightly earlier than nontreponemal tests and patients remain seroreactive for life, even if successfully treated. False-positive treponemal tests can be seen in various conditions, particularly spirochetal infections, including Lyme disease (in which the nontreponemal test shows negative results).

EIAs are over 98% sensitive and over 99% specific. Nontreponemal tests, on the other hand, may result in false-negatives, particularly in very early or late syphilis, in patients with reinfection or those who are HIV positive. The PPV of nontreponemal tests is poor when used alone in low-prevalence populations. In general, treponemal tests are 98% sensitive at all stages of syphilis (except early primary syphilis) and more specific (98–99%) than nontreponemal tests. None of these serologic tests will detect syphilis in its incubation stage, which may last for an average of 25 days[28].

The tests used to define seroreactivity vary across settings and over time, from the Wasserman and Kahn tests (for which sensitivity and specificity data are not available) in early studies to the VDRL or RPR tests (sensitivity, 71–100%; specificity, 98%), the FTA-ABS test (sensitivity, 84–100%; specificity, 97%) and the MHA-TP (sensitivity, 76–100%; specificity, 99%) in more recent studies[39].

The UK-recommended screening procedure for syphilis includes a highly sensitive test to detect antibodies (EIA), followed by a highly sensitive and specific confirmatory treponemal test (TPPA) or *T. pallidum* hemagglutination (TPHA). The use of EIAs in the UK has been reported to have the advantage of producing objective results, since there is linkage of EIA plate readings directly to laboratory computer systems. The reported sensitivity and specificity of treponemal EIAs is high, ranging from 85–99.5% and 98.3–100%, respectively[39].

Routine screening of pregnant women is not offered for the following infections in the UK:

- asymptomatic bacterial vaginosis (BV)
- chlamydia trachomatis
- group B *Streptococcus* (GBS)
- hepatitis C virus (HCV)
- toxoplasma
- CMV.

Asymptomatic bacterial vaginosis

BV is not a sexually transmitted infection and is the most common cause of vaginal discharge and malodour. It arises from relative deficiency of normal *Lactobacillus* species and relative overgrowth of anaerobic bacteria, such as *Mobiluncus* species, *Gardnerella vaginalis*, *Prevotella* species and *Mycoplasma hominis* resulting in reduction of the normal vaginal acidity. About half of women with BV during pregnancy will be asymptomatic. The diagnosis of BV is undertaken by either Amsel's criteria or Nugent's criteria.

BV is said to be associated with preterm birth. Many trials have been undertaken to investigate efficacy of treatment of BV and its effect on reducing preterm birth. These treatments included yoghurt, vaginal metronidazole, oral metronidazole, oral metronidazole plus erythromycin, amoxicillin, vaginal metronidazole cream, vaginal clindamycin cream and oral clindamycin. Systematic review of randomized controlled trials have shown no significant differences in rates of preterm birth or perinatal death between the two groups – treatment and no treatment or placebo, although oral or vaginal antibiotics were found to be highly effective in eradicating BV in pregnancy. Antibiotic treatment was also associated with a reduction in the risk of preterm premature rupture of membranes.

The evidence, therefore, does not support screening and treating healthy low-risk pregnant women.

Chlamydia trachomatis

Chlamydia is the most common sexually transmitted infection in England and the majority of people infected with *C. trachomatis* are not aware of their infection because they remain asymptomatic. During pregnancy, chlamydia infection has been associated with low birthweight, preterm delivery, preterm rupture of membrane, neonatal respiratory infection and conjunctivitis. However, a causal link between the organism and these adverse outcomes has not been established. There are also concerns regarding the implementation of adequate counseling, contact tracing, partner testing and follow-up in the antenatal period.

Chlamydia screening should not be offered routinely, but because 1 in 10 men and women under the age of 25 years are positive for the disease, pregnant women under the age of 25 years should be informed of the National Chlamydia Screening Programme.

Group B *Streptococcus*

GBS resides in the genital and gastrointestinal tract of pregnant women without producing any symptoms or harmful effects to the women. Maternal intrapartum GBS colonization is a risk factor for early onset GBS disease in infants within their first week of life. Such infants can suffer from sepsis, pneumonia and meningitis. The prevalence of early onset GBS infant disease in England and Wales is estimated to range from 0.4/1,000 to 1.4/1,000 live births, which is equivalent to approximately 340 babies per annum. Trials have indicated that with intrapartum antibiotic treatment, an 80% reduction in early onset GBS disease could be achieved. With this assumption, the number of babies affected each year will decrease from an estimated 340 to 68. This means that for every 1,000 women treated with intrapartum antibiotics for GBS, approximately 1.4 cases of early onset GBS disease could be prevented. However, this estimate assumes that screening will identify all GBS carriers and therefore, in practice, the number of women treated to prevent one case is most likely to be much higher.

There are several missing crucial data about true prevalence of GBS, prevalence of early onset disease in screen-positive women, prevalence of screen-negative women and the prevalence of GBS among the women with risk factors. Without good quality data on these parameters, it becomes impossible to calculate the overall number of cases of early onset GBS avoided, and costs of implementing such a screening strategy.

Hepatitis C virus

HCV infection is a major public heath concern as it remains one of the major causes of liver cirrhosis, hepatocellular carcinoma and liver failure. The virus can be acquired through blood borne routes, e.g., injection of drugs, body piercing and across the placental barrier (mother to child). The risk of mother-to-child transmission in the UK is estimated to be between 3% and 5%. There is evidence that the risk of mother-to-child transmission of HCV increases with increasing maternal viral load, but it is unknown whether there exists any threshold level for transmission to occur. Consistent evidence showing significant difference in the proportion of infected babies among women delivered vaginally and those delivered by cesarean section is lacking. Moreover, the clinical course of HCV in infants who acquire the disease through mother-to-child transmission is unclear. It has been suggested that a proportion of infected children subsequently become HCV-RNA negative. However, given the long latency of HCV infection in adults, it is possible that infected infants may develop disease manifestations after long durations.

When HCV infection is confirmed the women should be referred to a hepatologist for appropriate counseling and management of the infection.

Toxoplasma

Toxoplasma gondii is the causative organism (parasite) for this infection. Primary infection is usually asymptomatic and life-long antibody response provides immunity from further infection. Toxoplasma infection can be acquired through the following routes:

- ingestion of viable tissue cysts in undercooked meat or infected milk
- ingestion of food (unwashed fruits or vegetables) or drinks containing oocytes as a result of contamination with cat excreta
- organ transplant or blood transfusion from infected host
- mother-to-child transmission when primary infection occurs in pregnancy.

Due to a lack of symptoms following primary infection, pregnant women at risk of transmitting infection to their fetus can only be recognized by serologic tests. Susceptible women could still be infected during pregnancy. Available tests to determine seroconversion cannot distinguish between infection acquired during pregnancy or up to 12 months beforehand. Infection acquired before conception does not give rise to mother-to-child transmission.

Pregnant women should be provided with information on how to prevent a primary infection. In addition to measures taken to avoid the above mentioned methods of transmission, hand washing before handling food items is essential.

Cytomegalovirus

CMV is type of herpes virus and remains latent in the host after primary infection. During periods of compromised immunity, the virus may become active again. Under the current understanding, it remains impossible to accurately determine the following:

- which pregnancies might result in the birth of an infected child
- which of the infected infants might have disease sequelae

- how best to prevent maternal infection
- how to prevent a mother to child transmission
- how to detect an infected fetus when mother to child transmission has occurred.

References

1. Wilson JMG, Jungner G. Principles and practice of screening for disease. Public Health Papers No. 34. Geneva: World Health Organization, 1968. http://whqlibdoc.who.int/php/WHO_PHP_34.pdf (accessed March 3, 2014).

2. Shepperd S, Farndon P, Grainge V, et al. DISCERN – Genetics: quality criteria for information on genetic testing. *Eur J Hum Genet* 2006; 14: 1179–88.

3. Norem CT, Schoen EJ, Walton DL, et al. Routine ultrasonography compared with maternal serum alpha-fetoprotein for neural tube defect screening. *Obstet Gynecol* 2005; 106(4): 747–52.

4. Benn PA, Horne D, Craffey A, et al. Maternal serum screening for birth defects: results of a Connecticut regional programme. *Connecticut Medicine* 1996; 60(6): 323–7.

5. Nicolaides KH, Snijders RJM, Sebire N. *The 11–14 week Scan: The Diagnosis of Fetal Abnormalities.* New York: Parthenon Publishing Group; 1999.

6. Kagan KO, Avgidou K, Molina FS, et al. Relation between increased fetal nuchal translucency thickness and chromosomal defects. *Obstet Gynecol* 2006; 107(1): 6.

7. Snijders RJ, Noble P, Sebire N, et al. UK multicentre project on assessment of risk of trisomy 21 by maternal age and fetal nuchal translucency thickness at 10–14 weeks of gestation. Fetal Medicine Foundation First Trimester Screening Group. *Lancet* 1998; 352(9125): 343–46.

8. Wald NJ, Rodeck C, Hackshaw AK, et al.; SURUSS Research Group. First and second trimester antenatal screening for Down's syndrome: the results of the Serum, Urine and Ultrasound Screening Study (SURUSS). *Health Technol Assess* 2003; 7: 1–77.

9. Malone FD, Canick JA, Ball RH, et al. First-trimester or second-trimester screening, or both, for Down's syndrome. *N Engl J Med* 2005; 353: 2001–11.

10. Sotiriadis A, Papatheodorou S, Eleftheriades M, et al. Nuchal translucency and major congenital heart defects in fetuses with normal karyotype: a meta-analysis. *Ultrasound Obstet Gynecol* 2013; 42(4): 383.

11. Alamillo CM, Fiddler M, Pergament E. Increased nuchal translucency in the presence of normal chromosomes: what's next? *Curr Opin Obstet Gynecol* 2012; 24(2): 102–8.

12. Hyett J, Nicolaides K. First trimester ultrasound screening with nuchal translucency. In: Evans M, Johnson MP, Yaron Y, Drugan A, eds. *Prenatal Diagnosis*, 1st edn. New York: McGraw-Hill, 2005; 289–309.

13. Bianchi DW, Crombleholme TM, D'Alton ME. Second trimester screening for aneuploidy. In: *Fetology: Diagnosis and Management of the Fetal Patient*, 2nd edn. New York: McGraw-Hill, 2010; 18–26.

14. Moreno-Cid M, Rubio-Lorente A, Rodríguez MJ, et al. Systematic review and meta-analysis of performance of second-trimester nasal bone assessment in detection of fetuses with Down syndrome. *Ultrasound Obstet Gynecol* 2014; 43: 247–53.

15. Kagan KO, Valencia C, Livanos P, et al. Tricuspid regurgitation in screening for trisomies 21, 18 and 13 and Turner syndrome at 11+0 to 13+6 weeks of gestation. *Ultrasound Obstet Gynecol* 2009; 33: 18–22.

16. Malone FD, D'Alton ME. First-Trimester Sonographic Screening for Down Syndrome. *Obstetrics & Gynecology* 2003; 102(5): 1066–79.

17. Wapner RJ. First trimester screening: the BUN study. *Semin Perinatol* 2005; 29: 236–9.

18. National Health Service UK National Screening Committee (UK NSC). Screening for Down's syndrome: UK NSC Policy recommendations 2011–2014 Model of Best Practice. NHS Fetal Anomaly Screening Programme (FASP).

19. Newby D, Aitken DA, Crossley JA, et al. Biochemical markers of trisomy 21 and the pathophysiology of Down's syndrome pregnancies. *Prenat Diagn* 1997; 17(10): 941.

20. Speroff L, Glass R, Kase N. *Textbook of Clinical Gynaecologic Endocrinology and Infertility*, 6th edn. Lippincott Williams & Wilkins, 1999; 275–339.

21. Palomaki GE, Haddow JE, Knight GJ, et al. Risk-based prenatal screening for trisomy 18 using alpha-fetoprotein, unconjugated oestriol and human chorionic gonadotropin. *Prenat Diagn* 1995; 15(8): 713.

22. Devore GR. Genetic sonography to assess the risk of aneuploidy combination of serum and ultrasound screening): the historical and clinical role of fetal echocardiography. *Ultrasound Obstet Gynecol* 2010; 35: 509–21.

23. Orzechowski KM, Berghella V. Isolated fetal pyelectasis and the risk of Down syndrome: a meta-analysis *Ultrasound Obstet Gynecol* 2013; 42: 615–21.

24. Simon-Bouy B, Satre V, Ferec C, et al. French Collaborative Group. Hyperechogenic fetal bowel: a large French collaborative study of 682 cases. *Am J Med Genet A* 2003; 121A(3): 209.

25. Scotet V, Duguépéroux I, Audrézet MP, et al. Focus on cystic fibrosis and other disorders evidenced in fetuses

with sonographic finding of echogenic bowel: 16-year report from Brittany, France. *Am J Obstet Gynecol* 2010; 203(6): 592.e1–e6.

26. Patel Y, Boyd PA, Chamberlain P, et al. Follow-up of children with isolated fetal echogenic bowel with particular reference to bowel-related symptoms. *Prenat Diagn* 2004; 24(1): 35.

27. Nyberg DA, Souter VL, El-Bastawissi A, et al. Isolated sonographic markers for detection of fetal Down's syndrome in the second trimester of pregnancy. *J Ultrasound Med* 2001; 20: 1053–63.

28. National Collaborating Centre for Women's and Children's Health; commissioned by the National Institute for Health and Clinical Excellence. *Antenatal Care: Routine Care for the Healthy Pregnant Woman*, 2nd edn. RCOG Press, March 2008.

29. Agathokleous M, Chaveeva P, Poon LCY, et al. Meta-analysis of second-trimester markers for trisomy 21. *Ultrasound Obstet Gynecol* 2013; 41: 247–61.

30. Nicolaides KH. Screening for chromosomal defects. *Ultrasound Obstet Gynaecol* 2003; 21; 313–21.

31. Kirwan D and the National Health Service Fetal Anomaly Screening Programme (NHS FASP). 18+0 to 20+6 weeks Fetal Anomaly Scan National Standards and Guidance for England, January 2010.

32. American College of Obstetricians and Gynecologists Committee on Genetics. Noninvasive prenatal testing for fetal aneuploidy. Committee Opinion No. 545, 2012; 120: 1532–4.

33. Benn P, Cuckle H, Pergament E. Non-invasive prenatal testing for aneuploidy: current status and future prospects. *Ultrasound Obstet Gynecol* 2013; 42: 15–33.

34. Chiu RW, Akolekar R, Zheng YW. Non-invasive prenatal assessment of trisomy 21 by multiplexed maternal plasma DNA sequencing: large scale validity study. *BMJ* 2011; 342: c7401.

35. Boat TF. Cystic fibrosis. In: Behrman RE, Kliegman RM, Jenson HB, eds. *Nelson Textbook of Paediatrics*. WB Saunders Company, 2000; 1315–27.

36. Smail F. Antibiotic treatment for symptomatic bacteriuria, antibiotic vs no treatment for asymptomatic bacteriuria in pregnancy. *CDSR* 2002(3); 1–5.

37. Smail F, Vazquez JC. Antibiotics for asymptomatic bacteriuria in pregnancy. *CDSR*, 2007, Apr 18; (2): CD 000490.

38. van Doornum GJJ, Buimer M, Gobbers E, et al. Evaluation of an expanded two ELISA approach for confirmation of reactive serum samples in an HIV-screening programme for pregnant women. *J Med Virol* 1998; 54: 285–90.

39. National Health Service UK National Screening Committee (UK NSC). The UK NSC recommendation on syphilis screening in pregnancy. http://www.screening.nhs.uk/syphilis (accessed February 12, 2014).

Chapter

4

Embryology for fetal medicine

Manju Nair and Bidyut Kumar

'He who sees things grow from the beginning will have the finest view of them.' Aristotle 384–322 B.C. (1)

In modern day obstetrics, the demand for ultrasound examination in pregnancy is on the rise. High-resolution abdominal and transvaginal scans have helped reveal detailed views of the embryo and the fetus. To interpret these early pregnancy ultrasound images and to appropriately counsel women, it is essential to have an accurate knowledge of human embryology.

Stages of development

The average duration of pregnancy is 266 days (38 weeks) after ovulation or 280 days (40 weeks) after the first day of the last menstrual period. This equates to a period of just over 9 calendar months. Traditionally, the age of a pregnancy is calculated from the first day of the last menstrual period (LMP) but it is easy to appreciate that this cannot be the same as the age of the embryo or the fetus as conception does not occur until after ovulation has taken place about fourteen days after the LMP. Those involved with in-vitro fertilization usually refer to the age of embryo as being equivalent to the number of days elapsed since fertilization, and this is commonly referred to as 'gestational days.' Thus, a traditionally defined 10 weeks' pregnancy is equivalent to 8 weeks or 56 gestational days.

There are three stages of development prior to birth: the cleavage stage, which is the 1st week following fertilization; the embryonic period, which includes the 2nd to 8th week following fertilization; and the fetal period from the 9th week to birth.

Cleavage stage

By a series of rapid mitotic cell divisions, the fertilized ovum is converted from the diploid stage to the 16-cell

morula stage. The morula undergoes differentiation and changes into a blastocyst, which consists of a central cavity (blastocoele) surrounded by a single layer of cells lining it called the *trophoblast*. The central group of cells move to one pole and form the inner cell mass or the embryoblast, which later on develops into the whole embryo.

The inner cell mass changes into a flattened bilaminar embryonic disc composed of the epiblast and the hypoblast. The trophoblast differentiates into the cytotrophoblast and synctitiotrophoblast. Cells of synctitiotrophoblast penetrate the maternal capillaries to form sinusoids, which interconnect with the synctitial lacunae forming the foundation for the uteroplacental circulation. The blastocyst thus gets embedded in the endometrial stroma.

Two main spaces develop in the embryo during this period, the amniotic cavity within the epiblast and the primary yolk sac below the hypoblast. The yolk sac is lined by the exocoelomic membrane and contains fluid that provides nutrition to the embryo until the placenta is formed. A layer of connective tissue, called the *extraembryonic mesoderm*, fills the space between the exocoelomic membrane and the cytotrophoblast. Between the 12th and 14th day, spaces appear in this layer forming the extra embryonic coelom. This later on develops into the chorionic cavity (Figure 4.1).

By the end of this period, the embryo is connected to the cytotrophoblast by the connecting stalk of the extra embryonic mesoderm, which later forms the umbilical cord.

Embryonic period

The most important event in this period is gastrulation, which is a process of formation of the three primary germ cell layers (ectoderm, mesoderm and endoderm) and formation of the body axis.

Fetal Medicine, ed. Bidyut Kumar and Zarko Alfirevic. Published by Cambridge University Press. © Cambridge University Press 2016.

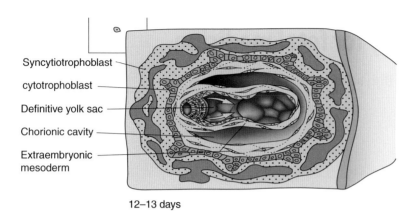

Syncytiotrophoblast

cytotrophoblast

Definitive yolk sac

Chorionic cavity

Extraembryonic
mesoderm

12–13 days

Figure 4.1 Day 12–13 embryo with the bilaminar embryonic disc and definitive yolk sac.
Reproduced from Schoenwolf G et al. *Larsen's Human Embryology*, 4th edn. Philadelphia: Churchill Livingstone Elsevier 2009, with permission.

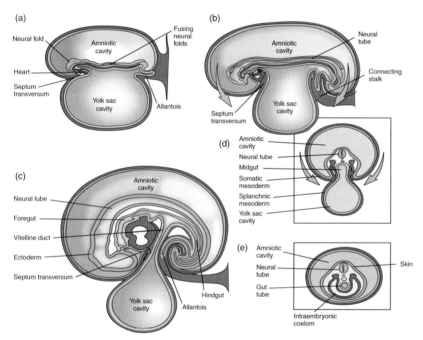

Figure 4.2 An illustration of the lateral and longitudinal folding of embryo and formation of the neural tube. (a) Septum transversum anterior to the cardiogenic area. (b, c) Allantois and connecting stalk combine with the yolk sac and vitelline duct. (d) Fusion of the ectoderm, mesoderm, endoderm and future coelomic cavities, except in the vicinity of the vitelline duct.
Reproduced from Schoenwolf G et al. *Larsen's Human Embryology*, 4th edn. Philadelphia: Churchill Livingstone Elsevier 2009, with permission.

The cells from the epiblast spread out laterally and beneath it forming the mesoderm, which occupies the space between the epiblast above and the hypoblast below. Thus, the bilaminar germ disc is now converted into a trilaminar disc. The epiblast and hypoblast layers are now called the *ectoderm* and *endoderm*, respectively, and are separated from each other throughout their extent by the mesoderm, except at the prochordal plate at the cephalic end and the cloacal plate at the caudal end. The prochordal plate forms the future buccopharyngeal membrane and the cloacal plate forms the future cloacal membrane.

The ectoderm gives rise to the skin and nervous system. The skeletal system, connective and muscle tissue are derived from the mesoderm and the endoderm forms the lining of the visceral organs.

By the 4th week the embryo develops a three-dimensional shape due to lateral and longitudinal folding (Figure 4.2).

The table in Figure 4.3 indicates the chronology of development of the important embryonic structures.

Nervous system

The development of the nervous system starts in the 3rd week. It originates from the thickened plate of embryonic ectoderm called the *neural plate*. Lateral edges of the neural plate elevate to form the neural folds, which

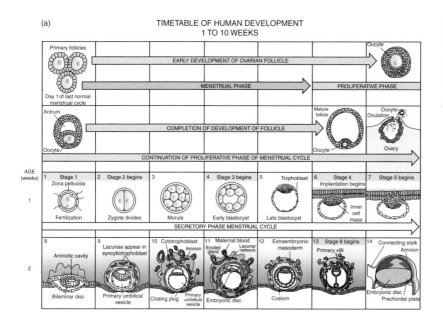

(a)

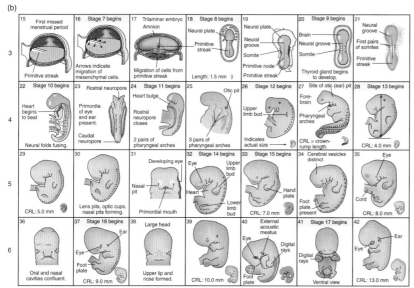

(b)

Figure 4.3 Timetable of human prenatal development Reproduced from Moore KL, Persaud TVN. The Developing Human: Clinically Oriented Embryology, 9th edn. Philadelphia: Elsevier/Saunders 2013, with permission.

fuse with each other in a craniocaudal fashion to form the neural tube. The anterior and posterior ends of the neural tube are originally open and are called the *cranial* and *caudal neuropores*, respectively. Final closure of cranial or anterior neuropore happens on the 25th day. The caudal or posterior neuropore closes on day 27.

Brain

The cephalic end of the neuropore develops three dilatations – prosencephalon, mesencephalon and rhombencephalon. It forms two flexures – a cephalic flexure at midbrain level and a cervical flexure at the junction of brain and spinal cord (Figure 4.4).

Prosencephalon has two divisions – the telencephalon and the diencephalon. The telencephalon develops into the cerebral hemispheres, olfactory bulbs and the hippocampus. The diencephalon develops into the thalamus and the optic tract. The cavity of the diencephalon forms the third ventricle and that of the lateral cerebral hemispheres forms the lateral ventricles.

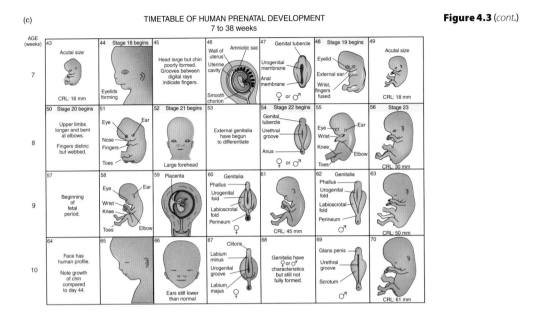

Figure 4.3 (cont.)

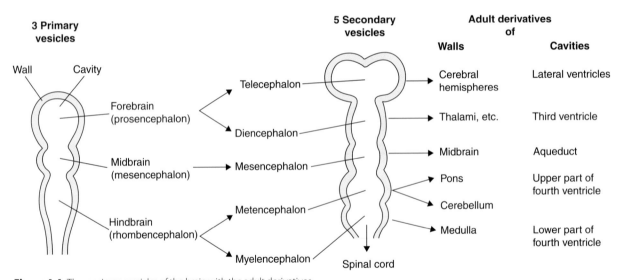

Figure 4.4 Three primary vesicles of the brain with the adult derivatives.
Reproduced from Moore KL, Persaud TVN. *The Developing Human: Clinically Oriented Embryology*, 9th edn. Philadelphia: Elsevier/Saunders 2013, with permission.

The mesencephalon forms the midbrain and its cavity forms the aqueduct of sylvius.

Rhombencephalon consists of metencephalon, which gives rise to pons and cerebellum, and myelencephalon, which gives rise to the medulla. The cavity of the rhombencephalon forms the fourth ventricle.

Sulcation and gyration of the brain begins from approximately 23 weeks of gestation. Secondary and tertiary sulci begin to develop after 32 weeks.

Spinal cord

Spinal cord develops from the neural tube caudal to the fourth pair of somites. Somites are segments of the paraxial mesoderm that develop on either side of the neural tube. The wall of the neural tube consists of neuroepithelial cells that rapidly proliferate and give rise to a mantle layer consisting of primitive germ cells or neuroblasts. This forms the gray matter of the spinal cord. Originating from this layer externally is the marginal layer consisting of myelinated nerve fibres, which forms the white matter of the spinal cord.

Skull

The neurocranium, constituting the skull vault, develops from the neural crest cells, except for the basilar part of the occipital bone, which develops from the mesoderm of the occipital sclerotome. Paraxial mesoderm (somites) forms a large portion of the membranous and cartilaginous portion of skull.

Clinical relevance

- Anencephaly occurs due to abnormal cranial vault ossification.
- Cranial meningiocele occurs due to defect in the squamous part of the occipital bone.
- Porencephaly occurs due to brain destruction in early gestation.
- The primitive streak normally disintegrates in the sacrococcygeal region of the embryo by the end of the 4th week. If it persists, it can give rise to a sacrococcygeal teratoma.
- Neuronal migration disorders occur due to insult to the developing brain at the time of neuronal migration along the glial fibres from the germinal matrix to the brain surface. Depending upon the timing of the insult, the cortex will completely lack gyri and sulci (lissencephaly), have a few coarse gyri (pachygyria), may have multiple small gyri (microgyria or polymicrogyria) or have fragments of gray matter present in an abnormal location of the brain (heterotopias).
- Agenesis of the corpus callosum can be complete or partial, depending upon the stage of development at which growth was arrested. In partial agenesis, the posterior portion of the corpus callosum is the part that is usually absent, since the corpus callosum develops in an anterior-to-posterior direction.
- Holoprosencephaly occurs when the prosencephalon fails to divide. Usually associated with facial defects, as development of face takes place at the same time. Depending on failure of partial or complete cleavage it can range from lobar (posterior failure), semilobar (anterior failure) or alobar (complete absence).

- Neurocristopathy describes the diseases related to maldevelopment of neural crest cells and the resulting abnormality in all the associated derivatives. For example, association with coloboma, heart anomalies, choanal atresia, retardation of growth and development, and genital and ear anomalies (CHARGE) is usually due to an insult in the second month of gestation.

Skeletal system

Vertebral column

During the process of gastrulation, some of the mesodermal cells migrate cranially from the primitive node forming a solid cord of cells called the *notochord*, around which the future vertebral column forms. The majority of the notochord disintegrates, except the part forming the nucleus pulposus of each intervertebral disc. The intraembryonic mesoderm on either side of the notochord forms the paraxial mesoderm, which divides into paired bodies called *somites* located on either side of the developing neural tube. The somite differentiates into the sclerotome, myotome and dermatome.

Mesodermal cells from the sclerotome migrate and condense around the notochord to form the vertebral body and arches.

Further development takes place by the chondrification of the vertebral bodies at 6 weeks followed by ossification 2 weeks later. There are three primary ossification centers, one in the body and two in the neural arch. The ossification of the body begins at the thoracolumbar region and proceeds in the cephalic and caudal direction. The neural arch ossification is independent of the vertebral body ossification, and proceeds in the caudal direction at the lumbar and sacral level and bidirectional at the other levels.

- Neural tube defects (NTDs) occur due to improper formation of the vertebral arches mainly in the lumbosacral region, resulting in the spectrum of spina bifida.
- Upper NTD occurs due to failure of closure of the anterior neuropore.
- Hemivertebra occurs either due to failure of unilateral chondrification of the vertebral body due to unilateral lack of vascularization or due to lack of synchrony in the development of each component of the somite pair. Normally each of these somites position themselves opposite to one

another prior to fusion in the midline to form a normal vertebra.

- Congenital spondylolisthesis (L5–S1) occurs due to failure of the pedicles of vertebral arches to fuse with the vertebral body.
- Diastematomyelia occurs due to persistence of the neuroenteric canal from the primitive node. This is filled with mesenchyme forming a fibrous tract, which can split the neural tube.

Axial system

The axial system is derived from the paraxial and lateral plate mesoderm on either side of the neural tube, which have the capacity to differentiate to osteoblasts, fibroblasts or chondroblasts.

Ossification of the extremities begins by the end of the embryonic period. The ossification starts from the center of the shaft or diaphysis and progresses to the end or epiphysis. Development of the lower limbs is 1–2 weeks behind that of the upper limb.

Abnormal ossification is noted in skeletal dysplasias.

Face and pharyngeal arches

The embryology of the face and neck is not complete without understanding the development of the pharyngeal arches. They appear between the 4th and 5th week and contribute to the external appearance of the embryo. They consist of mesenchymal tissue in the center, ectoderm externally and endoderm internally. In addition to the original mesenchymal tissue, there is further contribution to the mesenchymal matrix by the neural crest cells. There are six arches of which the last two are rudimentary. Each arch has its own artery, vein, nerve, muscular and cartilaginous elements, and are separated from each other by pharyngeal pouches and clefts.

Abnormality in the development of the pharyngeal arches causes a conglomerate of anomalies of all the organs developing from the particular arch. Defect in the first pharyngeal arch is hence associated with anomalies of the eyes, ear, mandible and palate. Some examples are the Robin syndrome (triad of micrognathia, cleft palate and glossoptosis), Treacher Collin syndrome/mandibulofacial dysostosis (deformities with malformed ears, small mandible and facial bones).

Face

During the 4th week, five facial prominences develop from the mesenchyme around the stomodeum, which is a depression on the ventral surface of the embryo at the site of the future mouth. These facial prominences consist of single frontonasal prominence, paired maxillary and mandibular prominences. The paired prominences are derived from the first pharyngeal arch. Two nasal placodes develop as thickenings on either side of the frontonasal prominence. These subsequently invaginate to form nasal pits with a ridge of tissue around them forming the lateral and medial nasal prominences (Figure 4.5).

The nose is thus formed by five facial prominences – the bridge by nasofrontal prominence, the tip by merged medial prominences and the alae by lateral prominences.

- Upper lip: formed by two medial nasal prominences and two maxillary prominences.
- Lower lip and jaw: formed by the mandibular prominences that merge across the midline.
- Cheek: formed from the maxillary prominences.
- Palate: the two merged maxillary prominences form the intermaxillary segment, which gives rise to the philtrum, premaxillary alveolar ridge and the primary plate. The secondary palate is formed by the fusion of palatine shelves, which are shelf-like outgrowths from the maxilla. The nasal septum grows downwards and fuses with the newly formed palate.

Anterior facial clefts occur due to partial or complete failure of fusion of maxillary prominences with medial nasal process. Posterior defects in the palate occur due to failure of fusion of palatine shelves, either due to shortness or inhibition of the process. Cleft palates occur more in females as the palatine shelves fuse 1 week later compared to males.

Heart

Cardiac activity can be visualized by transvaginal scanning as early as 40 menstrual days or in embryos as small as 2 mm.

There are two cardiogenic areas in the embryo – the primary and secondary heart fields. The progenitor heart cells that originate from the epiblast at the cranial end of the primitive streak form the primary heart field. The secondary heart field is located at the splanchnic mesoderm ventral to the pharynx. Along with the lateral folding of the embryo, the primary and secondary heart fields fuse in the middle to form the endocardial tube. The tubular heart elongates and forms alternate dilatations and constrictions as noted below.

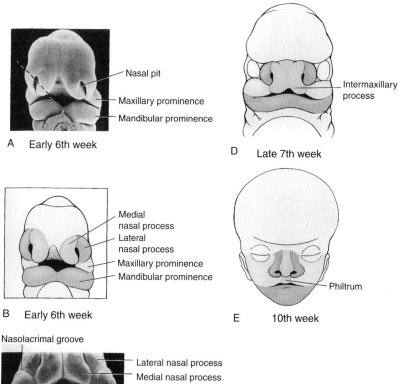

A   Early 6th week

B   Early 6th week

D   Late 7th week

E   10th week

Nasal pit

Maxillary prominence

Mandibular prominence

Intermaxillary process

Medial nasal process

Lateral nasal process

Maxillary prominence

Mandibular prominence

Philtrum

Figure 4.5 Development of the face. (a, b) The 6th week showing nasal pits with lateral and medial nasal prominences. (c, d) The 7th week showing the medial and lateral nasal processus fuse to form intermaxillary process. (e) By the 10th week, intermaxillary process forms the philtrum of the upper lip.
Reproduced from Schoenwolf G et al. *Larsen's Human Embryology*, 4th edn. Philadelphia: Churchill Livingstone Elsevier 2009, with permission.

Nasolacrimal groove

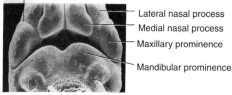

Lateral nasal process

Medial nasal process

Maxillary prominence

Mandibular prominence

C   Early 7th week

Table 4.1

Embryonic dilatations	Derivatives
Truncus ateriosus	Aorta, pulmonary trunk
Bulbus cordis	Smooth part of right and left ventricle
Primitive ventricle	Trabeculated part of right and left ventricle
Primitive atrium	Trabeculated part of right and left atrium
Sinus venosus	Smooth part of right atrium, coronary sinus, oblique vein of left atrium

The main stages in the development of the heart are: formation of the endocardial tube, looping of the tube, formation of the atrioventricular septum, aorticopulmonary septum and interventricular septum.

- The heart tube undergoes rightward looping to change from anterior/posterior polarity to left/right polarity.
- The atrioventricular septum is formed by the fusion of bulges from the dorsal and ventral wall of the atrioventricular canal.
- Neural crest cells migrate from the hindbrain region through pharyngeal arches 3, 4 and 6, and invade the truncal and bulbar ridges. These ridges grow in a spiral fashion and fuse with each other to form the aorticopulmonary septum, which divides the truncus into the aorta and pulmonary trunk.
- The muscular portion of the interventricular septum develops from the floor of the ventricle and grows towards the atrioventricular cushion. The membranous portion originates by proliferation and fusion of tissue from three sources – the right and left bulbar ridges, and atrioventricular cushions (Figure 4.6).

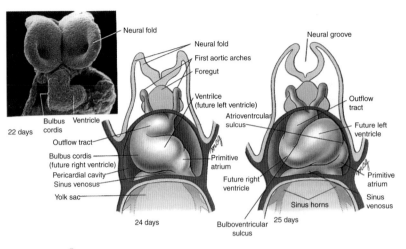

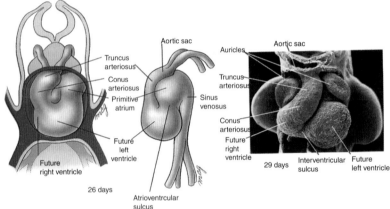

Figure 4.6 Looping of the heart tube with the bulbus cordis anteriorly and to the right, ventricles on the left, atrium posteriorly and superiorly.
Reproduced from Schoenwolf G et al. *Larsen's Human Embryology*, 4th edn. Philadelphia: Churchill Livingstone Elsevier 2009, with permission.

Clinical relevance

- The 22q11.2 deletion or velocardiofacial syndromes are related to abnormality in the neural crest. Neural crest cells contribute to development of the craniofacial region and the cronotruncal endocardial cushions, which contribute to the development of cardiac outflow tracts. Hence, these syndromes are characterized by facial anomalies and anomalies related to the outflow tract.
- Abnormality in cardiac looping can cause dextrocardia. Situs inversus occurs, which is a defect in gastrulation, as a result of which the laterality can be completely reversed.
- Persistent truncus aretriosus is due to abnormal neural crest migration and partial development of atrioventricular septum; hence, there is no division of outflow tracts.

- Transposition of the great arteries occurs due to nonspiral development of the atrioventricular septum, hence, the aorta arises from the right ventricle and the pulmonary trunk from the left ventricle.
- Membranous defect of the ventricular septum occurs due to faulty fusion of bulbar ridges and atrioventricular cushions. Muscular defect occurs due to multiple perforations in the muscular septum.

Fetal circulation

Fetal circulation is different from adult circulation in the following ways (Figure 4.7).

- The placenta provides the necessary nutrients and oxygenation to the fetus via oxygenated blood in the umbilical vein. The deoxygenated blood is returned to the placenta via the umbilical artery.

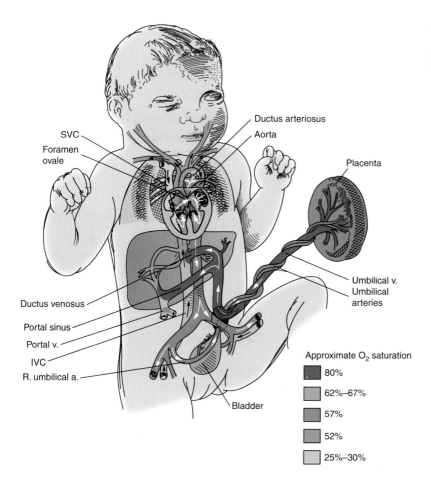

Figure 4.7 Fetal circulation. Reproduced from Schoenwolf G et al. *Larsen's Human Embryology*, 4th edn. Philadelphia: Churchill Livingstone Elsevier 2009, with permission.

SVC
Foramen ovale
Ductus arteriosus
Aorta
Placenta
Ductus venosus
Portal sinus
Portal v.
IVC
R. umbilical a.
Bladder
Umbilical v.
Umbilical arteries

Approximate O$_2$ saturation
80%
62%–67%
57%
52%
25%–30%

- There are three main fetal shunts: (1) the foramen ovale, which shunts blood from the right atrium to the left atrium; (2) the ductus arteriosus, which shunts blood from the pulmonary artery to the aorta; and (3) the ductus venosus, which shunts oxygenated blood through the liver to the inferior vena cava and then to the right atrium of the heart.
- Changes at birth occur whereby the ductus arteriosis and the ductus venosus constrict, and aeration of the lungs causes a fall in the pulmonary vascular resistance and an increase in the pulmonary blood flow. This causes an increase in the left atrial pressure, which causes the closure of the foramen ovale.

Diaphragm

The diaphragm originates from the septum transversum, pleuroperitoneal membranes, dorsal mesentery of the esophagus and muscular growth from the lateral body walls.

The septum transversum is developed around the end of the 3rd week, from the mesoderm cranial to the pericardial cavity. It is deficient on either side of the esophagus at the region of the pleuropericardioperitoneal canals. The pleuroperitoneal membranes are a pair of membranes that separate the pleural and peritoneal cavities, and their free edges project into the lower end of the pericardioperitoneal canal. They fuse with the dorsal mesentery of the esophagus and the septum transversum (Figure 4.8).

During the 4th week, the septum transversum lies opposite the cervical somites. The nerve components of the 3–5th segments of spinal cord therefore grow into the septum. Hence, the motor innervation of the diaphragm is from the phrenic nerve, which originates from the ventral rami of C3, 4 and 5 cervical spinal nerves. By the 6th week the developing diaphragm moves down to the level of the thoracic somites due to

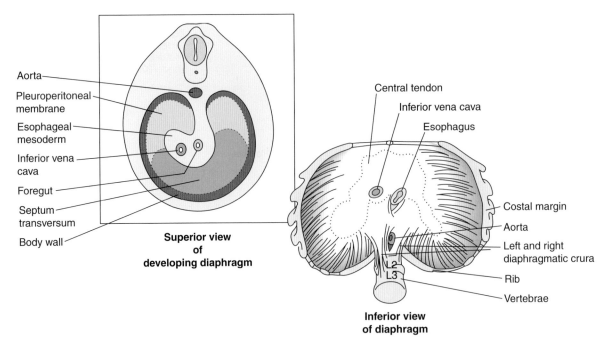

Figure 4.8 Formation of the diaphragm.
Reproduced from Schoenwolf G et al. Larsen's Human Embryology, 4th edn. Philadelphia: Churchill Livingstone Elsevier 2009, with permission.

the rapid growth of the dorsal part of the embryo compared to the ventral side.

Diaphragmatic hernia occurs due to failure of fusion of the pleuroperitoneal membranes in the midline. This closure normally occurs at the end of the 6th week. As a result, at the time of the return of the intestines into the abdominal cavity at the 10th week, there can be herniation of the bowel into the thoracic cavity.

Respiratory system

The larynx, trachea and bronchi develop around the 4th week from the ventral wall of the endodermal lining of the foregut as an outpouching into the splanchnopleuric mesoderm. A trachea-esophageal septum separates the larynx, trachea and bronchi from the pharynx and esophagus.

A respiratory diverticulum develops at the junction of the cranial and caudal foregut.

This gives rise to two lung buds, which further divide to form the bronchial tree. These divisions are not completed until after birth.

Lung maturation occurs in four phases.

(1) Pseudoglandular (5–17 weeks). The gas exchange elements of the lungs are not developed.

(2) Canalicular (16–25 weeks). The terminal bronchioles and alveolar ducts are formed and the lungs become vascular.

(3) Terminal sac (24 weeks to birth). There is intimate contact between the epithelial cells of the terminal alveoli and the endothelial cells of the capillaries. Type 2 alveolar cells begin to secrete surfactant, which continues up to term.

(4) Alveolar phase (from 32 weeks). There is formation of thin-walled alveolar sacs, thus establishing a thin alveolocapillary membrane in order to promote gaseous exchange.

- In oesophageal atresia, the oesophagus ends blindly and does not continue at the distal gut tube, thereby causing a connection between the trachea and distal gut tube.

- Tracheoesophagial fistula results from the incomplete division of the cranial part of the foregut into the trachea and esophagus, or due to a defective tracheoesophagial septum. It is usually associated with esophageal atresia (Figure 4.9).

Respiratory distress syndrome is associated with premature delivery due to the absence of surfactant production until late gestation. The severity is dependent on the stage of lung development.

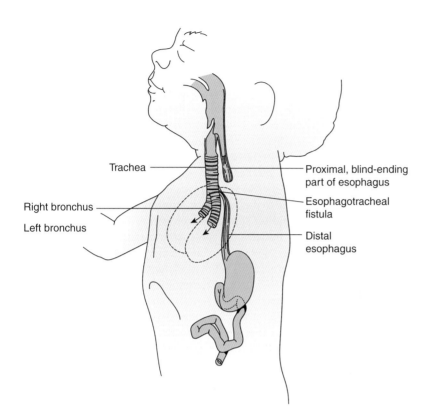

Figure 4.9 Demonstration of esophageal atresia and trachea-esophageal fistula. Reproduced from Schoenwolf G et al. *Larsen's Human Embryology*, 4th edn. Philadelphia: Churchill Livingstone Elsevier 2009, with permission.

Trachea

Right bronchus

Left bronchus

Proximal, blind-ending part of esophagus

Esophagotracheal fistula

Distal esophagus

Abdominal wall

During the 3rd and 4th weeks of embryo development, the endoderm folds down ventrally to form the gut tube. The embryo now has a dorsal neural tube and ventral gut tube with the mesoderm in between. The lateral plate of mesoderm splits into a parietal and visceral layer. The space between the two forms the primitive body cavity, which is continuous in the beginning but slits later into pericardial, pleural and peritoneal cavities. The parietal mesoderm fuses with the ectoderm to form the lateral body folds. The two lateral folds join ventrally to form the ventral body wall. This closure is aided by the growth of the head and tail folds, which causes the embryo to curve in a fetal position. The closure of the ventral body wall is complete except in the region of the connecting stalk and at the region of the vitelline duct, which connects to the yolk sac. This gets incorporated with the umbilical cord and degenerates with the yolk sac by the 2nd and 3rd month of gestation.

Ventral body wall defects, including ectopia cordis, bladder exstrophy and abdominal wall malformations such as gastroschisis and omphalocele, occur as one or both lateral body folds fail to progress ventrally.

Gastrointestinal system

The primitive gut tube is formed by the dorsal and lateral folding of the embryo. It extends from the oropharyngeal membrane to the cloacal membrane, and is divided into foregut, midgut and hindgut.

The foregut divides into the cranial part forming the pharynx and a caudal portion, which forms the esophagus dorsally and trachea ventrally. The esophagus and the trachea are seperated by the tracheoesophageal septum. The other foregut derivatives are the stomach and part of duodenum.

The midgut extends from the duodenum to the transverse colon. The hindgut extends from two-thirds of the length of transverse colon to the anal canal. It opens into the cloaca, which is divided by the urorectal septum into the urogenital sinus anteriorly and rectum posteriorly.

- Physiologic umbilical hernia occurs between the 6th to the 10th week when the midgut tube rapidly enlarges and herniates into the umbilical cord due to limited space in the abdominal cavity. It returns when there is more space as the embryo grows.
- Omphalocoele occurs due to failure of the return of the midgut after the physiologic herniation.

- One of the theories to explain the development of gastroschisis is the vascular disruption theory, which suggests that ischemia of the anterior abdominal wall occurs due to thrombosis of the umbilical vein or omphalomesenteric artery, thereby resulting in a visceral hernia.
- Initially, the gut is a hollow organ, but in the 2nd month it is converted into a solid organ due to proliferation of cells of its lining. This is followed by a recanalization process. Failure of this process results in intestinal stenosis. Polyhydramnios is noted more with proximal atresia compared with distal atresia.
- Hirschsprung's disease occurs due to failure of the development of sympathetic ganglia in the intestinal wall due to abnormal neural crest cells migration.
- Imperforate anus results from failure of the breakdown of the anal membrane.
- Esophageal atresia occurs when the tracheoesophagial septum deviates too much dorsally, thereby causing the esophagus to end as a closed tube.

Urogenital system

The development of the renal system is closely linked with the genital system, especially in the male. The urogenital system develops from the urogenital ridge, which is a longitudinal elevation of the intra-embryonic mesoderm on either side of the dorsal aorta. This ridge has two parts – the nephrogenic cord, which gives rise to the urinary system, and the genital ridge, which contributes to the development of the genital system.

There are three stages of development of the fetal renal system. In a craniocaudal and chronologic order of the development these are: the pronephros (rudimentary and nonfunctional, disappears by the end of the 4th week), the mesonephros (functional in early fetal life) and the metanephros (forms the permanent kidney). The purpose of the pronephros is to induce the development of the mesonephros. During the 5th week of development, the mesonephros lengthens rapidly and forms a longitudinal collecting duct called the *mesonephric duct*. Some of the cranial tubules degenerate and disappear by the 2nd month. In the male, a few of the caudal tubules of the mesonephric duct persist and contribute to the ductus deferens.

The metanephros starts development by the 5th week and starts to function around 9 weeks. The permanent kidney develops from two parts – the ureteric bud and the metanephric mass of intermediate mesoderm. The ureteric bud develops as an outgrowth of the mesonephric duct and penetrates the metanephric tissue. It gives rise to the ureter, major and minor calyces of the renal pyramid and the collecting tubules. The distal end of the collecting ducts induces clustering of mesenchymal cells in the metanephric mass of mesoderm to form the metanephric vesicles. The proximal ends of these tubules are invaginated by glomeruli, which rapidly increase in number from the 10th week until the 32nd to the 36th week. Continuous development of the nephrons continues even after birth (Figure 4.10).

Initially the metanephric kidneys are positioned near the sacrum. They attain the adult position at the level of L1 by the 9th week due to the growth of the abdomen and pelvis. They gradually rotate anteriorly so that the renal pelvis is anteromedial in the third trimester.

The urinary bladder develops from the urogenital sinus and is continuous with the allantois, which regresses in adult life to form the urachus and median ligament.

Table 4.1 summarizes the embryologic origin of the renal system.

Genital system

Indifferent gonad develops from the intermediate mesoderm on the gonadal ridges, which are on the medial part of the paired urogenital ridges. The primordial germ cells migrate from the yolk sac via the dorsal mesentery of hindgut, and induce the cells in the gonadal ridges to form the primitive sex cords. By the 8th week, the gonad differentiates into male and female.

In males, the testis determining factor – a protein produced by the sex determining gene on the Y chromosome – causes differentiation of the primate sex cords into testicular cords, sertoli cells and seminiferous tubules, and the gonadal mesenchymal cells into Leydig cells. Testosterone produced by the Leydig cells stimulates the mesonephric duct to develop into the ductus deferens, epididymis and seminal vesicle. Simultaneously, there is regression of the paramesonephric duct by the antimullerian hormone secreted by the sertoli cells.

In the female, the primitive sex cords extend into the medulla of the gonad, undergo degeneration and form the vascular stroma of the ovary. In the 4th month, they invest the primordial germ cell to form the ovarian follicles, and there is regression of the mesonephric ducts. Paramesonephric ducts, lateral to the mesonephric ducts, fuse at the lower end

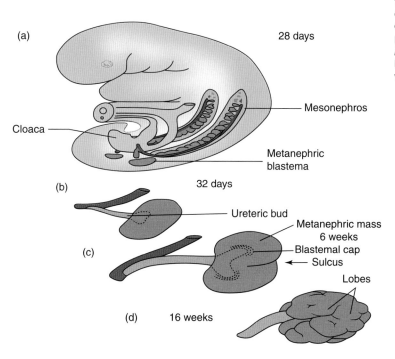

(a)

28 days

Mesonephros

Cloaca

Metanephric
blastema

(b)

32 days

Ureteric bud

Metanephric mass
6 weeks

(c)

Blastemal cap

Sulcus

Lobes

(d)   16 weeks

Figure 4.10 (a) Metanephric blastema from the intermediate mesoderm. (b–d) Bifurcation of ureteric bud which induces further differentiation of metanephric blastema. Reproduced from Schoenwolf G et al. *Larsen's Human Embryology*, 4th edn. Philadelphia: Churchill Livingstone Elsevier 2009, with permission.

Table 4.2 Embryologic origin of the renal system

Structure	Embryologic origin
Nephrons (excretory apparatus – Bowman's capsule, proximal convoluted tubule, loop of Henle and distal convoluted tubule)	Metanephric blastema from the intermediate mesoderm
Renal pelvis, calyces, collecting tubules	Ureteric bud
Renal parenchyma	Metanephric blastema
Ureter	Ureteric bud
Urinary bladder	Urogenital sinus, part of the allantois
Urethra – female	Mainly by the pelvic portion of urogenital sinus
Urethra – male	Pelvic portion of urogenital sinus forms the membranous and prostatic urethra. The phalic portion of the urogenital sinus forms the penile urethra

to form the uterovaginal canal. This gives rise to the uterus, cervix and upper part of the vagina. A pair of sino vaginal bulbs develops where the uterovaginal canal contacts the urogenital sinus. These form the lower two-thirds of the vagina. It is initially solid and canalizes later.

There is no difference in the appearance of the external genitalia until the 5th week. In the male, the production of androgen causes the genital tubercle to enlarge. The penis forms from the genital tubercle and the urethral folds. Lateral to the genital tubercle are the labioscrotal swellings. These fuse in the male and form the scrotum. In the female, the lack of androgenic effect causes the genital tubercle to remain small and this forms the clitoris. The labioscrotal swellings do not fuse and form the labia majora. The urethral folds remain separate in the female and form the labia minora.

Clinical relevance

• Renal agenesis occurs due to failure of the development of the ureteric bud or a defective interaction between the metanephric blastema and the ureteric bud.

- Multicystic dysplastic kidney results due to failure of branching of the ureteric bud and failure of the mesonephric blastema to form nephrons.
- In polycystic renal disease, cysts develop from all segments of the nephron, and is due to a mutation in the cilia-related protein. Examples of ciliopathies include Bardet Biedel Syndrome (renal cysts, obesity, intellectual disability, limb defects) and Meckel Gruber syndrome (renal cysts, hydrocephalus, microphthalmia, cleft palate, absence of olfactory tract, polydactyly).
- Duplex ureter occurs due to duplication of the ureteric bud. It can be complete, with each having its own pelvis and corresponding metanephric tissue, or it can be partial. Rarely, there can be development of two ureteric buds, one of which will be in the normal position and the other moves downward with the mesonephric duct, which normally opens into the urogenital sinus. Hence, one ureter opens into the bladder and the other can have an ectopic opening in the vagina, urethra or vestibule.

- A horseshoe kidney is found in the region of the abdomen below the inferior mesenteric artery. The caudal poles of the kidney fuse in the pelvis and cannot migrate past the inferior mesenteric artery. There is restriction of the normally occurring anterior rotation.
- Definitive kidney, which develops from the metanephros, becomes functional at 12 weeks. Hence, in bilateral renal agenesis oligohydramnios, it may not be apparent prior to 12 weeks.

Bibliography

1.   Moore KL, Persaud TVN. *The Developing Human: Clinically Oriented Embryology*, 9th edn. Philadelphia: Elsevier/Saunders, 2013.

2.   Schoenwolf GC, Bleyl SB, Brauer PR, et al. *Larsen's Human Embryology*, 4th edn. Philadelphia: Churchill Livingstone Elsevier, 2009.

3.   Dudeck RW. *High-Yield Embryology*, 3rd edn. Philadelphia: Lippincott Williams & Wilkins, 2004.

4.   Sadler TW. *Langman's Medical Embryology*, 12th edn. Philadelphia: Lippincott Williams & Wilkins, 2011.

5.   Mitchell B, Dudek RS. *Embryology – An Illustrated Colour Text*, 1st edn. Churchill Livingstone/Elsevier, 2009.

Chapter

5

Ultrasound assessment of normal fetal anatomy

Manju Nair and Bidyut Kumar

In recent years, ultrasound screening for fetal anomalies and diagnostic testing have shifted from the second trimester to the first, providing women and their care providers with more reproductive choices and better risk assessment. Ever increasing experience in the assessment of fetal anatomy in the first trimester has been made possible by the use of high-resolution transabdominal and transvaginal transducers, and with a better understanding of early fetal development.

Prerequisites for an ultrasound examination

Women should be offered verbal and written information about the objective, advantages and limitations of the ultrasound examination. All scanning equipment should have certain basic standards like real time gray-scale ultrasound, transabdominal transducer (3–5MHz range) and transvaginal probe (5–10 MHz), power output controls with display standards, capacity for digital storing and printing, magnification facility, Doppler and harmonic function, good precision and resolution facility[1]. There should be appropriate documentation of the results and storing of the images in line with local protocols and ultrasound governance framework. Safety principles should be followed at all times and the thermal index (TI), mechanical index (MI) and fetal exposure times should be minimized[2]. The TI reflects the temperature rise in the tissue and can vary with the nature of the tissue. It is the ratio of the acoustic power emitted by the transducer to the acoustic power required to produce a one-degree rise in temperature at a particular equipment setting. The MI gives an estimate of the mechanical effects of the ultrasound beam like the cavitation effect. The values for MI and TI should not exceed 1. Unless clinically indicated, it is advisable to avoid Doppler ultrasound in the first trimester due to the risk of increased power and thermal effect, especially with spectral pulsed Doppler[3].

First-trimester fetal anatomy scan

An early pregnancy scan is routinely offered for assessment of fetal viability, reliable dating of the pregnancy, confirmation of site of the pregnancy and for determination of chorionicity in multiple pregnancy.

The optimal gestational age for a first-trimester scan for fetal anatomy is between 11–13 weeks as the majority of the organogenesis is complete by this gestation[1,4].

Safety

The use of brightness mode (B-mode) and motion mode (M-mode) prenatal ultrasonography is safe for all stages of pregnancy. However, the use of Doppler examination of fetal vessels in early pregnancy should be limited and should not be performed without a clinical indication[1,6].

A stepwise approach for a routine scan at 11–13+6 weeks is listed below.

(1) Confirm viability.

(2) Order of pregnancy.

(3) Dating of pregnancy. The crown–rump length (CRL) is most accurate, with a margin of error of 2.1 days, and should be used for the dating of the pregnancy (15–60 mm)[5]. For CRL measurements exceeding 84 mm, head circumference (HC)[1] is more accurate for pregnancy dating (Figure 5.1).

(4) Measurements. Biparietal diameter (BPD) and HC need to be measured in a routine

Fetal Medicine, ed. Bidyut Kumar and Zarko Alfirevic. Published by Cambridge University Press. © Cambridge University Press 2016.

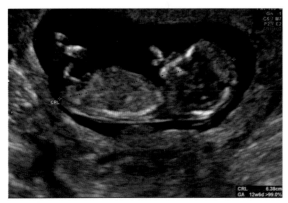

Figure 5.1 Sagittal section of a fetus showing measurement of crown–rump length.

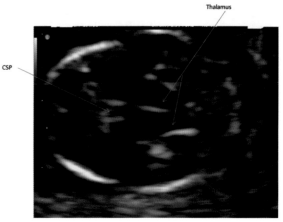

Figure 5.2 Transverse section through fetal head showing midline echo, thalamus and cavum septum pellucidi (CSP).

first-trimester scan. These can be measured on the largest true symmetrical axial view of the fetal head. Abdominal circumference and femur length need not be routinely measured. (Refer to the section on second trimester anomaly scan for details on the measurement techniques).

(5) Systematic structural survey.

(6) Chromosomal anomaly assessment.

(7) Assessment of the uterine adnexa.

Algorithm for a structural survey in early pregnancy

Brain

Cranial bone ossification and the integrity of the skull should be noted to exclude severe anomalies like acrania. The hemispheres should appear symmetrical and separated by a clear midline falx cerebri and interhemispheric fissure. By 7 weeks, a sonolucent area can be seen in the cephalic pole. By 9 weeks, a convoluted pattern of three primary cerebral vesicles is noted, followed by the appearance of brightly echogenic choroid plexus filling the lateral ventricles by 11 weeks. It is difficult to assess the integrity of the cerebellum, cavum septum pellucidum and corpus callosum at this gestation (Figures 5.2 and 5.3).

A BPD measurement less than the 10th centile may be a subtle sign of open spina bifida[7].

Neck

One of the biggest advances in prenatal diagnosis is the measurement of nuchal translucency (NT). The correct NT should be obtained by adopting and ensuring the following criteria are met.

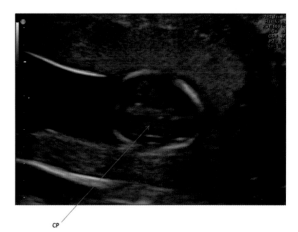

Figure 5.3 Transverse section through brain ventricles demonstrating relatively prominent-appearing choroid plexus (CP).

- Obtain a sagittal section of the fetus and magnify the image in order to include only the fetal head and upper thorax. The true sagittal section will demonstrate an echo from the tip of the nose, a second echo from the nasal bone and a square and well-defined echo from the maxilla.

- Fetal spine and neck should be in a neutral position with a pool of amniotic fluid between the chin and the upper chest. Hyperflexion or hyperextension will lead to erroneous measurement.

- Calipers should be placed correctly, with the horizontal portion of the + marker exactly on the inner borders of the lines demarcating the nuchal space or NT. It should be placed perpendicular to

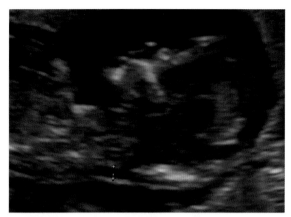

Figure 5.4 A midline sagittal section showing measurement of nuchal translucency.

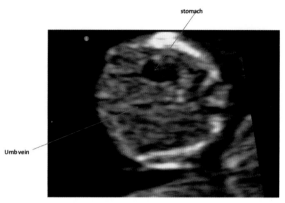

Figure 5.5 Transverse section through fetal abdomen shows the stomach and an oblique section of the umbilical vein. Longitudinal section of a single rib on either side and a cross-section of the spine is also visible.

the long axis of the fetus at the widest portion of the NT space. The amnion should be seperately identified to avoid mistaking it for the fetal skin (Figure 5.4).

- If more than one measurement meeting all the criteria is obtained, the maximum one should be recorded and used for aneuploidy risk assessment.

Face

An attempt should be made to look at the face in coronal plane. If clear views are not obtained, it should be re-assessed at the second-trimester scan[1].

Heart

A four-chamber view of the heart can be obtained starting from 10 to 13 weeks[8]. Complete examination of the fetal heart in the first trimester can be challenging due to the smaller size. As a minimum, the position of the heart and the four-chamber view should be noted. In case of any suspected abnormality, a detailed scan is warranted in the second trimester for further evaluation.

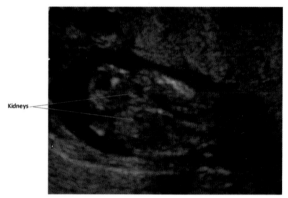

Figure 5.6 Coronal section through fetal trunk showing a section of the spine and longitudinal section of the fetal kidneys.

Abdomen

The physiologic umbilical hernia is present up to 11 weeks, and should be differentiated from gastroschisis and omphalocoele. Kidneys and bladder should be noted. Kidneys appear in the paraspinal region as bean-shaped structures. The bladder can be visualized in the normal site as a hypoechoic area (Figures 5.5–5.8).

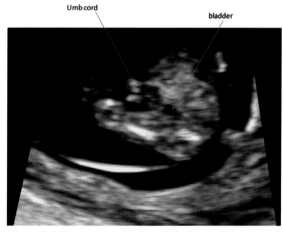

Figure 5.7 Transverse section through fetal lower abdomen showing umbilical cord insertion and the bladder.

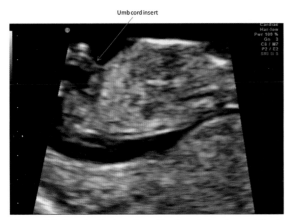

Figure 5.8 Longitudinal section of fetal trunk showing umbilical cord insertion and the anterior abdominal wall.

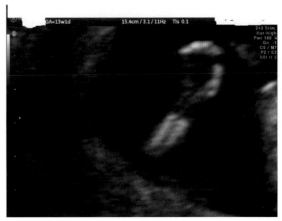

Figure 5.10 Longitudinal section through fetal forearm and hand showing both long bones and five digits.

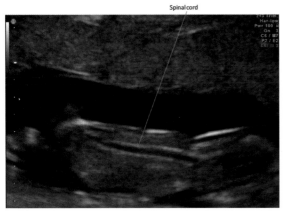

Figure 5.9 Longitudinal section through fetal spine to show skin covering. The spinal cord is visible as a tubular sonolucent structure. Faint echogenic vertebrae are also visible.

Spine

The role of the first-trimester scan in detecting small defects of the spine is limited; however, severe cases of spinal abnormalities may be detected by a systematic examination[9]. Careful observation should be undertaken to visualize an intact skin covering over the spine (Figure 5.9).

Limbs

Note the presence of four limbs with three bony segments in each of the upper and lower limbs with normal orientation of the two hands and feet (Figure 5.10).

Limitations

One of the limitations of the first-trimester anomaly scan as a routine screening method in a low-risk

Checklist for examination of fetal anatomy in the first trimester[1]

Brain	Integrity of skull
	Midline falx
	Choroid plexus – filled
	Ventricles
Face	Eyes with lens
	Nasal bone
	Normal profile/mandible
	Intact lips
Neck	Nuchal translucency thickness
	Any fluid-filled collections
Spine	Longitudinal and axial view of vertebrae
	Skin integrity
Chest	Symmetrical lung fields
	No effusions or masses
	Regular cardiac activity
	Four-chamber view
	Check situs visceralis with stomach and heart on the left side of the abdomen
	Diaphragm
Abdomen	Stomach in left upper quadrant
	Intact abdominal wall
	Normal cord insertion after 12 weeks
	Kidney and bladder
Extremities	Four limbs each with three segments
	Hands and feet with normal orientation
	Femoral length
Placenta and amniotic fluid volume	

population is the poor sensitivity for certain anomalies like those of the heart, spine and brain due to the stages of embryologic development. Therefore, even if an early fetal anomaly scan were offered, the second-trimester scan should not be abandoned. Secondly, in women with raised body mass index, the image quality in the transabdominal scan may be compromised. A transvaginal approach will improve the sensitivity, but the patient's acceptance may be a limiting factor.

The routine second-trimester scan

The second-trimester anomaly scan is offered between 18+0 weeks to 20 weeks and 6 days of gestation in most countries. The timing is appropriate for detailed evaluation of most of the anatomical structures. Although not the ideal gestation for dating the pregnancy, it can be useful in dating in the case of a missed opportunity for a first-trimester scan.

Diagnostic value of routine ultrasound scan in the second trimester

(a) Lethal anomalies[10]

Anencephaly	97.6%
Trisomy 18	68.4%
Trisomy 13	50.0%
Hypoplastic left heart	54.5%
Bilateral renal agenesis	90.0%
Lethal musculoskeletal disorders	33.3%

(b) Possible survival and long-term morbidity[10]

Spina bifida	66.3%
Hydrocephalus	68.9%
Encephalocele	90.9%
Holoprosencephaly	72.7%
Down's syndrome	14.6%
Complex cardiac malformations	21.3%
Atrioventricular septal defect	12.9%
Nonlethal dwarfism	100%
Anterior abdominal wall defect	89.5%
Gastroschisis	94.1%
Exomphalos	84.6%
Congenital diaphragmatic hernia	47.9%
Tracheoesophageal atresia	7.4%
Small bowel obstruction/atresia	40.6%
Congenital cystic adenomatoid malformation	100%
Renal dysplasia (bilateral)	84.2%
Multiple abnormality/syndrome	77.8%

(c) Anomalies amenable to intrauterine therapy[10,11]

Obstructive uropathy	100%
Pleural effusion or hydrothorax	100%

(d) Anomalies associated with possible short term/ immediate morbidity[10]

Facial clefts	13.8%
Talipes	20.1%
Atrial/ventricular septal defect	6.3%
Isolated valve anomalies	22.7%
Renal dysplasia (unilateral)	86.7%

A stepwise approach for a routine second-trimester anomaly scan is listed below.

(1) Confirm viability.
(2) Order of pregnancy.
(3) Placentation.
(4) Fetal biometry.
(5) Systematic structural survey.
(6) Amniotic fluid assessment.

Fetal biometry

For assessment of the fetal size and growth, the standard measurements used are the HC, BPD, abdominal circumference and femoral length.

Head circumference and biparietal diameter

Both the HC and BPD measurements can be obtained from the same plane; the transventricular plane or the transthalamic plane can be used for obtaining these measurements. The HC can be measured by using the ellipse method by placing the ellipse around the outside of the skull bone echoes. HC measurement is more reliable than the BPD in cases of abnormal shape of the head.

The BPD can be measured by two techniques – the outer-edge to inner-edge technique or the outer-edge to outer-edge by placing the calipers at the widest part of the skull. It is important to ensure that the placement of the calipers corresponds to the technique described on the reference chart, especially for the BPD (outer-to-outer or outer-to-inner) (Figures 5.11 and 5.12).

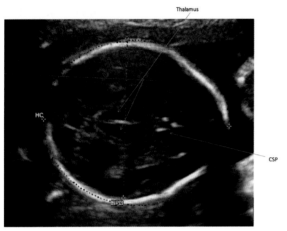

Figure 5.11 Transthalamic section of fetal head showing measurement of head circumference (HC) and biparietal diameter (BPD).

A cross-sectional view of the head is obtained at the level of thalami with a short midline echo equidistant from the proximal and distal skull echoes. The structures that should be identified in the midline anteriorly to posteriorly are the cavum septum pellucidum (CSP), the thalami and basal cisterns[12].

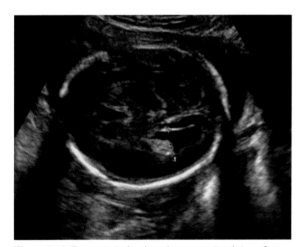

Figure 5.12 Transventricular plane. A cross-sectional view of the head is obtained at the level of lateral ventricles with a long midline echo equidistant from the proximal and distal skull echoes. The structures that should be identified in the midline anteriorly to posteriorly are the anterior horn of the lateral ventricles, cavum septum pellucidum and posterior horns of the lateral ventricles.

Algorithm for structural survey in the second trimester

Brain

Examine the brain in the three planes as described in Figures 5.11, 5.12 and 5.15–5.18. Assess the integrity of

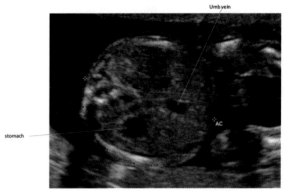

Figure 5.13 Measurement of abdominal circumference. Transverse section through fetal upper abdomen demonstrating the cross-section of a vertebrae, an unbroken rib, stomach, cross-section of the umbilical vein, which should be one-third of the distance between the anterior abdominal wall and fetal spine and midway between the lateral abdominal walls[12]. AC, abdominal circumference.

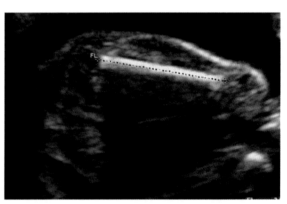

Figure 5.14 Longitudinal section through fetal thigh showing measurement of femur length (FL). The longest axis of the ossified diaphysis of the upper femur is measured. Each caliper is placed at the ends of the ossified diaphysis without including the distal femoral epiphysis. It is important to exclude artifacts at the end as this might give falsely raised values.

the skull, midline structures, lateral ventricles, cavum septum pellucidum, cerebellum and cisterna magna.

Face

Two-dimensional ultrasound screening for cleft lip and palate in a low-risk population has a relatively low detection rate (DR)[14]. The generally reported rates of prenatal recognition of cleft lip range between 21% and 30%. However, this can be increased when the face is examined in three planes, i.e., sagittal, coronal and axial, and by using three-dimensional ultrasound[15].

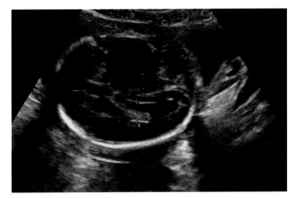

Figure 5.15 Transverse section through fetal brain showing measurement of the lateral ventricle width distal to the ultrasound probe. Once the transventricular plane is obtained, the calipers are placed at the level of the glomus of the choroid plexus along the inner edges of the ventricular walls at the widest part of the atrium. Values of more than 10 mm are considered abnormal. Due to the physical properties of ultrasound, the proximal ventricle is always more difficult to delineate when scanning from the lateral aspect. Readjusting the ultrasound machine controls and angulating the probe may provide a better view.

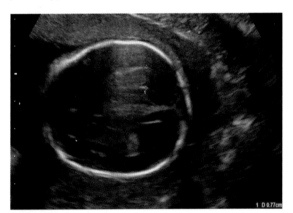

Figure 5.16 Measurement of the proximal cerebral ventricular width.

Thorax

Assessment of the thorax is important to exclude any abnormalities in the heart, lungs, diaphragmatic hernia, hydrops and lethal skeletal dysplasias.

Checklist for assessment of the thorax

- Shape of the chest. Normal shape is circular to an ellipse in the axial section.
- Lungs appear as low level homogeneous echoes.
- The diaphragm appears as a thin echo, poor concave line separating the thorax and abdomen.
- Exclude any chest wall edema.
- Assess the shape of the ribs and integrity of the thoracic spine.

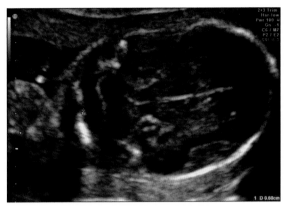

Figure 5.17 Transcerebellar section showing measurement of cisterna magna width, which is the horizontal distance between the outer border of the vermis of cerebellum to the inner border of the skull. It should normally measure ≤10 mm.

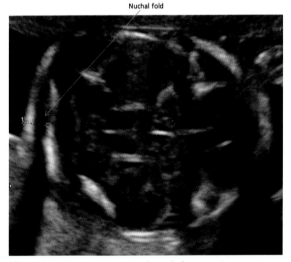

Figure 5.18 Transverse section through the posterior aspect of fetal skull showing measurement of nuchal fold thickness. The antero-posterior width is measured from the outer border of the skull to the outer border of the skin and normally should not be more than 6 mm. Part of the cerebellum and cisterna magna is also visible.

- Measurement of the thoracic circumference at the level of the four-chamber view of the heart in cases of suspected skeletal dysplasia.
- Position of the heart. The heart occupies one-third of the thoracic area with the cardiac axis pointed to left by 45° ± 20°.

Heart

Checklist for assessment of the fetal heart[8,16]

- Position of the heart. The apex of the heart and stomach should be on the left side of the fetus and

(e) Checklist for a midtrimester scan[13]

Structure	Routine screening
Skull	Integrity, shape Measurement of biparietal diameter, head circumference
Brain	Cavum septi pellucidi Midline falx Thalami Cerebral ventricles (atrial width measurement of lateral ventricles) Cerebellum (measurement of transcerebellar diameter) Cisterna magna
Face	Both orbits, lips, mouth Median facial profile Coronal view of nostrils and both lips
Neck	Absence of masses Nuchal fold thickness
Spine	Transverse, coronal, sagittal views Check integrity, overlying skin
Heart	Normal situs, rate, rhythm Four-chamber view Aortic and pulmonary outflow tracts Three-vessel view
Thorax	Regular shape of thorax and ribs Exclude any increased echogenicity in the lungs and mediastinal shift Diaphragm
Abdomen	Abdominal wall, stomach, any bowel dilatation, umbilical cord insertion
Genitourinary tract	Kidneys, renal pelvis, bladder Assessment of the external genitalia is optional, dependent on parental consent and local policy
Limbs	Arms with radius, ulna, humerus, both hands with normal relationship Legs with femur, tibia and fibula, both feet with normal relationship
Placenta	Placental position and amniotic fluid volume assessment

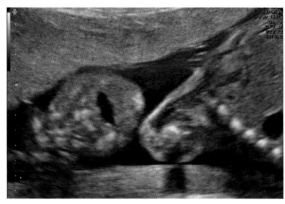

Figure 5.19 Coronal section through the lower face showing the chin, opening of mouth, faint view of upper jaw, nasal bone and the lower margin of orbits.

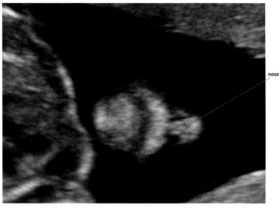

Figure 5.20 Coronal section through fetal lips and nostrils.

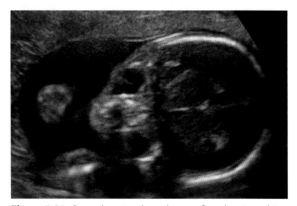

Figure 5.21 Coronal section through upper face showing orbits.

the liver on the right side. The laterality should be decided by assessing orientation of the fetal lie and position, and not on the basis of the position of the stomach or the heart.

- Four-chamber view of the heart. The two atria and the two ventricles, with the foramen ovale in the interatrial septum and the intact interventricular septum, should be visualized.

Both the atria and the ventricles should be of the same size. The tricuspid and mitral valves form an offset cross at the atrioventricular (AV) junction as the septal leaflet of the tricuspid

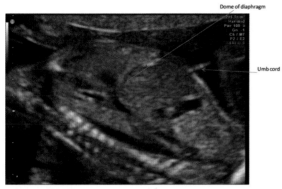

Figure 5.22 Midline sagittal section through fetal trunk showing the dome of diaphragm. Faint echo of umbilical cord insertion is also visible.

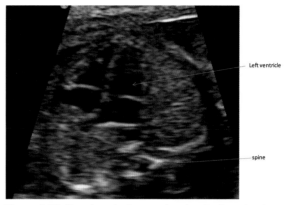

Figure 5.23 Transthoracic close-up view showing four-chamber view of the heart and foramen ovale. Note the offset valve leaflets. Ultrasound fall-off at the interventricular septum near the crux of the heart gives a false impression of a ventricular septal defect.

valve inserts slightly lower than the mitral valve. Observe the contractility of the atria and the ventricles. An isolated finding of a small echogenic rim around the heart usually represents a normal variation and should not be mistaken for a pericardial effusion.

- The AV valves and the flap valve of the foramen ovale should be freely opening and closing.
- Venous drainage. The pulmonary venous connection can be seen on the back of the left atrium by scanning up and down horizontally at the back of left atrium.
- Origin of the great vessels. This is best done by moving the probe cranially from the four-chamber view. On angling towards the right shoulder, the left ventricular outflow tract can be demonstrated. The transverse section cranial to this will demonstrate the origin of the pulmonary artery from the right ventricle.
- Crossover of the great vessel at right angles to each other at their respective origins.
- Three-vessel views demonstrate from left to right, and anterior to posterior, the pulmonary artery, the aorta and the superior vena cava (SVC). The pulmonary artery is the largest in diameter, followed by the aorta and the SVC.
- In the three-vessels and tracheal view, which is more cephalad from the three-vessel view, the aortic arch, the ductal arch and the trachea can be visualized. For the right ventricular connections, obtain a longitudinal view of the left ventricle and angulate the transducer slightly in the opposite direction. This will demonstrate the inferior vena cava entering the right atrium, the origin of

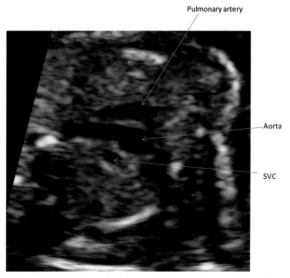

Figure 5.24 Oblique view through the heart demonstrating the three-vessel view, pulmonary artery, aorta and the superior vena cava (SVC) from above below.

pulmonary artery from the right ventricle and its connection to the ductus arteriosus.

- The aortic arch can be examined in the longitudinal axis view.
- Observe the cardiac rhythm and exclude pericardial effusion.

Abdomen

Systematic examination of the abdomen is important to exclude anterior abdominal wall defects (gastroschisis and exomphalos), bowel atresia or obstruction, diaphragmatic hernia, tracheoesophageal fistula. It is also an important landmark for fetal biometry.

The following are the structures that need to be routinely identified.

- The normal insertion of the umbilical cord should be documented after 12 weeks. The physiologic umbilical hernia is present up to 11 weeks and should be differentiated from gastroschisis and omphalocoele.
- Presence of the stomach. Absence of the stomach could be due to anhydramnios or a tracheoesophageal fistula.
- The position of the stomach on the left side of the abdomen together with levocardia helps to confirm normal situs visceralis.

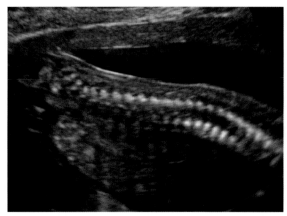

Figure 5.27 Midline sagittal section through fetal spine showing normal curvature and continuous skin covering.

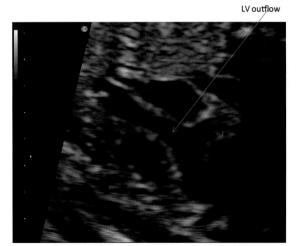

Figure 5.25 Oblique view through fetal heart showing left ventricular (LV) outflow tract.

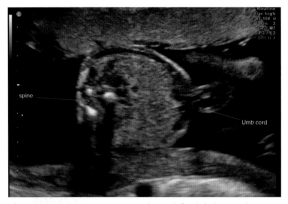

Figure 5.26 Transverse section through fetal abdomen showing cross-section of the spine and umbilical cord insertion.

Spine

To improve the detection rate of spinal abnormalities, the spine should be viewed in three planes – sagittal, coronal and transverse.

- In the sagittal plane, the spine has a double railway appearance and it should enable one to appreciate the soft tissue over it.
- In the coronal plane, the three ossification centers of the vertebrae should be seen. The neural arch should be examined from the cervical segment to the sacrum in all three planes.
- In the transverse/axial plane, the vertebrae have different shapes at different levels. The cervical vertebrae are quadrangular in shape, the thoracic and lumbar vertebrae have a triangular shape with the ossification centers surrounding the neural canal, and the sacral vertebrae appear flat.

Extremities/appendicular skeleton

In a routine midtrimester scan, examine the presence of the upper limbs with the humerus, radia, ulna and hands, and the lower limbs with femur, tibia and fibula. The fingers and toes need not be counted. The only bone that needs to be measured in a routine scan is the femur.

Renal system

The following points are useful in assessing the fetal renal system.

- The fetal kidneys should be noted in their expected paraspinal location by 12 weeks of gestation.

- Assessment of renal pelvis. The renal pelvis appears as a hypoechoic area in the kidney. It is measured in the transverse section of the kidneys with the calipers placed on the inner-to-inner side of the renal pelvis. There is wide variation in the literature regarding the maximum cut-off for the renal pelvic diameter at each gestation. A value of 5 mm in the second trimester and 7–10 mm in the third trimester can be used as a cut-off to increase the sensitivity of detection for significant postnatal renal pathology[8].
- Echogenicity of the kidneys.
- Assess for any parenchymal abnormality (e.g., renal cortical thinning, lack of corticomedullary differentiation).

- Imaging of fetal bladder. By 12–13 weeks of gestation, the fetal bladder should be visible as a median hypoechoic round structure in the lower abdomen. In case of difficulty in visualizing the bladder, color Doppler can be used to demonstrate the two umbilical arteries encircling the bladder. Changes in the size of the bladder can be observed during the course of the examination because the fetus empties its bladder every 30 to 45 min.
- Assessment of the adrenal gland. The normal adrenal glands can be imaged with ultrasound as early as 9½ weeks of gestation. They appear as bilateral midecho structures located immediately above the fetal kidneys.

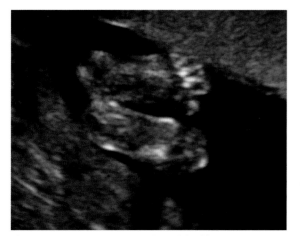

Figure 5.28 Transverse section through fetal feet showing normal orientation of feet.

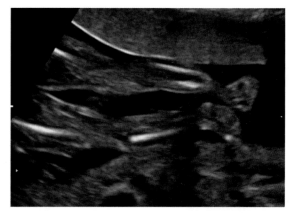

Figure 5.30 Longitudinal section through lower limbs showing normal relation of feet to lower legs. The three long bones of each leg are visible.

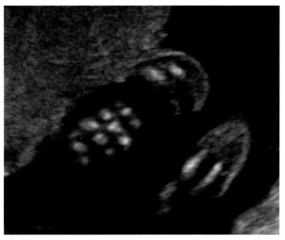

Figure 5.29 Coronal section through four fingers. The thumb usually lies in a slightly different plane in the resting position.

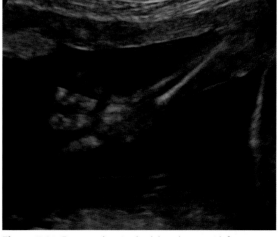

Figure 5.31 Forearm showing both long bones with fingers.

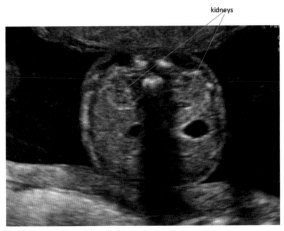

Figure 5.32 Transverse section through fetal abdomen showing hypoechoeic kidneys situated on either side of the spine.

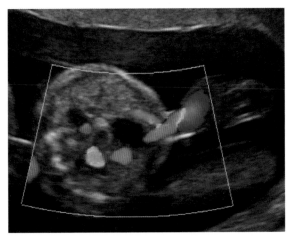

Figure 5.34 Transverse section through fetal lower abdomen demonstrating the two umbilical arteries around the bladder.

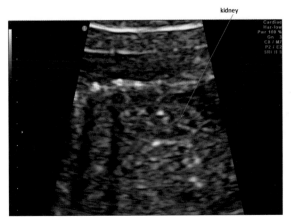

Figure 5.33 Section through long axis of the spine. The renal length should be measured in this plane.

External genitalia

Reporting of gender is not a part of the routine midtrimester scan. It should be considered only with parental consent and in the context of local practice and clinical need, for example, to assist in managing an X-linked disorder.

Extended examination

An extended examination may be required for further evaluation in case of suspected anomalies. Some of the additional measurements are briefly outlined below and will be covered in detail in the relevant chapters.

Brain

Examination of the corpus callosum is useful in certain conditions, such as ventriculomegaly. It can be imaged in the coronal and sagittal planes. Applying color Doppler to identify the pericallosal artery is useful in the imaging of the corpus callosum. The artery can be demonstrated in the mid-sagittal plane and forms a semicircular course over the superior surface of the corpus callosum[17].

Face

The interorbital distance is useful to rule out hyper- or hypotelorism. It is the distance between the medial borders of the two orbits.

Thorax

Normograms are available for thoracic circumference[15]. Values less than 5th centile and a thoracic and abdominal circumference ratio less than 0.79 are associated with lethal skeletal dysplasia and pulmonary hypoplasia[18].

Kidneys

Measurement of renal size in anteroposterior (AP), transverse and longitudinal diameter in cases of suspected renal anomaly. Longitudinal diameter is measured in the sagittal image, the AP and transverse diameters are measured in the transverse section image. All these measurements are obtained by using the outer-to-outer placement of the calipers along the renal outline. Normograms are available for renal size[19].

Abdomen

Measurement of the bowel diameter is useful in suspected bowel obstruction. Multiple fluid-filled areas in the abdomen can indicate bowel obstruction. In this case, measure the diameter, assess the peristalsis and echogenicity. The diameter is measured from the inner wall to inner wall at the point of maximum dilatation in a cross-section of the fetal abdomen. A clue to differentiate the large bowel from the small bowel is the peripheral location and presence of haustrae. There are no standardized normograms for bowel diameters. A prospective study by Lap et al. has produced a reference chart for small and large bowel diameters in normal fetuses at varying periods of gestation.

Extremities

A femoral length less than 5th centile for the gestation or less than three standard deviations is a strong predictor of skeletal dysplasia. In this case, it is useful to measure all the other long bones and feet, assess the contour of the bones and the mobility of the joints. The views of the tibia and fibula are obtained by rotating the probe from the lower end of the femur. In this view, only the cross-section of the talus of the foot should be seen. Normally, only one bone can be measured at a time. A sagittal view of the foot can be obtained in the lateral view image of the lower limb. By rotating the probe 90° from the lateral view, the plantar view of the foot can be obtained[12]. Three features should be noted in the foot – the carrying angle, shape of the heel and the sole of the foot. The normal femur/foot ratio should be 1, irrespective of the gestational age.

References

1. Salomon LJ, Alfirevic Z, Bilardo CM, et al. ISUOG Practice Guidelines: performance of first-trimester fetal ultrasound scan. *Ultrasound Obstet Gynecol* 2013; 41: 102–13.

2. British Medical Ultrasound Society. Guidelines for the safe use of diagnostic ultrasound equipment. London: BMUS; 2009.

3. Salvesen K, Lees C, Abramowicz J, et al. on behalf of the Board of the International Society of Ultrasound in Obstetrics and Gynaecology (ISUOG). ISUOG statement on the safe use of Doppler in the 11 to 13 + 6-week fetal ultrasound examination. *Ultrasound Obstet Gynecol* 2011; 37(6): 628.

4. Souka AP, Nicolaides KH. Diagnosis of fetal abnormalities at the 10–14-week scan. *Ultrasound Obstet Gynecol* 1997; 10: 429–42.

5. Bogota-Ángel SP, Bega G. Ultrasound in pregnancy: if, when, what. In: *Obstetric Evidence-Based Guidelines*. Vincenzo Bergh E (ed). London: Informa Health Care; 2007: 23–9.

6. Duck FA. Is it safe to use diagnostic ultrasound during the first trimester? *Ultrasound Obstet Gynecol* 1999; 13: 385–88.

7. Khalil A, Coates A, Papageorghiou A, et al. Biparietal diameter at 11–13 weeks gestation in foetuses with open spina bifida. *Ultrasound Obstet Gynaecol* 2013; 42(4): 409–15.

8. Twining P, McHugo JM, Pilling DW. *Textbook of Fetal Abnormalities*. London: Churchill Livingstone; 2000.

9. Sepulveda W, Wong AE, Fauchon DE. Fetal spinal anomalies in a first-trimester sonographic screening program for aneuploidy. *Prenat Diagn* 2011; 31(1): 107–14.

10. National Collaborating Centre for Women's and Children's Health. NICE Clinical Guideline: Antenatal care – routine care for the healthy pregnant woman. London: RCOG Press; 2008: 134–79.

11. Chudleigh P, Thilaganathan B. *Obstetric Ultrasound: How, Why and When*, 3rd edn. London: Churchill Livingstone/Elsevier; 2004.

12. Salomon J, Alfirevic Z, Berghella V, et al. ISUOG Clinical Standards Committee. Practice guidelines for performance of the routine mid-trimester fetal ultrasound scan. *Ultrasound Obstet Gynecol* 2011; 37: 116–26.

13. Maarse W, Bergé SJ, Pistorius L, et al. Diagnostic accuracy of transabdominal ultrasound in detecting prenatal cleft lip and palate: a systematic review. *Ultrasound Obstet Gynecol* 2010; 35(4): 495–502.

14. Rotten D, Levaillant JM. Two- and three-dimensional sonographic assessment of the fetal face. 2. Analysis of cleft lip, alveolus and palate. *Ultrasound Obstet Gynecol* 2004; 24(4): 402–11.

15. Carvalho JS, Allan LD, et al. ISUOG practice guidelines (updated): sonographic screening examination of the fetal heart. *Ultrasound Obstet Gynecol* 2013; 41: 348–59.

16. ISUOG. Sonographic examination of the fetal central nervous system: guidelines for performing the 'basic examination' and the 'fetal neurosonogram'. *Ultrasound Obstet Gynecol* 2007; 29: 109–16.

17. D'Alton M, Mercer B, Riddick E, et al. Serial thoracic versus abdominal circumference ratios for the prediction of pulmonary hypoplasia in premature rupture of the membranes remote from term. *Am J Obstet Gynecol* 1992; 166: 658–63.

18. Chitty LS, Altman DG. Appendix: Charts of fetal measurements. In: Rodeck CH, Whittle MJ (eds). *Fetal Medicine Basic Science and Clinical Practice*, 2nd edn. London: Churchill Livingstone/Elsevier; 2009: 738–44.

19. Lap C, Manten G, Mulder E, et al. A prospective longitudinal ultrasound study of the fetal small bowel and colon diameters. *Ultrasound Obstet Gynecol* 2012; 40: 294.

Chapter

6

Fetal central nervous system anomalies

Gianluigi Pilu and Zarko Alfirevic

Central nervous system (CNS) malformations are some of the most common congenital abnormalities encountered at birth. The true incidence of these anomalies is, however, probably underestimated as most epidemiologic surveys are based upon clinical examinations performed in the neonatal period, whereas many cerebral malformations will only be discovered later on in life. Indeed, long-term population based studies suggest that the incidence may be as high as 1%[1].

Detection of CNS anomalies was one of the most compelling motivations for the routine use of sonography in pregnancy. It is now clear that open neural tube defects, including anencephaly, open spina bifida and large cephaloceles, as well as other severe malformations such as major holoprosencephaly, are readily identified in early gestation. In fact, the major challenge for the fetal medicine specialist is more to interpret findings of uncertain clinical significance than to detect serious cerebral malformations. Many subtle anomalies that are poorly understood, like ventriculomegaly, agenesis of the corpus callosum and posterior fossa cysts, are now detected antenatally. As there is not a clear-cut correlation between abnormal anatomy and long-term cerebral function, the consequences of these anomalies are difficult to predict. This causes anxiety to the couples, requires difficult decisions and may eventually lead to the loss of normal fetuses.

Ventriculomegaly

Enlargement of the lateral cerebral ventricles, commonly referred to as ventriculomegaly (Figure 6.1), is a nonspecific marker of abnormal brain development. The presence of normal fetal lateral ventricles on ultrasound examination decreases the risk of a CNS anomaly, whereas ventriculomegaly carries a much increased risk. Although many different approaches to

the evaluation of the integrity of lateral ventricles have been proposed, measurement of the internal width of the atrium (or posterior horn) of the lateral ventricle is currently favored. Under normal conditions, the measurement is <10 mm between 15 and 40 weeks' gestation. In most cases with significant enlargement, both lateral ventricles are symmetrically affected. Less pronounced enlargement is frequently unilateral.

A value of >15 mm indicates *severe ventriculomegaly*. This is almost always associated with an intracranial malformation, although the outcome is variable and depends largely upon the underlying etiology of the ventricular dilatation. The available studies suggest that fetuses with isolated severe ventriculomegaly have an increased risk of perinatal death and a probability of severe long-term neurologic sequelae in approximately 50% of survivors[2].

An intermediate value of the atrial width, 10–15 mm, is commonly referred to as *mild ventriculomegaly* and is less frequently associated with many CNS anomalies, including agenesis of the corpus callosum and open neural tube defects[2,3]. Mild ventriculomegaly is associated with chromosomal aberrations: the risk of trisomy 21 is increased 3.8 times when ventricular enlargement is an isolated finding[4]. Fetal infections, such as cytomegalovirus, may result in ventricular enlargement, although usually with other sonographic abnormalities (cerebral echogenicities, microcephaly and porencephaly). When associated anomalies are ruled out, most infants are completely asymptomatic after birth. However, several reports have indicated that some fetuses develop severe cerebral anomalies in advanced gestation or after birth (hydrocephalus, white matter injury and cortical plate abnormalities) and have suggested an increased risk of neurologic compromise. Studies that have investigated

Fetal Medicine, ed. Bidyut Kumar and Zarko Alfirevic. Published by Cambridge University Press. © Cambridge University Press 2016.

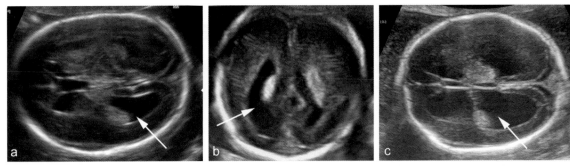

Figure 6.1 Fetal lateral cerebral ventriculomegaly (arrows). (a) Mild ventriculomegaly; (b) unilateral mild ventriculomegaly; (c) severe ventriculomegaly.

the prognosis of mild ventriculomegaly have been limited by the lack of standardized follow-up protocols and difficulty in defining 'normality.' However, most fetuses develop normally, and only about 10% demonstrate neurodevelopmental abnormalities of variable types and magnitude[3].

It is commonly accepted that when mild ventriculomegaly is encountered, all efforts must be made to rule out associated anomalies. A detailed expert sonographic survey of fetal anatomy is mandatory and invasive testing for cytogenetic analysis should be considered. Detailed ultrasound assessment may necessitate scanning by the vaginal route. There is debate as to whether fetal magnetic resonance imaging (MRI) is indicated in all cases of apparently isolated ventriculomegaly[3]. This technique may provide significant diagnostic information, particularly in the last trimester of gestation. In continuing pregnancies, there is no indication to modify the standard obstetric management.

Key counseling points

(1) Offer an expert sonography survey of fetal anatomy, karyotype and serial scans to assess progression.
(2) Consider a maternal infection screen (cytomegalovirus, toxoplasomsis).
(3) Consider fetal MRI to exclude subtle intracranial pathology, including neuronal migration disorders and intracranial bleeding.
(4) In mild (10–12 mm), nonprogressive ventriculomegaly, abnormal neurodevelopmental outcome is rare (<10%).

Neural tube defects

Anencephaly is characterized by the absence of the cranial vault and telencephalon. The diagnosis is easy in the second and third trimester, and relies upon the demonstration of the absence of the cranial vault. However, most cases can be confidently identified at the 11–13 weeks' scan. At this time, a cephalic pole is usually present, but appears overtly abnormal because of the lack of an ossified calvarium[5] (Figure 6.2). The terms *acrania* and *excencephaly* have also been used to describe such an appearance, which represents an early stage in the development of anencephaly. The outcome is uniformly fatal.

Spina bifida is commonly subdivided into open and closed forms. Open spina bifida is characterized with a full-thickness defect of the skin, underlying soft tissues and vertebral arches exposing the neural canal. The defect may vary considerably in size. The lumbar, thoracolumbar or sacrolumbar areas are most frequently affected. Leakage of cerebrospinal fluid through the defect causes an increased concentration of alpha-fetoprotein and acetylcholinesterase in the amniotic fluid and maternal serum, but these are no longer used for diagnostic purposes. Open spina bifida can be identified sonographically by demonstrating the opening of the neural tube and the defect of the overlying soft tissues. A cyst formed by the fusion of the malformed cord and meninges (myelomeningocele) is usually found. In a minority of cases, there is no covering membrane (myelocele). The diagnosis of a neural tube defect may be difficult and always requires meticulous scanning. Examination of the fetal head is useful, as open spina bifida is consistently associated with easily recognizable cranial lesions. Leakage of cerebrospinal fluid leads to displacement of the cerebellum and medulla oblongata through the foramen magnum inside the upper cervical canal (Chiari type II or Arnold–Chiari malformation). Sonographically, this results in small head measurements at midgestation, obliteration of the cisterna magna, small size and abnormal shape of the cerebellum that is impacted deep

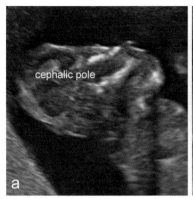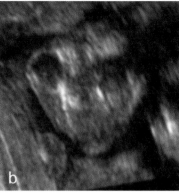

cephalic pole

a   b

Figure 6.2 Anencephaly. (a) At 12 weeks' gestation, a cephalic pole, albeit abnormal, is visible. (b) From midgestation, the cephalic pole is usually completely absent.

into the posterior fossa (banana sign), frontal bossing (lemon sign) and ventriculomegaly. The detection rate of a midtrimester scan is in the range of 90%[6,7]. Abnormalities of the posterior fossa and lateral ventricles have also been described at the 11–13 weeks' scan, but the diagnostic accuracy of these findings to screen for spina bifida is still being assessed.

There is a correlation between the site and extension of the spinal lesion and the neurologic outcome. Indeed, the lower and smaller the defect, the less severe the neurologic compromise. Fetal medicine experts often record the level of the lesion by counting the affected vertebrae either from the most distal one, the fourth sacral vertebra (S4), or from the 12th thoracic vertebra in the rib cage (T12). Antenatal ultrasound assessments correlate reasonably well with postnatal assessment (75%) and MRI adds little in this respect, but it is impossible to predict with precision motor functions, morbidity and developmental milestones[8]. On the other hand, ventricular enlargement does correlate with the need for postnatal shunting[9]. Antenatal counseling is complex and should involve a multidisciplinary team, including pediatric neurosurgeons. Postnatal hydrocephalus requiring shunting and incontinence, and motor weakness requiring wheelchair support are common. Most women will chose termination of pregnancy, although an increasing number may choose expectant management and even contemplate intrauterine treatment (see Chapter 28). It has been suggested that cesarean section may ameliorate the neurologic outcome of infants with open spina bifida, but the evidence is weak. As a rule, a cesarean section is only performed for obstetric indications.

Closed spina bifida is characterized by a vertebral schisis covered by skin. Most defects are small, involving only few veretebral segments, and the classical intracranial signs (lemon-shaped skull, banana-shaped cerebellum) are always absent. As a consequence of this, diagnosis with sonography is difficult and, in practice, is only possible in those cases associated with a subcutaneous mass, a meningocele or lipoma, overlying the defect[6]. The outcome of closed spina bifida is difficult to predict. These infants do not develop Arnold–Chiari malformation and hydrocephalus. Particularly those with subcutaneous masses, however, may suffer from neurologic sequelae of variable entity, including weakness or paralysis of the legs and incontinence, which are usually a consequence of tethering or compression of the spinal cord.

The term *cephalocele* indicates a protrusion of intracranial contents through a bony defect of the skull. In most cases, the lesion arises from the midline, in the occipital area, less frequently from the parietal or frontal bones. Encephaloceles are characterized by the presence of brain tissue inside the lesion. When only meninges protrude, the term *cranial meningocele* is used. Cephaloceles often cause impaired cerebrospinal fluid circulation and hydrocephalus, and massive encephaloceles may be associated with microcephaly. Associated anomalies are frequent. Fetal cephaloceles are suspected when a paracranial mass is observed on sonography. The diagnosis of encephalocele is easy, as the presence of brain tissue inside the sac is striking on ultrasound. Differentiation of a cranial meningocele from soft tissue edema or a cystic hygroma of the neck may be difficult. The diagnosis of cephalocele is favored when it is possible to demonstrate a defect in the cranial vault or cerebral abnormalities, such as ventriculomegaly. The pediatric literature suggests that the outcome of cephaloceles is mainly related to the presence or absence of brain tissue inside the lesion. However, the largest available antenatal series reports a dismal prognosis for both varieties[10], with the

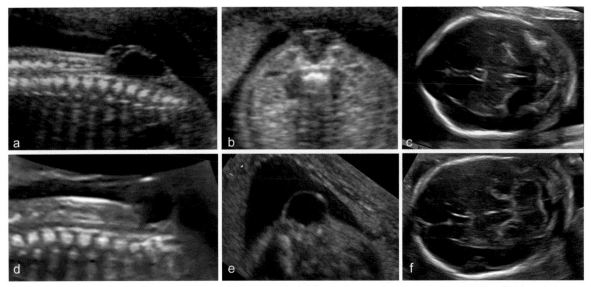

Figure 6.3 (a–c) Open spina bifida (myelomeingocele): large vertebral defect with an overlying septated cyst associated with typical findings of Arnold–Chiari malformation, cranial bossing and obliteration of the cisterna magna. (d–f) Closed or skin-covered cystic spina bifida (meningocele): a small vertebral defect with an overlying nonseptated cyst, and normal intracranial anatomy.

possible exception of small lesions in the presence of a normal intracranial anatomy (Figure 6.3).

Key counseling points

(1) Fetal karyotyping is not indicated in apparently isolated neural tube defects.
(2) With open spina bifida, correlation between the level of the defect and postnatal function is relatively poor.
(3) Closed spina bifida has a better outcome than open spina bifida, but neurologic compromise is possible and is difficult to predict.
(4) Large cephaloceles, particularly in the presence of abnormal intracranial anatomy, have a poor outcome.
(5) Multidisciplinary counseling is strongly advised.

Midline anomalies

The *holoprosencephalies* are complex abnormalities of the forebrain that share in common an incomplete separation of the cerebral hemispheres and formation of diencephalic structures. They are rarely seen at birth. However, they have a high intrauterine fatality rate and are a relatively common group in the series of antenatally detected CNS anomalies. The etiology is heterogeneous. In most cases, the anomaly is isolated and sporadic. In other cases, chromosomal abnormalities

(trisomy 13 and polyploidy) and/or anatomic abnormalities are found.

The most widely accepted classification of these disorders recognizes three major varieties: the alobar, semilobar and lobar types. More recently, middle interhemispheric variant has been added. The alobar, semilobar and middle interhemispheric variant types have a similar appearance on antenatal ultrasound – there is no midline echo anteriorly and there is a single ventricular cavity (Figure 6.4). Gross facial abnormalities (cyclopia, hypotelorism and absence of the nose) are frequent. In most cases the diagnosis is possible at the 11–13 weeks' scan. The lobar variety is associated with more subtle findings (absence of the septum pellucidum with central fusion of the frontal horns) and the diagnosis is rarely made prior to 20 weeks' gestation[11].

The invariably poor prognosis for infants affected by a lobar and semilobar holoprosencephaly is well established. Termination of pregnancy should be offered. Even cases with antenatally diagnosed lobar holoprosencephaly have an extremely poor postnatal neurodevelopment.

Agenesis of the corpus callosum (ACC) is an anomaly of uncertain prevalence and clinical significance. The best estimates suggest prevalence of around 1.4 per 10,000 live births in the general population and 2–3% in the developmentally disabled. The etiology is heterogeneous. Genetic causes are predominant, and the anomaly is frequently a part of many different syndromes.

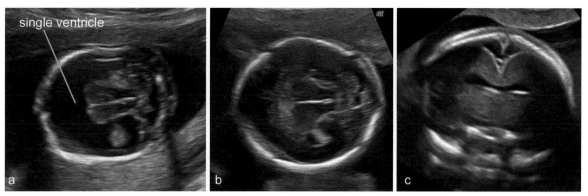

Figure 6.4 (a) A typical case of fetal holoprosencephaly: a large single ventricular cavity is seen and there is no midline in the anterior part of the brain. (b) A case with less obvious findings. (c) The anterior midline is absent but the single ventricular cavity can only be clearly demonstrated with a transvaginal coronal scan.

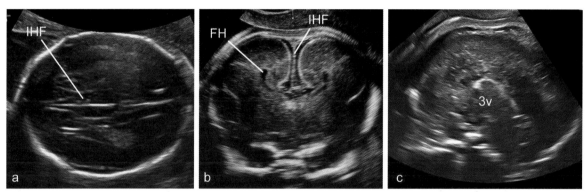

Figure 6.5 Complete agenesis of the corpus callosum (CC). (a) The axial plane reveals mild enlargement of the lateral ventricles that have a typical tear-drop shape, absence of the cavum septi pellucidi (CSP) and distension of the interhemispheric fissure (IHF) that is centrally partitioned by the falx cerebrii. (b) The coronal plane demonstrates the large IHF, the absence of any bridging structure connecting the two hemispheres, and the lateral separation of the frontal horns that appear medially concave. (c) The sagittal plane demonstrates the absence of complex formed by CC and CSP over the third ventricle. FH, frontal horns.

The high frequency of associated malformations and chromosomal aberrations suggest that ACC is often part of a widespread developmental disturbance. ACC may be either complete or partial. In the latter case, also referred to as dysgenesis, the caudad portion is missing to varying degrees. Hypoplasia refers to a corpus callosum (CC) of normal length but with much decreased thickness, and is rarely identified prenatally.

Although the anatomy of complete ACC is variable, this condition is usually suspected in routine examinations at midgestation because of the absence of the *cavum septi pellucidi* (CSP) and the presence of a peculiar configuration of the lateral ventricles characterized by an increased separation of the frontal horns and a mild enlargement of the posterior horns (tear-drop ventricles), frequently associated with mild ventriculomegaly. The definitive diagnosis is made by demonstrating the absence of the CC in coronal and/or sagittal scans (Figure 6.5)[12]. Diagnosis of partial agenesis is also possible, but the sonographic findings are more elusive than with the complete form. The CSP is usually present and the axial sections may be completely unremarkable. The diagnosis requires a sagittal section demonstrating that the CC shorter than normal and does not form a complete arch over the third ventricle (Figure 6.6). Normal charts of the size of the CC are available, but should be used with caution because partial agenesis is a rare condition and it has not been possible thus far to establish a clear threshold for pathologic appearance. Most cases diagnosed antenatally have shown a reduction in size of 50% or more. We have seen many cases with measurements <5th centile and, as expected, most resulted in the birth of normal children (Figures 6.5 and 6.6).

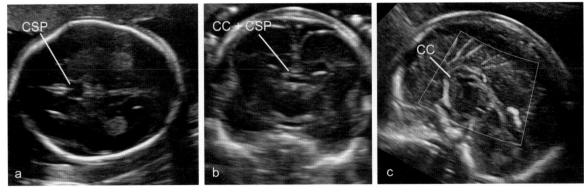

Figure 6.6 A panel of images highlighting the difficulties in the diagnosis of partial agenesis of the corpus callosum. (a) The axial plane reveals a rather normal-looking cavum septi pellucidi (CSP). (b) The coronal plane demonstrates the presence of the complex formed by the corpus callosum (CC) and CSP bridging between the two hemispheres. (c) Only the sagittal plane demonstrates a CC that is at the same time quite short (the arch does not cover entirely the area of the third ventricle, and the measurement is about 50% the expected size at this gestational age) and irregular in shape.

ACC, be it complete or partial, is frequently a part of syndromes or multiple malformations. A recent systematic review assessed the rate of neurodevelopmental outcome in 132 fetuses (16 studies) with isolated ACC[13]. The authors reported neurodevelopmental outcome as: normal; borderline or moderate disability; or severe disability. In complete ACC, the respective figures were 74.3%, 14.3% and 11.4%. The outcome was slightly less favorable, although not significantly different, for partial ACC (65.5%, 6.9% and 27.6%, respectively). When taking into account only those studies using MRI and standardized tools of neurodevelopmental assessment, in complete ACC, the rates were 83.7%, 8.2% and 8.2% for normal, borderline/moderate and severe disability, respectively. The corresponding rates for partial ACC were not reported due to the small number of cases. The authors of the review highlighted many limitations in existing studies, including limited and inconsistent data that prevented subgroup analyses. Providing a precise estimate of the risk of neurodevelopmental delay is difficult. One important limitation of the available studies is the time of follow-up. In most cases, assessment was made in the preschool period. This may represent an important shortcoming as in one series a progressive decline of intellect was noted, with a considerable number of infants demonstrating learning difficulties in school.

The septum pellucidum, with the inferior fornix, forms the medial border of the lateral ventricles. It contains two leaves that in fetal life are separated by a fluid-filled cavity, the CSP. The leaves fuse in late gestation or immediately after birth and the cavity is seen only in a minority of adults. *Absence of the septum pellucidum* in fetuses is frequently associated with a number of cerebral anomalies, including ACC, holoprosencephaly, destruction secondary to raised intraventricular pressure, schizencephaly and septo-optic dysplasia (deMorsier syndrome). Isolated absence of the septal leaves with central fusion of the frontal horns is possible, and is usually of no consequence (Figure 6.7). The greatest challenge is to differentiate isolated absence from septo-optic dysplasia. Visualization of the optic chiasma by either Magnetic resonance or three-dimensional ultrasound is useful, although it does not seem to allow a definitive diagnosis. The available experience is limited, but thus far, two-thirds of fetuses with absent CSP were reported to be normal at birth. If a normal optic chiasma can be demonstrated, the probability increases to 90%[14].

Key counseling points

(1) Holoprosencephaly is frequently associated with trisomy 13 and, in general, has a very poor prognosis. The lobar type, although associated with an equally poor prognosis, may be difficult to diagnose antenatally.

(2) ACC is frequently a part of syndromes or multiple anomalies. Offer a detailed scan, MRI and karyotype, including microarray testing. There is no need, however, to test for infections.

(3) Three out of four children with complete isolated ACC will have normal neurodevelopmental outcome, at least at pre-school age; partial agenesis may represent a different clinical entity

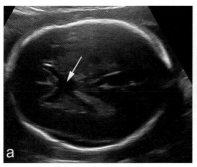 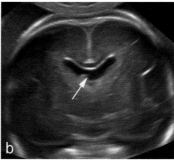

Figure 6.7 Absence of the septum pellucidum demonstrated in (a) an axial and (b) transvaginal coronal plane. The two frontal horns communicate centrally and there is no evidence of the leaves of the septum pellucidum (arrows).

Table 6.1 Sonographic findings of posterior fossa cyst and cyst-like anomalies

Anomaly	Findings
Megacisterna magna	Intact cerebellum; cisterna magna >10 mm
Blake's pouch cyst	Cerebellum of normal size, intact vermis with mild rotation (usually <30°)
Dandy–Walker malformation	Cerebellum of normal or diminished size, normal to small vermis with significant rotation (usually >45°), large cisterna magna
Vermian hypoplasia	Cerebellum of normal or diminished size, small dysmorphic vermis with or without moderate rotation (usually <45°), normal cisterna magna
Joubert syndrome	Cerebellum and cisterna magna of normal size, extremely small or absent vermis, typical configuration of fourth ventricle and cerebellar peduncles
Posterior fossa arachnoid cyst and other extra-axial cysts	Cystic asymmetric enlargement of the cisterna magna with a mass effect on the cerebellum

than complete agenesis, but the available data are limited.

(4) Isolated agenesis of the septum pellucidum is asymptomatic in two out of three cases; the risk can be further decreased if the optic chiasma and tracts appear normal either on ultrasound or MRI.

Cystic and cyst-like abnormalities of the posterior fossa

Abnormal fluid collections in the fetal posterior fossa encompass a wide spectrum of different entities, ranging from normal variants to severe anomalies (Table 6.1).

In the late first trimester, the fourth ventricle is large and a relatively small cerebellum is found on top of it. In the following weeks, the cerebellum grows to enfold completely the fourth ventricle. However, a small finger-like appendage of the fourth ventricle, the Blake's pouch, is frequently seen protruding into the cisterna magna, caudally to the cerebellum. It has been suggested that there is a continuum of anatomic anomalies involving the fourth ventricle–Blake's pouch

complex (Figure 6.8)[15]. The mildest of these anomalies is the *Blake's pouch cyst*, an isolated persistence of the Blake's pouch. This term was originally introduced in pediatric neuroradiology to indicate a compressive cyst of the posterior fossa displacing superiorly the cerebellar vermis and causing obstructive hydrocephalus. More recently, the same term has become popular in fetal imaging studies to indicate cases with a posterior fossa cyst displacing superiorly an intact cerebellar vermis, typically in association with a normal ventricular system and a normal size of the posterior fossa. The entity described in the original neonatal studies and the one later described in fetal studies are likely to be different, as the latter has typically a normal outcome and appears to be rarely associated with ventriculomegaly. *Megacisterna magna* may be a variation of the Blake' pouch cyst that does not result in superior displacement of the vermis.

In the largest available series, Blake's pouch cyst and megacisterna magna were the two most common entities observed antenatally, representing about 50% of all cystic anomalies of the fetal posterior fossa[16]. These two conditions share in common many clinical

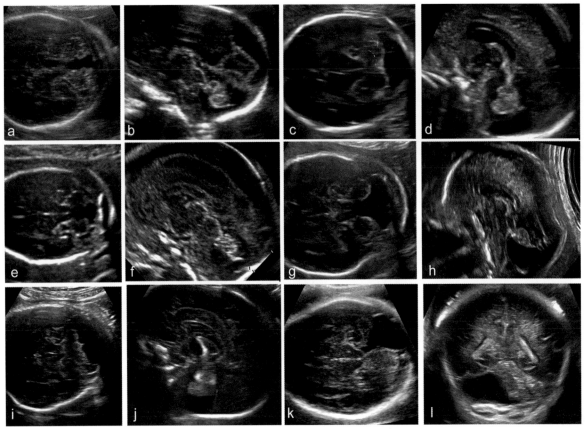

Figure 6.8 Categorization of posterior fossa fluid collections (see Table 6.1). (a, b) Blake's pouch cyst; (c, d) megacisterna magna; (e,f) vermian hypoplasia; (g, h) Dandy–Walker malformation; (i, j) cerebellar hypoplasia; (k, l) arachnoid cyst of the posterior fossa.

similarities. Although they may be associated with other anomalies, when isolated, they undergo spontaneous resolution throughout gestation in one-third of cases, and result in a normal postnatal neurodevelopment in about 90% of cases[16].

Dandy–Walker malformation is rare, with an estimated incidence of about 1:30,000 births and 4–12% of infantile hydrocephalus. The main features are enlargement of the cisterna magna and superior displacement of the cerebellar vermis that can be intact or incompletely formed. Hydrocephalus was classically considered an essential diagnostic element of this condition, but more recent evidence suggests that it is not present at birth in most patients, although it may develop in later life. Dandy–Walker malformation is frequently associated with other neural defects (ACC, holoprosencephaly, encephaloceles), chromosomal aberrations and extraneural anomalies (polycystic kidneys, cardiovascular defects and facial clefting). When isolated, the outcome is variable. In antenatal studies,

only 50% of surviving infants were found to have a normal intelligence[16].

Vermian agenesis/hypoplasia is characterized by a small or absent vermis with a normal cisterna magna. This condition was originally labelled *Dandy–Walker variant*, a term no longer in use. Follow-up studies of antenatally diagnosed children had conflicting results, spanning from a mainly normal outcome to a high prevalence of neurological compromise[16,17].

Joubert syndrome and related disorders are a group of conditions that share in common hypoplasia of the cerebellar vermis with the characteristic neuroradiologic "molar tooth sign" – the elongated superior cerebellar peduncles giving an appearance reminiscent of a molar or wisdom tooth. These features are associated with extraneural anomalies to constitute different syndromes that share in common an unfavorable outcome[18].

Arachnoid cysts of the posterior fossa are exceedingly rare, and most frequently cause a mass effect on the cerebellar structures, but at times they may be

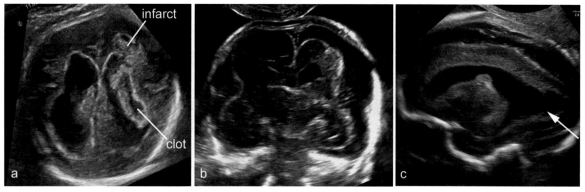

Figure 6.9 Intrauterine cerebral injuries. (a) Intracranial hemorrhage grade IV (see Table 6.2): within one of the enlarged lateral ventricles a blood clot is visible, and there is evidence of an infarct into the white matter. (b) Fetal stroke after the death of a monochorionic twin: one of the cerebral hemispheres is diminutive with irregular morphology and echogenicity following acute ischemia. (c) Cerebral cytomegalovirus sequelae: the images suggests a septum within the cavity of the lateral ventricle, but in reality the finding is the consequence of a cavitation of the white matter in the occipital lobe close to the ventricular cavity.

difficult to differentiate from megacisterna magna or Dandy–Walker malformation.

With the exception of megacisterna magna, whose diagnostic criteria are clear-cut (the widely accepted definition is a cisterna magna depth >10 mm), the appearance of the other cystic anomalies of the fetal posterior fossa is similar and differential diagnosis is difficult. Blake's pouch cyst, Dandy–Walker malformation, vermian hypoplasia/agenesis and Joubert syndrome share in common a similar finding: the impression in an axial plane of a communication between the fourth ventricle and the cisterna magna (open fourth ventricle sign). In reality, the image is conjured by the presence of a cystic structure extending from the roof of the fourth ventricle into the cisterna magna beneath the cerebellar vermis. This finding is frequent in early gestation and becomes significant only when it is demonstrated after 20 weeks' gestation. After this time, the most valuable diagnostic information is obtained from a mid-sagittal view of the brain. Antenatal studies combining the use of ultrasound and MRI report a diagnostic precision in the range of 90%. Differentiating a Blake's pouch cyst from a Dandy–Walker malformation, and diagnosing vermian hypoplasia in early gestation, are the greatest difficulties encountered thus far[16].

Key counseling points

(1) A cisterna magna >10 mm or a posterior opening of the fourth ventricle in fetuses after 20 weeks may indicate the presence of a cerebral anomaly but are more frequently normal anatomic variants.

(2) A detailed examination of the entire fetal anatomy is indicated; the posterior fossa should be studied with a combination of axial and sagittal views, with special attention to the cerebellar vermis: fetal karyotyping and MRI should be considered.

(3) In the absence of associated anomalies, a cerebellar vermis of normal size and morphology, with or without a mild rotation, usually indicates a normal outcome.

Destructive cerebral lesions

Many congenital anomalies of the brain are not the consequence of an embryogenetic malformative process but are due to a destructive process (Figure 6.9). The pathophysiology is frequently unclear and the conditions remain idiopathic. A link with obstetric complications of a different nature is, however, frequently found.

Intracranial hemorrhage (ICH) is a frequent complication in premature infants. Rarely, it may occur antenatally, as a consequence of fetal thromobocytopenia and other coagulopathies, trauma, or other yet unexplained factors. The sonographic appearance is extremely variable depending upon the type (Table 6.2), the severity and the time since it occurred. Blood appears initially as an echogenic collection. With time, the blood clot retracts and demonstrates an anechoic core, and is frequently associated with ventricular dilatation. Large intraventricular hemorrhagic collections may be complicated by infarct and destruction of the surrounding white matter. There is

Table 6.2 Categorization of fetal intracranial hemorrhage

Type of hemorrhage	Findings
Intraventricular hemorrhage, grade 1	Hemorrhage limited to the germinal matrix
Intraventricular hemorrhage, grade 2	Intraventricular spill with ventricles <15 mm, intact brain parenchyma
Intraventricular hemorrhage, grade 3	Intraventricular spill with ventricles >15 mm, intact brain parenchyma
Intraventricular hemorrhage, grade 4	Intraventricular spill and periventricular lesions
Cerebellar hemorrhage	Hemorrhage within the cerebellar parenchyma
Subarachnoid hemorrhage and subdural hematoma	Accumulation of blood external to the hemispheres, the two entities are difficult to discriminate antenatally

a correlation between the outcome and the grade of the hemorrhage (Table 6.2). The prognosis is favorable with grade 1 and 2 hemorrhages, which at times may even resolve in utero, and is severe with grade 3 and 4 lesions. Most cases identified prenatally belong to grade 3 and 4, and in a review of the literature, 50% died perinatally and 50% of survivors were neurologically compromised[19]. If intracranial hemorrhage is suspected, fetalalloimmune thrombocytopenia must be excluded (see Chapter X). Fetal MRI is particularly helpful in distinguishing hemorrhage from other intracranial pathologies.

Fetal stroke has been documented antenatally[20]. The etiology is heterogeneous, but thus far most cases have been identified in monochorionic twin gestation, usually as a consequence of fetal demise of a cotwin or severe hemodynamic compromise following twin-to-twin transfusion. The appearance is variable. Following the insult, discrete cerebral echogenicity is observed. In the following stages, microencephaly, cystic intraparenchymal cavities (porencephaly, schizencephaly, periventricular leukomalacia) and cortical malformations will develop. The outcome is dictated by the size and location of the lesion. Microcephaly and extensive porencephaly have a severe prognosis.

Intrauterine infection in general is one of the major causes of congenital brain lesions. Fetuses with cytomegalovirus (CMV) infection affecting the brain may present with a wide range of intracranial abnormalities, including periventricular and intraparenchymal echogenicity, ventriculomegaly, cerebellar hypoplasia, microcephaly and cortical abnormalities. The most specific findings include an echogenic periventricular halo and septations within the occipital horns. The main value of fetal neurosonograms in patients with recent CMV infection lies in its very high positive predictive value. Specific cerebral findings predict a symptomatic infection virtually in all cases. The negative

predictive value is limited. Recent series suggest that false-negative scans (a normal scan when the fetus is affected) are rare in the third trimester, but do happen in the second trimester[21].

Microcephaly

Microcephaly indicates the association of abnormal neurologic development and a small head. The smaller the head dimensions, the greater the probability of microcephaly. However, there is not an absolute quantitative cut-off. The incidence is estimated to be 1.6 per 1,000 single-birth deliveries, but only a minority of microcephalic infants diagnosed by the first year of age are detected at birth. Microcephaly can result from primary cerebral malformations or exposure to teratogens. It is part of a wide variety of syndromes and can also be transmitted with Mendelian inheritance, usually as an autosomal recessive trait. Association with abnormal intracranial anatomy is common.

Microcephaly is a progressive condition, and therefore definitive prenatal diagnosis is impossible in most cases. About 80% of affected infants have a normal head circumference (HC) at birth, and about 90% of those diagnosed at birth have normal cranial measurements in the second trimester. Cases diagnosed in utero represent the exception, and include fetuses with extreme reduction of head dimensions, usually with multiple anomalies.

Traditional teaching is that microcephaly is suspected if the head perimeter is two standard deviations (SD) below the mean for gestational age, but only when the measurement is ≥5 SD below the mean, the diagnosis is certain[22]. In those cases in which the head measurement is in the intermediate zone, a detailed neurosonographic examination and/or cerebral MRI may be of use as two-thirds of microcephalic infants have abnormal cerebral anatomy, including mostly holoprosencephaly, anomalies of the CC or cortical malformations.

The outcome is different depending on the presence of associated anomalies. For infants without associated malformations, the prognosis is related to head size. The pediatric literature suggests that the risk of mental retardation with a HC between –2 and –3 SDs is in the range of 10–30%, rising to 50–60% for measurements below –3 SDs. Prenatal data are limited. In the largest available series, none of the 20 infants that were found in utero to have a HC between –2 and –3 SD had mental retardation or neurocognitive problems at long-term follow-up[23].

Intracranial cysts and tumors

Intracranial *arachnoid cysts* are accumulations of clear cerebrospinal-like fluid between the dura and the brain substance. The histologic diagnosis is not always available, and the term is frequently used to indicate any intracranial cyst located in the subarachnoid space (Figure 6.10a).

Arachnoid cysts may be found anywhere in the CNS, including the spinal canal. Most of the cases diagnosed antenatally involve supratentorial cysts in the midline, or between the skull and the hemispheres. They appear as well-defined anechoic lesions occasionally associated with ventriculomegaly, which usually develop only in late gestation. They should be differentiated from other cystic lesions with different prognostic implications, and the most important clue is that they are external to the hemispheres. Porencephalic cysts occur within the brain substance and frequently communicate with the ventricular cysts. Arachnoid cysts may be asymptomatic, but they may cause epilepsy, mild motor or sensory abnormalities, or hydrocephalus. In general, the neurosurgical series suggests a good prognosis, with the absence of symptoms in more than 70% of cases.

Choroid plexus cysts appear as round sonolucent areas in the context of the choroid plexus of lateral ventricles, which are found in 1–3% of midtrimester fetuses (Figure 6.10b). They may be unilateral or bilateral, or sometimes multiple, and are typically found at the level of the atrium of lateral ventricles, less frequently within the bodies. They are benign findings that are, however, associated with an increased likelihood of trisomy 18. The available data do not indicate an association with other chromosomal aberrations, including trisomy 21. As fetuses with trisomy 18 usually have severe malformations readily detectable with ultrasound, the consensus is that isolated choroid plexus cysts do not warrant an invasive procedure for fetal karyotyping. Isolated choroid plexus cysts do not modify standard obstetrical management. As no deleterious effect on the fetus has been thus far reported with this finding, there is no need for follow-up scans. A handful of cases with very large cysts of the choroid plexuses causing intracranial hypertension have been described in the neurosurgical literature, but these represent probably a separate clinical entity.

Fetal *intracranial tumors* are rare, with about 3–4 cases per million live births. Teratomas account for most cases. In the remaining minority, neuroepithelial tumors, lipomas and craniopharyngiomas are found. Ultrasound will rarely allow a specific diagnosis because teratomas, astrocytomas and craniopharyngiomas have a similar appearance: a complex mass distorting the brain architecture, possibly associated with macrocephaly, ventriculomegaly and intracranial

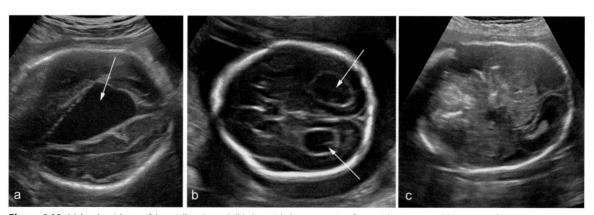

Figure 6.10 (a) Arachnoid cyst of the midline (arrow); (b) chorioid plexus cysts in a fetus with trisomy 18; (c) intracranial teratoma.

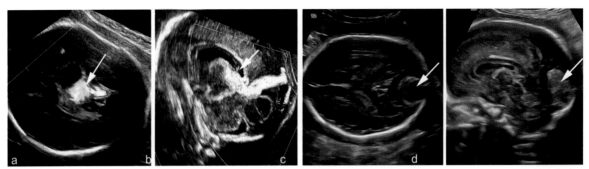

Figure 6.11 Vascular anomalies of fetal brain. (a, b) Aneurysm of the vein of Galen: color Doppler demonstrates gross enlargement of the vein of Galen with turbulent flow (arrows). (c, d) Thrombosis of the sinus confluence: a large sonolucent collection containing an echogenic core suggestive of a thrombus is visible in the occipital area, posterior to the brain (arrows).

calcifications (Figure 6.10c)[24]. Only intracranial lipomas and choroid plexus papillomas have a specific sonographic appearance: the former well-defined echogenic areas, usually located in the midline, in the position normally occupied by the CC, and/or within the bodies of lateral ventricles; the latter large choroid plexuses, most frequently in association with ventriculomegaly and subarachnoid space enlargement. Cerebral tumors typically develop rapidly in late gestation. Several cases have been reported in which midtrimester sonograms were unremarkable. The differential diagnosis includes other space occupying intracranial lesions. At times, it may be particularly challenging to distinguish between a tumor and a fresh intraparenchymal hemorrhage.

The prognosis of congenital tumors is poor. The overall mortality rate is in the range of 75%. No clear data are available with regard to the degree of neurologic impairment in survivors, but this is also expected to be high. Large complex mass distorting intracranial anatomy (usually teratomas, astrocytomas or craniopharyngiomas) were found to have a particularly dismal prognosis, with overall survival of only 14%[24]. Intracranial lipomas represent an exception, in that the survival rate is 100% and the developmental handicap rare.

Tuberous sclerosis is a syndrome featured by multiorgan involvement transmitted as an autosomal dominant trait, but frequently arising from a spontaneous mutation. Mental retardation is present in 50–80% of cases and appears to be more frequent when the diagnosis is made prenatally or in early infancy. The most typical brain lesions are the tubers, nodules of variable size composed with poorly differentiated neurons and glial cells disseminated in the neural plate or periventricular area. However, these are extremely difficult to identify antenatally. The condition is usually suspected

when cardiac tumors are identified. About 90% of these tumors are rabdomyoma and about 75% of these fetuses will be affected by tuberous sclerosis[25]. Therefore, whenever cardiac tumors, particularly multiple ones, are identified, a search for cerebral lesions is warranted. Sonographic diagnosis is possible, although MRI is generally considered to be more accurate.

Vascular abnormalities

Vascular anomalies of the fetal brain are rare, and only a handful of cases have been described thus far. The majority of reports concentrate upon the vein of Galen vascular malformations.

The term *aneurysm of the vein of Galen* indicates a spectrum of arteriovenous malformations, ranging from a single large aneurysmal dilatation of the vein of Galen to multiple communications between the vein and the carotid and vertebrobasilar systems. The typical finding is an elongated anechoic area at the level of the cistern of the vein of Galen, with color and pulsed Doppler evidence of turbulent venous and/or arterial blood flow (Figure 6.11a, b). The cerebral architecture may be intact or it may be distorted due to the associated ventriculomegaly, porencephaly and/or brain edema presenting by increased echogenicity of the cortex. Large arteriovenous shunts may increase cardiac work and result in high-output heart failure and hydrops. The available experience with prenatal diagnosis suggests a mortality rate in the range of 50%, and a normal development in about 50% of survivors[26]. However, the outcome is strongly dependent upon the antenatal evidence of other intracranial abnomalities (hydrocephalus, brain edema, porencephaly) and/or hydrops. When any of these have been found, the prognosis was always poor. In general, cases with a normal postnatal development had

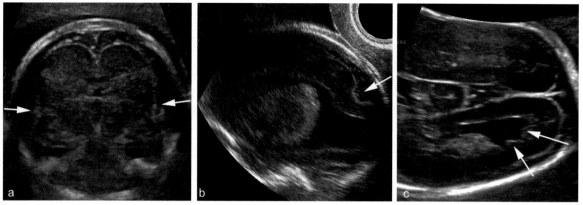

Figure 6.12 Examples of cortical malformations (see Table 6.3). (a) Lissencephaly: in this fetus at the third trimester of pregnancy, the brain contour appears smooth, without evidence of convolutions and without any development of the Sylvian fissure (arrows). (b) An irregular sulcus is noted in this fetus that was diagnosed after birth with polymicrogyria. (c) The irregular contour of the lateral ventricle suggests periventricular nodular heterotopia.

isolated vascular lesions, without cerebral or cardiovascular compromise in utero, and were treated after birth with angiographic embolization.

It may be difficult to distinguish an aneurysm of the vein of Galen from a pial arteriovenous malformation[27]. This is a vascular malformation within the brain parenchyma, which results in an enlargement of the cerebral venous system, and the vein of Galen in particular. However, the outcome is similar, and the prognosis is poor when there are associated abnormal cerebral findings or signs of cardiac overload.

Several cases of *thrombosis of the dural sinuses* have been described recently. The sonographic findings are typical: the enlarged sinuses result in a posterior fluid-filled structure displacing anteriorly the fetal brain, and usually contain an echogenic core, probably representing the thrombus (Figure 6.11c, d). The etiology of antenatal cases is uncertain. Thrombophilias may be found, but usually the condition is an idiopathic one. Despite that the intrauterine appearance may be quite dramatic, complete remission is frequent[28]. Indeed, if there are no signs of cerebral compromise, the outcome is good in most cases.

Cortical malformations

The neuronal cells that form the gray matter originate from the surface of the lateral ventricles and only later migrate along radially aligned glial cells to the surface of the brain. The migration occurs in different waves that last for several weeks. Most of the process takes place between 8 and 16 weeks' gestation, but continues up to 25 weeks. Once the neuronal cells have reached their destination on the surface of the brain, they undergo a process of maturation and differentiation, grow axons and dendrites and develop synapses with other neurons, giving rise to a well-ordered, six-layer cortex. Cortical malformations are characterized by the incomplete formation of the cortical layers, with abnormal locations of neurons that have failed to reach their final destination. The migrational process may be arrested by environmental factors (ischemia, teratogens), but a genetic predisposition is clearly present at least for some anomalies. Although the anatomy is variable, the cortex is frequently thickened by a large, disorganized layer of neurons and the white matter underneath thinned. Macroscopically, the main finding is an alteration in the convolutional pattern of the brain, which may be associated with modifications in brain mass and size of the ventricles. Cortical malformations should be considered in the differential diagnosis of ventriculomegaly, microcephaly and macrocephaly, and are suspected when an anomalous pattern of cerebral convolutions is present[29]. A detailed description of these rare and heterogeneous anomalies is beyond the scope of this chapter. The entities most frequently described in antenatal studies are summarized in Table 6.3 and Figure 6.12. The technique of choice for the diagnosis of these anomalies postnatally is MRI because it allows a clear discrimination between white and gray matter. Antenatally, however, fast sequences are used that have limited resolution, and most of all, the neural plate is incompletely formed. However, MRI does provide a panoramic view of the fetus and a better visualization of the cerebral surface, and therefore has

Table 6.3 Sonographic findings associated with cortical malformations

Anomaly	Sonographic findings
Lissencephaly	Smooth brain contour without recognizable convolutions; ventriculomegaly and/or microcephaly may be present
Unilateral megalencephaly	Macrocephaly; shift of the midline with overgrowth of one hemisphere; thick abnormal convolutions and ventriculomegaly frequently present in the largest hemisphere
Schizencephaly	Clefts of the brain connecting the subarachnoid space with the cavity of lateral ventricles; unilateral or bilateral
Periventricular nodular heterotopia	Irregular outline of the lateral ventricles with square shaped frontal horns; cystic cisterna magna may be present
Polymicrogyria	Multiple small sulci
Pachygyrias	Large deep sulci

many advantages over ultrasound. Early prenatal diagnosis is rarely made because cortical malformations are progressive lesions, usually detectable only in late gestation.

Summary

When abnormal fetal cerebral anatomy is identified, counseling the parents regarding sensible obstetric management is exceedingly difficult. Some cerebral anomalies have outcomes that can be predicted with reasonable precision. This is certainly the case with catastrophic lesions such as anencephaly and severe holoprosencephaly. However, a large number of conditions that can be accurately identified in utero have an unclear natural history and a wide range of long-term outcomes. MRI is often helpful, particularly if other specialists are involved in counseling, as they will be much more familiar with MRI than antenatal ultrasound images. Such multidisciplinary counseling involving pediatric neurologists and neurosurgeons, and clinical genetics does represent a gold standard that most tertiary fetal medicine teams should strive to provide.

References

1. Myrianthopoulos NC. Epidemiology of central nervous system malformations. In: Vinken PJ, Bruyn GW, eds. *Handbook of Clinical Neurology*. Amsterdam: Elsevier; 1977: 139–71.

2. Gupta JK, Bryce FC, Lilford RJ. Management of apparently isolated fetal ventriculomegaly. *Obstet Gynecol Surv*. 1994; 49(10): 716–21.

3. Melchiorre K, Bhide A, Gika AD, et al. Counseling in isolated mild fetal ventriculomegaly. *Ultrasound Obstet Gynecol* 2009; 34(2): 212–24.

4. Agathokleous M, Chaveeva P, Poon LC, et al. Meta-analysis of second-trimester markers for trisomy 21. *Ultrasound Obstet Gynecol* 2013; 41(3): 247–61.

5. Johnson SP, Sebire NJ, Snijders RJ, et al. Ultrasound screening for anencephaly at 10–14 weeks of gestation. *Ultrasound Obstet Gynecol* 1997; 9(1): 14–6.

6. Ghi T, Pilu G, Falco P, et al. Prenatal diagnosis of open and closed spina bifida. *Ultrasound Obstet Gynecol* 2006; 28(7): 899–903.

7. Van den Hof MC, Nicolaides KH, Campbell J, et al. Evaluation of the lemon and banana signs in one hundred thirty fetuses with open spina bifida. *Am J Obstet Gynecol* 1990; 162(2): 322–7.

8. Appasamy M, Roberts D, Pilling D, et al. Antenatal ultrasound and magnetic resonance imaging in localizing the level of lesion in spina bifida and correlation with postnatal outcome. *Ultrasound Obstet Gynecol* 2006; 27(5): 530–6.

9. Khalil A, Caric V, Papageorghiou A, et al. Prenatal prediction of need for ventriculoperitoneal shunt in open spina bifida. *Ultrasound Obstet Gynecol* 2014; 43(2): 159–64.

10. Goldstein RB, LaPidus AS, Filly RA. Fetal cephaloceles: diagnosis with US. *Radiology* 1991; 180(3): 803–8.

11. Blaas HG, Eriksson AG, Salvesen KA, et al. Brains and faces in holoprosencephaly: pre- and postnatal description of 30 cases. *Ultrasound Obstet Gynecol* 2002; 19(1): 24–38.

12. Santo S, D'Antonio F, Homfray T, et al. Counseling in fetal medicine: agenesis of the corpus callosum. *Ultrasound Obstet Gynecol* 2012; 40(5): 513–21.

13. Sotiriadis A, Makrydimas G. Neurodevelopment after prenatal diagnosis of isolated agenesis of the corpus callosum: an integrative review. *Am J Obstet Gynecol* 2012; 206(4): 337 e1–5.

14. Bault JP, Salomon LJ, Guibaud L, et al. Role of three-dimensional ultrasound measurement of the optic tract in fetuses with agenesis of the septum pellucidum. *Ultrasound Obstet Gynecol* 2011; 37(5): 570–5.

15. Robinson AJ. Inferior vermian hypoplasia – preconception, misconception. *Ultrasound Obstet Gynecol*. 2014; 43(2): 123–36.

16. Gandolfi Colleoni G, Contro E, Carletti A, et al. Prenatal diagnosis and outcome of fetal posterior fossa fluid collections. *Ultrasound Obstet Gynecol* 2012; 39(6): 625–31.

17. Limperopoulos C, Robertson RL, Estroff JA, et al. Diagnosis of inferior vermian hypoplasia by fetal magnetic resonance imaging: potential pitfalls and neurodevelopmental outcome. *Am J Obstet Gynecol* 2006; 194(4): 1070–6.

18. Quarello E, Molho M, Garel C, et al. Prenatal abnormal features of the fourth ventricle in Joubert syndrome and related disorders. *Ultrasound Obstet Gynecol* 2014; 43(2): 227–32.

19. Ghi T, Simonazzi G, Perolo A, et al. Outcome of antenatally diagnosed intracranial hemorrhage: case series and review of the literature. *Ultrasound Obstet Gynecol* 2003; 22(2): 121–30.

20. Govaert P. Prenatal stroke. *Semin Fetal Neonatal Med* 2009; 14(5): 250–66.

21. Picone O, Teissier N, Cordier AG, et al. Detailed in utero ultrasound description of 30 cases of congenital cytomegalovirus infection. *Prenat Diagn* 2014; 34(6): 518–24.

22. Chervenak FA, Rosenberg J, Brightman RC, et al. A prospective study of the accuracy of ultrasound in predicting fetal microcephaly. *Obstet Gynecol* 1987; 69(6): 908–10.

23. Stoler-Poria S, Lev D, Schweiger A, et al. Developmental outcome of isolated fetal microcephaly. *Ultrasound Obstet Gynecol* 2010; 36(2): 154–8.

24. Schlembach D, Bornemann A, Rupprecht T, et al. Fetal intracranial tumors detected by ultrasound: a report of two cases and review of the literature. *Ultrasound Obstet Gynecol* 1999; 14(6): 407–18.

25. Tworetzky W, McElhinney DB, Margossian R, et al. Association between cardiac tumors and tuberous sclerosis in the fetus and neonate. *Am J Cardiol* 2003; 92(4): 487–9.

26. Sepulveda W, Platt CC, Fisk NM. Prenatal diagnosis of cerebral arteriovenous malformation using color Doppler ultrasonography: case report and review of the literature. *Ultrasound Obstet Gynecol* 1995; 6(4): 282–6.

27. Garel C, Azarian M, Lasjaunias P, et al. Pial arteriovenous fistulas: dilemmas in prenatal diagnosis, counseling and postnatal treatment. Report of three cases. *Ultrasound Obstet Gynecol* 2005; 26(3): 293–6.

28. Laurichesse Delmas H, Winer N, Gallot D, et al. Prenatal diagnosis of thrombosis of the dural sinuses: report of six cases, review of the literature and suggested management. *Ultrasound Obstet Gynecol* 2008; 32(2): 188–98.

29. Malinger G, Kidron D, Schreiber L, et al. Prenatal diagnosis of malformations of cortical development by dedicated neurosonography. *Ultrasound Obstet Gynecol* 2007; 29(2): 178–91.

Fetal face and neck anomalies

Manish Gupta

Face and neck anomalies are some of the hardest abnormalities to detect and diagnose antenatally, but are very important due to associated chromosomal and syndromic conditions. Facial abnormalities, in particular, may have a major psychologic and emotional impact.

Cleft lip and palate

The most common facial abnormality is a cleft lip, with or without cleft palate, with an overall incidence of about 1 in 700 births. There is, however marked ethnic variation with an incidence of 1.5–2.0 per 1,000 in Asian populations and 0.5 per 1,000 in African and Caribbean populations. There also seems to be a sex difference with cleft lip, with or without cleft palate, being twice as common in males as females[1]. Detection rates (DR) vary from 17.5% to 75% in a low-risk population. The UK Fetal Anomaly Screening Programme has set a target DR of 75%. Cleft lip and cleft palate are distinct anomalies, but they frequently occur together. In all cases of orofacial cleft, 60–75% involve cleft lip, with or without palate, and 25–40% are isolated cleft palate. The majority are unilateral, occurring twice as commonly on the left side as on the right side. Among orofacial clefts, isolated cleft palate is more frequently associated with other anomalies. Isolated cleft palate has a different pathophysiology than either cleft lip or cleft lip associated with cleft palate.

Diagnosis

A coronal section through the face reveals the lips, chin prominence and nostrils, often in the same plane. A sagittal profile view may show a 'proboscis'-like appearance of the upper lip. This appearance is caused by the lack of attachment of the unpaired frontonasal process to the paired bilateral maxillary processes.

In the case of cleft palate, color Doppler examination during fetal swallowing or breathing movement may reveal mixing of fluid in the nasal and buccal cavity.

The advent of three-dimensional (3D) scanning has allowed a better representation of the defect and may be helpful for the maxillofacial surgeons in advising parents on prognosis and the type of surgery required.

Cause

The majority of cases are multifactorial in nature. However, there is a strong association with chromosomal and syndromic malformations. A variety of chromosomal abnormalities have been reported in 3–4% of cases of cleft lip and cleft palate, and 1–2% of cases of cleft palate alone. Hence, prenatal karyotyping should be considered in all cases following the diagnosis of orofacial cleft. However, even isolated cleft lip and palate does show a familial tendency, although this is likely to be multifactorial rather than a single gene defect. Some evidence is coming to light that folic acid deficiency may play a role in cleft lip and palate[2–4].

Smoking and alcohol consumption have been implicated in the incidence of cleft lip and palate, with smoking increasing the risk by twofold. The antiepileptic medications phenytoin and carbamazepine are associated with cleft lip and palate. Other drugs include methotrexate and retinoids, such as vitamin A. Rarely, amniotic band syndrome can cause bizarre patterns of facial clefts.

Management

Once a diagnosis of cleft lip or palate is made, a search should be performed for associated abnormalities, particularly congenital heart disease; 5–12% of cases

Fetal Medicine, ed. Bidyut Kumar and Zarko Alfirevic. Published by Cambridge University Press. © Cambridge University Press 2016.

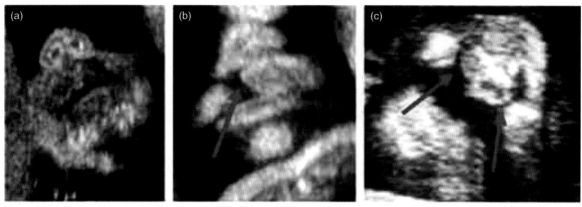

Figure 7.1 (a) Normal face and lips, (b) unilateral and (c) bilateral cleft lips.

with cleft lip and palate have an associated congenital heart defect[5]. Karyotyping should be offered, particularly if the cleft lip or palate is midline or bilateral or there are associated abnormalities, as these have a higher chance of a chromosomal issue.

A further ultrasound scan can be performed in the third trimester to detect further abnormalities that may become more obvious in later pregnancy or fetal growth restriction. Mild polyhydramnios may be noted but is usually of no clinical consequence.

The parents should be referred to a specialist cleft team and offered support through a specialist organization. A multidisciplinary approach to neonatal management with neonatologists and specialist cleft surgeons should be discussed with the parents.

Outcome

If the cleft lip or palate is isolated, there is no need to deliver at a tertiary level center unless there are associated abnormalities. The main issue after delivery will be the establishment of feeding, and there are multiple specialized devices available, such as bottles with longer teats.

The majority of cleft lip and palates have a good outcome if isolated, and modern cosmetic surgery is associated with a good result. All cleft lips and palates will need some form of surgical repair. Three surgical procedures are usually required. The first operation is usually performed at around 10 weeks to close the external lip and facial soft tissues. The second operation is usually performed at 6–12 months and involves the closure of deeper palatal and alveolar defects to allow speech and language development. A third procedure is performed at 6–10 years to correct alveolar

Table 7.1 Recurrence rates for cleft lip and palate[7]

Relationship to index case	Recurrence risk (%)
Sibling unilateral cleft lip	2–3
Sibling unilateral cleft lip and palate	4
Sibling bilateral cleft lip and palate	5–6
Two affected siblings	10
Affected sibling and parent	10
Affected parent	4

bony defects. A final procedure may be required in the late teen period to revise the jaw, lip or nose.

Recurrence

Recurrence depends on the underlying cause, but if isolated, varies from 2–5% if one first-degree relative is affected and up to 10% if a parent and sibling are affected (Table 7.1). Folic acid prenatally may reduce this risk[6].

Micrognathia (small jaw)

Micrognathia is characterized by a small mandible and a receding chin. It has an incidence of 1 in 5,000 to 1 in 10,000 deliveries. There are a large number of syndromes and chromosomal abnormalities that can be associated with micrognathia.

Diagnosis

Micrognathia can be difficult to assess as it is largely subjective. It can only truly be assessed in the profile view. It is worth noting that it is very easy to create false

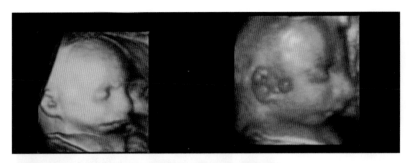

Figure 7.2 (a–c) Three- and two-dimensional ultrasound images of micrognathia in a fetus with Pierre Robin syndrome.

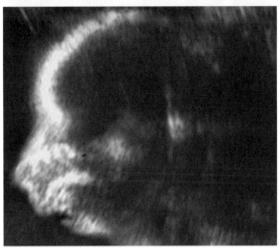

micrognathia if an oblique profile view is obtained. Again, as in facial clefts, the use of 3D scanning may help to visualize the facial profile and may be used in counseling the parents on outcome.

Micrognathia is associated with a wide range of chromosomal abnormalities, in particular, trisomies 18 and 13. In fact, about 60% will have some form of chromosomal issue. There are also a wide range of syndromic abnormalites associated with micrognathia, which include Treacher–Collins syndrome, an autosomal dominant condition with micrognathia and hearing loss, Pierre Robin syndrome, which has an associated cleft palate, Stickler syndrome, which is a collagen gene disorder, as well as a strong association with cardiac abnormalities due to its association with other syndromes, such as DiGeorge or 22q11 deletion syndrome[8].

Management

In cases of micrognathia, full karyotyping is essential due to the wide range of chromosomal associations. A careful secondary survey looking for other abnormalities should be performed, and a fetal echocardiogram is also important, with the aim to establish an underlying genetic problem or syndrome. If other abnormalities are detected, a geneticist should be involved to determine the underlying diagnosis.

The main antenatal issue is that of polyhydramnios, which may be severe due to the inability of the jaw to open and swallow fluid, causing preterm delivery, and may require amniodrainage. Further scanning should be performed at regular intervals throughout the pregnancy to detect polyhydramnios, as well as to search for other structural abnormalities that may become apparent later in pregnancy, and to diagnose fetal growth restriction due to the underlying chromosomal or syndromic issue[9].

When diagnosed prenatally, a discussion with neonatalogists and pediatric ear, nose and throat surgeons is essential. Delivery should occur at a center with the ability to provide expertise in dealing with difficult intubations and with the ability to perform emergency tracheostomy. It may be that the fetus needs to be delivered electively by cesarean section so that the appropriate pediatric team are available to deal with a difficult intubation.

Outcome

There is a risk of airway obstruction at birth and this can be related to the degree of polyhydramnios antenatally. A pediatrician skilled in neonatal airway management should attend the delivery and emergency tracheostomy is rarely required. After delivery, there may be difficulty in feeding, particularly with Pierre Robin syndrome where there is a posteriorly displaced tongue, and rarely a gastrostomy may be required.

Nuchal translucency, nuchal thickness and cystic hygroma

The nuchal translucency (NT) is a measurement performed in the first trimester, which measures the amount of fluid in the neck in a mid-sagittal section of the fetus[10]. See chapter 3 for more details on NT based screening for aneuploidy.

The nuchal fold or thickness is very different. It is a measurement of the amount of fluid in the skin posterior to the skull at the anomaly scan, with the image taken in the transcerebellar plane. The normal value at this stage is <6 mm 3.

A cystic hygroma is a septated lesion with increased fluid around the neck and sometimes head of the fetus. They are thought to arise due to a delay in development of the communication between the jugular lymphatic system and the internal jugular veins.

Diagnosis

The NT is measured in the first trimester, usually between 11 and 14 weeks, and when the fetal crown–rump length is between 45 and 84 mm in a mid-sagittal section. There are many common pitfalls in performing an ultrasound for the NT and adequate training must be completed before performing this type of ultrasound. Common errors include measuring a nuchal cord or measuring the amnion rather than the NT. Both of these may increase the false-positive rate. However, a measurement is achievable in over 95% of cases[10].

The nuchal fold or thickness is measured at the anomaly scan in the transcerebellar plane and a cystic hygroma appears as increased fluid in either scan, but is septated.

The presence of a raised NT in the first trimester is associated with a number of abnormalities. The association is size dependent: the greater the NT, the higher the chance of abnormality (Table 7.2)[11].

(1) Chromosomal. A raised NT is associated with a wide range of chromosomal and syndromic abnormalities, particularly trisomy 21 and karyotyping should be offered.

(2) Structural abnormalities, particularly cardiac defects. A raised NT is associated with almost any structural abnormality and developmental delay, but in particular cardiac defects, and fetal echocardiography should be performed. The risk is size dependent (Table 7.3).

(3) Fetal loss <20 weeks. However, it is worth noting that after 20 weeks, if the karyotype is normal and the fetus is structurally normal, then the outcome is not much different for a pregnancy where the NT was normal[12].

A cystic hygroma constitutes a far greater risk to the fetus of chromosomal and structural abnormalities

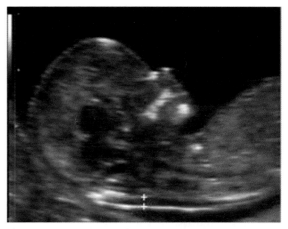

Figure 7.3 Measurement of nuchal translucency.

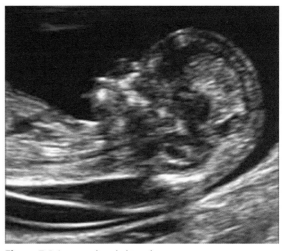

Figure 7.4 Increased nuchal translucency.

Table 7.2 Outcome of NT measurements at the 11–14 week scan[10,11]

Nuchal translucency (mm)	Chromosomal abnormality	Normal karyotype with pregnancy loss <20 weeks	Normal karyotype but major structural abnormality	Alive and well
<95th centile	0.2	1.3	1.6	97
3.5–4.4 mm	21.1	2.7	10.0	70
4.5–5.4 mm	35.3	3.4	18.5	50
5.5–6.4 mm	50.5	10.1	24.2	30
≥6.5 mm	64.5	19.0	46.2	15

Table 7.3 Risk of CHD dependent on NT thickness[13]

Nuchal translucency (mm)	Risk of congenital heart disease (%)
3.5–4.4	3.5
4.5–5.4	6.4
>5.5	12.7

and demise than a raised NT alone. The FASTER study showed 51% of cases had a chromosomal abnormality, the most common being trisomy 21, Turner syndrome and trisomy 18. Of those who were chromosomally normal, 34% had a major structural abnormality, mainly cardiac or skeletal issues, 8% had an in-utero fetal death, and only 17% who survived to term were normal[14].

An increased nuchal fold or thickness is considered a marker of chromosomal issues, particularly trisomy 21, and a karyotpye should be offered.

Hypertelorism and hypotelorism

The orbit lies between the face and the cranium and is formed by seven different bones – frontal, zygomatic, sphenoid, ethmoidal, maxillary, lacrimal and palatine.

In hypertelorism, a larger-than-average distance exists between the orbits and is defined as an increased distance between the medial orbital walls. Fetal sonographic measurements are obtained from either the outer-to-outer or inner-to-inner bony orbital margins. It is rare and is associated with median facial and brain defects, such as encephalocele, facial cleft, and craniosynostosis, as well as syndromes, such as Waardenburg, Opitz or Noonan. Karyotyping and fluorescence in-situ hybridization analysis for 22q11.2 deletion is indicated.

Orbital hypotelorism is defined as a shortened distance between the medial aspects of the orbital walls

with reduced inner and outer canthal distances, and results from developmental abnormalities of the telencephalon, which is a derivative of the forebrain. It is associated with midline craniofacial defects and major cerebral anomalies, such as holoprosencephaly. Because of its association with aneuploidy, commonly trisomy 13, fetal karyotyping should be offered.

References

1. Nyberg DA, Sicjkler GK, Hegg F, et al. Fetal cleft lip with or without cleft palate: ultrasound classification and correlation with outcome. *Radiology* 1995; 195: 677–84.
2. Cockell A, Lees M. Prenatal diagnosis and management of orofacial clefts. *Prenat Diagn* 2000; 20(2): 149–51.
3. Bergé SJ, Plath H, Van de Vondel PT, et al. Fetal cleft lip and palate: sonographic diagnosis, chromosomal abnormalities, associated anomalies and postnatal outcome in 70 fetuses. *Ultrasound Obstet Gynecol* 2001; 18(5): 422–31.
4. Bergé SJ, Plath H, von Lindern JJ, et al. Natural history of 70 fetuses with a prenatally diagnosed orofacial cleft. *Fetal Diagn Ther* 2002; 17(4): 247–51.
5. Geis N, Seto B, Bartoshesky L, et al. The prevalence of congenital heart disease among the population of a metropolitan cleft lip and palate clinic. *Cleft Palate J* 1981; 18(1): 19–23.
6. Wilcox AJ, Lie RT, Solvoll K, et al. Folic acid supplements and risk of facial clefts: national population based case-control study. *BMJ* 2007; 334(7591): 464.
7. Firth H, Hurst J. *Oxford Desk Reference Clinical Genetics*, ch 2: p. 77. Oxford University Press, 2007.
8. Bromley B, Benacerraf BR. Fetal micrognathia: associated anomalies and outcome. *J Ultrasound Med* 1994; 13(7): 529–33.
9. Vettraino IM, Lee W, Bronsteen RA, et al. Clinical outcome of fetuses with sonographic diagnosis of isolated micrognathia. *Obstet Gynecol* 2003; 102(4): 801–5.

10. Nicolaides K. The 11–13^{+6} week scan. The Fetal Medicine Foundation, 2004.

11. Souka AP, Von Kaisenberg CS, Hyett JA, et al. Increased nuchal translucency with a normal karyotype. *Am J Obstet Gynecol* 2005; 192(4): 1005–21.

12. National Health Service. Nuchal translucency greater than or equal to 3.5 mm. FASP, 2010.

13. Atzei A1, Gajewska K, Huggon IC, et al. Relationship between nuchal translucency thickness and prevalence of major cardiac defects in fetuses with normal karyotype. *Ultrasound Obstet Gynecol* 2005; 26(2): 154–7.

14. Malone FD, Ball RH, Nyberg DA, et al; FASTER Trial Research Consortium. First-trimester septated cystic hygroma: prevalence, natural history, and pediatric outcome. *Obstet Gynecol* 2005; 106(2): 288–94.

Chapter

8

Congenital heart disease in the fetus

Orhan Uzun

Fetal cardiovascular anomaly scan

Fetal cardiac assessment should start with the situs determination in the subxiphoid transverse plane[1–5]. The location of the fetal spine should be determined in relation to the maternal spine in order to work out the left and right sides of the fetus and to assess the position of its thoracic and abdominal organs. A two-dimensional echocardiography should be employed in special scanning planes to identify diagnostic features of normal cardiac structures (Table 8.1). Although a four-chamber view may be helpful in detecting up to 40% of cardiac anomalies, it may appear entirely normal in some major outflow tract anomalies. Inclusion of the outflow tract view in routine anomaly screening improves the rate of detection of cardiac anomaly to 60–80%, but would still fail to identify some important congenital heart defects[6–13].

Therefore, methodical application of other multiple scanning views should be utilized for accurate detection of all congenital heart anomalies (Table 8.2). In addition, M-mode, color flow, and pulse wave Doppler modalities (as deemed appropriate) should be employed when assessing integrity and function of those structures[14,15]. Measurement of cardiac structures should be performed in systole and diastole (Table 8.3 and Figure 8.1), and their values should be compared with established normal ranges in the corresponding gestation (Table 8.4)[15–18].

Ultrasound appearance of major cardiac anomalies and differential diagnosis

Normal fetal circulation

The placenta is the main blood supply for the fetus. Its main function is to provide oxygenation for fetal venous blood. There are three unique fetal cardiovascular connections: the ductus venosus (DV) (a connection between the umbilical vein and the inferior vena cava (IVC)), the foramen ovale (FO) (a communication between the right (RA) and the left atrium (LA)) and the ductus arteriosus (DA) (a connection between the pulmonary artery and the aorta) (Figure 8.2). Increased oxygen tension in the ductal tissue promotes closure of the DA within a few days after birth. As the pulmonary vascular resistance drops, pulmonary arterial blood flow increases significantly, which in turn leads to increased pulmonary venous return to the LA. Due to increased left atrial pressure, the flap valve of the FO moves rightward onto the septum secundum resulting in functional closure of the FO.

Outline of antenatal and postnatal management of major cardiac abnormalities

From the sonographic diagnostic point of view, it is more logical to describe heart defects by their diagnostic anatomic features in specific scanning views (Table 8.5). Congenital heart defects can also be classified according to their clinical importance as severe, moderately severe and minor anomalies (Table 8.6). Clinical classification of cardiac anomalies determines the need for prostaglandin infusion or requirement of surgery at birth or in the infancy, thereby allowing the fetal medicine specialist to decide place of delivery. Generally, half of congenital heart defects are major (severe) requiring surgery within the first year of life. There is also a subgroup of life-threatening severe congenital heart defects, so called "ductus arteriosus dependent congenital heart anomalies" (Table 8.7), which most certainly require delivery at a surgical center and infusion of prostaglandin-E immediately after birth. If such anomalies escape detection antenatally or after birth, they may lead to cardiovascular collapse and sudden death following closure of the DA. Between 35% and 65% of pregnancies with major (severe) cardiac anomalies are

Fetal Medicine, ed. Bidyut Kumar and Zarko Alfirevic. Published by Cambridge University Press. © Cambridge University Press 2016.

Table 8.1 Anatomical features of normal cardiac structures and their ultrasound scanning views

Structure	Defining features	Best scanning view
Right atrium	1. Receives IVC and SVC	1. Sagittal
	2. Broad based appendage	2. Sagittal
	3. Receives coronary sinus	3. Four chamber
	4. Connects to TV	4. Four chamber
Left atrium	1. Receives pulmonary veins	1. Four chamber
	2. Finger-like long narrow-based appendage	2. Parasternal short axis
	3. Flap valve of FO floats inside	3. Four chamber
	4. Connects to MV	4. Four chamber
Right ventricle	1. Receives TV	1. Four chamber
	2. TV attachment to septum	2. Four chamber
	3. TV more apically positioned	3. Four chamber
	4. Moderator band	4. Four chamber
	5. Coarse trabeculation	5. Four chamber
	6. Connects to a bifurcating pulmonary artery	6. Parasternal short axis
Left ventricle	1. Receives MV	1. Four chamber
	2. MV more basally positioned	2. Four chamber
	3. MV attaches to the free wall only	3. Parasternal long axis
	4. Apex is wide open	4. Four chamber
	5. Fine trabeculation	5. Four chamber
	6. Connects to a non-bifurcating aorta with head and neck vessels arising from it	6. Parasternal long axis
Pulmonary artery	1. Arises from an anterior ventricle	1. Parasternal short axis
	2. Bifurcates within first centimeter of its origin	2. Parasternal short axis
	3. Continues with DA into DAO	3. Sagittal ductal arch
Aorta	1. Arises from a posterior ventricle	1. Parasternal long axis
	2. Branches out superiorly towards neck	2. Sagittal aortic arch view
	3. In continuity with MV	3. Parasternal long axis
Ductal arch	1. Arises anteriorly with horizontal golf club appearance	1. Sagittal ductal arch
	2. Trifurcates with LPA and RPA, and DA	2. Sagittal ductal arch
	3. In continuity with DA and DAO	3. Sagittal ductal arch
Aortic arch	1. Round "walking-stick" appearance	1. Sagittal aortic arch
	2. Gives off head and neck vessels	2. Sagittal aortic arch
	3. Arises from the middle of chest	3. Sagittal aortic arch

DA, ductus arteriosus; DAO, descending aorta; FO, foramen ovale; IVC, inferior vena cava; LPA, left pulmonary artery; MV, mitral valve; RPA, right pulmonary artery; SVC, superior vena cava; TV; tricuspid valve.

medically terminated (Table 8.5), which might affect the postnatal frequency of a specific congenital heart defect (Table 8.8) [19–24]. Antenatal and postnatal management of major congenital cardiac anomalies are summarized in Tables 8.6 to 8.9 [25–39]. We will now describe each cardiac anomaly and its diagnostic features and long-term outlook in the following section.

Intracardiac shunts that can be detected in four-chamber view

Ventricular septal defect

Ventricular septal defect (VSD) is a communication between the left and right ventricles (Figure 8.3). It is the most common of all congenital heart lesions and usually occurs as an isolated abnormality. It can also be associated with coarctation of the aorta (CoA), atrio-ventricular septal defect (AVSD), tetralogy of Fallot (TOF) and truncus arteriosus.

There are three major locations: underneath the inlet valves (perimembranous-inlet), in the middle of ventricular septum (muscular) and underneath outflow tracts (outlet). Muscular and perimembranous-inlet type defects can be detected in the four-chamber view, but the five-chamber, long-axis and short views are all needed to demonstrate the outflow defects. Color flow or pulse wave Doppler may aid in diagnosing smaller

Table 8.2 The five fetal scanning views and likely cardiac anomalies detectable in each plane

Scanning view	Cardiac anomalies
A. Four-chamber view	1. Primum ASD 2. VSD 3. AVSD 4. Mitral or tricuspid atresia 5. Ebstein's anomaly of the tricuspid valve 6. Enlargement of atriums and ventricles 7. Hypoplastic left or right ventricle 8. Atrial septal aneurysm 9. Double inlet left ventricle 10. Abnormal connection of pulmonary veins 11. Congenitally corrected TGA 12. Left superior vena cava to coronary sinus connection
B. Outflow tract views	
I. Left ventricular outflow tract (parasternal long axis)	1. Aortic stenosis or atresia 2. TGA 3. Double outlet right ventricle 4. Truncus arteriosus 5. VSD 6. Left SVC to coronary sinus connection
II. Right ventricular outflow (parasternal short axis)	1. Pulmonary stenosis or atresia 2. Absent pulmonary valve syndrome 3. TOF 4. VSD
C. Three-vessel and trachea view	1. CoA 2. Vascular ring, double aortic arch or right aortic arch 3. Left SVC to coronary sinus connection 4. Pulmonary artery hypoplasia 5. Aortic hypoplasia 6. Ductal anomalies, abnormal, restricted or reversed ductal flow 7. TGA 8. TOF
D. Bicaval long-axis view	1. Interrupted IVC 2. Vein of Galen 3. Abnormal connection of pulmonary veins 4. Absent ductus venosus 5. Sinus venosus ASD 6. Restrictive FO
E. Ductal and aortic arch view	1. CoA 2. TGA 3. Hypoplasia of aorta or pulmonary artery 4. Interrupted aortic arch

ASD, atrial septal defect; AVSD, atrioventricular septal defect; CoA, coarctation of the aorta; FO, foramen ovale; IVC, inferior vena cava; SVC, superior vena cava; TGA, transposition of the great arteries; TOF, tetralogy of Fallot; VSD, ventricular septal defect.

Table 8.3 Cardiac structures and measurement sites

Cardiac Structures	Measurement Sites
Aortic annulus	At valve level, long-axis view
Ascending aorta	Above sinus of Valsalva, long-axis view
Descending aorta	Below entrance of ductus arteriosus, long-axis view
Ductus arteriosus	At its middle, short-axis view
Superior vena cava	At the entry into the RA
Inferior vena cava	At the entry into the RA
Aortic valve width	Aortic valve, short and long-axis view
Ascending ortic width	Aortic annulus, long-axis view
Main pulmonary artery	Above the annulus, short-axis view
Left and right pulmonary arteries	At origin, short axis view
Left and right ventricular width	Below coapted AV leaflets, four-chamber view
Ventricular free wall and septal thickness	Below coapted AV leaflets, four-chamber view
Left and right ventricular length	From the apex to the point of the coapted valve leaflets, four-chamber view
Left and right atrial width	From the lateral wall to the line between the two portions of the FO, four-chamber view
Left and right atrial length	From the coapted AV valve leaflet to the posterior wall, four-chamber view
Left ventricular width	Below coapted AV valve, from the septum to the posterior wall, long-axis view
Left ventricular length	From the apex to the point of coapted valve leaflets, long-axis view
Left atrial width	From the anterior to the posterior wall, long-axis view
Left atrial length	From the coapted MV leaflets to the top of the atrium
Right atrial width	From the lateral wall to the line between the 2 portions of the FO, short-axis view
Right atrial length	From the coapted TV leaflets to the posterior wall, short-axis view

AV; atrioventricular; FO, foramen ovale; MV, mitral valve; RA, right atrium.

defects by showing bidirectional flow pattern across the ventricular septum. False-positive and negative rates are high.

The fetal clinical course is uncomplicated. The majority of small VSDs close spontaneously either in utero or after birth. It is important to exclude commonly associated defects such as CoA, TOF and truncus arteriosus.

Amniocentesis should be recommended for large VSDs located in inlet or outlet septum, to exclude 22q11 microdeletion and trisomy 21[38]. Delivery can take place at a local hospital if the VSD is an isolated anomaly regardless of its size.

Postnatally, no special precaution is needed in the newborn other than routine pediatric and cardiac review. A large VSD may lead to faltering growth and heart failure in infancy.

Treatment involves either stitch or patch closure of the defect with surgery. Some anatomically suitable defects may be amenable to device closure via percutaneous transcatheter approach. VSD has an excellent late functional and survival outcome after treatment.

Complete atrioventricular septal defect

AVSD has an atrial and ventricular communication with a common atrioventricular (AV) valve (Figure 8.4). In the incomplete form, there is an ostium primum atrial septal defect and a cleft mitral valve without a defect in the ventricular septum. This abnormality can be suspected from the four-chamber view by showing the left and right inlet valves being at the same level instead of having a normal off-setting appearance.

Fetuses with this defect are commonly asymptomatic, but due to its frequent associations with chromosome abnormalities, amniocentesis is strongly recommended. Approximately 40–50% of fetuses with AVSD will have trisomy 21, 18 or 13. Likewise, 40–50% of fetuses with trisomy 21 will have AVSD. AVSD may also coexist with pulmonary stenosis in 2–10% of cases[36].

Postnatally, neonates with AVSD may be totally asymptomatic or only slightly cyanosed, and diagnosis in some cases may be overlooked. Any newborn with AVSD should have a careful pediatric, cardiac and if necessary, genetics review. Percutaneous oxygen saturation should be monitored after birth. Once the pulmonary vascular resistance drops, the neonates with a large VSD may develop respiratory symptoms, faltering growth and heart failure generally beyond 2 weeks of age.

Surgical repair of complete AVSD is usually undertaken before 6 months of age. After surgical repair, reasonable quality of life is expected, but there is a 20% re-operation rate for leaky inlet valves. However, if there is disproportionate ventricular size (unbalanced

Table 8.4 Normal dimensions of cardiac structures at 20 weeks

Examined cardiac structure	Normal value
Cardiac size	
Cardiac/thoracic area ratio	0.25–0.35
Cardiac/thoracic circumference ratio	<0.5
Foramen ovale	
FO diameter	0.28 ± 0.05 cm
FO Doppler velocity	<0.5 m/s
FO/right atrium diameter ratio	0.45 ± 0.01
FO/aorta diameter ratio	0.96 ± 0.16
FO/atrial septum length ratio	0.33 ± 0.04
Right heart	
Atrial septal length	0.88 ± 0.13 cm
Right atrium transverse diameter	0.73 ± 0.08
Left/right atrium transverse diameter ratio	0.94
Tricuspid valve annulus	0.59 ± 0.11 cm
Tricuspid valve Doppler	0.52 ± 0.07 m/s
Tricuspid valve E/A ratio	0.64 ± 0.07
Right ventricle diastole	0.62 ± 0.11 cm
Right/left ventricle diameter ratio	1–1.2
Right ventricular free wall	0.23 ± 0.05
Pulmonary artery	
Pulmonary valve	0.3 ± 0.05 cm
Pulmonary valve Doppler	0.55 ± 0.19 m/s
Main pulmonary artery	>0.3 ± 0.01 cm
Right pulmonary artery	>0.23 cm
Pulmonary/aorta size ratio	1–1.2
Left heart	
Left atrium transverse diameter	0.68 ± 0.08
Mitral valve annulus	0.56 ± 0.09 cm
Mitral valve Doppler	0.45 ± 0.07 m/s
Mitral E/A ratio	0.63 ± 0.07
Left ventricular posterior wall	0.23 ± 0.05 cm
Interventricular septum	0.22 ± 0.05 cm
Left ventricle diastole	0.61 ± 0.12 cm
Left/right ventricle size ratio	0.97 ± 0.1
Fractional shortening	>28%
Aorta	
Aortic valve	0.3 ± 0.05 cm
Aortic valve Doppler	0.6 ± 0.26 m/s
Ascending aorta	>0.3 ± 0.05 cm
Isthmus/ductus ratio	>0.74
Descending aorta	>0.25 cm

Ductus arteriosus	
Three-vessel trachea view	>0.21 cm
Sagittal view	>0.21 cm
Ductus arteriosus velocity	0.6–0.8 m/s
Ductus/pulmonary artery diameter ratio	0.67 ± 0.1
Aorta/pulmonary artery ratio	0.92
Cardiac output	
Right ventricular stroke volume	0.8 mL
Right ventricular output	110 mL/min
Left ventricular stroke volume	0.65 mL
Left ventricular output	88 mL/min
Right/left ventricular output ratio	1.2

E/A, early ventricular filling velocity/late ventricular filling velocity; FO, foramen ovale.

AVSD), the postnatal outlook is less unfavorable as the corrective two-ventricle repair cannot be achieved.

Anomalous pulmonary venous connection

In total anomalous pulmonary venous connection (TAPVC), some or all pulmonary veins fail to connect to the LA (Figure 8.5). Instead they may connect to the superior vena cava (SVC), RA, or into the liver either directly or indirectly via a common channel. An obstructed venous channel should be excluded. This abnormality is notoriously difficult to detect antenatally with no more than 6–10% detection rates. Presence of nonpulsatile pulmonary vein Doppler flow may alert the sonographer to this diagnosis.

Fetuses with this abnormality are asymptomatic. TAPVC is rarely associated with chromosome abnormality. Usual prenatal follow-up at 4–6 weeks' intervals is required.

Postnatally some of these patients may exhibit very little in the way of cyanosis, and diagnosis can easily be overlooked. If there is pulmonary venous obstruction, cyanosis will be accompanied by respiratory difficulties, which may frequently mimic persistent pulmonary hypertension of the newborn.

Surgical treatment involves re-implantation of pulmonary veins into the LA. Once corrected, most patients remain asymptomatic with no major long-term issues.

Outflow tract abnormalities

TOF and double outlet right ventricle

TOF has four features: severe narrowing of the right ventricular outflow (infundibular pulmonary

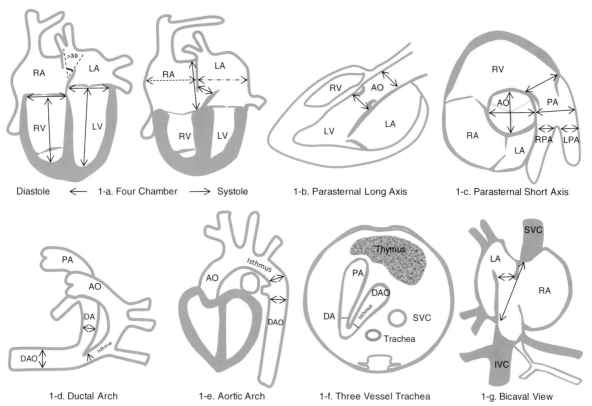

Diastole ⟵ 1-a. Four Chamber ⟶ Systole   1-b. Parasternal Long Axis   1-c. Parasternal Short Axis

1-d. Ductal Arch   1-e. Aortic Arch   1-f. Three Vessel Trachea   1-g. Bicaval View

Figure 8.1 Measurement of cardiac structures. a) Measurement point of the four-chamber view in diastole and systole; b) from parasternal long axis view shows measurement of aortic valve and root; c) from parasternal short axis view shows aortic and pulmonary artery measurement points; d) from the ductal arch view shows ductus arteriosus, isthmus and descending aortic measurement points; e) from the aortic arch view shows isthmus and descending aortic measurement points; f) from the three vessel and trachea view shows measurement points of ductus arteriosus and the isthmus; g) from bicaval view shows measurement point of foramen ovale, IVC and SVC. LA, left atrium; RV, right ventricle; LV, left ventricle; AO, ascending aorta; PA, pulmonary artery; RPA, right pulmonary artery; LPA, left pulmonary artery; DA, ductus arteriosus; DV, ductus venosus; DAO, descending aorta; IVC, inferior vena cava; SVC, superior vena cava; FO, foramen ovale.

stenosis), a large subaortic VSD, overriding of the aortic outlet above the ventricular septum and right ventricular hypertrophy (Figure 8.6). The 22q11 chromosome microdeletion is not infrequently (5–10%) associated with this anomaly. The four-chamber view may be completely normal, but an extended apical five-chamber view should demonstrate the VSD and the aortic override. The parasternal short-axis view is necessary to show the site of pulmonary stenosis.

Fetuses are commonly asymptomatic with this condition. Management involves offering amniocentesis to exclude chromosome abnormalities, such as 22q11 microdeletion and trisomy 21.

Postnatally, the most important element is the narrowing in the right ventricular outflow tract, which determines the degree of cyanosis. Some tetralogy patients may develop so-called "tetralogy spells" (blue spells) where hypoxia becomes profound. Some

infants may have a so-called "pink Fallot" where a large VSD dominates the clinical picture and the pulmonary stenosis is relatively mild; in such cases, dyspnea is the main symptom and the oxygen saturation is usually normal.

The term "double outlet right ventricle" (DORV) is used if the aortic override is more than 50% or when both outflow tracts arise from the right ventricle. In such cases, cyanosis dominates if there is severe pulmonary stenosis, or when the VSD is in a subpulmonary location and the aorta is situated to the right of the pulmonary artery and further away from the ventricular septum. In infants with unrestrictive pulmonary blood flow, the main features are breathlessness, poor feeding, failure to thrive and congestive heart failure.

Total surgical correction is usually performed in infancy before the child's first birthday unless tetralogy spells develop earlier, in which case an interim

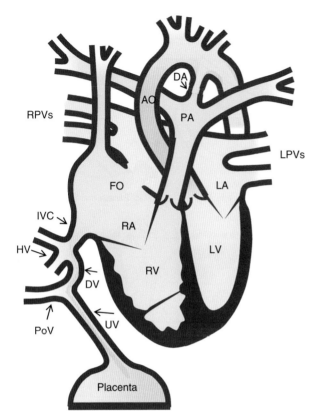

Figure 8.2 Normal fetal circulation. UV, umbilical vein; PoV, portal vein; DV, ductus venosus; HV, hepatic vein; IVC, inferior vena cava; RA, right atrium; LA, left atrium; RV, right ventricle; LV, left ventricle; AO, ascending aorta; PA, pulmonary artery; DA, ductus arteriosus; DV, ductus venosus; DAO, descending aorta; IVC, inferior vena cava; RPVs, right pulmonary veins; LPVs, left pulmonary veins; FO, foramen ovale.

aortopulmonary shunt procedure may be required. After total correction, children should have a reasonable quality of life, but 10–25% will require repeat operations, such as pulmonary valve replacement, by early adulthood.

Pulmonary atresia

Pulmonary atresia (PAt) describes a total obstruction of flow from the right ventricle to the pulmonary artery (Figure 8.7). It may coexist with or without a VSD. Other features include varying degrees of tricuspid valve and right ventricular hypoplasia.

Fetuses are commonly asymptomatic with this condition. Although rare, a restrictive FO or a restrictive DA may result in fetal cardiovascular compromise in some cases. Amniocentesis is recommended. Delivery should take place at a surgical center.

After birth, cyanosis is the main symptom and since this is a duct-dependent lesion, prostaglandin-E infusion is mandatory at birth to maintain ductal patency. Surgical correction depends on the patency and size of the tricuspid valve and the dimensions of the right ventricular cavity. Complete surgical repair of PAt usually includes placement of a conduit between the right ventricle and pulmonary artery. If the right ventricular cavity size is diminutive, then a series of palliative operations (Fontan route) will be contemplated with less favorable long-term outcomes.

Transposition of the great arteries

In simple transposition of the great arteries (TGA), the atriums and ventricles are arranged normally, but the aorta and the pulmonary arteries arise from the opposite ventricles, i.e., the aorta comes off the anterior right ventricle and pulmonary artery arises from the posterior left ventricle (Figure 8.8).

The presence of other congenital anomalies, such as DORV, single ventricle and pulmonary stenosis constitute complex transposition of the aorta, which requires special management according to the dominant lesion.

During fetal life, this anomaly does not have any ill effect on fetal development unless premature closure of the FO or DA develops. TGA is rarely associated with chromosomal abnormality and amniocentesis is usually not undertaken. Delivery should be planned at a surgical center.

Postnatally, there has to be adequate mixing either through the FO or via the arterial duct, otherwise this condition cannot be compatible with life. Prostaglandin E infusion at birth is therefore required to keep the arterial duct open and the newborn baby alive.

Balloon atrial septostomy needs to be carried out to create a reliable communication for adequate mixing at atrial level. Balloon septostomy provides interim palliation before the total correction with arterial switch operation can be performed. Surgery involves re-implanting of the pulmonary artery and the aorta onto their correct ventricles. The long-term outlook after surgical correction is favorable.

Truncus arteriosus

Truncus arteriosus describes a single arterial trunk arising from both ventricles (Figure 8.9). A single artery then divides into the pulmonary artery and aorta. A single semilunar valve is shared between these two arteries. Almost universally, there is a VSD below the truncal valve that provides mixing of venous and

Table 8.5 Diagnostic features of major cardiac anomalies, scanning views and detection and termination rates

Heart anomaly	Diagnostic features	Scanning views	Detection rate (%)	Termination rate (%)
Atrioventricular septal defect	1. Atrioventricular valves at the same level 2. Primum atrial septal defect 3. Common inlet valve 4. Most common abnormality inlet VSD 5. Left/right inlet valve regurgitation 50% 6. With tetralogy of Fallot 10–25% 7. With isomerism 15–20%	1. Four chamber 2. Short axis 3. Long axis	56–70	6–40
Ventricular septal defect	1. Communication between LV and RV 2. 75% perimembranous type: tetralogy, DORV 3. 10–15% muscular 4. 5% outlet: truncus 5. 5–8% inlet type: AVSD	1. Four chamber 2. Long axis	7–50	0–5
Hypoplastic left heart syndrome	1. Small LA and LV 2. Hypoplastic/stenosed/atretic aorta 3. Hypoplastic or atretic mitral valve 4. Check foramen ovale restriction 5. Check aortic arch coarctation 6. Check endocardial fibroelastosis	1. Four chamber 2. Five chamber 3. Long axis 4. Sagittal	63–95	36–63
Tricuspid atresia	1. Atretic right inlet valve 2. Small RV 3. VSD or intact ventricular septum 4. 25% TGA, 3% CCTGA	1. Four chamber	40–80	30–59
Total anomalous pulmonary venous connection	1. Small left-sided structures 2. Enlarged right heart 3. Increased flow from SVC, IVC	1. Four chamber 2. Long axis 3. Bicaval view 4. Sagittal view	0–12	0–10
Ebstein's anomaly	1. Enlarged right atrium/enlarged heart 2. Apically displaced tricuspid valve 3. Severe tricuspid regurgitation 4. 30% VSD or PS 5. 30–50% accessory pathways/arrhythmias	1. Four chamber 2. Five chamber 3. Short axis	59–80	6–44
Double inlet left ventricle	1. Mitral and tricuspid valves open into a large single LV 2. RV hypoplastic 3. RV usually give rise to both great arteries 4. VSD	1. Four chamber 2. Five chamber 3. Short axis	30–50	51–55

Table 8.5 (cont.)

Tetralogy of Fallot	1. VSD, 10% AVSD 2. PS/regurgitation 3. Hypertrophied right ventricle 4. Aortic override <50% 5. Right aortic arch >25% 6. Small ductus in 70% and not visualized in 30%, LSVC in 10%	1. Four chamber 2. Five chamber 3. Short axis 4. Long axis 5. Three-vessel trachea	15–69	0–17
Truncus arteriosus	1. Single artery arises from both ventricles and overrides VSD 2. Truncal valve either narrow or leaky in more than 50% 3. Biventricular hypertrophy 4. VSD, right aortic arch 33%, interrupted aortic arch 10–20% 5. PA arises from the main trunk	1. Four chamber 2. Five chamber 3. Short axis 4. Long axis	18–50	20–35
Double outlet right ventricle	1. Both great arteries arising from RV 2. VSD subaortic 47%, subpulmonary 23% 3. PS 4. TGA	1. Four chamber 2. Five chamber 3. Short axis 4. Long axis 5. Three-vessel trachea	50–65	31–56
Pulmonary stenosis or atresia	1. Pulmonary valve atretic or severely stenosed 2. RV hypoplastic or hypertrophied 3. VSD or intact ventricular septum 4. Major aortopulmonary collateral circulation	1. Four chamber 2. Short axis 3. Three-vessel and trachea	31–50	13
Transposition of the great arteries	1. Aorta arises from RV 2. PA arises from LV 3. Failure to show crossover of great arteries 4. VSD 40–45% 5. PS 30–50% 6. Coarctation or interruption 5%	1. Five chamber 2. Short axis 3. Long axis 4. Three-vessel and trachea	72–85	0–14
Coarctation/interruption of aorta	1. Small ascending aorta, VSD, bicuspid aortic valve 2. Small aortic isthmus (coarctation) 3. Discontinuity between transverse arch and descending aorta (interruption) 4. Large RV and PA compared with small LV	1. Five chamber 2. Long axis 3. Sagittal ductal arch 4. Sagittal aortic arch 5. Three-vessel and trachea	16–42	0–4

AVSD, atrioventricular septal defect; CCTGA; congenitally corrected transposition of the great arteries; DORV, double outlet right ventricle; IVC, inferior vena cava; LA, left atrium; LV, left ventricle; PA, pulmonary artery; PS, pulmonary stenosis; RV, right ventricle; SVC, superior vena cava; TGA, transposition of the great arteries; VSD, ventricular septal defect.

Table 8.6 Classification and ideal delivery place of babies with severe, moderate and mild CHD

Category	Anomaly
I. Severe CHD This category includes heart anomalies that require prostaglandin-E infusion at birth or operation in the newborn period. Therefore, delivery of a baby with such an anomaly should take place at a surgical center.	1. TGA 2. Pulmonary atresia 3. Absent pulmonary valve syndrome with severe stenosis 4. Hypoplastic right heart with severe PS 5. TA with restrictive FO, restrictive ventricular septum, severe PS 6. Hypoplastic left heart 7. Aortic atresia 8. Mitral atresia with restrictive FO, restrictive ventricular septum, severe PS or AS 9. Single ventricle (double inlet left ventricle) with severe PS or AS 10. Critical PS 11. Critical AS 12. TAPVC 13. Truncus arteriosus 14. Critical–severe CoA 15. Interrupted aortic arch 16. DORV with unrestricted pulmonary flow, severe PS or AS 17. Ebstein's anomaly with severe tricuspid regurgitation and PS 18. TOF with absent pulmonary valve syndrome
II. Moderately severe CHD These anomalies do not require prostaglandin infusion at birth but some of them are expected to require surgery in the infancy. These babies need to be delivered at a tertiary cardiac center with or without surgical facility.	1. TOF 2. DORV with balanced pulmonary and systemic flow 3. Ebstein's anomaly with mild-to-moderate tricuspid regurgitation 4. Double outlet left ventricle 5. CCTGA 6. AVSD 7. Large VSD 8. Mild-to-moderate AS or incompetence 9. Mild-to-moderate PS or incompetence 10. Noncritical coarctation 11. Vascular ring, double aortic arch
III. Mild CHD These patients do not require prostaglandin infusion at birth or surgery within neonatal period or in infancy. Therefore, these babies can be delivered locally. They are usually asymptomatic, and their cardiac anomaly may undergo spontaneous resolution, remain static or their progression is rather gradual over the years.	1. Small VSD 2. Atrial septal defect – primum or sinus venosus types

AS, aortic stenosis; AVSD, atrioventricular septal defect; CHD, congenital heart disease; CoA, coarctation of the aorta; DORV, double outlet right ventricle; FO, foramen ovale; PS, pulmonary stenosis; TA, tricuspid atresia; TAPVC, total anomalous pulmonary venous connection; TGA, transposition of the great arteries; TOF, tetralogy of Fallot; VSD, ventricular septal defect.

arterial blood. Truncal valve is either stenotic or regurgitant in half of the cases. In up to 10% of cases there may also be an interrupted aortic arch.

Fetuses are commonly asymptomatic with this anomaly. Usual follow-up at 3–4 week intervals would suffice. Amniocentesis is recommended to exclude 22q11 chromosome microdeletion, which is frequently associated with this anomaly. Absent thymus may offer a clue in identifying cases of 22q11 microdeletion.

Newborn babies with this condition are mainly breathless but are also mildly cyanosed. This condition is not duct dependent, and surgery invariably involves the use of a prosthetic conduit to connect the pulmonary arteries to the right ventricle in addition to patch repair of the main arterial trunk. Following repair, some patients may have residual truncal valve regurgitation or stenosis, or narrowing of the right ventricle to pulmonary artery conduit. Repeat surgical procedures

Table 8.7 Ductus dependent cardiac anomalies and their management

Cardiac anomaly	Antenatal management	Postnatal management
A. DA dependent systemic and pulmonary circulation	The DA must remain open therefore avoid the use of ibuprofen, indomethacin, and discourage excess consumption of polyphenol rich food and drinks.	Normal planned delivery with induction at 39 weeks in a surgical center if local facilities are away from a tertiary surgical center.
1. Transposition of the great arteries.		
B. DA dependent systemic circulation	The FO must remain open, hence monitor patency of the interatrial communication with bi-weekly ultrasound.	Delivery at a nonsurgical center may be feasible if there is local pediatric cardiology service, local neonatal intensive care and neonatal transfer facilities are available.
1. Hypoplastic left heart syndrome	Monitor pulmonary vein Doppler to help identify FO restriction in HLHS.	Prostaglandin infusion at 5–10 ng/kg/min should be started after birth.
2. Critical aortic stenosis,	Discuss at MDT meeting with neonatologist and pediatric cardiologist.	Avoid excess use of oxygen or unnecessary intubation.
3. Aortic atresia	Check karyotype to exclude 22q11 microdeletion in IAA, PS with VSD; Noonan syndrome in critical PS; Turner syndrome in coarctation; and William's syndrome in supravalvar aortic stenosis.	Oxygen saturations between 70–90% are acceptable.
4. Coarctation of the aorta		Nil by mouth until diagnosis is established and management plan is drawn
5. Interrupted aortic arch		
C. Ductus arteriosus dependent pulmonary circulation		
1. Critical pulmonary stenosis		
2. Pulmonary atresia		

CoA, coarctation of the aorta; DA, ductus arteriosus; FO, foramen ovale; HLHS, hypoplastic left heart syndrome; IAA, interrupted aortic arch; MDT, multidisciplinary team; TGA, transposition of the great arteries.

Table 8.8 Major congenital heart anomalies, their frequency, birth incidence and outcomes

Heart anomaly	Fetal frequency among CHD %	Incidence in per 1,000 live birth	Outcome
Atrioventricular septal defect	5–16	0.19–0.35	1. <2% operative mortality 2. 95% survival at 20 year 3. 25% reoperation rate for AV valve regurgitation 4. 40% associated with Down's syndrome, 20% trisomy 13 and 18
Ventricular septal defect	15–35	1.1–3.57	1. <2% operative mortality 2. Risk of complete heart block postoperatively 3. Excellent long term outlook
Hypoplastic left heart syndrome/critical aortic stenosis	4–16	0.14–0.27	1. 20% IU death 2. >85% survival after stage 1 Norwood and >98% survival after Glenn and Fontan 3. 50% survival in 10 years 4. 15% association with chromosome abnormalities, Turner most common 5. Isolated aortic stenosis 25-year survival >70% 6. Need for repeat operation to replace aortic valve
Tricuspid atresia	1–3	0.03–0.5	1. >90% survival with arterial shunt, >98% survival with Glenn operation and >98% survival with Fontan operation. 2. 85% survival at 10 years 3. 8% associated with 22q11 deletion
Total anomalous pulmonary venous connection	0.6–3	0.06–0.09	1. Excellent long term outlook 2. 2% risk of pulmonary vein stenosis
Ebstein's anomaly	0.3–0.7	0.06–0.11	1. IU mortality up to 45–100 % in severe cases, up to 90% survival in mild cases 2. May be associated with trisomy 21
Double inlet left ventricle	0.07–0.1	N/A	1. 10 year survival >70%
Tetralogy of Fallot	3–7	0.42	1. 8–23% 22q11 deletion, up to 75% if absent pulmonary valve syndrome 2. Tetralogy has excellent long term survival but up to 30% reoperation for PS or regurgitation 3. 30–50% mortality in absent pulmonary valve syndrome
Truncus arteriosus	3–4.8	0.05–0.11	1. 40% 22q11 deletion 2. 50% truncal valve regurgitation or stenosis 3. Early pre-operative death 5–10%, early survival 90% at 5 years
Double outlet right ventricle	2.4–12	0.16	1. Survival 70–80% at medium term
Severe pulmonary stenosis or atresia	2.4–6.5	0.16–0.26	1. PA-VSD 8–23% associated with 22q11 deletion 2. PS may be associated with Noonan's, Alagille, and Leopard syndromes 3. Outlook is good in PS and tripartite right ventricle 4. PA-IVS survival 65% at 5 years and PA-VSD 70% survival at 10 years
Transposition of the great arteries	4.3–11	0.24–0.32	1. Excellent long term survival 97% at 10 years 2. Branch pulmonary artery stenosis 5–30%
Coarctation/interruption of aorta	8.9	0.14–0.41	1. 50% of interruption has 22q11 and 35% of Turner has coarctation 2. 25% associated with noncardiac anomalies 3. Excellent survival 4. 4% recurrence rate and reoperation risk, 25% risk of hypertension

AV, atrioventricular; CHD, congenital heart disease; IU, intrauterine; PA-VSD, pulmonary artery-ventricular septal defect.

Table 8.9 Antenatal and postnatal management of major heart anomalies

Cardiac defect	Frequency of antenatal scans	Antenatal management	Place of delivery	Postnatal management
Ventricular septal defect	20 weeks and 32 weeks	No special intervention	Cardiac center	No special intervention at birth. Monitor growth and signs of heart failure. Corrective surgery commonly within first year.
Atrioventricular septal defect	20 weeks and 32 weeks	Exclude trisomy 13, 18, 21, monitor size of right and left ventricles	Cardiac center	No special intervention at birth. Genetic review. Monitor growth and signs of heart failure. Corrective surgery mostly within 6 months.
Aorta-pulmonary window	20 weeks and every 4 weeks	No special intervention	Cardiac center	No special intervention at birth. Monitor growth and signs of heart failure. Corrective surgery within first few months.
Transposition of the great arteries	20 weeks and every 4 weeks	Monitor FO-DA patency, exclude PS and interrupted aortic arch	Surgical center	Prostin infusion and balloon atrial septostomy at birth. Corrective surgery-arterial switch within first few weeks of life.
Truncus arteriosus	20 weeks and every 2–4 weeks	Monitor truncal valve size, exclude truncal valve stenosis, regurgitation or interrupted aortic arch; offer amniocentesis to exclude 22q11 microdeletion	Surgical center	Prostin infusion if there is interrupted aortic arch. Check neonate calcium levels, monitor immunity and give Irradiated blood for when needed if 22q11 deletion present. Corrective surgery within first few weeks.
Total anomalous pulmonary venous connection	20 weeks and every 4 weeks	Determine site of connection of pulmonary veins, and presence of venous obstruction	Surgical center	No special intervention at birth. Corrective surgery within first few weeks.
Hypoplastic left heart	20 weeks and every 2–4 weeks	Monitor foramen ovale-ductus arteriosus patency, exclude CoA	Surgical center	Prostin infusion at birth. Three-stage palliative surgery (Fontan route): either Norwood, or Sanno or hybrid procedure as stage one at birth; SVC to-pulmonary artery shunt (Glenn) operation as second stage beyond 6 months of age and finally total cavo-pulmonary shunt (Fontan) operation at 5 years of age as the third stage.
Aortic atresia	20 weeks and every 2–4 weeks	Monitor FO-DA patency, size and function of left ventricle	Surgical center	Prostin infusion at birth. Corrective surgery within first few weeks of life.
Coarctation of the aorta	20 weeks and every 4 weeks	Monitor DA patency	Surgical center	Prostin infusion at birth. Blood pressure monitoring. Corrective surgery within first few weeks of life.
Interrupted aortic arch	20 weeks and every 4 weeks	Monitor DA patency; offer amniocentesis to exclude 22q11 microdeletion	Surgical center	Prostin infusion at birth. Blood pressure monitoring. Corrective surgery within first few weeks of life. Check neonate calcium levels, monitor immunity and give Irradiated blood for when needed if 22q11 deletion present.

Condition	Timing	Monitoring	Center	Management
Tetralogy of Fallot	20 weeks and 32 weeks	Monitor pulmonary artery size and growth; offer amniocentesis to exclude 22q11 microdeletion	Cardiac center	No special intervention at birth. Airway management and prevention of hypoxic spells. Check neonate calcium levels, monitor immunity and give Irradiated blood for when needed if 22q11 deletion present. Corrective surgery within first year.
Pulmonary atresia	20 weeks and every 4 weeks	Monitor FO-DA patency, pulmonary artery size and growth, size and function of right ventricle	Surgical center	Prostin infusion at birth. Three-stage palliative surgery within first few years: first few weeks of life aortopulmonary shunt operation; SVC-to-pulmonary artery shunt (Glenn) operation as second stage beyond 6 months of age and finally total cavo-pulmonary shunt (Fontan) operation at 5 years of age as the third stage. Corrective surgery may be possible if the right ventricle and pulmonary artery are of adequate size and they are in a connectable position.
Tricuspid atresia	20 weeks and every 4 weeks	Monitor FO-DA patency, pulmonary artery size and growth, size of VSD; determine origins of great vessels	Surgical center	Prostin if there is duct dependent heart defect or atrial septectomy if the foramen ovale is restrictive. Three-stage palliative surgery within first 5 years of life: first stage is at birth, aorto-pulmonary shunt operation if PS is severe or pulmonary artery banding if pulmonary flow is unrestricted; SVC-to-pulmonary artery shunt (Glenn) operation as second stage beyond 6 months of age and finally total cavopulmonary shunt (Fontan) operation at 5 years of age as the third stage.
Mitral atresia	20 weeks and every 4 weeks	Monitor FO-DA patency, pulmonary artery size and growth, size of VSD; determine origins of great vessels	Surgical center	Prostin if there is duct dependent heart defect or atrial septectomy if the FO is restrictive. Three-stage palliative surgery within first five years: first few weeks of life aorto-pulmonary shunt operation if PS is severe or pulmonary artery banding if pulmonary flow is unrestricted; SVC-to-pulmonary artery shunt (Glenn) operation as second stage beyond 6 months of age and finally total cavo-pulmonary shunt (Fontan) operation at 5 years of age as the third stage.
Ebstein's anomaly	20 weeks and every 4 weeks	Monitor fetal heart rate and rhythm; size of right atrium, ventricle and pulmonary artery; pulmonary flow; severity of tricuspid regurgitation; cardiac function	Cardiac center	No special intervention at birth but prostin may be needed if pulmonary flow is not adequate. Surgery is determined by adequacy of pulmonary flow and degree of tricuspid regurgitation.

CoA, coarctation of the aorta; DA, ductus arteriosus; FO, foramen ovale; PS, pulmonary stenosis; SVC, superior vena cava; VSD, ventricular septal defect.

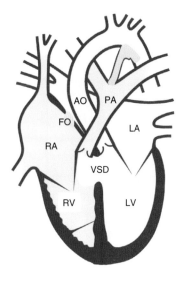
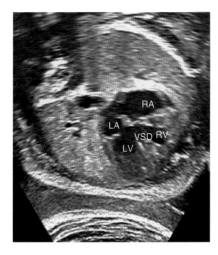

Figure 8.3 Ventricular septal defect. Left: from the four-chamber view shows a ventricular septal defect. Echocardiography on the right from the four-chamber view shows a ventricular septal defect. RA, right atrium; LA, left atrium; RV, right ventricle; LV, left ventricle; VSD, ventricular septal defect; FO, foramen ovale; PA, pulmonary artery; AO, aorta.

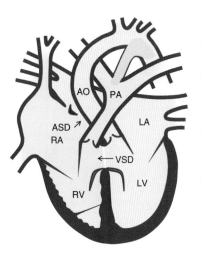
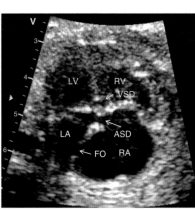

Figure 8.4 Atrioventricular septal defect. Diagram on the left from the four-chamber view shows atrioventricular septal defect. Echocardiography on the right from the four chamber view shows atrioventricular septal defect. RA, right atrium; LA, left atrium; RV, right ventricle; LV, left ventricle, ASD, atrial septal defect; VSD, ventricular septal defect; PA, pulmonary artery; AO, aorta.

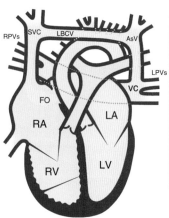
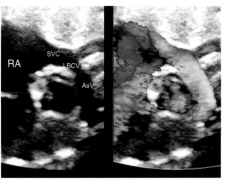

Figure 8.5 Total anomalous pulmonary venous connection. Diagram on the left from the four chamber view shows supracardiac total anomalous pulmonary venous connection to the left brachiocephalic vein. Echocardiography on the right from the four-chamber view shows total anomalous venous connection to the left brachiocephalic vein. RA, right atrium; LA, left atrium; RV, right ventricle; LV, left ventricle; AV, ascending vein; LBCV, left brachiocephalic vein; SVC, superior vena cava; PV, pulmonary vein.

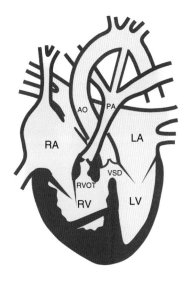
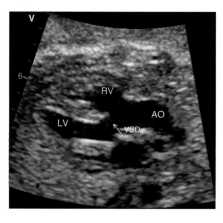

Figure 8.6 Tetralogy of Fallot. Diagram on the left from the four-chamber view shows right ventricular hypertrophy, right ventricular outflow tract obstruction, ventricular septal defect and an overriding aorta. On the left, echocardiography from the parasternal long axis view shows an overriding aorta and ventricular septal defect. This view does not demonstrate pulmonary stenosis which can be obtained from the parasternal short axis view. RA, right atrium; LA, left atrium; RV, right ventricle; LV, left ventricle; RVOT, right ventricular outflow tract; VSD, ventricular septal defect; AO, aorta; PA, pulmonary artery.

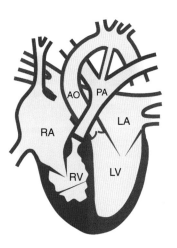
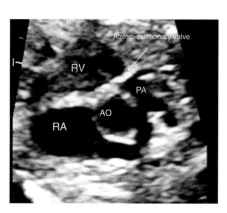

Figure 8.7 Pulmonary atresia with intact ventricular septum. Diagram on the left from the four-chamber view shows an atretic pulmonary valve and hypertrophied right ventricle. Echocardiography on the right from the parasternal short axis view shows the atretic pulmonary valve. RA, right atrium; LA, left atrium; RV, right ventricle; LV, left ventricle; AO, aorta; PA, pulmonary artery.

are a norm in the childhood and adolescent years to replace the narrow conduit.

Stenotic (obstructive) lesions

Hypoplastic left heart syndrome

Hypoplastic left heart syndrome encompasses an underdeveloped LA, diminutive and noncontractile left ventricle, critically narrowed or atretic aortic and mitral orifices, and hypoplasia of the ascending aorta (Figure 8.10). The left ventricle may have a bright and noncontractile appearance, described as "endocardial fibroelastosis."

If the FO becomes restrictive, fetal wellbeing can be threatened; therefore, continuing biweekly surveillance until the end of pregnancy is required. Amniocentesis is recommended. CoA may also coexist. All cardiac views need to be expedited to document associated abnormalities.

This is a duct-dependent cardiac abnormality and requires prostaglandin E infusion immediately after birth to keep the baby alive. Newborn infants with this condition are very sick, and exhibit profound cyanosis and signs of congestive heart failure once the DA is closed, and the majority will die within the first few days of life unless palliative surgery is performed.

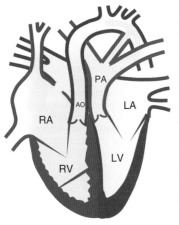
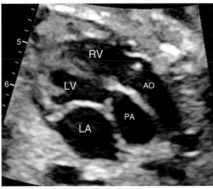

Figure 8.8 Transposition of the great arteries. Diagram on the left from the four chamber view shows transposed great arteries with the aorta arising from the right ventricle and the pulmonary artery arising from the left ventricle. Echocardiography on the right from the parasternal long axis view shows similar arrangement. RA, right atrium; LA, left atrium; RV, right ventricle; LV, left ventricle; AO, aorta; PA, pulmonary artery.

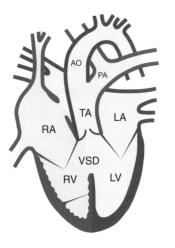
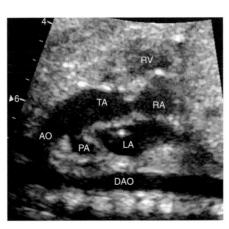

Figure 8.9 Truncus arteriosus. Diagram on the left from the four chamber view shows a ventricular septal defect and a single arterial trunk arising from both ventricle. The main pulmonary artery arises beyond the truncal valve and underside of the main arterial trunk. Echocardiography on the right from the sagittal arch view shows a single arterial trunk giving rise to the pulmonary artery from its underside. RA, right atrium; LA, left atrium; RV, right ventricle; LV, left ventricle; VSD, ventricular septal defect; TA, truncus arteriosus; AO, aorta; DAO, descending aorta; PA, pulmonary artery.

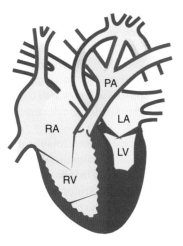
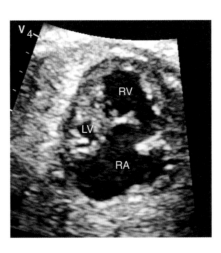

Figure 8.10 Hypoplastic left heart syndrome. Diagram on the left from the four chamber view shows an atretic mitral valve, an atretic aortic valve, hypoplastic left ventricle and an hypoplastic ascending aorta. Echocardiography on the right from the four chamber view shows an atretic mitral valve, and a hypoplastic left ventricle. RA, right atrium; LA, left atrium; RV, right ventricle; LV, left ventricle.

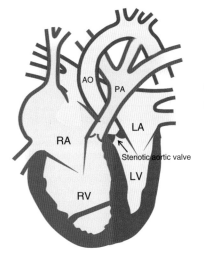

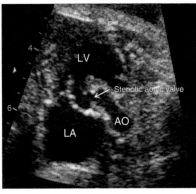

Figure 8.11 Aortic stenosis. Diagram on the left shows a thickened and stenosed aortic valve with a dilated right ventricle. Echocardiography on the right shows an enlarged left atrium, small and stenosed aortic valve. RA, right atrium; LA, left atrium; RV, right ventricle; LV, left ventricle; AO, aorta; PA, pulmonary artery.

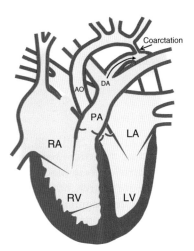

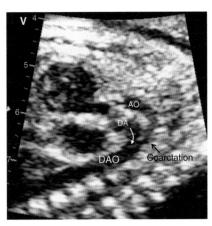

Figure 8.12 Coarctation of the aorta. Diagram on the left from the four chamber view shows a dilated right ventricle, pulmonary artery, and ductus arteriosus. Aortic isthmus is hypoplastic with discrete coarctation of the aorta. Echocardiography from the sagittal aortic arch view shows very narrow aortic isthmus just above the insertion of the ductus arteriosus. RA, right atrium; LA, left atrium; RV, right ventricle; LV, left ventricle; AO, aorta; DAO, descending aorta; PA, pulmonary artery; DA, ductus arteriosus.

A three-stage Norwood operation and its modifications are the main palliative procedures in the management of this severe anomaly.

Aortic stenosis or atresia

Arterial exit from the left ventricle is either narrowed (stenosis) or totally obstructed (atresia); the left ventricle may be hypertrophied, dilated or underdeveloped (hypoplastic) (Figure 8.11). VSD or mitral valve abnormality may also coexist. Parasternal long-axis or apical five-chamber views would be the most helpful planes to demonstrate this anomaly.

If the FO becomes restrictive, fetal wellbeing can be threatened, therefore biweekly fetal cardiac surveillance until the end of pregnancy is required. Amniocentesis is recommended to exclude particularly Williams and Turner syndromes.

Following birth, in critical aortic stenosis or atresia, right ventricular output alone is unable meet the metabolic demand of peripheral tissues. Prostaglandin infusion is mandatory in such cases in order to maintain effective circulation.

Rapid intervention with balloon dilatation or surgery to relieve aortic obstruction is required. If the

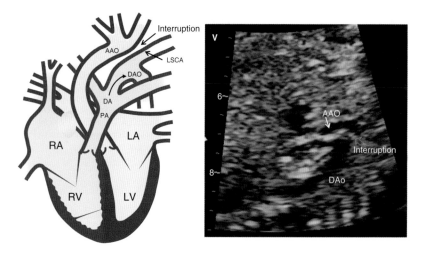

Figure 8.13 Interrupted aortic arch. Diagram on the left from a four chamber and great vessel view shows the ascending aorta being disconnected from its descending portion. The descending aorta is supplied by the pulmonary artery via the ductus arteriosus. Echocardiography on the left from the sagittal aortic arch view shows discontinuity between the transverse arch and the descending aorta. RA, right atrium; LA, left atrium; RV, right ventricle; LV, left ventricle; AO, aorta; PA, pulmonary artery; DA, ductus arteriosus; LSCA, left subclavian artery; DAO, descending aorta; AAO, ascending aorta.

left ventricle is too small and unable to sustain the systemic circulation, similar complex surgical interventions as in hypoplastic left heart syndrome may be necessary.

Coarctation of the aorta

In CoA, the descending aorta is narrowed at the junction of the DA and the left subclavian artery (Figure 8.12). Although it is a congenital lesion, it may also develop after birth following closure of the ductus arteriosus. Up to 60% of patients with CoA may have an associated defect in the form of a bicuspid aortic valve, VSD, or mitral stenosis. The sagittal view is the best plane to document this abnormality. The three-vessel view may also offer help in showing a small aorta and a large pulmonary artery. There is frequent association of left SVC to coronary sinus connection in fetuses with CoA.

Monthly fetal cardiac surveillance until the end of pregnancy is adequate. Amniocentesis is recommended to exclude Turner syndrome in female fetuses.

Severe CoA is a duct-dependent lesion, and therefore corrective surgery is necessary within the first few weeks of life. Surgery involves resection of the constricted area and end-to-end anastomosis of normal segments. Occasionally, a subclavian arterial flap may be utilized to enlarge the narrow segment. In older children, coarctation may be managed with balloon dilatation or stent implantation. Gore-Tex interposition grafts are infrequently used in children in the modern era. The long-term outlook is favorable with only 4% requiring repeat operations and 25% exhibiting hypertension.

Interrupted aortic arch

There is a complete discontinuity between the ascending and descending aortic segments (Figure 8.13). The left ventricle ejects blood into the proximal segment of the aortic arch, but the distal aorta beyond the interrupted segment receives blood from the right ventricle through the ductus arteriosus. Sagittal view is necessary to document this abnormality.

Monthly fetal cardiac surveillance until the end of pregnancy is adequate. Absent thymus and 22q11 microdeletion are commonly associated with this anomaly. Amniocentesis is recommended to exclude Turner syndrome in female fetuses.

This is a duct-dependent lesion, and therefore, life is incompatible without surgery. Infants with interrupted aorta exhibit signs of left ventricular failure and circulatory collapse due to progressive tissue hypoxia. Surgery involves an end-to-end anastomosis of normal segments after resection of the ductal tissue. Rarely, subclavian arterial flap may be utilized to cover the interrupted segment. A Gore-Tex interposition graft may be required in difficult cases. The long-term outlook is favorable.

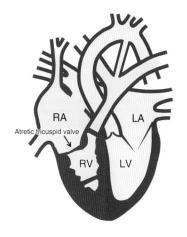

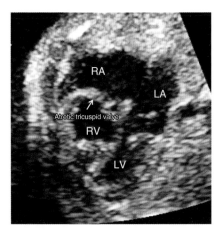

Figure 8.14 Tricuspid atresia intact ventricular septum and pulmonary stenosis. Diagram on the left from the four-chamber view shows an atretic tricuspid valve with a hypoplastic right ventricle and intact ventricle septum. Echocardiography from the four-chamber view shows an atretic tricuspid valve, hypertrophied right ventricle and intact ventricular septum. RA, right atrium; LA, left atrium; RV, right ventricle; LV, left ventricle.

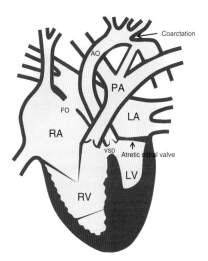

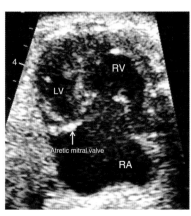

Figure 8.15 Mitral atresia, ventricular septal defect and coarctation. Diagram on the left from the four-chamber view shows an atretic mitral valve with a hypoplastic left ventricle and VSD. There is also coarctation of the aorta. Echocardiography from the four-chamber view shows an atretic mitral valve, hypertrophied left ventricle and VSD. RA, right atrium; LA, left atrium; FO, foramen ovale; RV, right ventricle; LV, left ventricle; VSD, ventricular septal defect; AO, aorta; PA, pulmonary artery; DA, ductus arteriosus; DAO, descending aorta.

Inlet valve abnormalities

Tricuspid atresia

Tricuspid atresia describes total obstruction to right ventricular inflow from the RA. Tricuspid atresia is commonly associated with a VSD and pulmonary stenosis or pulmonary artresia. Four-chamber view offers diagnostic clues but outflow tract view is also necessary to document any additional pulmonary stenosis or artresia (Figure 8.14).

The FO must remain open throughout the pregnancy and after birth in all cases. If the FO becomes restrictive, fetal wellbeing can be threatened; therefore, biweekly fetal cardiac surveillance until the end of pregnancy is required. Amniocentesis is recommended.

Surgical intervention may not be necessary at birth if there is an adequate-sized VSD and balanced blood flow to the lungs through a patent pulmonary valve.

Depending on the degree of pulmonary blood flow either an aortopulmonary shunt (restricted flow) or pulmonary artery band (unrestrictive flow) procedures may be required during the neonatal period. This is followed by a SVC-to-pulmonary artery shunt (Glenn) operation between 6 and 12 months of age, and then finally the Fontan completion (total cavopulmonary shunt) can be contemplated at the age of five. The long-term outlook is guarded.

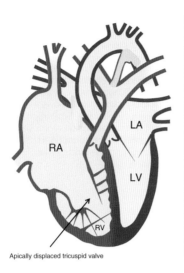

Apically displaced tricuspid valve

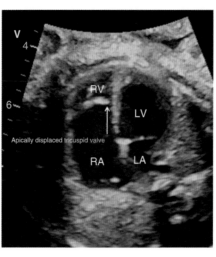

Apically displaced tricuspid valve

Figure 8.16 Ebstein's anomaly of tricuspid valve. Diagram on the left from a four-chamber view shows an apically displaced tricuspid valve and an atrialised right ventricle. Echocardiography from the four chamber view shows a large right atrium due to apically displaced tricuspid valve. RA, right atrium; LA, left atrium; RV, right ventricle; LV, left ventricle.

Mitral atresia

Mitral atresia is characterized by total obstruction to left ventricular inflow from the LA (Figure 8.15). The FO must remain open throughout the pregnancy and after birth in all cases. This anomaly may be associated with pulmonary or aortic stenosis, and VSD.

If the FO becomes restrictive, fetal wellbeing can be threatened; therefore, biweekly fetal cardiac surveillance until the end of pregnancy is required. Amniocentesis is recommended.

Depending on the degree of pulmonary blood flow, either an aortopulmonary shunt or pulmonary artery banding may be carried out during the neonatal period, as in tricuspid atresia. This is followed by a SVC-to-pulmonary artery shunt (Glenn) operation between 6 and 12 months of age, and then finally the Fontan completion (total cavopulmonary shunt) is performed by the age of five.

Ebstein's anomaly

In Ebstein's anomaly, the tricuspid valve opening is displaced down from its usual basal position towards the cardiac apex (Figure 8.16). Tricuspid valve leaflets are tethered onto right ventricular walls. The base of the right ventricular cavity becomes part of the enlarged RA and the contractile portion of the right ventricle is confined to the apex. Tricuspid valve regurgitation and globally enlarged heart are the usual ultrasound features. VSD and pulmonary stenosis can also occur with Ebstein's anomaly. Lithium and marijuana use are pathologically linked with the occurrence of this anomaly.

A half of babies with Ebstein's anomaly may develop tachycardia due to the presence of accessory pathways. Noncompaction cardiomyopathy, fetal heart failure, severe tricuspid regurgitation, pericardial effusion and significant cardiomegaly may occur in some cases.

Amniocentesis is recommended in selected cases with left ventricular noncompaction to exclude the myosin heavy chain (MYH7) mutation. A three-to-four weekly follow-up in fetal medicine is necessary in most cases and biweekly ultrasound may be required in severe cases.

Long-term prognosis varies depending on the severity of tricuspid regurgitation, left ventricular and right ventricular function.

Double inlet left ventricle

Both inlets, mitral and tricuspid valves open into a common chamber of left ventricular morphology (Figure 8.17). The right ventricle is hypoplastic and most commonly located on the left side of the morphological left ventricle. Other abnormalities associated with this condition include VSD, aortic stenosis, pulmonary stenosis and interrupted aortic arch.

Fetuses are commonly asymptomatic with this anomaly. However, if there is aortic coarctation or interruption, or severe pulmonary stenosis, i.e., ductus-dependent anomaly, close follow-up is necessary to ensure the DA patency. Otherwise, usual follow-up at 3–4 week intervals would suffice. Amniocentesis is recommended to exclude 22q11 chromosome microdeletion in cases with interrupted aortic arch. Absent thymus may offer a clue in identifying cases of 22q11 microdeletion.

Newborn babies with this condition may be breathless but are also mildly cyanosed. This condition may be

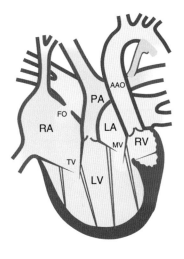 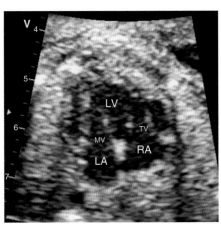

Figure 8.17 Double inlet left ventricle. Diagram on the left shows that both mitral and tricuspid valves open into a single left ventricle. Right ventricle is hypoplastic and connected to the left via a ventricular septal defect. Aorta arises from the hypoplastic right ventricle. Echocardiography on the right shows a single left ventricle receiving both mitral and tricuspid valves. RA, right atrium; LA, left atrium; RV, right ventricle; LV, left ventricle.

duct dependent, and the severity of left and right heart obstruction should be carefully assessed after birth.

Surgical intervention may not be necessary at birth if there is an adequate-sized VSD, unrestrictive systemic flow, and balanced blood flow to the lungs through a patent pulmonary valve. If there is left ventricular outflow tract obstruction, further operations, such as enlargement of VSD, Damus–Kay–Stansel operation, aortic arch repair may be required. Depending on the degree of pulmonary blood flow, either an aorta-pulmonary shunt (severe pulmonary stenosis) or pulmonary artery band (unrestrictive flow) procedures may be required during the neonatal period. These are followed by a SVC-to-pulmonary artery shunt (Glenn) operation between 6 and 12 months of age, and then finally the Fontan completion (total cavopulmonary shunt) can be contemplated at the age of five. The long term outlook is guarded.

Pathology and epidemiology

Pathology and incidence of major cardiac anomalies, risk factors (including family history) and associated chromosomal or genetic anomalies (including 22q11 microdeletion)

CHD is the most common congenital anomaly occurring with a frequency of 5–12 in 1,000 live births (Table 8.8)[19–24]. In addition, congenital heart defects also constitute the most common cause of death among congenital anomalies[25–27]. Approximately,

20–30% of congenital heart defects involve cardiac outflow tracts and 60–70% involve cardiac four chambers. The prenatal incidence of congenital heart defects may range from 0.5% to 39.5% (median, about 7.9%) with up to 40–65% of fetuses with a cardiac anomaly spontaneously aborting (Table 8.8).

Approximately 50% of the congenital heart cases are minor or can be surgically corrected; however, the remaining major heart defects account for over half of deaths from congenital abnormalities in childhood[25–40]. Antenatal and perinatal management of major heart anomalies are summarized in Table 8.9.

Congenital heart disease occurs most commonly as a result of unknown interactions between environmental factors (Table 8.10) and genetic predispositions (Table 8.11)[41–54]. Less commonly, single gene (Mendelian) and chromosomal defects may cause cardiovascular abnormalities (Table 8.11). Chromosomal abnormalities cause only 10% of congenital heart disease and often these are recognizable as distinct multiple malformation syndromes (Table 8.12). Chromosome aberrations commonly include aneuploidies (trisomy 21, 18 and 13) or microdeletion (22q deletion/Di George and Williams/7q deletion) syndromes (Tables 8.11 and 8.12)[47].

Several of these apparent nongenetic factors relevant to the polygenic/multifactorial inheritance include micronutrients (e.g., folic acid) and toxic substances (e.g., alcohol). It is likely that intrauterine infections (e.g., maternal rubella) and immunologic challenges (maternal autoimmune disease) may also play a part in the development of some congenital heart diseases (Table 8.10). Most polygenic/mutlifactorial

Table 8.10 Maternal and environmental risk factors for congenital heart defects

Maternal, environmental and fetal risk factors	Frequency of CHD	Type of defect
Diabetes mellitus	3–5	VSD, TGA, HCM
Connective tissue disorder	2–20	Heart block, cardiomyopathy
Phenylketonuria	12–50	TOF
Rubella	6–58	PDA, PPS, VSD, TOF, PS
Alcohol	20–30	VSD, TOF, ASD
Hydantoin	2–3	VSD, PS, AS, CoA
Lithium, marijuana, solvents	10	Ebstein's anomaly
Retinoic acid, vitamin A	10–25	Conotruncal defects
Trimethadione	15–30	TGA, TOF, HLHS
Central nervous system	2.5–15	VSD, TOF, CoA, HRH
Gastrointestinal system	5–39	VSD, HLHS, TOF, CAT
Renal system	2–42	VSD, CoA, TOF, AVSD, TAPVC, DORV, HRH
Mediastinum	10–40	VSD, TOF, CoA, PS, PAt, TA, DORV
Abdominal wall	14–30	VSD, HLHS, PA, PS, CAT, HRH, TA, AS
Vascular	5–21	VSD, AVSD, TA, TOF, HLHS

AS, aortic stenosis; ASD, atrial septal defect; AVSD, atrioventricular septal defect; CAT, common arterial trunk; CHD; congenital heart disease. CoA, coarctation of the aorta; DORV, double outlet right ventricle; HCM, hypertrophic cardiomyopathy; HLHS, hypoplastic left heart syndrome; HRH, hypoplastic right heart; PA, pulmonary artery; PAt, pulmonary atresia; PDA, patent ductus arteriosus; PPS, peripheral pulmonary artery stenosis; PS, pulmonary stenosis; TA, tricuspid atresia; TAPVC, total anomalous pulmonary venous connection; TGA, transposition of the great arteries; TOF, tetralogy of Fallot; VSD, ventricular septal defect.

etiologies result in either single or complex congenital heart defects with low recurrence risk (2–3%).

Molecular diagnosis for some of these genes is now available in clinical practice. As the identification of a pathogenic mutation in an affected child or parent could help in genetic counseling and assist the parent in managing a future conception (pre-implantation genetic diagnosis) or pregnancy (prenatal diagnosis).

Recurrence risk of heart defects

If the cardiac lesion is part of a syndrome due to a single gene mutation, the autosomal dominant genes will be expected to appear in 50% of children [48–54]. An autosomal recessive gene produces disease in 25% of children. The risk of occurrence of a cardiac abnormality varies with the specific chromosomal defect (Table 8.12).

The overall recurrence risk of a congenital heart defect may be influenced by having an affected parent or sibling (Table 8.13)[49–51, 53]. If the mother is affected, the recurrence risk in a child is 5–10%. If the previous child is affected, the risk of recurrence is 2–5% in the next child, and in the case of the father being affected, the risk remains at 2–4%. As the number of individuals in a family with congenital heart defects

increases, so does the risk of recurrence. If a father and child both had congenital heart defects, the risk to a future child would be 4–10%.

Congenital heart defects often occur in association with multiple congenital anomalies, including abnormal facial features, limb anomalies, other organ malformations, developmental abnormalities or growth abnormalities (Table 8.14)[55]. There are now a number of genetic tests that can assist clinicians in diagnosing genetic alterations in the child with congenital heart defects including cytogenetic techniques, fluorescence in situ hybridization, DNA mutation analysis, and microarray-comparative genome hybridization.

Specific genetic disorders associated with CHD

These specific genetic disorders include trisomy 21 (Down's syndrome), trisomy 18 (Edward syndrome), trisomy 13 (Patau syndrome), Turner syndrome, Williams–Beuren syndrome, Alagille syndrome, DiGeorge syndrome (22q11 deletion), Holt-Oram syndrome, Ellis–van Creveld syndrome and Noonan syndrome[47] (Table 8.11).

Table 8.11 Genetic syndromes and CHD

Genetic syndrome	Prevalence	Chromosome abnormality	Responsible gene	Frequency of CHD %	Type of CHD
Marfan	1:5,000	15q21.1	Fibrillin1 (FBN1)	70–80	AR, MR, AO aneurysm
Turner	1:2,500	XO	Sex chromosome	20–45	AS, BCAV, CoA, PS, MVP, AR
William	1:8,000	7q11.23	Elastin	53–85	AS, PS, PPS
Noonan	1:1–2,500	12q24, 12p1.21	PTPN11, KRAS, SOS1, 2p21	50–60	PS, HCM, PDA, ASD, PPS
DiGeorge	1:2–4,000	22q11		75	TOF, VSD, DORV, PA–VSD, IAA, APVS, CAT
Down	1:700	Trisomy 21	DSCAM, Collagen VI	50	VSD, AVSD, ASD
Edward	2.3:10,000	Trisomy 18		90–100	VSD, ASD, PDA, TOF, DORV, TGA, BCAV, CoA, PVND
Patau	1.4:10,000	Trisomy 13		80	VSD, ASD, PDA
Ellis–van Creveld	1:60,000–200,000	4p16	EVC, EVC2	60	ASD
Alagille	1:20,000–70,000	20p12	JAG1	85–94	ASD, VSD, AVSD, PPS, PS, TOF, PDA, R-ARCH, CoA
Holt Oram	1:100,000	12q24	TBX5	18	ASD, VSD, AVSD, TOF, HLHS, TOF, CAT, TA, DORV, TAPVC
Klinefelter	1:500–1,000	XXY	XXY	50	MVP, PDA, ASD
Cri du Chat	1:20,000–50,000	del(5p-)		25	ASD, VSD, TOF, PDA, DORV
Neurofibromatosis type 1	1:2,000–3,000	17q11.2	Neurofibromin	0.4–6.4	PS, AS coarctation

AO, ascending aorta; APVS, *absent pulmonary valve syndrome*; AR, aortic regurgitation; AS, aortic stenosis; ASD, atrial septal defect; AVSD, atrioventricular septal defect; BCAV, brachiocephalic artery/vein; CAT, common arterial trunk; CHD, congenital heart disease; CoA, coarctation of the aorta; DORV, double outlet right ventricle; HCM, hypertrophic cardiomyopathy; HLHS hypoplastic left heart syndrome; IAA, *interrupted aortic arch*; MR, mitral regurgitation; MVP, mitral valve proplaspe; PA–VSD, pulmonary atresia with ventricular septal defect; PDA, patent ductus arteriosus; PPS, peripheral pulmonary artery stenosis; PS, pulmonary stenosis; PVND; polyvalvular nodular dysplasia; R-ARCH, right-sided aortic arch; TA, tricuspid atresia; TAPVC, total anomalous pulmonary venous connection; TGA, transposition of the great arteries; TOF, tetralogy of Fallot; VSD, ventricular septal defect.

Table 8.12 Major congenital heart anomalies, causative genes, and frequency of associated chromosome abnormalities

Heart anomaly	Causative gene/chromosome locus	Chromosome abnormality	Frequency of chromosome abnormalities %
Atrioventricular septal defect	CRELD1/3p21, ZIC3	Maternal disomy 16; 8p23 microdeletion; trisomy 13, 18, 21	35–47
Ventricular septal defect	GATA4/8p23, TBX5, NKX2-5, FOXH1, ACTC1	Mosaic trisomy 10; paternal disomy 10; maternal disomy 16; trisomy 21, microdeletion 1p36; 1q44-qter; 4q35; 5q35; 6p25; 9q34; 17q25; 19p13; 22q11	37–48
Hypoplastic left heart syndrome	NKX2-5, GJA1, HAND1	Microduplication 22q11.2; microdeletion 1p36, 8p23, 11q26, 15q24-q26; 20q11	4–10
Tricuspid atresia	NKX2-6, GATA6		2–9
Total anomalous pulmonary venous connection	TBX5, ZIC3		0
Ebstein's anomaly	NKX2-5, MYH7		0–12
Double inlet left ventricle			N/A
Tetralogy of Fallot	ZFPM2/8q23, NKX2-5/5q34-q35, JAG1/JAG1, TBX5, VEGFA, GJA5, CITED2, GATA4, GATA6, FOXH1	Microdeletion 5q11.2; 9q34; 22q11; 22q11.2 microduplication; trisomy 21	11–27
Truncus arteriosus	TBX5	22q11 microdeletion	4–33
Double outlet right ventricle	CFC1/2q21, NKX2-5, GATA4	8p23 microdeletion	11–38
Pulmonary stenosis or atresia	GATA4, PTPN11, JAG1, ZIC3	22q11 microdeletion	4–5
Transposition of the great arteries	CFC1/2q21, ZIC3, PROSIT240/12q24, NKX2-5, CITED2, NODAL,		0–3
Coarctation/interruption of aorta	TBX1	Mosaic chromosome 16; maternal disomy 16; 6p25 microdeletion; 22q11 microdeletion; 22q11.2 microduplication; 45X Turner	20–30

Table 8.13 Major congenital heart anomalies, recurrence risk and associated chromosome anomalies

Heart anomaly	Incidence in per 1,000 live births	Recurrence risk one sibling affected %	Two siblings or mother affected %	Father affected %
Atrioventricular septal defect	0.35	3–4	10–14	1
Ventricular septal defect	1.1–3.57	3	6–10	2–3
Hypoplastic left heart syndrome	0.14–0.27	2–3	6–10	N/A
Tricuspid atresia	0.03–0.08	1	3	N/A
Total anomalous pulmonary venous connection	0.06–0.09	0	N/A	N/A
Ebstein's anomaly	0.06–0.11	1	3–6	N/A
Double inlet left ventricle	N/A	0	N/A	N/A
Tetralogy of Fallot	0.42	2.5	8	1–2
Truncus arteriosus	0.05–0.11	1	3	N/A
Double outlet right ventricle	0.16	2.5	8	N/A
Pulmonary stenosis or atresia	0.16–0.26	1–2	3–6	N/A
Transposition of the great arteries	0.24–0.32	1.5	5	N/A
Coarctation/interruption of aorta	0.14–0.41	2	4–6	2–3

Antenatal management and outcome of arrhythmia

Normal fetal heart rate is between 110–160 bpm. Bradycardia is defined as a rate below 110 bpm. Pathological tachycardia is more likely if the fetal heart rate is over 160 bpm. The differential diagnosis of fetal arrhythmia (Table 8.15) requires systematic acquisition of necessary Doppler tracings in all recommended scanning views (Table 8.16) and correct interpretation of Doppler recordings (Figure 8.18) [56–66].

Premature atrial contractions

The most frequent cause of irregular fetal heart rhythm is premature atrial contractions. The frequency of premature atrial contractions is reported to be approximately 5–14% of all fetuses referred for detailed cardiac scan [56–63, 66]. Postulated mechanisms for premature atrial contractions generation are enhanced automaticity of the atrial myocardium, atrial muscle re-entry, atrial dilatation due to restrictive FO and mechanical irritation of the atrial wall due to atrial septal aneurysm.

Fetal arrhythmia can be an unsettling finding for obstetricians. For instance, some non-conducted PACs may result in postectopic pause that could lead to a misdiagnosis of bradycardia, or even heart block. Since slow heart rate is also a warning sign for fetal distress, on some occasions obstetricians may resort to performing early delivery to avoid fetal demise.

Premature atrial contractions can be differentiated from true bradycardia by simple Doppler interrogation of simultaneous mitral and aortic flow during a cardiac ultrasound examination (Figure 8.18b, c). Although most premature atrial contractions can initiate ventricular response in a one-to-one manner, some early atrial beats may fail to conduct to ventricles; hence, such premature atrial contractions result in irregular heart rhythm, which can be perceived as bradycardia.

Premature atrial contractions have a high spontaneous resolution rate of 50% during the first visit and over 90% by the end of pregnancy[50, 60, 64]. Structural and functional heart disease (1%), cardiomyopathy, AV conduction disease, congenital long QT syndrome (2.5%) and atrial tumor (1–9%) can be demonstrated in some

Table 8.14 Frequency of associated systemic anomalies in selected congenital heart defects (%)

Heart anomaly	Total system anomalies	Craniofacial	Respiratory	Gastrointestinal	Genitourinary	Central nervous	Musculoskeletal
Atrioventricular septal defect	15–50	10	10	10	20	10	20
Ventricular septal defect	30–62	38.3	14.9	31.9	25.5	19.1	27.6
Hypoplastic left heart syndrome	4–35	5	10	10	5	5	10
Tricuspid atresia	15–30	16.6	0	16.6	0	0	16.6
Total anomalous pulmonary venous connection	0–37.5	0	25	0	25	0	0
Ebstein's anomaly	0–17.6	0	0	0	0	0	0
Double inlet left ventricle	38.9–62	14.3	9.5	14.3	19	9.5	8.7
Tetralogy of Fallot	26.8–48	11.1	16.6	11.1	16.6	5.5	11.1
Truncus arteriosus	17–50	12.5	12.5	0	0	0	12.5
Double outlet right ventricle	25–71	28.5	28.5	0	14.3	14.3	0
Pulmonary stenosis or atresia	10–50	25	12.5	0	25	12.5	50
Transposition of the great arteries	9–33	0	6.6	0	0	3.3	3.3
Coarctation/interruption of aorta	12–68	34.8	13	13	30.4	17.4	8.7

Table 8.15 Differential diagnosis of fetal arrhythmias

Differential diagnosis	Atrial rate	Atrial rhythm	Ventricular rate	Ventricular rhythm	Atrioventricular or ventriculoatrial relationship
Normal sinus rhythm	Normal 130–150	Regular	Same as atrial rate	Regular	1:1
Sinus tachycardia	High 150–180	Regular but varying	Same as atrial rate	Same as atrial rhythm	1:1
Sinus bradycardia, junctional rhythm	Low 70–110	Regular	Same as atrial rate	Regular	1:1
PAC or PVC	Low 70–130 or normal	Irregular	Same as atrial rate, slower or faster	Irregular	1:1 or variable
Chaotic atrial tachycardia, atrial flutter/fibrillation	High 180–200	Irregular or "chaotic"	Same as atrial rate	Irregular	Variable
AV re-entry SVT, or AV node re-entry SVT	High 200–300	Regular	Same as atrial rate	Regular	1:1
Atrial flutter	High 300–450	Regular	Faster than atrial rate 150–225	Regular or irregular	1:1, 2:1, 3:1, or variable
Permanent junctional reciprocating tachycardia	High 180–300	Regular but varying	Same as atrial rate	Same as atrial rhythm	1:1
Accelerated ventricular or junctional rhythm	Normal 130–150	Regular	Faster than atrial rate 180–200	Regular	Dissociated or intermittent 1:1
Ventricular tachycardia, or junctional tachycardia	Normal 130–150	Regular	Faster than atrial rate 210–400	Regular or irregular	Dissociated or 1:1
Second-degree AV block	Normal 130–150	Regular	Faster than atrial rate 70–110	Irregular	Intermittent dissociated
Third-degree AV block	Normal 130–150	Regular	Faster than atrial rate 40–110	Regular	Dissociated

PAC, premature atrial contractions; PVC, premature ventricular contractions; SVT, supraventricular tachycardia.

Table 8.16 Fetal arrhythmia detection methods

Echocardiographic methods	Irregular rhythm PAC or PVC	Atrioventricular block	Supraventricular or ventricular tachycardia	Atrial flutter	PR interval
M-mode Doppler	Easy to obtain Reliable but difficult to interpret in detail	Easy to obtain Reliable, most useful and easy to interpret	Easy to obtain Reliable and most easy to interpret	Easy to obtain Reliable, most useful and easy to interpret	Easy to obtain Difficult to ascertain accurate PR interval
Aortic outflow–mitral inflow pulse wave Doppler	Easy to obtain Most useful and easy to interpret Not obtainable if aortic or mitral atresia	Easy to obtain Reliable and easy to interpret Not obtainable if aortic or mitral atresia	Easy to obtain Reliable and easy to interpret Not obtainable if aortic or mitral atresia	Easy to obtain Unreliable and difficult to interpret in detail Not obtainable if aortic or mitral atresia	Easy to obtain Reliable and easy to interpret Not obtainable if aortic or mitral atresia
Aorta–superior vena cava pulse wave Doppler	Difficult to obtain Difficult to interpret in detail Not obtainable if aortic atresia or aortic atresia	Difficult to obtain Difficult to interpret in detail Not obtainable if aortic atresia	Difficult to obtain Reliable but difficult to interpret in detail Not obtainable if aortic atresia	Difficult to obtain Difficult to interpret in detail Not obtainable if aortic atresia	Difficult to obtain Difficult to interpret in detail Not obtainable if aortic atresia
Pulmonary vein–pulmonary artery pulse wave Doppler	Difficult to obtain Reliable and helpful but requires skills to interpret Not obtainable if anomalous pulmonary veins or pulmonary atresia	Difficult to obtain Reliable and helpful but requires skills to interpret Not obtainable if anomalous pulmonary veins or pulmonary atresia	Difficult to obtain Reliable and easy to interpret Not obtainable if anomalous pulmonary veins or pulmonary atresia	Difficult to obtain Reliable and helpful but requires skills to interpret Not obtainable if anomalous pulmonary veins or pulmonary atresia	Difficult to obtain Reliable and helpful but requires skills to interpret Not obtainable if anomalous pulmonary veins or pulmonary atresia
Tissue Doppler	Easy to obtain Reliable and helpful but requires specialists skills to interpret	Easy to obtain Reliable and helpful but requires specialists skills to interpret	Easy to obtain Reliable and helpful but requires specialists skills to interpret	Easy to obtain Reliable and helpful but requires specialists skills to interpret and offline measurements	Easy to obtain Reliable and helpful but requires specialists skills to interpret

PAC, premature atrial contractions; PVC, premature ventricular contractions.

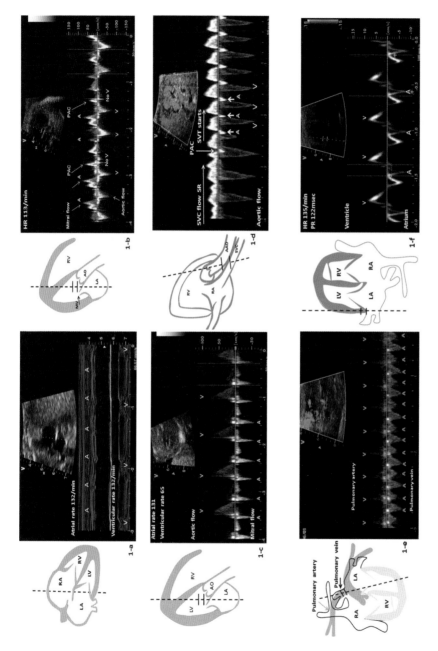

Figure 8.18 Doppler assessment of fetal heart rhythm. a) M-mode assessment of atrial and ventricular rates in a fetus with heart block; b) simultaneous pulse wave Doppler assessment of mitral inflow and aortic outflow in a fetus with irregular heart rhythm; c) simultaneous pulse wave Doppler assessment of mitral inflow and aortic outflow in a fetus with heart block; d) simultaneous pulse wave Doppler assessment of SVC and aortic flow in a fetus with SVT; e) simultaneous pulse wave Doppler assessment of pulmonary artery and vein in a fetus with atrial flutter; f) tissue Doppler interrogation of lateral mitral valve annulus in a fetus with sinus rhythm. PAC, premature atrial contraction; A, atrial beat; V, ventricular beat; PVC, premature ventricular contractions; RA, right atrium; LA, left atrium; LV, left ventricle; RV, right ventricle; MV, mitral valve; AO, aorta; AAO, ascending aorta; SVC, superior vena cava.

Table 8.17 Irregular heart rhythm due to premature atrial and ventricular contractions, treatment protocol. PAC, premature atrial contractions; PVC, premature ventricular contractions; U&Es, urea and electrolytes; LFTs, liver function tests; LQTS, long QT syndrome; HCM, hypertrophic cardiomyopathy; ARVC, arrhythmogenic right ventricular cardiomyopathy; CPVT, catecholaminergic polymorphic ventricular tachycardia; PPM, permanent pacemaker; ECG, electrocardiography; HR, heart rate; TID, ter in die (three times per day); BID, bis in die (twice per day)

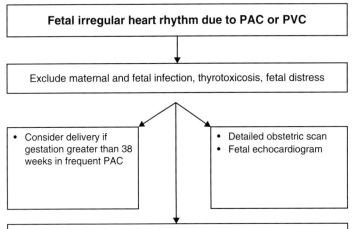

Fetal irregular heart rhythm due to PAC or PVC

Exclude maternal and fetal infection, thyrotoxicosis, fetal distress

- Consider delivery if gestation greater than 38 weeks in frequent PAC

- Detailed obstetric scan
- Fetal echocardiogram

Maternal assessment
- Baseline U&Es, LFTs, viral screen, and urine catecholamines if necessary
- Thyroid function
- Exclude stimulant medications
- Maternal Lupus or Sjögren
- Detailed maternal and paternal medical history to exclude any inherited arrhythmic syndromes such as LQTS, Brugada, HCM, ARVC, CPVT or family history of cot death and sudden cardiac death
- Obtain 12 lead ECG from the mother if there is LQTS, Brugada, HCM, ARVC, CPVT

Fetal medicine followup
- Twice weekly fetal heart rate auscultation by a midwife to ensure HR is not below 110 at all times or above 180 at all times
- Weekly ultrasound examination of fetal and placental well-being by a fetal medicine specialist to exclude fetal distress or placental insufficiency
- Fortnightly fetal echocardiogram by a fetal cardiologist
- When there is frequent ectopic activity or blocked PACs or PVCs, fetal cardiology review should be intensified at weekly intervals to facilitate early recognition and treatment of sustained arrhythmia
- Start digoxin 250 mcg BID if there is cardiac dysfunction

Delivery decision
Normal delivery if there is no obstetric or fetal concern. Even in the presence of irregular rhythm.

Advice to pregnant women
- Abstain from excess consumption of caffeine, stimulant beverages or food
- Stop smoking
- Avoid use of excess beta stimulant
- Avoid use of excess antihistaminic
- Avoid excess consumption of polyphenol rich food or herbal remedies
- Monitor fetal movement by kick count, if there is any concern seek immediate help

fetuses with atrial extrasystole. However, the presence of a heart anomaly, underlying placental insufficiency, fetal compromise or myocarditis, but not the premature atrial contractions per se, has an unfavorable effect on the overall outcome. In some cases, premature atrial contractions may initiate supraventricular tachycardia (SVT) (0.5–5%). Blocked premature atrial contractions can lead to a significant arrhythmia more frequently (13–44%) than conducted premature atrial contractions.

The fetuses presenting with premature atrial contractions or irregular heart rhythm should have a thorough assessment of fetoplacental unit, fetal cardiovascular system, and AV conduction properties (Table 8.17). Fetuses exhibiting frequent or blocked premature atrial contractions and cardiac dysfunction should be kept under close surveillance by a midwife check twice a week, and by weekly obstetric and cardiac ultrasound assessments. Pregnant women should be advised to count fetal kicks, and in case of reduced

count should be instructed to seek immediate medical advice. Common triggers for premature atrial contractions, such as the use adrenergic stimulants, medications with known arrhythmic side effects, consumption of excess caffeine containing food and beverages, and smoking by the mother should be limited or completely avoided. Following delivery, newborn infants exhibiting an irregular pulse should undergo electrocardiographic, and if necessary, echocardiographic assessment.

Bradycardia and heart block

Short periods of bradycardia occur in normal fetuses with no serious consequences. However, sustained bradycardia is a rare but significant rhythm abnormality in fetal life, and its detection should prompt detailed maternal and fetal cardiac evaluation[56–58]. Bradycardia as a result of AV block is associated with a high risk of hydrops and also increased mortality in fetal life. Persistent

Table 8.18 Atrioventricular block treatment protocol. U&Es, *urea and electrolytes*; LFTs, *liver function tests*; LQTS, *long QT syndrome*; CMP, *cardiomyopathy*; PPM, *permanent pacemaker*; ECG, *electrocardiography*; HR, *heart rate*; TID, *ter in die (three times per day)*; BID, *bis in die (twice per day)*; ECG, electrocardiography; TID, ter in die (three times per day).

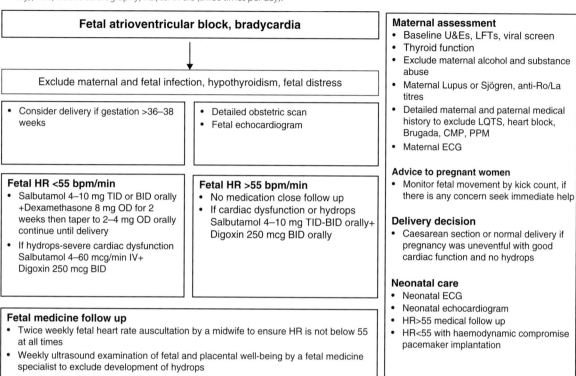

bradycardia can also occur with nonconducted premature atrial contractions, sick sinus syndrome, central nervous system abnormalities, maternal beta-blocker treatment, prominent vagal tone, long QT syndrome, hydrops and intrauterine growth retardation[60, 64–66].

Fetuses with AV block and a structurally normal heart usually exhibit higher titers of maternal anti-Ro or anti-La antibodies (60–90%)[56–64]. Many asymptomatic mothers who have a fetus with isolated complete heart block may develop connective tissue disorder in the next 10 years. Mothers with lupus or Sjogren syndrome have a 2–5% risk of producing a baby with complete heart block in their first pregnancy. In the second pregnancy, this risk increases to 16–20%. Structural heart disease accounts for the remaining 10% of the fetal heart block cases[56–64].

In addition to structural heart disease, atrial isomerism, slower fetal heart rates of less than 55 bpm, and the presence of hydrops are all suggested to be poor prognostic indicators[56–64].

In-utero therapeutic trials with beta stimulants, digitalis, and steroids have been attempted with mixed results. In some fetuses with first- or second-degree AV block, recovery of sinus rhythm has been reported to occur with or without medication. In-utero therapeutic trails with beta-stimulants, digitalis, and steroids have been attempted with mixed results but it is generally recommended that a trial of beta mimetic and dexamethasone combination may be considered in fetuses showing cardiac dysfunction and heart rates of below 55 bpm (Table 8.18).

Supraventricular tachycardia and atrial flutter

SVT is the most common cause of fast heart rhythm in the fetus. Atrial flutter (AF) constitutes the second most common type of tachycardia[56–58]. Ventricular dysrhythmia is rarely encountered. Fetal SVT is usually noted incidentally at a later stage in

Table 8.19 Supraventricular tachycardia (SVT) treatment protocol. IUV, intraumbilical vein; ECG, electrocardiography; TID, ter in die (three times per day); BID, bis in die (twice per day); U&Es, urea and electrolytes; LFTs, liver function tests.

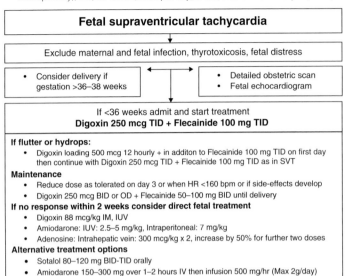

Fetal supraventricular tachycardia

↓

Exclude maternal and fetal infection, thyrotoxicosis, fetal distress

- Consider delivery if gestation >36–38 weeks
- Detailed obstetric scan
- Fetal echocardiogram

If <36 weeks admit and start treatment
Digoxin 250 mcg TID + Flecainide 100 mg TID

If flutter or hydrops:
- Digoxin loading 500 mcg 12 hourly + in additon to Flecainide 100 mg TID on first day then continue with Digoxin 250 mcg TID + Flecainide 100 mg TID as in SVT

Maintenance
- Reduce dose as tolerated on day 3 or when HR <160 bpm or if side-effects develop
- Digoxin 250 mcg BID or OD + Flecainide 50–100 mg BID until delivery

If no response within 2 weeks consider direct fetal treatment
- Digoxin 88 mcg/kg IM, IUV
- Amiodarone: IUV 2.5–5 mg/kg, Intraperitoneal: 7 mg/kg
- Adenosine: Intrahepatic vein: 300 mcg/kg x 2, increase by 50% for further two doses

Alternative treatment options
- Sotalol 80–120 mg BID-TID orally
- Amiodarone 150–300 mg over 1–2 hours IV then infusion 500 mg/hr (Max 2g/day)
- Amiodarone oral 600–800 mg BID–TID loading for 7 days (Max 2.4g/day)
- Maintenance amiodarone oral 200–800 mg/day

Fetal assessment
- Fetal heart auscultation twice a week
- Fetal ultrasound weekly by fetal medicine
- Fetal echocardiogram weekly by fetal cardiologist

Delivery decision
- Normal delivery if sinus rhythm and there is no maternal or fetal concern
- Caesarean section if tachycardia persists

Maternal assessment
- Baseline maternal ECG, U&Es, LFTs, viral screen, thyroid function
- Urine catecholamines if necessary
- Check flecainide and digoxin serum levels on day 3 and weekly thereafter
- Keep drug levels close to top end of normal
- Weekly ECG and U&Es, keep PR interval <240 ms, QTc interval <480 ms and QRS prolongation <25%
- Monitor maternal and neonatal thyroid function, liver function, QTc with amiodarone
- Renal function, QTc monitoring with sotalol

Advice to pregnant women
- Abstain from smoking, excess consumption of caffeine, stimulant beverages or food
- Monitor fetal movement by kick count, if there is any concern seek immediate help

Side effects
Digoxin
- Dizziness and sickness
- Visual disturbance, yellow vision
- PR interval prolongation
- T wave inversion
- Bidirectional tachycardia
- Atrial tachycardia

Flecainide
- Fatigue
- Metallic taste, loss of appetite
- Gastrointestinal disturbance
- ST segment elevation-Brugada
- QRS prolongation
- Proarrhythmia

pregnancy. It may lead to hydrops fetalis when it is incessant or in earlier gestations, with fast heart rates above 250 bpm. On the other hand, intermittent tachycardia has also been shown to be associated with complications[60–64, 66].

Multiple ultrasound methods, such as M-mode, pulse wave, tissue Doppler and direct recording of fetal electrocardiogram can be used to tease out the nature of irregular rhythms (Figure 8.18). Each of these modalities has its own advantages and limitations (Table 8.16). M-mode can help diagnose AV relationship in any rhythm but interval measurements are a little less accurate with this method compared to pulse wave or tissue Doppler assessment. M-mode is also helpful in assessing how well the atria and ventricles are contracting. Pulse wave Doppler can also be used if the operator positions the ultrasound beam between the mitral valve and aortic outflow tract. Newer technologies involving recording of fetal electrocardiogram are still evolving.

There are numerous complicated treatment algorithms for SVT or AF either proposing digoxin,

propranolol, sotalol, amiodarone, and flecainide alone or in combination[56–64]. Mortality rates as high as 30% and with up to 8% neurological morbidity remain attached to some of these treatment regimens.

Digoxin has been commonly used as the first-line agent in nonhydropic fetuses with varying success rates of between 46% and 62%. If there is hydrops, digoxin exhibits lower success rates of 0–10%. As a single agent or in combination with digoxin, flecainide has been shown to have an up to 95% efficacy and no mortality. Sotalol has been used as a second-line agent with low conversion rates of 40–60%, and disappointingly higher fetal mortality rates of 19% in fetal SVT. Amiodarone has been shown to be effective but with a slower action. One preferred approach has been a combination treatment with digoxin and flecainide from the onset of the diagnosis of tachycardia until delivery (Table 8.19) [62]. This particular approach in our practice had resulted in survival of all fetuses with high conversion rates (95% in atrioventricular re-entry tachycardia and 50% in AF) and successful rate control of AF (100%). Maternal side effects are mild and commonly resolve with reduction

Table 8.20 Treatment protocol for ventricular tachycardia. U&Es, urea and electrolytes; LFTs, liver function tests; LQTS, long QT syndrome; HCM, hypertropic cardiomyopathy; ARVC, arrhythmogenic right ventricular cardiomyopathy; ECG, echocardiography; HR, heart rate; TID, ter in die (three times per day); IV, intravenous; D5W, 5% dextrose in water; BP, blood pressure.

Fetal ventricular tachycardia	Maternal assessment

Fetal ventricular tachycardia

Exclude maternal and fetal infection, hyperthyroidism, fetal distress

- Consider delivery if gestation >36–38 weeks
- Detailed obstetric scan
- Fetal echocardiogram

Admit and keep until sinus rhythm restored
No long QT syndrome, cardiac dysfunction or hydrops:
- Amiodarone 150–300 mg over 1–2 hours IV then infusion 500 mg/hr (Max 2g/day), or 15mg/kg/day IV or 500–2000 mg /day
- Amiodarone oral 600–800 mg TID loading for 7 days (Max 2.4g/day)
- Add Propranolol 80 mg TID if no response
- Maintenance amiodarone oral 200–800 mg/day
- Sotalol 80–120 mg TID orally
- Flecainide 100 mg TID orally

If hydrops or cardiac dysfunction
- IV magnesium 1–2 g given in 100 mL of D5W over 30–60 min; may be repeated q4h

Torsade de pointes and long QT syndrome suspected
- IV magnesium 1–2 g IV given in 100 mL of D5W over 1–2 min (4–8 mmol or 25–50 mg/kg); may be repeated every 4h (watch BP and deep tendon reflexes)
- Lidocaine loading dose 1.0–1.5 mg/kg IV over 15 minutes followed by 1–3 mg/min IV
- Continue with Propranolol 80 mg TID orally

Maternal assessment
- Baseline U&Es, LFTs, calcium and magnesium, viral screen
- Thyroid function
- Exclude maternal alcohol and substance abuse
- Detailed maternal and paternal medical history to exclude LQTS, HCM, ARVC, Brugada, CMP, heart block
- Maternal ECG

Advice to pregnant women
- Monitor fetal movement by kick count, if there is any concern seek immediate help

Fetal medicine follow up
- Twice weekly fetal heart rate auscultation by a midwife to ensure HR is not above 180 at all times
- Weekly ultrasound examination of fetal and placental well-being by a fetal medicine specialist to exclude hydrops development

Fetal cardiology review
- Weekly echocardiogram to monitor cardiac function, fetal heart rate

Delivery decision
- Sinus rhythm, normal delivery if there are no maternal or fetal concerns.
- If ventricular tachycardia, Caesarean section.

of dose. So-called "long RP tachycardias" (atrial tachycardia or permanent junctional re-entry tachycardia) are more resistant to antiarrhythmic treatment, and direct fetal treatment may be required in such cases. Early delivery before 34 weeks of gestation should be avoided; however, in some difficult cases this may be the only option.

Ventricular tachycardia

Ventricular tachycardia is the rarest arrhythmia in the fetus and its diagnosis remains challenging due to the fact that the presence of atrioventricular dissociation may be difficult to ascertain. The choice of antiarrhythmic treatment varies dependent on the mechanism and etiology of ventricular arrhythmia (Table 8.20) [62]. In cases with long QT syndrome, treatment may include lidocaine (administered directly into the fetal umbilical vein) or with oral maternal administration of propranolol or mexiletine. Sotalol or amiodarone can be tried in more difficult cases of ventricular tachycardia, but the prognosis of this arrhythmia remains guarded[58–60, 66].

References

1. Carvalho JS, Allan LD, Chaoui R, et al. ISUOG Practice Guidelines (updated): sonographic screening examination of the fetal heart. *Ultrasound Obstet Gynecol* 2013; 41: 348–59.
2. The American Institute of Ultrasound in Medicine. AIUM practice guideline for the performance of fetal echocardiography. *J Ultrasound Med* 2011; 30: 127–36.
3. Cardiac screening examination of the fetus: guidelines for performing the 'basic' and extended basic' cardiac scan. *Ultrasound Obstet Gynecol* 2006; 27(1): 107–13.
4. Yagel S, Cohen SM, Achiron R. Examination of the fetal heart by five short axis views: a proposed screening method for comprehensive cardiac evaluation. *Ultrasound Obstet Gynecol* 2001; 17(5): 367–9.
5. Rychik J, Ayres N, Cuneo B, et al. American Society of Echocardiography guidelines and standards for performance of the fetal echocardiogram. *J Am Soc Echocardiogr* 2004; 17: 803–10.
6. Vergani P, Mariani S, Ghidini A, et al. Screening for congenital heart disease with the four chamber view of the fetal heart. *Am J Obstet Gynecol* 1992; 167: 1000–3.

7. Buskens E, Grobbee DE, Frohn-Mulder IM, et al. Efficacy of routine fetal ultrasound screening for congenital heart disease in normal pregnancy. *Circulation* 1996; 94: 67–72.

8. Copel JA, Pilu G, Green J, et al. Fetal echocardiographic screening for congenital heart disease: The importance of the four-chamber view. *Am J Obstet Gynecol* 1987; 157: 648.

9. Oggè G, Gaglioti P, Maccanti S, et al. Prenatal screening for congenital heart disease with four-chamber and outflow-tract views: A multicenter study. *Ultrasound Obstet Gynecol* 2006; 28: 779.

10. Chaoui R. The four-chamber view: four reasons why it seems to fail in screening for cardiac abnormalities and suggestions to improve detection rates. *Ultrasound Obstet Gynecol* 2003; 22: 3.

11. DeVore GR. The aortic and pulmonary outflow tract screening in the human fetus. *J Ultrasound Med* 1992; 11: 345.

12. Carvalho JS, Mavrides E, Shinebourne E, et al. Improving the effectiveness of routine prenatal screening for major congenital heart defects. *Heart* 2002; 88: 387.

13. Kirk JS, Riggs TW, Comstock CH, et al. Prenatal screening for cardiac anomalies: The value of routine addition of the aortic root to the four chamber view. *Obstet Gynecol* 1994; 84: 427.

14. Allan L, Hornberger L, Sharland G (eds). *Textbook of Fetal Cardiology*. London: Greenwich Medical Media, 2000.

15. Yagel S, Silverman N, Gembruch U (eds). *Fetal Cardiology*. London: Martin Dunitz, 2003.

16. Schneider C, McCrindle BW, Carvalho JS, et al. Development of Z-scores for fetal cardiac dimensions from echocardiography. *Ultrasound Obstet Gynecol* 2005; 26: 599.

17. DeVore G. The use of Z-scores in the analysis of fetal cardiac dimensions. *Ultrasound Obstet Gynecol* 2005; 26: 596.

18. Firpo C, Hoffman J, Silverman N. Evaluation of fetal heart dimensions from 12 weeks to term. *Am J Cardiol* 2001; 87: 594.

19. Khoshnood B, De Vigan C, Vodovar V, et al. Trends in prenatal diagnosis, pregnancy termination, and perinatal mortality of newborns with congenital heart disease in France, 1983–2000: a population-based evaluation. *Pediatrics* 2005; 115: 95.

20. Hoffman, JI, Kaplan, S. The incidence of congenital heart disease. *J. Am. Coll. Cardiol* 2002; 39: 1890–1900.

21. Ferencz C, Rubin JD, McCarter RJ, et al. Congenital heart disease: Prevalence at live birth. The Baltimore-Washington Infant Study. *Am J Epidemiol* 1985; 121: 31.

22. Garne E, Stoll C, Clementi M; Euroscan Group. Evaluation of prenatal diagnosis of congenital heart diseases by ultrasound: experience from 20 European registries. *Ultrasound Obstet Gynecol* 2001; 17: 386.

23. Ariane J, Marelli AS, Mackie RII, et al. Congenital heart disease in the general population changing prevalence and age distribution. *Circulation* 2007; 115: 163–172.

24. van der Linde D, Konings EE, Slager MA, et al. Birth prevalence of congenital heart disease worldwide: a systematic review and meta-analysis. *J Am Coll Cardiol* 2011; 58(21): 2241–7.

25. Hoffman J, Christianson R. Congenital heart disease in a cohort of 19,502 births with long-term follow-up. *Am J Cardiol* 1978; 42: 641.

26. Allen H, Gutgesell H, Clark E, et al. (eds). *Moss and Adams' Heart Disease in Infants, Children and Adolescents Including the Fetus and Young Adult*, 6th ed. Philadelphia: Lippincott Williams & Wilkins, 2001.

27. Keane J, Lock J, Fyler D, et al. (eds). *Nadas' Pediatric Cardiology*, 2nd edn. Philadelphia: Saunders, 2006.

28. Rajiah P, Mak C, Dubinksy TJ, et al. Ultrasound of fetal cardiac anomalies. *AJR Am J Roentgenol* 2011; 197(4): W747–60.

29. Burch M. Congenital heart disease. *Medicine* 2006; 34; 7: 274–281.

30. Jaeggi ET, Sholler GF, Jones OD, et al. Comparative analysis of pattern, management and outcome or pre versus postnatally diagnosed major congenital heart disease: A population-based study. *Ultrasound Obstet Gynecol* 2001; 17: 380.

31. Kirklin JW, Barratt-Boyes BG. *Cardiac Surgery*, 2nd edn. New York: Churchill Livingstone, 1993.

32. Anderson RH, Macartney FJ, Shinebourne EA, et al. *Paediatric Cardiology*. Edinburgh: Churchill Livingstone, 2001.

33. Uzun, O Ethical dilemmas in Fetal Cardiology: improving outcomes or reducing incidence. *Welsh Paed J* 2008; 24: 22–25.

34. Gopalakrishnan PN, Sinha A, Uzun O. Change in referral and diagnostic trends in fetal cardiac screening over 7 years in South Wales. *Arch Dis Child Fetal Neonatal Ed* 2011; 96: Fa66–Fa67.

35. Sinha A, Gopalakrishnan PN, Tucker D, et al. Outcome after prenatal diagnosis of hypoplastic left heart syndrome (HLHS) in South Wales over a 7-year period. *Arch Dis Child Fetal Neonatal Ed* 2011; 96: Fa67.

36. Sinha A, Gopalakrishnan PN, Tucker D, et al. Outcome of all antenatally diagnosed cases of complete atrioventricular septal defect (CAVSD) in South Wales over a 7 year period: impact of associated chromosomal

anomalies. *Arch Dis Child Fetal Neonatal Ed* 2011; 96: Fa69.

37. Uzun O, Sinha A. Outcome of hypoplastic left and right heart syndrome (HLHS and HRHS) after antenatal diagnosis in South Wales over a seven year period. *Cardiol Young* 2011; 21 (Suppl. 1): S1–S167.

38. Uzun O. Outcome of congenital heart defects associated with 22q11.2 Deletion. AEPC 2012, Istanbul. *Cardiol Young* 2012; 22 (Suppl. S1): S3–S176.

39. Uzun O, Ofoe V, Worrall S. Changing trends in tetralogy of Fallot: impact of improved antenatal detection rate, earlier catheter and surgical intervention. *Cardiol Young* 2014; 24 (Suppl. 1): S148.

40. Uzun O, Babaoglu K, Bendapudi P, et al. Total anomalous pulmonary venous connection: clinical presentation and long term outcome of 60 patients at a single institution in 32 years. AEPC 2014 Helsinki. *Cardiol Young* 2014; 24 (Suppl. 1): S60–61.

41. Pierpont ME, Craig T, Basson D. Genetic basis for congenital heart defects: current knowledge. A scientific statement from the American Heart Association Congenital Cardiac Defects Committee Council on Cardiovascular Disease in the Young. *Circulation* 2007; 115: 3015–38.

42. Peter J, Gruber PJ, Epstein JA. Development gone awry: congenital heart Disease. *Circ Res* 2004; 94: 273–83.

43. Kyle Niessen K, Karsan A. Notch signaling in cardiac development. *Circ Res* 2008; 102: 1169–81.

44. Stankunas K, Shang C, Twu KY, et al. Pbx/Meis deficiencies demonstrate multigenetic origins of congenital heart disease. *Circ Res* 2008; 103: 702–9.

45. James J, Noba JJ. Multifactorial inheritance hypothesis for the etiology of congenital heart diseases: the genetic-environmental interaction. *Circulation* 1968; 38: 604–17.

46. Goldmuntz E. The genetic contribution to congenital heart disease. *Pediatr Clin N Am* 2004; 51: 1721–37.

47. Marino B, Digilio MC. Congenital heart disease and genetic syndromes: Specific correlation between cardiac phenotype and genotype. *Cardiovasc Pathol* 2000; 9: 303–15.

48. Nora JJ, Nora AH. Maternal transmission of congenital heart diseases: new recurrence risk figures and the questions of cytoplasmic inheritance and vulnerability to teratogens. *Am J Cardiol* 1987; 59: 459.

49. Allan LD, Crawford DC, Chita SK, et al. Familial recurrence of congenital heart disease in a prospective series of mothers referred for fetal echocardiography. *Am J Cardiol* 1986; 58: 334.

50. Boughman JA, Berg KA, Astemborski JA, et al. Familial risks of congenital heart defect in a population-based epidemiological study. *Am J Med Genet* 1987; 26: 839.

51. Whittemore R, Wells J, Castellsague X. A second-generation study of 427 probands with congenital heart defects and their 837 children. *J Am Coll Cardiol* 1994; 23: 1459.

52. Hyett J, Perdu M, Sharland G, et al. Using fetal nuchal translucency to screen for major congenital cardiac defects at 10–14 weeks of gestation: population based cohort study. *BMJ* 1999; 318: 81.

53. Burn J, Brennan P, Little J, et al: Recurrence risks in offspring of adults with major heart defects: Results from first cohort of British collaborative study. *Lancet* 1998; 351: 311.

54. Garne E, Stoll C, Clementi M; Euroscan Group. Evaluation of prenatal diagnosis of congenital heart diseases by ultrasound: experience from 20 European registries. *Ultrasound Obstet Gynecol* 2001; 17: 386.

55. Copel JA, Pilu G, Kleinman CS. Congenital heart disease and extracardiac anomalies: Associations and indications for fetal echocardiography. *Am J Obstet Gynecol* 1986; 154: 1121.

56. Kleinman C, Nehgme R, Copel J. Fetal cardiac arrhythmias: diagnosis and therapy. In: Creasy R, Resnik R, Iams J (eds). *Maternal-Fetal Medicine*, 5th edn. Philadelphia: Saunders, 2003.

57. Kleinman CS, Nehgme RA. Cardiac arrhythmias in the human fetus. *Pediatr Cardiol* 2004; 25: 234.

58. Simpson J. Fetal arrhythmias. *Ultrasound Obstet Gynecol* 2006; 27: 599.

59. Respondek M, Wloch A, Kaczmarek P, et al. Diagnostic and perinatal management of fetal extrasystole. *Pediatr Cardiol* 1997; 18: 361.

60. Strasburger J, Huhta J, Carpenter R, et al. Doppler echocardiography in the diagnosis and management of persistent fetal arrhythmias. *J Am Coll Cardiol* 1986; 7: 1386.

61. Uzun O, Sinha A, Beattie B. Comparison of transplacental treatment of fetal supraventricular tachyarrhythmias with digoxin, flecainide, and sotalol: Results of a nonrandomized multicenter study. *Circulation* 2012; 125: e956.

62. Uzun O, Babaoglu K, Sinha A, et al. Rapid control of foetal supraventricular tachycardia with digoxin and flecainide combination treatment. *Cardiol Young* 2011; 29: 1–9.

63. Uzun O, Babaoglu K, Ayhan YI, et al. Maternal serum antiarrhythmic drug levels do not predict fetal supraventricular tachycardia response time. AEPC 2013, London. *Cardiol Young* 2013; 23 (Suppl. 1): S57.

64. Babaoglu K, Uzun O, Ayhan YI, et al. 10-year review of outcome of fetal arrhythmias in Wales. AEPC 2012, Istanbul. *Cardiol Young* 2012; 22 (Suppl. S1): S3–S176.

65. Uzun O. Outcome of heart block diagnosed during fetal and postnatal life. AEPC 2012, Istanbul. *Cardiol Young* 2012; 22 (Suppl. S1): S3–S176.

66. Donofrio MT, Moon-Grady AJ, Hornberger LK, et al; American Heart Association Adults with Congenital Heart Disease Joint Committee of the Council on Cardiovascular Disease in the Young and Council on Clinical Cardiology, Council on Cardiovascular Surgery and Anesthesia, and Council on Cardiovascular and Stroke Nursing. Diagnosis and treatment of fetal cardiac disease: a scientific statement from the American Heart Association. *Circulation* 2014; 129(21): 2183–242.

Chapter

9

Fetal thoracic anomalies

R. Bryan Beattie

Embryology and normal lung development

Normal lung development is dependent upon the presence of normal fetal breathing, an adequate intrathoracic space, adequate levels of amniotic fluid, normal amounts of lung fluid within the lungs and airways and normal pulmonary blood flow. Other factors that may adversely affect it include maternal health and nutrition, local and systemic endocrine factors, smoking, and other diseases. Although not required for intrauterine survival, it is essential that there is normal fetal lung development prior to birth. It is also an important source of amniotic fluid contributing about 15 mL per kg body weight.

There are five main phases of intrauterine lung development, as shown in the schematic below, and the phases in which some of the thoracic malformations develop are listed below.

- Embryonic: laryngeal, tracheal stenosis, tracheal/esophageal fistula, pulmonary sequestration, bronchogenic cysts.
- Pseudoglandular: pulmonary hypoplasia, malacia, congenital cystic adenomatoid malformation.
- Canalicular; pulmonary hypoplasia, arteriovenous malformation.
- Saccular: pulmonary hyperplasia.
- Alveolar: lobar emphysema, lymphatic anomalies.

At birth

The amniotic fluid and lung secretions fill the airways prior to birth. During early labor, the production of fetal adrenaline and maternal thyrotrophin-releasing hormone cause the fetal pulmonary epithelial cells to absorb lung fluid. Active pulmonary fluid absorption

is increased and most of the lung fluid is cleared within the first 2 hrs of extrauterine life. There is active transport of sodium ions from the alveolar spaces into the interstitial tissues. Tactile stimulation and changes in temperature are potent stimulants to fetal breathing. The inflation of the lungs leads to a fall in pulmonary vascular arteriolar resistance and increased pulmonary blood flow. The alveoli become aerated and are lined with surfactant, and the lungs become much easier to aereate at lower negative intrathoracic pressures.

Normal healthy lungs are composed of an orderly system of tubes (airways) and sacs (airspaces or alveoli) in a strict relationship to pulmonary blood vessels (arterial from the right ventricle and venous return to the left atrium) with a normally developed systemic blood supply (aorta to superior vena cava) and lymphatic drainage. Congenital lung malformations arise whenever one or more of these structures are abnormal or when their relationships are altered.

Congenital lung malformations represent 5–19% of all congenital anomalies. This range may be an underestimate because of the high frequency of undetected or asymptomatic lesions.

Ultrasound of the normal thorax

The main views used to assess the thorax are the four-chamber view of the heart and the saggital view of the diaphragm. The heart usually occupies about one-third of the chest and the axis should be about 45° to the anteroposterior midline. The position within the chest should also be noted to identify any mediastinal shift. Other important observations include the presence of polyhydramnios, which may reflect a mass or pressure effect if a lung lesion, mass or abnormality is identified.

Fetal Medicine, ed. Bidyut Kumar and Zarko Alfirevic. Published by Cambridge University Press. © Cambridge University Press 2016.

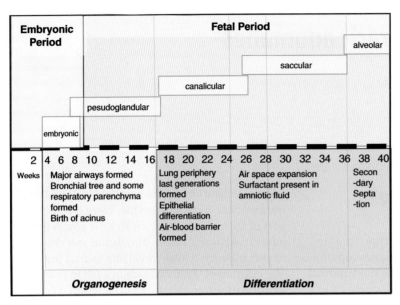

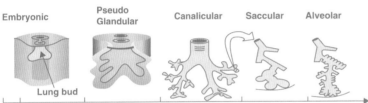

Figure 9.1 Schematic diagram showing the timeline for embryologic and fetal lung development, with pictorial representation below.

Ultrasound of thoracic malformations

Lung malformations are rare but are an important cause of morbidity and mortality from infection, hemorrhage and hypoxia. The overall outcome is dependent on their size, local pressure effects and effect on lung function[1]. Small lesions are often asymptomatic and easily missed. Most fetal parenchymal lung pathology appears as an echogenic lung mass, which may be unilateral (congenital diaphragmatic hernia (CDH), congenital cystic adenomatoid malformation of the lung (CCAML), pulmonary sequestration) or bilateral (laryngeal atresia), but lesions may apparently resolve later in the pregnancy or be complicated by cystic components often seen in CDH and CCAML. Large fluid-filled lobes may be present in congenital lobar emphysema. Indeed postnatal X-rays and ultrasound scans may appear normal and computed tomography (CT) or magnetic resonance imaging (MRI) may be indicated.

In the case of pulmonary hypoplasia, there may be other clues to their aetiology, such as oligohydramnios or renal pathology as the principle etiology, ultrasound markers for fetal chromosomal abnormalities, skeletal dysplasia or central nervous system malformations, or abnormal movements or posture due to neuromuscular disease.

Lung biometry and blood flow studies

Lung growth is linear from about 16–40 weeks.

Ratios between thoracic circumference (TC) or diameter and reference measurements such as abdominal circumference (AC), head circumference, femur length and end-diastolic biventricular cardiac diameter remain constant with a high correlation coefficient in normal pregnancy[2–4].

The TC:AC ratio is normally >0.8 after 20 weeks; absolute and relative TC measurements are useful in predicting subsequent pulmonary hypoplasia and serial TC:AC ratios are predictive in early premature rupture of membranes[5].

Lung:head ratios (LHR) have also been shown to correlate with subsequent prognosis[6].

- LHR ≤1, the prognosis is poor.
- LHR 1.0–1.4, extracorporeal membranous oxygenation (ECMO) is often needed.
- LHR >1.4, the prognosis is better.

Prenatal MRI is a useful adjunct to ultrasound imaging and also allows assessment of the nature and the size of lungs and lung lesions. Whilst pulmonary artery blood flow can be measured using Doppler ultrasound, it is of limited value in assessing the likelihood pulmonary hypoplasia, although color Doppler imaging is useful in differentiating CCAML from pulmonary sequestration.

Congenital diaphragmatic hernia

Congenital diaphragmatic hernia (CDH) affects around 1:4,000 births and occurs when the diaphragm fails to form a complete barrier in the pleuroperitoneal canal between the thoracic and abdominal cavities (usually around 10 weeks). This leads to the presence of any combination of bowel, stomach and other herniated organs into the thoracic cavity causing significant morbidity and mortality from the compounded effects of pulmonary hypoplasia, abnormal lung development, pulmonary hypertension and cardiac compression.

There is a high incidence of associated abnormalities (30–60%), chromosomal abnormalities (10–20%) and other genetic syndromes (e.g., Beckwith–Wiedemann syndrome), and thus a careful search for other anomalies and the offer of karyotyping is appropriate. CDH is often identified at the routine 20-week anomaly scan when the fetal stomach cannot be found in its normal position in the abdomen below the diaphragm. The stomach and other herniated viscera, such as the bowel, liver and spleen, are found in the chest. Some CDHs are variable in appearance with the stomach and bowel sliding in and out of the chest. Other differential

diagnoses include CCAML, bronchopulmonary sequestration and thoracic teratomas.

Pressure effects within the chest can cause esophageal compression leading to polyhydramnios and cardiac compression leading to hydrops. Thus, in all cases of CDH, serial scans are required to monitor for these features.

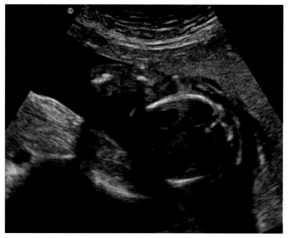

Figure 9.3 Transverse ultrasound scan through fetal thorax showing fetal heart and stomach in the same plane. Note the appearance of a single rib on either side confirms that this is not an oblique view.

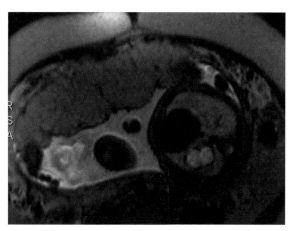

Figure 9.4 Transverse magnetic resonance imaging of left-sided congenital diaphragmatic hernia with the stomach seen in the middle of the left hemithorax. The right lung is normal. Axial, sagittal and coronal T2-weighted sequences were obtained through the fetal thorax and abdomen. The stomach and several loops of bowel are lying posteriorly within the lower left thorax. On the sagittal images, there is suggestion that the anterior part of the diaphragm is intact but cannot differentiate between this being a posterior diaphragmatic hernia or an eventration. There is, however, a good lung volume bilaterally and the heart lies centrally with no mediastinal shift. Normal abdominal organs.

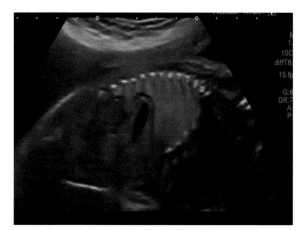

Figure 9.2 Saggital ultrasound scan section through fetal trunk showing congenital diaphragmatic hernia, with the stomach clearly seen within the thoracic cavity.

Prognosis

Various factors have been assessed to try to predict the prognosis in cases of CDH, with liver herniation a predictor of poor outcome and LHR ratio being shown to be of prognostic value[6]. The LHR is measured at the level of the heart in the four-chamber view and compared with the HC. Low LHR values of <1 are associated with poor survival rates around 10%. The LHR is gestation dependent and gestation specific charts should be used rather than a fixed threshold value.

Attempts to assess lung volume using two-(2D) and three-dimensional (3D) ultrasound and MRI have had variable success.

Initial management

Following a diagnosis of CDH, referral should be made to a tertiary fetal medicine unit for a detailed anatomic survey, including an assessment of fetal anatomy, identification of ultrasound markers, amniotic fluid index, a fetal echo, karyotyping and more recently microarray-comparative genome hybridization studies. Amniotic fluid is preferred to fetal blood as conditions like Pallister–Killian syndrome can be missed by analyzing fetal blood. Fetal MRI or 3D ultrasound may be of value to evaluate lung volume. Counseling should be offered with involvement of a multidisciplinary team, including a pediatric surgeon and/or a neonatologist regarding the neonatal and long-term implications, and neonatal and surgical management. Termination of pregnancy would also be an option and should be discussed in view of the high mortality and morbidity. Subsequent management includes serial scans to identify polyhydramnios, which increases the risk of preterm labor and may require specific management, and for fetal hydrops, which may warrant early delivery.

In utero treatment

Treatment in utero has been successful in some cases using ultrasound and then fetoscopic-guided tracheal occlusion. This technique has been shown to improve lung mass, airway branching and pulmonary vascular development. The main benefit seems to be preventing the escape of lung fluid, which distends the airways, and importantly the distal airways, during the critical canalicular and secular phases of lung development. For this reason, it is of minimal value in late pregnancy. Although the evidence from randomized controlled trials has shown little benefit in terms of overall survival from in utero treatment (73% treated in utero compared to 77% controls), a subgroup with potentially the worst prognosis who had liver herniation and LHR <1 did show a marked improvement in survival from 10% to 40–50% when treated in utero[7]. An unresolved challenge is the morbidity and mortality of premature delivery.

Delivery and neonatal care

In general, delivery would be at term in a tertiary unit with access to on-site neonatal surgery and neonatal intensive care unit (NICU) facilities. A senior pediatrician should be present with early elective intubation. There is no advantage to cesarean section and the mode of delivery would be on the basis of normal obstetric grounds. Following delivery, stabilisation is essential prior to surgery with major challenges from pulmonary hypoplasia and pulmonary hypertension. In some cases, ECMO may need to be considered. Prostacyclin and nitrous oxide may also be of benefit. Surgery will usually be with primary closure or in cases of a large defect, a mesh may be required. Resumption of normal feeding is often slow, and prolonged total parenteral nutrition may often be required.

Congenital cystic adenomatoid malformation of the lung

Cystic congenital adenomatoid malformation of the lung (CCAML) affects 1 in 1,100–3,500 live births, is more common in males than females and accounts for about 25% of all lung malformations. Abnormal lung development is thought to be due to aberrant HOXB-5, FGF-7 and PDGFB genes. The affected parts of the lung are deficient in normal alveoli, and there is both proliferation and abnormal branching and cystic dilatation of the terminal respiratory bronchioles. The cysts that result from the overgrowth of the terminal bronchioles may be small and give an echogenic appearance (microcystic) or may coalesce into larger visible cysts (macrocystic), which can be seen on ultrasound.

Most are unilateral (85%) and they are commoner on the left side (60%). CCAML will often be identified at the routine 20-week anomaly scan as a unilateral or bilateral echogenic lung mass with or without visible cysts. Local pressure effects can occur causing pulmonary hypoplasia of the surrounding and indeed contralateral lung and the risk of esophageal compression and polyhydramnios and cardiac compression and hydrops. The risk of hydrops is greatest for those

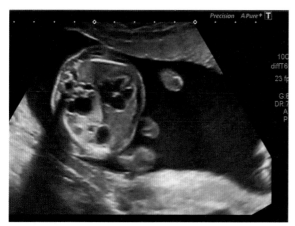

Figure 9.5 Transverse ultrasound scan section through fetal thorax showing extensive macrocystic congenital cystic adenomatoid malformation of the lung, echogenic lung and large lung cysts on the right side.

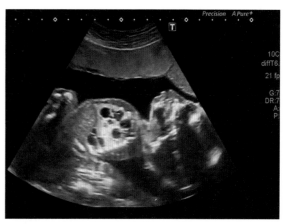

Figure 9.6 Ultarsound saggital section through fetal body showing extensive macrocystic congenital cystic adenomatoid malformation of the lung and echogenic lung.

with large lesions and high CCAML:HC ratios have been shown to be predictive of subsequent development of hydrops. Generally, the maximum growth is in midtrimester, with reduced growth towards the end of the pregnancy. The echogenicity is also often reduced in late pregnancy and the lesion may no longer be visible on ultrasound giving the false reassurance that it has resolved.

Differentiation from bronchopulmonary sequestration may be difficult as the vascular supply and drainage is derived from the pulmonary system and lesions may have a systemic arterial blood supply similar to that seen in bronchopulmonary sequestration. These are referred to as hybrid lesions. Some authorities suggest that since it is not possible to distinguish CCAML from these hybrid lesions, the term "congenital pulmonary airway malformation" (CPAM) should be used instead.

After birth, the ventilation of the abnormal alveolar tissue, which can often be seen on a chest X-ray, poses a significant risk of respiratory distress and pneumothorax. Unilateral solid or cystic lung masses on a neonatal X-ray should always arouse suspicion of a possible CCAML.

Prognosis

In general, about 45–85% of antenatally diagnosed CCAML will spontaneously regress; however, large macrocystic or solid lesions can cause local pressure effects leading to polyhydramnios and preterm delivery, hydrops, pulmonary hypoplasia, cardiac

dysfunction and perinatal death. Assessment of CPAM volume ratio (CVR), based on comparison with HC on ultrasound and fetal MRI, has been shown to be prognostic with smaller lesions with a CVR <1.6 having a better outcome[8–10].

Classically there are three described types of CCAML.

(1) Macrocystic (13%). Best prognosis. One or more large cysts (>5 mm) lined with pseudostratified ciliated epithelium.

(2) Microcystic (73%). Small cysts giving the lungs a bright echogenic appearance, lined with ciliated columnar or cuboidal epithelium.

(3) Solid (13%). Worst prognosis. Cuboidal epithelium-lined bronchioles. This tissue is airless in postnatal life.

Although the macrocystic types have larger cysts, they tend to involve smaller volumes of lung than the microcystic or solid types, and hence their relatively better prognosis. Other pathologic classifications are based on a five-category system:

(1) type 0 – acinar dysplasia

(2) type I – multiple large cysts or a single dominant cyst

(3) type II – multiple evenly spaced small cysts – may be associated with other abnormalities

(4) type III – mainly solid mass

(5) type IV – mainly peripheral cysts.

It is thought that the appearance may relate to the abnormal phase of lung development with types I–III having bronchiolar epithelium due to abnormal pseudoglandular development and type IV having alveolar acinar epithelium. All types are usually in direct communication with the tracheobronchiolar tree.

Antenatal diagnosis and initial management

The main features of CCAML are often identified on the routine anomaly scan on the basis of either an echogenic lung mass or cystic areas within the lungs. More subtle findings, such as cardiac axis deviation or mediastinal shift, should prompt a careful search for other lung pathology, such as CCAML or CDH.

CCAML is usually an isolated abnormality but some may be associated with other structural abnormalities, particularly cardiac (tetralogy of Fallot (TOF) and truncus arteriosus). A detailed anatomic survey should therefore be undertaken including an assessment of fetal anatomy, amniotic fluid index and exclusion of hydrops and a fetal echo. The role for karyotyping is controversial as this is not usually a feature of CCAML, but the suspected diagnosis of CCAML may be incorrect. Following the diagnosis of any significant lung pathology, the patient should be referred to a tertiary fetal medicine center for multidisciplinary review, and subsequent management may include counseling by a pediatric surgeon and/or a neonatologist regarding the neonatal and long-term implications, and neonatal and surgical management. Termination of pregnancy would also be an option, particularly for larger or complex nonisolated lesions, and should also be discussed. A careful search for a feeding vessel, which would be suggestive of a bronchopulmonary sequestration as opposed to a hybrid lesion should be sought, but in hybrid cases they tend to arise from the descending aorta. Other differential diagnoses include a CDH, bronchogenic cyst or neuroblastoma.

Subsequent management

Subsequent management includes serial scans to identify polyhydramnios, which increases the risk of preterm labor and may require specific management, and fetal hydrops, which may warrant early delivery. The echogenicity of the lesions usually darkens in late pregnancy giving the false reassurance that the CCAML has apparently resolved. Mediastinal shift may be an indicator of a higher risk of pulmonary hypoplasia and respiratory failure.

In utero treatment

In type 1 or macrocystic CCAML, there may a single large cyst, which can cause significant pressure effects leading to polyhydramnios or hydrops. Pleuroperitoneal aspiration or drainage may be beneficial, particularly when hydrops is present. In such cases, shunting may be preferable as the fluid tends to reaccumulate following aspiration.

Delivery and neonatal care

In most cases, the multidisciplinary team is likely to advise delivery at term in a tertiary unit with access to on-site neonatal surgery and NICU facilities as antenatal assessment cannot accurately predict the likely degree of respiratory compromise in the newborn, although larger lesions and those with significant mediastinal shift pose a greater risk. A senior pediatrician should be present with recourse to early elective intubation. There is no advantage to cesarean section, and the mode of delivery would be on the basis of normal obstetric grounds. Admission to NICU for observation is advised and an early chest X-ray should be performed. In most cases (about 60%), cystic adenomatoid malformation manifests clinically with respiratory complications soon after the neonatal period. It also results in recurrent chest infections due to poor clearance of mucous and other lung secretions.

Many lesions will regress to some extent following birth but late effects, though rare, include malignancy in the form of pulmonary blastoma, rhabdomyosarcoma, and bronchoalveolar carcinoma. Whilst surgery may usually be deferred until about 2 years old, if the baby is well and there is no significant respiratory compromise or recurrent serious respiratory infections, because of the risk of recurrent infections and malignancy, the affected lung tissue is usually removed and the long-term outcome is then usually good. Early surgery may, however, sometimes be needed if there is significant early respiratory compromise.

Bronchopulmonary sequestration

Pulmonary sequestration accounts for 6% of all congenital lung malformations and affects 1:1,000 live births. It mostly affects the lower lobes. A sequestration is a bronchopulmonary mass without a normal bronchial communication, and is thought to be due to development of a primitive lung bud from the foregut during embryonic development. The affected part of the lung is not connected to the airways, although rarely, communication with the tracheobronchial tree may occur via fistulas. The vascular supply is usually also abnormal with the arterial blood supply coming from the systemic side of the circulation (and directly off the aorta in 80% of cases) rather than the pulmonary circulation. It is important to distinguish sequestration from Scimitar syndrome in which there is tracheobronchial communication and venous drainage.

The affected part of the lung may be intralobar (75%) or extralobar (25%) with no sex differentiation in the incidence of intralobar lesions but a 4:1 male-to-female ratio in those with extralobar lesions[11]. It is thought that intralobar lesions are due to abnormal early lung budding, which leads to an area of lung with no separate pleural covering, whereas extralobar sequestration forms a lung lesion consisting of lung parenchymal tissue with a distinct pleural covering, which delineates it from the normal surrounding lung.

Intralobar lesions

Intralobar or intrapulmonary lesions more commonly affect the posterior lung bases (99%). About 10% are associated with other structural abnormalities, such as CDH and eventration, tracheoesophageal fistula, cardiac defects, foregut abnormalities and chromosomal abnormalities. Despite the arterial supply being from the systemic circulation, the venous drainage is usually through the pulmonary circulation. One important differential diagnosis is an azygous lobe, which is a malformation of the right upper lobe caused by an aberrant azygous vein suspended by a pleural mesentery. An azygous lobe is a radiographic curiosity without clinical significance that occurs in 0.5% of the general population.

Extralobar lesions

Although most (90%) extralobar (extrapulmonary) lesions are above the diaphragm and on the left side (80%), they can also occur below the diaphragm and thus can be easily missed or misinterpreted. Associated structural abnormalities are more common than for intralobar lesions affecting over 60% of cases and may include CDH, gut duplication, vertebral abnormalities and pulmonary hypoplasia. Venous drainage is usually into the systemic circulation via the subdiaphragmatic veins via the azygous system into the right atrium. Pleural effusions may also be present in up to 10%, thought to be due to increased lymphatic transudate in the thorax. They may also connect with the gut.

Imaging

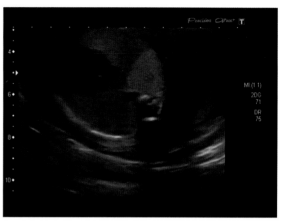

Figure 9.7 Transverse ultrasound scan section through fetal thorax showing intralobar bronchopulmonary sequestration showing an extensive right-sided echogenic lung mass and also normal lung tissue and normal left lung and cardiac axis (main differential diagnosis would be cystic congenital adenomatoid malformation of the lung).

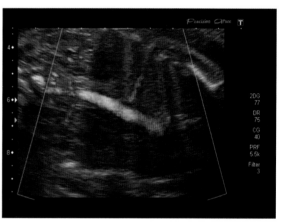

Figure 9.8 Longitudinal coronal ultrasound section with color Doppler imaging of intralobar bronchopulmonary sequestration showing typical features of an abnormal feeding vessel from a direct aortic blood supply.

Antenatal diagnosis and initial management

Sequestrations usually present at the anomaly scan with an echogenic lung mass with or without cardiac axis deviation or mediastinal shift. The main distinguishing diagnostic feature is the presence of a feeding blood vessel, which can be seen on color Doppler[12].

Referral should be made to a tertiary fetal medicine unit for a detailed anatomic survey, including an assessment of fetal anatomy, amniotic fluid index and exclusion of hydrops and a fetal echo. Karyotyping should be offered. Counseling should be offered by a pediatric surgeon and/or a neonatologist regarding the neonatal and long-term implications, and neonatal and surgical management. Termination of pregnancy would also be an option, particularly for larger or complex nonisolated lesions, and should also be discussed. Color or power Doppler may aid in identifying a feeding vessel and its source. The area under the diaphragm should be carefully inspected for abdominal components. Fetal MRI may be considered. Other differential diagnoses include CDH, CCAML, bronchogenic cyst, mediastinal hamartoma or neuroblastoma.

Subsequent management

Subsequent management is based on serial scans to identify changes in the size of the sequestration and in intrathoracic lesions to assess any pressure effects on the oesophagus (causing polyhydramnios) and heart (causing hydrops). Intra-abdominal lesions are unlikely to cause prenatal complications.

In utero treatment

There is no specific intrauterine treatment, but specific treatment may be required for associated pleural effusions (shunt or drainage) and polyhydramnios (amnioreduction or medical treatment), and steroids to mature the lungs if preterm delivery is planned. Hydrops can occur either due to a pressure effect or from vascular shunting and high output cardiac failure.

Delivery and neonatal care

In general, delivery would be at term in a tertiary unit with access to on-site neonatal surgery and NICU facilities. A senior pediatrician should be present and intubation may be required if there is significant respiratory compromise more typically seen in large intrathoracic lesions. There may be a flow murmur due to systemic arterial flow and shunts may lead to congestive cardiac failure

There is no advantage to cesarean section, and the mode of delivery would be on the basis of normal obstetric grounds. Admission to NICU for observation is advised and an early chest X-ray should be performed. Neonatal and early infant morbidity from extralobar sequestration (recurrent chest infections, reduced exercise intolerance due to vascular shunting)

is much higher than for those with intralobar lesions, which often are asymptomatic or present much later with cough, fever, wheeze, chest infections and rarely hemoptysis.

CT, MRI and angiography may be necessary to determine the full extent and blood supply of the lesion[13–15].

Lobectomy is often required for intralobar types as the masses are poorly defined, although segmental resection may be possible for smaller lesions. In extralobar cases, it is often possible to resect just the affected sequestered area with its distinct pleural covering, although the identification and ligation of the abnormal arterial supply is often a significant challenge. In pulmonary sequestration and arteriovenous malformation, systemic arterial blood supply can be embolised, although thoracotomy and resection is usually just as quick as and more effective than embolisation.

Whilst the overall prognosis is usually good, there is also well-recognized chronic morbidity from recurrent chest infections, asthma, gastro-esophageal reflux, pectus excavatum and pyloric stenosis.

Malignant change can also occur in affected lung tissue, such as squamous cell carcinoma, adenocarcinoma and rhabdomyosarcoma.

Congenital lobar emphysema

Congenital lobar emphysema (now sometimes referred to as congenital lobar overinflation (CLO)) is varied in its etiology and can be caused by absence or abnormality (bronchomalacia) of cartilaginous rings causing bronchial stenosis (50%), extrinsic compression causing malacia by structures such as a bronchogenic cyst, vascular abnormalities such as a large pulmonary artery, or mucus plugs. Congenital cytomegalovirus infection has also been implicated. CLO is more common in Caucasian infants and frequently involves the upper lobes (95%) and usually causes mediastinal shift. The left upper lobe is involved in 41% of patients, the right middle lobe in 34% and the right upper lobe in 21%. CLO may be associated with congenital heart defects, such as ventricular septal defect (VSD), patent ductus arteriosus (PDA) and TOF.

After birth, the airways become inflated, but the ball-valve effect of the collapsed softened proximal airways leads to over distension and hyperinflation. There is progressively incremental trapping of air, which leads to significant pressure damage to the surrounding lung tissue. In about 10% of cases, the aetiology is unknown.

Neonatal symptoms of respiratory distress and sometimes progressive cyanosis usually occur within a few days of birth but can be up to about 6 months[16]. It can therefore mimic other conditions, such as cyanotic congenital heart disease, bronchopneumonia and other lung malformations. It occurs more frequently in males with a 3:1 male:female ratio.

Antenatal diagnosis

This is rarely correctly diagnosed during pregnancy, and in most cases it follows the antenatal suspicion of an echogenic lung mass with or without mediastinal shift. As with following a diagnosis of any echogenic lung mass, including those which may turn out to be CLO, referral should be made to a tertiary fetal medicine unit for a detailed anatomic survey, including an assessment of fetal anatomy and amniotic fluid index. Fetal echo is important as associated cardiac malformations are found in about 10–15% (usually a VSD or PDA). Differential from other lung malformations should be possible on the basis of the echogenicicty and reflectivity but prenatal diagnosis is uncommon. Fetal MRI may be of value to make the diagnosis. Counseling should be offered by a pediatric surgeon and/or a neonatologist regarding the neonatal and long-term implications, and neonatal and surgical management.

Subsequent management

Subsequent management includes serial scans to identify polyhydramnios, which increases the risk of preterm labor and may require specific management, and fetal hydrops, which may warrant early delivery.

In utero treatment

This is usually not appropriate.

Delivery and neonatal care

Most cases of CLO can be identified on a neonatal chest X-ray, but can be confused with a tension pneumothorax with inappropriate attempts to treat with a chest drain. It is also important to remember that the area may be fluid-filled in neonates rather than air-filled, and thus appear dark on X-ray. As there is a high risk of misdiagnosis, various other modalities such as CT scan, bronchoscopy and pulmonary angiography (slow and poor arterial filling) ventilation/perfusion scans, MRI (to exclude an anomalous pulmonary artery) and barium studies (to exclude a pulmonary sling or

bronchogenic cyst) may be required in refining the diagnosis and impact.

In the absence of significant respiratory distress, the main morbidity is from recurrent respiratory infection.

The neonate is usually nursed in the decubitus position with the involved side dependent, and the noninvolved side is selectively intubated.

Surgical treatment with lobectomy is often required if conservative management fails. In cases of vascular anomalies causing constriction or pressure, these may need resection. The long-term outcome is usually good following surgery in over 85% cases.

Bronchogenic cysts

Bronchogenic cysts are relatively rare and are thought to be due to foregut duplication due to abnormal budding of the ventral foregut. Most occur very early around 4–8 weeks, and therefore do not communicate with the bronchiolar tree. The majority are right-sided, midline and close to the tracheobronchial tree, but whilst most are mediastinal (85%), the rest are actually within the lung itself. One classification has been proposed based on their location as follows:

- paratracheal
- carinal
- para-esophageal
- hilar
- other.

The cysts may contain normal tracheal tissue, including mucus glands, elastic tissue, smooth muscle and cartilage, are lined with ciliated epithelium and typically 20–100 mm in diameter. The contents may be serous or a protein-rich exudate.

Bronchogenic cysts are probably the most commonly found mediastinal cyst. The cysts are usually single but can be multiple and their location may be central or peripheral and most (70%) are now diagnosed antenatally. If they are suspected antenatally, a neonatal chest X-ray should not be relied upon and a CT scan would always be advised.

The cysts can be central or peripheral. The peripheral cysts are usually multiple and appear in late pregnancy. Postnatally they may be filled with air or fluid with air-fluid levels. The mediastinal cysts are commonly found near the carina and are often attached to, but not in communication with, the tracheobronchial tree. On rare occasions, they have also been found in other remote sites, such as the heart, neck and abdomen.

Imaging

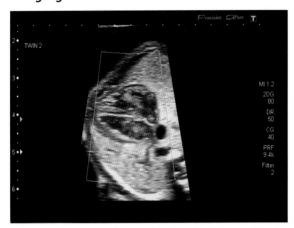

Figure 9.9 Transverse ultrasound section of fetal thorax with color Doppler imaging of a unilocular circular bronchogenic cysts just above the left atrium.

Antenatal diagnosis and initial management

Bronchogenic cysts usually present as well-defined, single, unilocular masses within the mediastinum or lung parenchyma. Their size varies up to 50 mm, increasing in size during the pregnancy, and they may be adherent to the bronchial or bronchiolar wall, or communicate via a pedicle. There is usually no mediastinal shift or mass effect causing polyhydramnios or hydrops. Adjacent lung compression can, however, cause pulmonary hypoplasia.

Following a diagnosis of bronchogenic cyst, referral should be made to a tertiary fetal medicine unit for a detailed anatomic survey, including an assessment of fetal anatomy and amniotic fluid index. Differential diagnosis includes esophageal duplication, cystic hygroma, thymic and thyroid tumors and thyroglossal duct cysts, dermoid cyst, congenital lung emphysema, pulmonary abscess, pneumatocele, bronchial duct cyst, teratomas, necrotic cervical lymphadenopathy, neurogenic tumors, primary malignancy, lipoma and leiomyoma and may be aided by fetal MRI. Counseling should be offered by a pediatric surgeon and/or a neonatologist regarding the neonatal and long-term implications, and neonatal and surgical management.

Subsequent management

Subsequent management includes serial scans to identify polyhydramnios, which increases the risk of preterm labor and may require specific management, and fetal hydrops, which may warrant early delivery.

In utero treatment

This is usually not appropriate, although if there are significant mass effects, aspiration or shunting could be performed.

Delivery and neonatal care

Many bronchogenic cysts are asymptomatic but the main complications are neonatal respiratory distress, infection and hemorrhage and rarely malignant change. Air trapping can also cause progressive atelectasis and emphysema. Conventional chest X-ray and chest CT are advised with additional information from barium swallow and MRI.

Surgical excision is usually advised (thorascopically if possible) as, if left untreated, they may cause respiratory complications or severe bleeding from rupture into the bronchus of pleura or recurrent chest infections, although these complications can occur both during and after surgery. Incomplete resection may lead to recurrence. In some cases, however, transparietal, transbronchial or mediastinal drainage may be useful if definitive surgery is not possible.

Although the prognosis for those who have undergone and survived surgery is good, there is a significant operative mortality up to 14%, but a much higher mortality for symptomatic infants who do not have surgery. Asymptomatic cases should therefore all be resected at around 3–6 months.

Pleural effusion and chylothorax

Pleural effusions occur in about 10,000–15,000 pregnancies and are usually unilateral. They are often associated with other structural and chromosomal abnormalities (10%), cardiac malformations (5%) and arrhythmias, fetal anemia, chylothorax and congenital viral infection[18].

Various viral infections have been implicated, such as adenovirus, parvovirus B19, herpes simplex virus type 1. They may be primary as in chylothorax or secondary as in cases of hydrops for other reasons. They have also been found in association with a congenital diaphragmatic hernia. Large persistent pleural effusions can have a major impact on lung development causing lung hypoplasia, and in extreme cases cardiac and caval compression, leading potentially to hydrops, both of which significantly increase the risk of fetal or neonatal demise. Prognosis is therefore dependent on etiology, pressure effects, the degree of pulmonary hypoplasia and gestation of onset and delivery.

Fetal chylothorax is thought to be due to the accumulation of chyle in the pleural cavity, and has a highly variable course with a 20–60% mortality rate depending on gestation of onset and delivery, the presence of hydrops and any other structural or chromosomal abnormalities. It is responsible for about 1 in 2,000 NICU admissions and has a major impact on respiratory function, immune function and nutrition. The course varies from complete spontaneous resolution to progressive enlargement causing significant intrathoracic pressure effects, hydrops, lethal pulmonary hypoplasia and stillbirth or neonatal death. Survivors may experience significant respiratory distress and require chest drain and intubation.

Whilst primary congenital chylothorax is due to an abnormality of the lymphatic duct, secondary types are usually due to trauma, thoracic surgery and thrombosis of the great vessels. Frequent associations include polyhydramnios, hydrops, lung masses (congenital cystic adenomatoid malformation and bronchopulmonary sequestration), mediastinal tumors (thyroid teratoma, congenital), superior vena caval obstruction, Turner syndrome, Down's syndrome and various genetic syndromes (Noonan and Opitz–Frias hypertelorism-hypospadias syndromes). Despite careful and extensive evaluation, the etiology may remain unknown even following delivery.

Imaging

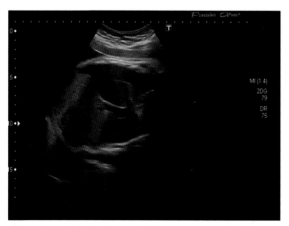

Figure 9.10 Oblique ultrasound scan section through fetal thorax showing bilateral pleural effusions with a clearly defined small right lung (top) and left-sided mediastinal shift.

Antenatal diagnosis and initial management

Pleural effusions are present as variable sized dark fluid-filled areas surrounding one or both lungs and may cause significant mediastinal shift. The pressure may cause cardiac compromise and hydrops, as well as polyhydramnios, from inadequate swallowing and potentially lethal pulmonary hypoplasia.

Following a diagnosis of a pleural effusion, referral should be made to a tertiary fetal medicine unit for a detailed anatomic survey, including an assessment of fetal anatomy, amniotic fluid index and fetal echo to exclude cardiac malformations[19]. Karyotyping is appropriate and middle cerebral Doppler studies should be undertaken to exclude fetal anemia. The size of the effusion, degree of mediastinal shift and any concurrent hydrops should be noted as a baseline and will need to be monitored. Fetal blood sampling may also be of value along with a maternal viral screen, maternal blood count, blood group and antibody status, and Kleihauer test.

A diagnostic pleural tap is useful to assess lymphocyte count (high in chylothorax) and can be used to identify viral infections and abnormal karyotype, and it may also be curative.

Once a definitive diagnosis is made, specific treatment may then be possible, e.g., treatment of fetal anemia or cardiac arrhythmia. Whilst some may resolve spontaneously, others may require drainage. Counseling should be offered by a paediatric surgeon and/or a neonatologist regarding the neonatal and long-term implications, and neonatal and surgical management. Termination of pregnancy should be offered, particularly in cases of significant chromosomal or structural abnormalities, progressive hydrops and failure of fetal therapy. Most isolated pleural effusions resolve after delivery.

Subsequent management

Subsequent management includes serial scans to monitor the size and the effects of the pleural effusions and to identify polyhydramnios, which increases the risk of preterm labor and may require specific management, and fetal hydrops, which may warrant early delivery. Drainage or shunting may promote normal lung development and may prevent hydrops. Initial treatment is usually by aspiration but often shunting is required if re-accumulation occurs. The development of hydrops carries a poor prognosis, with survival rates around 10% compared with about 60% in those cases without it.

In utero treatment

Small nonprogressive lesions may not require treatment. Pleurocentesis may sometimes be curative with no recurrence, but in many cases they re-accumulate and multiple aspirations or a pleuroamniotic shunt may need to be considered. Obviously each procedure carries a procedure-related risk and these would be cumulative. Early successful shunting results in drainage of the effusion, expansion of the lung and a reduction in cardiac pressure, and often resolution of hydrops. As with any invasive procedure, there is a recognized risk of miscarriage, preterm labor and delivery, preterm rupture of the membranes, infection and fetal trauma (including the heart).

Shunt complications, such as blockage, migration and displacement, can occur, but overall survival for successfully shunted cases is 80%[18]. Drainage may also be of value immediately predelivery to optimize initial neonatal resuscitation. Successful pleurodesis has been attempted using either blood or OK-432, which causes the two layers of the pleura to adhere. OK-432 is an avirulent derivative of *Streptococcus pyogenes*, which causes an inflammatory change and has been successful for use in treating adults with chylothorax and newborns with lymphangiomas, as well as fetuses with cystic hygromas and chylothorax. Polyhydramnios may need amnioreduction or medical treatment.

Delivery and neonatal care

In general, delivery for chromosomally normal fetuses without severe compromise should be beyond 32 weeks, but may need to be by cesarean section if significantly early. Delivery should be in a tertiary unit with access to on-site neonatal surgery and NICU facilities. A senior paediatrician should be present and intubation may be required if there is significant respiratory compromise. If a shunt is present, it needs to be clamped immediately to prevent an iatrogenically induced pneumothorax, although in some cases surgical removal is required if it has migrated into the thoracic cavity.

Pulmonary agenesis, aplasia and hypoplasia

Pulmonary agenesis is due to the lack of development of the lungs, and importantly the carina, whereas pulmonary aplasia is due to small underdeveloped lung with a bronchiolar tree and carina present. They are both often associated with renal abnormalities and cardiac defects (50%). True pulmonary agenesis is rarer than hypoplasia and predominantly affects the left lung (75%) with a 50% mortality rate overall and a higher mortality for right-sided lesions as the right lung is larger. Other associated structural abnormalities include components of the VACTERL (vertebral, anorectal, cardiac, tracheoesophageal, renal and limb anomalies) association. The findings may vary from complete failure of development of the entire lung and bronchiolar tree to just the failure of alveolar development with an intact bronchiolar tree. Pulmonary hypertension is common due to a combination of relatively high perfusion volume and vasoconstriction due to hypoxia.

Antenatal diagnosis and initial management

The absence of lung tissue causes cephalic displacement of the diaphragm and abdominal organs and can mimic a CDH. The true birth prevalence is about 1.4% of all births[20], but in cases of early prelabor preterm rupture of the membranes (PPROM) it ranges from 9–28%[21].

The differentiation from other lung pathology includes failure to image the airways on 2D ultrasound and vascular lung connections. Doppler imaging may assist in identifying the absence of the normal pulmonary artery branches[22], and also pulmonary veins as they enter the left atrium.

Pulmonary hypoplasia involves incomplete development of the distal lung tree, and the prognosis depends both on the degree of hypoplasia and gestation of delivery. Under 28 weeks' gestation, the incidence is about 20%. The underlying mechanism may be due to intrathoracic or extrathoracic pathology causing underdevelopment of the lung due to restricted growth.

Intrathoracic causes include:

- congenital diaphragmatic hernia: (most common)
- extralobar sequestration
- mediastinal masses
- decreased pulmonary vascular (arterial) perfusion:
  - from a congenital cardiovascular anomaly, e.g., TOF
  - unilateral absence of the pulmonary artery

Extrathoracic causes include:

- oligohydramnios (commonly PPROM)
- skeletal dysplasia
- large intra-abdominal mass compressing the thorax
- neuromuscular conditions, which affect fetal breathing.

One of the most common causes is secondary to oligohydramnios (e.g., in preterm rupture of the membrane or renal agenesis/dysplasia), as fetal breathing and swallowing of normal amounts of amniotic fluid are essential to normal lung growth. Serial amnioinfusions have been attempted to improve the amniotic fluid volume and lung development, but the outcome has been variable. In addition to the physical and mechanical effects on lung growth, amniotic fluid urinary proline is important in lung collagen formation, and thyroid transcription factors are also important in growth regulation.

Other well-recognized causes are abnormalities of the thoracic cage, such as in skeletal dysplasia, congenital diaphragmatic hernia (mechanical effect and pulmonary hypertension) and other space-occupying lung malformations and neuromuscular disease, which affects fetal breathing. There is a high incidence of associated abnormalities affecting the heart, gut and skeletal system, and rare conditions such as Fryns, Meckel–Gruber, Neu–Laxova and Pena–Shokeir syndromes.

In utero treatment

In utero treatment with fetal tracheal occlusion either by balloon or a clip has been attempted in the hope of improving lung growth by the entrapment of lung fluid, but the outcome has been variable and the treatment remains experimental.

Delivery and neonatal care

At birth there may be telltale signs, such as a small thoracic cage and, if unilateral, reduced air entry on the affected side with mediastinal shift towards it. Neonatal presentation may include respiratory distress, recurrent chest infections and scoliosis. ECMO is useful for short-term treatment of pulmonary hypoplasia with attempts to improve lung growth. Interventions such as positive pressure liquid ventilation using perfluorcarbons and nitrous oxide may be helpful in cases of significant pulmonary hypertension. Surgical procedures, such as thoracoplasty and sternotomy, to try

and improve the size of the thoracic cage have been described.

Other lung malformations

A number of other lung malformations have been described due to abnormal lung development, vascular and lymphatic malformations and lung tumors, and not all are amenable to prenatal diagnosis.

Abnormal lung development

Pulmonary isomerism

Usually the right lung has three lobes and the left has two lobes, but in cases of pulmonary isomerism there may be abnormal numbers of lobes in one or both lungs. Pulmonary isomerism may be isolated or can be associated with situs inversus, asplenia, polysplenia and total anomalous pulmonary drainage. The latter is identified on fetal echo.

Polyalveolar lobe

In a polyalveolar lobe, which may be associated with CLO, there is a massive increase in the number of alveoli, which can retain extra lung fluid causing early neonatal fetal distress following birth.

Vascular malformation

Pulmonary arteriovenous malformation

Pulmonary arteriovenous malformations are rare and are formed by noncapillary containing anastomoses between the arterial and pulmonary circulations. They can cause significant shunting and thus high-output cardiac failure and hydrops prior to birth, but may be asymptomatic prior to adult life when they may cause a range of effects from exercise-induced shortness of breath to significant respiratory compromise, and also hemoptysis. They are also found in association with cutaneous telangiectasia in Osler's disease (hereditary hemorrhagic telangiectasia). They may also cause respiratory infections and pulmonary emboli. The malformations may be seen using color Doppler antenatally and are usually clearly seen on a postnatal chest X-ray. They are usually confined to the lower lobes and may be single or multiple with up to 10% affecting both lungs. A neonatal CT scan is useful, and treatment is by resection or embolization.

Scimitar syndrome

Scimitar syndrome is a form of anomalous pulmonary venous malformation where the abnormal vein traces a curved path towards the inferior vena cava in the shape of a scimitar. There may be other associated abnormalities, such as dextrocardia, pulmonary hypoplasia, bronchiolar abnormalities and the abnormal systemic arterial supply to the right lung. Early presentation may be as congestive heart failure with associated pulmonary hypertension but many remain asymptomatic.

Alveolar capillary dysplasia

Alveolar capillary dysplasia is usually a lethal condition that cannot be cured, and is caused by reduced intra-alveolar mesenchymal tissue with reduced alveolar blood flow and thickened capillary endothelium. In neonates it presents as resistant pulmonary hypertension which does not respond to nitric oxide, and whilst ECMO may be effective, it does not solve the underlying problem. There may also be other associated renal and cardiac malformations.

Lymphatic malformation

Pulmonary lymphangiectasis

Pulmonary lymphangiectasis is a rare malformation characterized by dilatation of the pulmonary lymphatics. It may be associated with some types of congenital heart defects and pulmonary lympangiectasis due to abnormal overgrowth of the lymphatic system. There may be evidence of multiple lymphangiomas elsewhere. Neonates are rarely symptomatic, although they tend to cause respiratory problems in adulthood.

Lung tumors

Lung cyst

Parenchymal-derived lung cysts are rare and their impact depends on their size, location and pressure effects from them. Resection of significant cysts is usually curative. These appear as discreet black fluid-filled areas of variable shape and location within the lung.

Hamartoma /teratoma

These are lung solid tumors within the lung or within the bronchial tree air passages, which contain cartilage, respiratory epithelium and collagen. They may be in the lung tissue or within the bronchial lumen where they can cause obstruction and are usually resected.

Imaging

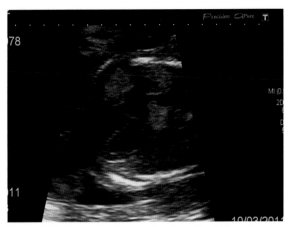

Figure 9.11 Transverse ultrasound section of fetal thorax showing four-chamber view of the heart and a mediastinal bronchogenic teratoma presenting as an echogenic mass above the left atrium.

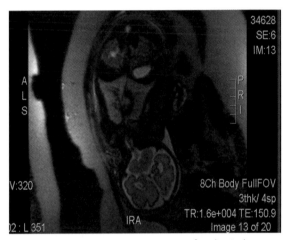

Figure 9.12 Magnetic resonance imaging of mediastinal bronchogenic teratoma presenting as an echogenic mass above the left atrium. Axial, coronal T1 and axial T2-weighted sequences through the fetal thorax. Superior/ middle mediastinal mass of high signal on T2 and low signal on T1 lying just superior to the heart, as seen on ultrasound. Signal intensity is very similar to that of the lung so this could represent lung tissue, however, it also has typical appearances of a mediastinal teratoma.

Laryngeal malformations

Laryngeal atresia

Laryngeal atresia is a rare and usually lethal malformation due to failure of canalization of the laryngotracheal tube resulting in complete airways obstruction. There are few reports of any survivors[23].

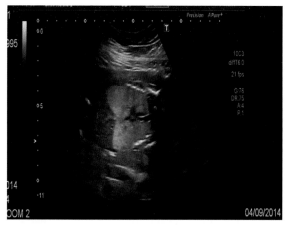

Figure 9.13 Oblique ultrasound scan image showing laryngeal atresia with bright echogencic lungs and relatively hypoechoic liver.

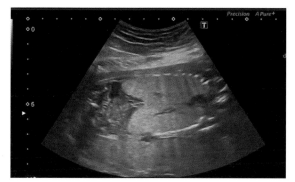

Figure 9.14 Longitudinal ultrasound section of thorax showing laryngeal atresia demonstrated by echogenic lungs, inverted domes of diaphragm and fluid-filled main, left (top) and right (bottom) main bronchi.

Antenatal diagnosis and initial management

In laryngeal atresia, the classical appearances on ultrasound are of hyperechogenic expanded lungs with tubular fluid-filled structures, which represent the dilated fluid-filled main-stem bronchi. The diaphragm is usually flattened or may even be inverted due to pressure from the extended lungs. Color Doppler flow may be useful to confirm no flow in the bronchial or tracheal segments.

Normally the lung echogenicity at the anomaly scan is similar to the echogenicity of the liver, but in many cases of laryngeal atresia, the echogenicity of the lungs exceeds that of the liver.

Laryngeal-tracheobronchial atresia results either from an obstructing lesion, such as a cartilaginous bar,

or an intrauterine vascular insult with atresia of the airways. Classically, the trachea and bronchi are filled with fluid and distended. Pressure effects from the distended lung can cause polyhydramnios due to esophageal compression.

Conditions associated with laryngeal atresia and inheritance

- Fraser syndrome – autosomal recessive
- Opitz–Frias syndrome (G syndrome or BBBG syndrome) – autosomal dominant
- Multiple congenital anomalies syndrome – unknown inheritance
- DiGeorge syndrome – 22q11.2 deletion
- Velo-cardio-facial syndrome – 22q11.2 deletion
- Marshall–Smith syndrome – unknown inheritance
- Laurence–Moon–Bardet–Biedl syndrome – autosomal recessive
- Short-rib polydactyly type II (Majewski) syndrome – autosomal recessive
- Oral-facial-digital type II (Mohr) syndrome – autosomal recessive
- Pallister–Hall syndrome – autosomal dominant
- Hydrolethalus syndrome – autosomal recessive
- Schinzel–Giedion syndrome – autosomal recessive
- Oculo-auriculo-vertebral spectrum (Goldenhar syndrome) – unknown inheritance
- VACTERL association – unknown inheritance
- Crouzon's syndrome – unknown inheritance
- Pfeiffer syndrome – unknown inheritance
- LEL syndrome (laryngeal atresia, encephalocele, limb deformities) – unknown inheritance

Delivery and neonatal care

At birth there is immediate respiratory distress due to airways obstruction, usually associated with significant respiratory efforts but no air entry into the lungs or crying. Intubation is unsuccessful. In cases with a high index of suspicion, an early resort to tracheotomy may be lifesaving. Occasionally, a tracheoesophageal fistula may be present, which allows some ventilation of the lungs.

Antenatal diagnosis or laryngeal atresia without a trachea-esophageal fistula may result from detailed fetal assessment of polyhydramnios or at the 20-week anomaly scan. This allows planned delivery and resuscitation with an ex utero intrapartum treatment (EXIT) procedure. This involves delivery of the fetal head, neck and shoulders at cesarean section and airway assessment and time for a tracheostomy whilst oxygenation is still possible from the placenta-fetal circulation. Alternatively, delayed cord clamping will buy some time for a tracheostomy if prenatal diagnosis has been made. ECMO may be required after delivery.

Laryngeal cysts

Laryngeal cysts are extremely rare with the most common being due to congenital saccular cysts. In such cases, obstruction of the laryngeal saccule orifice leads to mucus retention and cystic dilatation of the saccules. These cysts may occur in the vallecula, subglottis or vocal cords as a congenital malformation or following prolonged intubation. Most are diagnosed endoscopically following problems with airways obstruction or dysphagia. Needle aspiration may be useful transiently but definitive treatment is by endoscopic or open excision. Laser treatment has also been described.

Laryngeal lymphangioma

Laryngeal lymphangiomas are rare and are due to abnormalities of lymphatic vessel development. Many (50%) present in the neonatal period and most (75%) by a year old. Depending on the size and location, they may be asymptomatic or cause airways obstruction. They may also enlarge significantly during upper respiratory tract infections. Endoscopy is usually diagnostic in suspected cases.

Individuals with laryngeal lymphangioma may be asymptomatic or may present with significant airway obstruction when the lesions attain a large size. Upper respiratory tract infections may precipitate symptoms by causing a rapid increase in the size of these lesions. Complete excision is difficult and laser treatment or sclerosing agents may be necessary to prevent recurrence. Significant obstruction may require tracheostomy.

References

1. Kumar S. Thoracic Abnormalities. In: *Handbook of Fetal Anomalies*. Cambridge University Press, 2009: 45–54.

2. Fong K, Ohlsson A, Zalev A. Fetal thoracic circumference: a prospective cross sectional study with real time ultrasound. *Am J Obstet Gynecol* 1988; 158: 1154–60.

3. Nimrod C, Nicholson S, Davies D, et al. Pulmonary hypoplasia testing in clinical obstetrics. *Am J Obstet Gynecol* 1988; 158: 277–80.

4. DeVore GR, Horenstein J, Platt LD. Fetal echocardiography: assessment of cardiothoracic disproportion – a new technique for the diagnosis of thoracic hypoplasia. *Am J Obstet Gynecol* 1986; 155: 1066–74.

5. D'Alton M, Mercer B, Riddick E, et al. Serial thoracic versus abdominal circumference ratios for the prediction of pulmonary hypoplasia in premature rupture of membranes remote from term. *Am J Obstet Gynecol* 1992; 166: 658–63.

6. Lipshutz GS, et al. Prospective analysis of lung-to-head ratio predicts survival for patients with prenatally diagnosed congenital diaphragmatic hernia. *J Pediatr Surg* 1997; 32(11): 1634–6.

7. Kamal A, Grigoratos D, Cornelius V, et al. Outcome of CDH infants following fetoscopic tracheal occlusion – influence of premature delivery. *J Pediatric Surg* 2013; 48 (9): 1831–6.

8. Cass DL, et al. Prenatal diagnosis and outcome of fetal lung masses. *J Pediatr Surg* 2011; 46(2): 292–8.

9. Crombleholme TM. Cystic adenomatoid malformation volume ratio predicts outcome in prenatally diagnosed cystic adenomatoid malformation of the lung. *J Pediatr Surg* 2002; 37(3): 331–8.

10. Adzick NS, Flake AW, Crombleholme TM. Management of congenital lung lesions. *Sem Pediatr Surg* 2003; 12: 10–16.

11. Frazier AA, Rosado de Christenson ML, Stocker JT, et al. Intralobar sequestration: radiologic-pathologic correlation. *Radiographics* 1997; 17(3): 725–45.

12. Smart LM, Hendry GM. Imaging of neonatal pulmonary sequestration including Doppler ultrasound. *Br J Radiol* 1991; 64(760): 324–9.

13. Salmons S. Pulmonary sequestration. *Neonatal Netw* 2000; 19(7): 27–31.

14. Amitai M, Konen E, Rozenman J, et al. Preoperative evaluation of pulmonary sequestration by helical CT angiography. *AJR Am J Roentgenol* 1996; 167(4): 1069–70.

15. Ooi GC, Cheung CW, Lam WK, et al. Pulmonary sequestration: diagnosis by magnetic resonance angiography and computed tomography. *Chin Med J (Engl)* 1999; 112(7): 668–70.

16. Donoghue VB, Bjørnstad PG. *Radiological Imaging of the Neonatal Chest*. Springer Verlag, 2007.

17. Berrocal T, Madrid C, Novo S, et al. Congenital anomalies of the tracheobronchial tree, lung, and mediastinum: embryology, radiology, and pathology. *Radiographics* 2004; 24(1): e17.

18. Smith RP, Illanes S, Denbow ML, et al. Outcome of fetal pleural effusions treated by thoracoamniotic shunting. *Ultrasound Obstet Gynecol* 2005; 26(1): 63–6.

19. Rustico MA, Lanna M, Coviello D, et al. Fetal pleural effusion. *Prenat Diagn* 2007; 27: 793–9.

20. Knox WF, Barson AJ. Pulmonary hypoplasia in a regional perinatal unit. *Early Hum. Dev* 1986; 14 (1): 33–42.

21. Berrocal T, Madrid C, Novo S, et al. Congenital anomalies of the tracheobronchial tree, lung, and mediastinum: embryology, radiology, and pathology. *Radiographics* 24(1): e17.

22. Bromley B, Benacerraf BR. Unilateral lung hypoplasia: report of three cases. *J Ultrasound Med* 1997; 16: 599–601.

23. Onderoglu L, Karamursell S, Bulun A et al. Prenatal diagnosis of laryngeal atresia prenatal diagnosis. *Prenat Diagn* 2003; 23: 277–80.

Chapter

10

Fetal abdomen and abdominal wall anomalies

Manish Gupta

Abnormalities of the anterior abdominal wall are some of the most common anomalies to detect on ultrasound. The UK National Health Service Fetal Anomaly Screening Programme (FASP) gives detection rates and auditable standards of 98% and 80% for gastroschisis and exomphalos, respectively, as well as antenatal and postnatal pathways for these conditions.

Abnormalities within the gut are dependent on the site, upper intestinal abnormalities being far easier to detect than lower ones due to the fact that polyhydramnios ensues at an early stage, therefore facilitating ultrasound diagnosis.

The anterior abdominal wall

The majority of these abnormalities are detectable in the first trimester in either the sagittal or axial view.

It is useful to recall that during development the bowel herniates extraembryonically within the umbilical cord and undergoes rotation between 6 and 10 weeks. Therefore, a reliable diagnosis of an anterior abdominal wall abnormality cannot usually be made prior to 12 weeks. If in doubt, the ultrasound should be repeated after 12 weeks.

Exomphalos (omphalocoele)

Exomphalos is defined as the contents of the abdomen occurring outside the abdominal cavity but within a peritoneal sac. It is caused by failure of return of the herniated bowel in the first trimester. It is exomphalos major if the liver and bowel are contained within the sac and exomphalos minor if only the bowel is within the sac (10–25%).

The incidence is 1 in 4,000 births. There is a high association with chromosomal abnormalities (approximately 33–61% depending on gestational age)

mainly trisomy 18 (the most common) and trisomy 13; 30–50% will have some form of cardiac abnormality. Paradoxically, the larger the lesion the less likely there is to be a chromosomal abnormality(1–3).

Diagnosis

The diagnosis is usually made after 12 weeks and is often detected at the first trimester dating scan in places where nuchal translucency (NT)-based screening is in place. It is best observed in the sagittal and axial views. The umbilical cord will insert onto the anterior part of the peritoneal sac and blood flow can be seen passing around the sac. In places where the triple or quadruple blood test is offered for screening, a raised alpha-fetoprotein (AFP) should prompt a search for an anterior abdominal wall abnormality.

The sac may contain bowel, stomach and liver. The bladder and stomach are often "pulled" towards the sac. In large lesions, the heart may also be shifted towards the defect. As the abdominal anatomy is distorted it is often difficult to obtain a true abdominal circumference, which may lead to inaccuracies in estimation of fetal weight or the misdiagnosis of fetal growth restriction.

Common chromosomal abnormalities associated with exomphalos are trisomy 18 and trisomy 21. Other syndromes associated with an exomphalos are Beckwith–Weidemann syndrome (macrosomia and macroglossia with renal cysts), OEIS (omphalocoele, bladder exstrophy, imperforate anus and spinal defects) and pentalogy of Cantrell (exomphalos, congenital diaphragmatic hernia, ectopia cordis, sternal cleft and intracardiac defect, usually a ventricular septal defect). A repeat anatomic survey should focus on these areas as well as the heart and features of trisomy

Fetal Medicine, ed. Bidyut Kumar and Zarko Alfirevic. Published by Cambridge University Press. © Cambridge University Press 2016.

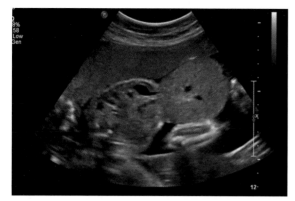

Figure 10.1 Exomphalos with stomach within peritoneal sac.

18 and 13. Cloacal and bladder extrophy can be associated with an exomphalos, and identification of the bladder is mandatory to exclude these conditions. Both are thought to be due to a defect in the development of the cloacal membrane.

Management

Karyotyping should be offered due to the high rate of chromosomal abnormalities, particularly trisomy 18. A full fetal echocardiogram should also be performed as approximately 30–50% will have some form of cardiac abnormality. Associated structural and/or chromosomal abnormalities worsen the prognosis. Counseling regarding the prognosis should be done in association with neonatalogists and pediatric surgeons.

The fetus should be monitored every 4 weeks with growth scans, but the true abdominal circumference may be difficult to measure, and so fetal growth restriction may be difficult to diagnose.

Delivery is best organized in a tertiary center with neonatal surgical facilities. A vaginal delivery is safe and cesarean section is not essential; cesarean section may be considered in certain cases where the exomphalos is very large. In general, the outcome is good with an 80–90% survival rate if there are no associated chromosomal or structural issues, but this depends upon the size of the lesion.

Neonatal management

A neonatal pediatrician should be present at the delivery of the baby. Initial management is focused on stabilization of the baby and the avoidance of trauma to the sac. The sac should have a moist covering to prevent evaporative heat and water loss. Neonatal

management is directed at fluid balance and blood sugar monitoring.

Repair depends upon firstly the exclusion of other structural abnormalities that may not have been detected antenatally, and the size of the peritoneal sac.

If the sac is small enough, then primary repair can be performed with excision of the sac and closure of the fascia and the abdominal wall. If the exomphalos is large, then a silastic pouch may be used to reduce the viscera into the abdominal cavity and closure performed when the sac is smaller.

Recurrence

The recurrence rate depends on the underlying cause but if isolated is rare.

Gastroschisis

Gastroschisis can be defined as herniation of the abdominal wall contents medial to the umbilical cord with no surrounding membrane. It occurs in approximately 1 in 4,000 births. The exact cause of gastroschisis is unknown but is believed to be caused by a disruption of the blood supply to the developing abdominal wall from the omphalomesenteric duct artery by the 8th week of gestation. There are no known genetic associations, and so karyotyping is not indicated[1–3].

Diagnosis

Gastroschisis can be diagnosed at the 11–14 week scan, and as there is an open defect the AFP levels are commonly raised. However, serum screening tests including AFP are not offered in most places, so the

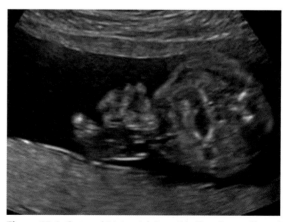

Figure 10.2 Gastroschisis in axial view with dilated internal bowel.

opportunity to find a raised AFP may not arise. The exposure of the bowel to the amniotic fluid leads to thickening of the bowel wall. As in exomphalos, the bladder and heart can be pulled towards the lesion distorting the internal anatomy.

The main issue is that of bowel atresias and necrosis that need to be resected after delivery, which if severe can lead to "short bowel" syndrome where long-term parenteral nutrition is required. Unfortunately, there do not seem to be any strong prognostic indicators. Bowel thickness (>2mm), hyperperistalsis, mesenteric arterial blood flow and bowel dilatation have all been evaluated. but none seem to be particularly good at predicting the need for surgery or the length of bowel that requires resection[4]. A recent review suggested that the only predictive factor was internal bowel dilatation greater than 14mm[5].

However, a ruptured exomphalos is a possibility, so a careful secondary survey is always necessary, in particular looking for a free-floating membrane in the amniotic fluid. There are other conditions that may appear to be a gastroschisis. Limb-body wall complex or body stalk anomaly, a large anterior thoracoabdominal wall abnormality with an associated myelomeningocoele. The contents of the abdomen, pelvis and chest lie outside the body cavities and can be attached to the uterine wall or placenta. This condition is lethal. Amniotic band syndrome, due to early amnion rupture, may cause disruption of the anterior abdominal wall and a gastroschisis.

Management

Gastroschisis is associated with fetal growth restriction and serial measurements of fetal biometry with umbilical cord Dopplers are required at least every 4 weeks, with delivery at around 37–38 weeks due to the risk of stillbirth. Ultrasonography underestimates the fetal abdominal circumference, and therefore there may be a false positive for diagnosis of fetal growth restriction.

Ultrasound evaluation of the bowel includes the measurement of internal and external bowel dilatation, the presence of intrabdominal peristalsis (which may indicate an area of stenosis) and blood flow within the extra-abdominal bowel. However, the only feature that may be predictive of bowel atresia or infarction is inflammatory bowel disease.

Multidisciplinary management and counseling are essential and should include pediatric surgeons and neonatalogists.

Delivery should occur at a facility with the appropriate neonatal surgical expertise, and vaginal delivery is not contraindicated because of the presence of a gastroschisis alone.

Neonatal management

In general, the outcome is good with a greater than 90% survival. A pediatrician should be present at the delivery, and immediate care involves keeping the bowel moist and covered, and careful fluid balance. Repair involves either immediate closure of the defect or delayed closure if there is a large amount of extra-abdominal bowel. If surgery cannot be performed immediately, the bowel is surrounded by a silastic (a plastic bag) to allow reduction of the bowel into the abdominal cavity. The baby may have intestinal ischemia with necrosis, and if required, may need either resection and primary anastomosis or the formation of temporary stomas. Following repair, the neonate requires 3 weeks of parenteral nutrition via central venous access.

Recurrence

The overall recurrence rate is low.

Gastrointestinal atresias

Atresia can occur anywhere in the bowel. In general, proximal atresias are easier to detect as the proximal bowel will fill up with fluid, and there will be a dilated segment and associated polyhydramnios.

Usually the small bowel cannot be seen as separate loops unless there is dilatation. Large bowel can be seen, particularly in the third trimester as meconium within the lumen has a different echogenicity, but if dilated can be recognized by its haustral pattern.

Esophageal atresia and tracheoesophageal fistula

These are rare conditions with an incidence of approximately 1 in 5,000. The most common abnormality is an esophageal atresia with a distal tracheoesophageal atresia. When the esophagus does not connect to the stomach, the esophagus appears very dilated, the stomach is absent and there is marked polyhydramnios. In the cases of a fistula, the stomach may appear small or normal and there may be no polyhydramnios.

The most common associations are chromosomal (trisomy 21 or 18) or the VACTERL (vertebral, anorectal, cardiac, tracheoesophageal, renal and limb anomalies) syndrome and karyotyping is recommended.

Due to the issues with polyhydramnios, amniodrainage may be required to prevent preterm labor, and cervical scanning may be useful in predicting this.

In the absence of other anomalies or chromosomal problems, the outcome is generally good with a 95% survival rate, and delivery should take place in a tertiary center with the appropriate neonatal surgical facilities.

Duodenal atresias

Doudenal atresia has an approximate incidence of 1 in 10,000. There is a strong association (33%) with trisomy 21 and invasive testing should be offered. The diagnosis is made by the appearance of a "double bubble" – the dilated duodenum proximal to the lesion and the dilated stomach proximal to this. There is often associated polyhydramnios.

Small bowel atresias

These occur in the jejunum or ileum and are most likely to occur due to vascular events or ischemic injury due to hypotension affecting the bowel wall or meconium ileus within the bowel lumen or secondary to cystic fibrosis.

On ultrasound, multiple dilated loops of bowel can be observed. Polyhydramnios is not as common as the more proximal lesions detailed above, as the bowel can dilate to accommodate the extra fluid.

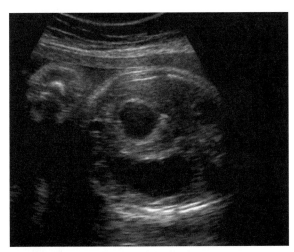

Figure 10.3 "Double bubble" of duodenal atresia.

In the absence of other abnormalities the prognosis is good.

Large bowel atresias

These are more difficult to detect as they do not appear on ultrasound until late in the third trimester due to the ability of the bowel to expand for the extra fluid. Polyhydramnios is rare because of this. Common causes are meconium ileus, Hirschprung's disease (lack of nervous innervation prevents relaxation of the bowel, and therefore an obstruction) and imperforate anus.

Intrabdominal cysts

A variety of cysts can occur within the abdominal cavity. The cause depends on the location[6].

Gastrointestinal tract
Mesenteric cyst
Enteric duplication cyst
Liver
Simple cyst
Gall bladder
Choledochal cyst
Adrenal
Hemorrhage
Neuroblastoma
Ovarian – determination of fetal sex is important
Follicular cyst – may undergo torsion

Intra-abdominal calcification

Intra-abdominal calfication is rare but can be indicative of fetal infection, particularly cytomegalovirus (CMV) and toxoplasmosis. However, in the absence of infection the outcome is good with no cause found.

Echogenic bowel

The true definition is that the bowel should be as "bright as bone," and there are multiple associations:

(1) chromosomal abnormalities, particularly trisomy 21, but in the context of screening this is only a minor marker of chromosomal anomalies

(2) first-trimester bleeding – the bloody amniotic fluid is swallowed and the iron from hemoglobin in the red blood cells precipitates in the bowel wall

(3) infection – CMV and toxoplasmosis

(4) cystic fibrosis – although this is rare

(5) fetal growth restriction – the most common issue is due to placental insufficiency caused by first-trimester bleeding.

References

1. Fratelli N, Papageorghiou AT, Bhide A, et al. Outcome of antenatally diagnosed abdominal wall defects *Ultrasound Obstet Gynecol* 2007; 30(3): 266–70.

2. Arnaoutoglou CI, Pasquini L, Abel R, et al. Outcome of antenatally diagnosed fetal anterior abdominal wall defects from a single tertiary centre. *Fetal Diagn Ther* 2008; 24(4): 416–9.

3. Rankin J, Dillon E, Wright C. Congenital anterior abdominal wall defects in the north of England, 1986–1996: occurrence and outcome. *Prenat Diagn* 1999; 19(7): 662–8.

4. Japaraj RP, Hockey R, Chan FY. Gastroschisis: can prenatal sonography predict neonatal outcome? *Ultrasound Obstet Gynecol* 2003; 21(4): 329–33.

5. Goetzinger KR, Tuuli MG, Longman RE, et al. Sonographic predictors of postnatal bowel atresia in fetal gastroschisis. *Ultrasound Obstet Gynecol* 2014; 43(4): 420–5.

6. Heling KS, Chaoui R, Kirchmair F, et al. Fetal ovarian cysts: prenatal diagnosis, management and postnatal outcome. *Ultrasound Obstet Gynecol* 2002; 20(1): 47–50.

Chapter

11

Sonographic diagnosis of fetal skeletal anomalies

Lyn S. Chitty, Thomas R. Everett and Fred Usakov

Fetal skeletal anomalies are relatively common, with etiologies including aneuploidy, teratogens, skeletal dysplasias, other genetic syndromes and idiopathic limb reduction deformities. The identification prenatally of skeletal abnormalities, the terminology of which is detailed in Table 11.1, can pose significant diagnostic challenges. However, recognition of the pattern of anomalies can facilitate targeted molecular genetic diagnosis, prediction of outcome, and thus parental counseling and informed decision making. The optimum approach to prenatal diagnosis requires a multidisciplinary approach, which should include a pediatric orthopaedic surgeon and, crucially, a clinical geneticist, since a molecular diagnosis is increasingly achievable. Where the pregnancy ends in fetal demise, an expert postmortem examination by a perinatal pathologist is recommended, although where parents decline full postmortem, the minimally-invasive approach[1] or one limited to external examination and radiology may enable diagnosis[2]. Here we will outline a structured approach to the diagnosis of generalized skeletal dysplasias before giving the suggested approach to the diagnosis of more localized limb anomalies (excluding isolated talipes), which may form part of a wider genetic syndrome.

Risk factors and clues to the diagnosis of skeletal anomalies

Family history

Although the majority of skeletal abnormalities are unexpected findings detected by ultrasound, some arise because of a relevant family history and others because of maternal drug use or maternal disease (Table 11.2).

Whilst diagnosis can be more straightforward in families where there is an affected child or when one parent is affected with a dominantly-inherited condition, parents do need to be aware that some conditions, e.g., achondroplasia[3], may present relatively late in pregnancy, and others may be more variable, e.g., hypochondroplasia, and thus not necessarily amenable to sonographic diagnosis. For these reasons, molecular genetic diagnosis may be the best option for definitive diagnosis, but in most cases this will necessitate a detailed genetic work-up prior to pregnancy in order to identify relevant mutations. Molecular genetic diagnosis requires fetal tissue or DNA for analysis, which in the past has required an invasive test (chorionic villus sampling or amniocentesis). However, this is increasingly possible using noninvasive prenatal diagnosis (NIPD) and analysis of cell-free fetal DNA (cffDNA) in maternal plasma[4, 5]. In view of the rapid advances in molecular genetics, genetic advice should be sought *before* pregnancy in families of known high risk to be sure of the optimum method of diagnosis.

Maternal drug ingestion or disease

There are a number of drugs that may be implicated in the etiology of fetal skeletal anomalies (Table 11.2). Maternal conditions, such as insulin-dependent diabetes, myasthenia gravis and myotonic dystrophy, can cause a variety of skeletal problems (Table 11.2), with other conditions, such as systemic lupus erythematosis and hypothyroidism also causing skeletal changes, but less commonly. In maternal myasthenia gravis, even when the mother is asymptomatic, transmission of acetycholine receptor antibodies to the fetus can result in generalized arthrogryposis and neonatal or infant death. In mothers with symptomatic myotonic

Fetal Medicine, ed. Bidyut Kumar and Zarko Alfirevic. Published by Cambridge University Press. © Cambridge University Press 2016.

Table 11.1 Glossary of terminology used in describing skeletal abnormalities

Achiria	Absent hand(s)
Achiropodia	Absent hand(s) and feet
Acromelia	Shortening of the distal segments of limbs, hands and feet
Adactyly	Absent fingers and/or toes
Amelia	Complete absence of one or more limbs from shoulder or pelvic girdle
Apodia	Absent foot (feet)
Arthrogryposis	Reduced mobility of multiple joints due to contractures causing fixation of the joints in extension or flexion
Brachydactyly	Short fingers
Camptomelia	Bent limb or bent fingers
Clinodactyly	Incurved 5th finger with short middle phalange
Ectrodactyly	Split hand(s) or feet (lobster claw deformity)
Hemimelia	Absence of the distal arm or leg below the elbow or knee
Kyphosis	Dorsal convex curvature of the spine
Kyphoscoliosis	Combination of lateral and antero-posterior curvature of the spine
Mesomelia	Shortening of the middle segment of a limb (radius/ulna and tibia/fibula)
Micromelia	Shortening of all long bones
Oligodactyly	Absent or partially absent finger(s) and toe(s)
Phocomelia	Grossly underdeveloped or absent limbs
Platyspondyly	Flattening of the vertebral bodies
Pre-axial polydactyly	Extra fingers or toes on the radial or tibial side
Post-axial polydactyly	Extra fingers or toes on the ulna of fibular side
Rhizomelia	Shortening of the proximal long bones (femur and humerus)
Syndactyly of the skin	Fusion of fingers +/- toes, skin only
Syndactyly bony	Osseous fusion of fingers +/- toes
Scoliosis	Lateral curvature of the spine
Talipes/club foot	Equinovalgus – foot twisted outwards Equinovarus – foot twisted inwards Equinus – extended foot

dystrophy (an autosomal dominant condition), there is an up to 50% chance of the baby having congenital myotonic dystrophy (Table 11.2), which carries a high neonatal mortality (around 20%), with most survivors having significant developmental delay and reduced life expectancy.

Fetal limb development and the timing of diagnosis

An understanding of the timing of the development of the fetal skeleton is essential for accurate sonographic diagnosis, particularly as there is an increasing tendency towards detailed anomaly scanning in early pregnancy. In the human, the upper limbs develop a few days in advance of the lower limbs, with the arm buds appearing at about $5\frac{1}{2}$ postmenstrual weeks. The clavicle begins to ossify at around 8 weeks' gestation, followed by the mandible, vertebral bodies and neural arches around 9 weeks, the frontal bones at 10–11 weeks and the long bones from 8 weeks (Figure 11.1) [6]. Of note, ossification of the cervical and sacral spine is not complete until around 20 weeks' gestation. Most skeletal structures can be identified by 12 weeks' gestation, but transvaginal scanning is recommended for accurate diagnosis at this gestation. In addition to sonographic expertise, accurate identification of skeletal anomalies requires aids such as charts of normal skeletal size, including length of long bones, clavicles, mandible, scapular, chest size, orbital diameters, renal

Table 11.2 Maternal factors associated with fetal skeletal abnormalities

Underlying etiology	Fetal skeletal anomalies	Other potential sonographic findings	Other aids to diagnosis
Maternal drug ingestion			
Warfarin	Rhizomelic shortening of limbs. Stippled epiphyses, 'disorganized spine', mid-face hypoplasia, depressed nasal bridge and small nose	Renal, cardiac and CNS anomalies	Maternal medication history
Sodium valproate	Forearm reduction deformity, polydactyly, oligodactyly, talipes	Cardiac and CNS anomalies	Maternal medical and medication history
Phenytoin	Stippled epiphyses	Micrognathia, cleft lip, cardiac anomalies	Maternal medication history
Methotrexate	Mesomelic shortening of long bones, hypomineralised skull, syndactyly, oligodactyly, talipes, micrognathia	CNS anomalies including neural tube defects,	Maternal medication history
Vitamin A	Hypoplasia or aplasia of arm bones	CNS and cardiac anomalies, spina bifida, cleft lip and palate, diaphragmatic hernia, exomphalos	Maternal history
Alcohol	Short long bones, forearm reduction deformity, pre-axial polydactyly of hands, oligodactyly, stippled epiphyses	IUFGR, cardiac anomalies	Maternal history
Cocaine	Reduction deformities of arms +/− legs, ectrodactyly, hemivertebrae, absent ribs	CNS, cardiac, renal anomalies, anterior abdominal wall defects, bowel atresias	Maternal history. Hair root analysis for drug metabolites
Maternal disease			
Insulin dependent diabetes	Femoral hypoplasia – often asymmetrical	Short spine/caudal regression	Glucose tolerance test
Myasthenia gravis	Multiple joint contractures	Decreased fetal movements	Maternal anticholinesterase antibodies
Myotonic dystrophy	Talipes	Decreased fetal movements, polyhydramnios	Maternal examination for signs of myotonia, facial appearance, family history, genetic referral
Systemic lupus erythematosus	Short limbs, stippled epiphyses, depressed nasal bridge		Autoantibody screen, maternal obstetric and medical history
Maternal hypothyroidism	Short limbs, stippled epiphyses, depressed nasal bridge, stippling of spine, hands and feet		Maternal obstetric and medical history, thyroid screen

CNS, central nervous system; IUFGR, intrauterine fetal growth restriction.

size, etc.[7–10]. Given knowledge of skeletal development, sonographic expertise and necessary aids, and with the technologic advances in ultrasound platforms, it is clear that scanning in the first and early second trimesters can be ideal for the detection of many serious skeletal dysplasias (Tables 11.3 and 11.4;[11]) as well as localized limb reduction defects (Table 11.5;[12]).

Sonographic approach: the diagnosis of generalized skeletal dysplasias

There are around 400 known generalized skeletal dysplasias, some of which can present with significant findings early in pregnancy[11], some do not have

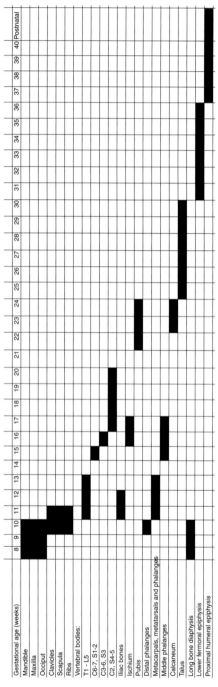

Figure 11.1 Chart demonstrating gestation at which ossification of the fetal skeleton commences as indicated from radiologic studies of fetuses after delivery (adapted from Calder and Offiah[6]).

Table 11.3 A structured approach to the sonographic examination of a fetus presenting with short long bones and suspected to have a skeletal dysplasia

Examination	Outcome	Common diagnoses	Other investigations[a]
Measure all long bones	All short	IUFGR	Maternal and fetal Dopplers. Review other biometry for small HC/AC. Serial scanning for growth velocity. Review maternal serum screening results for high hCG and MSAFP or low PAPP-A. Obstetric history for IUFGR, SB, PET, etc. Maternal medical history for autoimmune disease. Check for reduced AFI.
		Constitutional short stature	F/H, examine parents, normal long bone growth velocity, normal Dopplers.
		Aneuploidy	Detailed anomaly scan for markers of aneuploidy. Consider karyotyping.
		Skeletal dysplasia	See below
Assess the gestation at onset of shortening[b]	First trimester	Thanatophoric, OI IIA/C/B, achondrogenesis types 1 and 2, most SRPSs, diastrophic dysplasia, SEDC, hypophosphatasia, Ellis–van Creveld, Boomerang dysplasia	
	Second trimester	OI IIB/III/IV, Jeune's asphyxiating thoracic dystrophy, most chondrodysplasia punctatas	
	Third trimester	Achondroplasia	Exclude IUFGR, maternal blood for NIPD for *FGFR3* mutations.
Compare measurements of proximal and distal long bones to classify type of shortening	Rhizomelic – shortening most evident in proximal long bones (humeri and femora)	Diastrophic dysplasia, SEDC, Jeune's asphyxiating thoracic dystrophy	
	Mesomelic – shortening of the mid-section of a limb (radius/ulna, tibia/fibula)	Ellis–van Creveld, Achondroplasia, oral-facial-digital IV	
	Micromelic – all long bones are very short	Achondrogenesis type 1 and 2, Boomerang dysplasia	
Evaluate the structure of bones	Fractured/bowed	OI type IIA/B/C/III/IV. Hypophosphatasia, campomelic dysplasia (legs only)	Parental alkaline phosphatase levels, urinary phosphoethanolamine levels.
	Hypomineralized	OI type IIA/B/C/III Hypophosphatasia	
	Metaphyseal flaring	Kniest syndrome	
	Absent bones	Roberts syndrome	Chromosome analysis for centromeric puffing.
	Stippled epiphyses	Rhizomelic chondrodysplasia punctata, Conradi Hunermann, X-linked recessive chondrodysplasia punctate, warfarin embryopathy, maternal SLE/auto-immune disease	Maternal drug history, mutations in ARSE gene, metabolic investigations – very long chain fatty acids and sterol profile, maternal history of autoimmune disease.

Table 11.3 (cont.)

Examination	Outcome	Common diagnoses	Other investigations[a]
Examine the extremities	Polydactyly	Jeune's asphyxiating thoracic dystrophy, Ellis–van Creveld syndrome, SRPSs	Family history, check for consanguinity.
	Syndactyly	Apert syndrome	NIPD for *FGFR2* mutations.
	Polysyndactyly	SRPSs, oral-facial-digital IV	
	Oligodactyly	De Lange, Roberts syndrome	
	Radial club hand	VATER/VACTERL	
	Short fingers/trident hand	Achondroplasia, acromesomelic dysplasia, thanatophoric dysplasia	Screen for mutations in *FGFR3* gene.
	Talipes	Diastrophic dysplasia, campomelic dysplasia, Kniest, oral-facial-digital IV	
	Hitchhiker thumbs/toes	Diastrophic dysplasia	
Examine the skull – size and shape	Severe hypomineralisation	OI IIA/C, achondrogenesis type 1, hypophosphatasia (severe neonatal type), Boomerang dysplasia	
	Mild hypomineralisation	OI IIB (OI III), cleido-cranial dysostosis	Examine the parents for cleido-cranial dysostosis.
	Cloverleaf skull or craniosynostosis	Thanatophoric dysplasia II, occasionally in SRPSs, Apert, craniosynostosis syndromes	Maternal blood for NIPD to screen cfDNA for mutations in the *FGFR3* and 2 genes.
	Relative macrocephaly	Thanatophoric dysplasia, achondroplasia, achondrogenesis type 1	Maternal blood for NIPD to screen cfDNA for mutations in the *FGFR3*.
	Progressive microcephaly	Rhizomelic chondrodysplasia punctate	
Examine the clavicles and scapulae	Short/absent clavicles	Cleido-cranial dysostosis	Examine parents.
	Small scapula	Campomelic dysplasia	NIPT for fetal sex if genitalia are ambiguous or female.
Examine the face – profile and coronal views	Frontal bossing	Achondroplasia, thanatophoric dysplasia, acromesomelic dysplasia	Maternal blood for NIPD to screen cfDNA for mutations in the *FGFR3* gene.
	Micrognathia	SEDC, Stickler syndrome, campomelic dysplasia, diastrophic dysplasia, Kniest syndrome	Examine parents. Consider NIPD for fetal sex if genitalia are ambiguous or female.
	Cleft lip	SRPSs – Majewski syndrome, Verma–Naumoff and Beemer–Langer, Ellis–van Creveld, Roberts syndrome, oral-facial-digital IV	
	Absent/flat nasal bridge	Rhizomelic chondrodysplasia punctata, Binder phenotype, Warfarin embryopathy	Drug history, mutations in arylsulfatase E gene, metabolic investigations – very long chain fatty acids and sterol profile, maternal history of autoimmune disease.

Examination	Finding	Associated conditions
		Examine the parents.
	Mid-face hypoplasia	Rhizomelic chondrodysplasia punctata, Binder phenotype, Kniest
	Small nose	Rhizomelic chondrodysplasia punctata, Binder phenotype, Kniest
	Cataracts	Rhizomelic chondrodysplasia punctate
Examine the thorax – assess the size by measuring circumference by comparing with the abdomen in the axial plane or assessing lung:heart ratio. Examine the parasagittal view for the 'champagne-cork' appearance	Short	SEDC, Stickler, Kniest
	Very small and narrow with champagne cork appearance	Thanatophoric dysplasia, SRPSs, dystrophy achondrogenesis, OI IIA/C
	Long and narrow	Jeune's asphyxiating thoracic dystrophy. Occasionally achondroplasia and Ellis–van Creveld
Examine the ribs in the axial plane for length and sagittal/coronal plane for beading/fractures/missing ribs	Short straight ribs	Thanatophoric dysplasia, SRPSs, Jeune's asphyxiating thoracic dystrophy, achondrogenesis type 2, Ellis–van Creveld , achondrogenesis type 1
	Fractures/beaded ribs	OI IIA/C/B
	Absent/disorganized ribs	Jarcot–Levin, spondylocostal dysplasia, campomelic dysplasia (occasionally only 11 ribs).
Examine the spine for mineralization, disorganization, hemivertebrae	Hypomineralized vertebral bodies	Achondrogenesis type I
	Hemivertebrae	VATER/VACTERL Spondylocostal dysplasia
	Disorganization (may be confused with extra calcification)	Jarcot–Levin, spondylocostal dysplasia, some chondrodysplasia punctatas, dyssegmental dysplasia, VATER/VACTERL
Examine the skin for edema	Increased nuchal translucency	Thanatophoric, OI, SRPSs, SEDC and several others
Examine the fetal viscera	Hydrops	SRPSs, achondrogenesis type 1, Boomerang dysplasia
	CNS anomaly	SRPSs (Majewski, Beemer–Langer), thanatophoric dysplasia type II, occasionally achondroplasia
	Cardiac anomaly	Campomelic dysplasia, Ellis van Creveld, SRPSs, VATER/VACTERL

Table 11.3 (cont.)

Examination	Outcome	Common diagnoses	Other investigations[a]
	Renal tract anomaly	Jeune's asphyxiating thoracic dystrophy, SRPSs	
	Anterior abdominal wall defect	SRPS (Beemer–Langer)	
	Genital anomalies	Campomelic dysplasia, SRPSs	NIPD for fetal sex determination
Amniotic fluid volume	Polyhydramnios	Achondroplasia, thanatophoric dysplasia, paternal uniparental disomy 14, VATER/VACTERL	
	Oligohydramnios	SRPSs with renal anomalies.	

[a] Investigations recommended if other features are compatible with a diagnosis.

[b] There is variability for some dysplasias and the timings given here reflect the authors' personal experience. In addition, where there is a family history scanning may be targeted at certain features that may otherwise be overlooked on a routine scan facilitating earlier diagnosis.

AC: abdominal circumference; AFI: amniotic fluid index; cfDNA: cell-free DNA; CNS: central nervous system; *FGFR3*: fibroblast growth factor 3; HC: head circumference; hCG: human chorionic gonadotropin; IUFGR: intrauterine fetal growth restriction; MSAFP: maternal serum alpha-fetoprotein; SRPS: short-ribbed polydactyly syndrome; NIPT: noninvasive prenatal testing; OI: osteogenesis imperfecta; PAPP-A: pregnancy-associated plasma protein A; PET: pre-eclamptic toxemia; SB: stillbirth; SEDC: spondylo-epiphyseal dysplasia congenica; SLE: systemic lupus erythema; VATER/VACTERL: vertebral anal atresia tracheoesophageal fistula radial anomaly/vertebral anal atresia cardiac trachea-esophageal fistula radial limb anomaly.

Table 11.4 Early sonographic features of skeletal dysplasias potentially identifiable by ultrasound by 14 weeks' gestation[12]

Condition	↑NT	FL	HC	Thorax	Skull	Other features	Inheritance	Gene	Lethal (Y/N)	Aids to diagnosis
Achondrogenesis I	+	<5th	N	Small	N Poor ossification	Hydrops, hypomineralized vertebral bodies	AR	1A – *TRIP11* 1B – *DTDST* or *SLC26A2*	Y	
Achondrogenesis II	+	<5th	N	Narrow, short ribs	No ossification	No/minimal ossification of vertebral bodies, poorly ossified long bones, generalized oedema	AD	*COL2A1*	Y	
Ellis–van Creveld	+/–	<5th	N	Small	N	Cardiac anomaly, polydactyly, posterior fossa cyst	AR	*EVC1, EVC2*	N	
Osteogenesis imperfecta IIA/C	+	<5th	N	Small	Hypomineralized	Short ribs, crumpled long bones, acute angling of femora	AD (AR)	*COL1A1/COL1A2 and others*	Y	
Osteogenesis imperfecta IIB/III		N/<5th	N	N/ slightly small	May have slightly poor mineralization	Bowed long bones	AD (AR)	*COL1A1/COL1A2 and others*	Y/N	
Thanatophoric dysplasia	+	5th/<5th	N/ >95th	Narrow, short ribs	N/abnormal shape (cloverleaf)	Frontal bossing, bowed femora, short fingers	AD	*FGFR3*	Y	NIPD to screen cfDNA for FGFR3 mutations
Campomelic dysplasia	+	<5th bowed	N	Small	N	Club feet, tibial spikes, arms normal length and appearance	AD	*SOX9*	Y/N	
Diastrophic dysplasia	+	<5th	N	N	N	Hitchhiker thumb, clubfoot, all long bones <5th	AR	*SLC26A2*	N	
Congenital hypophosphatasia	+/–	<5th / 10th	N	N/ narrow, short ribs	Hypomineralized	Poorly ossified ribs, vertebrae and long bones, polyhydramnios, short long bones, talipes	AR	*TNSALP*	Y	Parental alkaline phosphatase levels

Table 11.4 (*cont.*)

Condition	↑NT	FL	HC	Thorax	Skull	Other features	Inheritance	Gene	Lethal (Y/N)	Aids to diagnosis
Greenberg skeletal dysplasia	+	<<3rd	N	Narrow	N	Hydrops, hepatomegaly, severe generalised micromelia	AR	*LBR*	Y	
Spondylo-epiphyseal dysplasia congenita	+	N – 5th	N	Short	N	Hypomineralized vertebral bodies	AD	*COL2A1*	N	
Boomerang dysplasia	+	<<5th		Short, small	Hypomineralized	Some long bones not visible	X-linked Unknown	*FLNB*	Y	
Jeune's asphyxiating thoracic dystrophy	+/–	<5th	N	Narrow, short ribs	N	Polydactyly	AR	*DTNCH2H1* *1FT80*	30%	
SRPS I (Saldino–Noonan)	+	<<3rd	N	Small	N	Generalized skin edema, severe micromelia, polydactyly	AR		Y	
SRPS II (Majewski)	+	5th/<<3rd	N	Small, short ribs	N/cloverleaf	Exomphalos, bladder outflow obstruction, polydactyly, generalized edema	AR	*DYNCH2H1, NEK1*	Y	
SRPS III (Verma-Naumoff syndrome)	+	<10th		Small	N	Postaxial polydactyly		*DTNCH2H1*	Y	
Blomstrand dysplasia	+	<5th				Flared metaphyses, generalized rhizo-meso-acromelic limb shortening	AR	*PTHR1*	Y	
Roberts syndrome	+	<5th			N	Oligodactyly, short long bones, talipes, facial cleft	AR	*ESCO2*	Y/N	Fetal chromosome 'puffing'
Cleido-cranial dysplasia	+	N/slightly short			Hypomineralized	Poor ossification of the vertebral spine, hypoplastic clavicle	AD	RUNX2	N	

Adapted from reference 12. AD, autosomal dominant; AR, autosomal recessive FL, femur length; HC, head circumference; NT, nuchal translucency; SRPS, short-ribbed polydactyly syndrome.

Table 11.5 Differential diagnosis for fetuses where the predominant skeletal abnormality is in the forearm or leg showing the variability of features, genetic associations where known and other prenatal diagnostic aids[11]

	Forearm abnormalities	Hands	Lower limbs	Other potential USS findings	Growth	Inheritance	Gene	Other diagnostic aids
Forearm anomalies								
Trisomy 18	Variable	Camptodactyly	Talipes	Cardiac, CNS, hydronephrosis, cystic kidneys etc	IUFGR	Usually sporadic	N/A	Fetal karyotype
Trisomy 13	Radial club hand	Polydactyly, absent thumbs	Rocker bottom feet, polydactyly					
Cornelia de Lange syndrome [13]	Variable	Absent fingers or oligodactyly, syndactyly	Small feet	Cardiac, microcephaly, diaphragmatic hernia, abnormal profile, long philtrum +/- micrognathia	IUFGR	AD	*NIPBL, SMC1A, SMC3*	Low PAPP-A
Thrombocytopenia Absent radius syndrome	Bilateral radial aplasia, ulnar hypoplasia	Thumbs always present, oligodactyly	Absent or abnormal tibia, fibula, femurs, talipes	Absent or abnormal humeri, CNS, renal,	Usually normal but short stature	+ (unclear, AR and AD suggested)	All patients have a 1q21.1 deletion	Fetal platelet count
Vertebrae anus trachea esophagus and renal (VATER) syndrome	Variable	Absent or hypoplastic thumbs	Normal	Cardiac, renal, hemivertebrae, tracheoesophageal fistula	Normal	Sporadic		
Holt–Oram syndrome	Variable	Oligodactyly, absent thumbs, triphalangeal thumbs	Normal	Cardiac (often ASD)	Normal	AD	*TBX5*	Examine parents +/- X-ray wrists and echocardiography
Fanconi anaemia	Variable	Hypoplastic thumbs, polydactyly, triphalangeal thumbs	Normal	Microcephaly, renal, cryptorchidism and others	IUFGR	AR	At least 15 genes (*FANCA, FANB, FANC, BRCA2*)	Chromosome breakage study
Baller–Gerold syndrome	Bilateral asymmetrical	Absent or hypoplastic thumbs	Normal	Cardiac, anal atresia, craniosynostosis	Normal	AR	*RECQL4*	Genetic counseling
Nager acrofacial dysostosis	Bilateral asymmetrical	Absent or hypoplastic thumbs, pre-axial polydactyly	Absent or abnormal fibula, occasional syndactyly of toes	Cardiac, cleft lip, microcephaly, micrognathia	Normal	Unclear, AD and AR suggested		Genetic counseling
Roberts syndrome	Bilateral	Absent thumbs, syndactyly	Absent or hypoplastic fibula	Cardiac, CNS, cleft lip and palate, craniosynostosis	Normal	AR	*ESCO2*	Chromosome puffing
Femur fibula ulna syndrome	Variable asymmetrical	Absent hands, oligodactyly, ectrodactyly	Absent or hypoplastic femur and/or fibula, bowed tibia	-	Normal	Uncertain, probably sporadic	-	-
Gollop syndrome	Variable	Oligodactyly, syndactyly, ectrodactyly	Bifid humerus, absent or hypoplastic femur and/or tibia	Hydronephrosis	Normal	Uncertain	-	-

Table 11.5 (*cont.*)

	Forearm abnormalities	Hands	Lower limbs	Other potential USS findings	Growth	Inheritance	Gene	Other diagnostic aids
Steinfeld syndrome	Bilateral	Absent thumbs	Normal	CNS, renal dysplasia, ectopic kidneys, cleft lip, abnormal ears	IUGR	Uncertain, likely AD with variable expression		-
Goldenhar syndrome	Variable	Absent or hypoplastic thumbs, triphalangeal thumbs	Normal	Absent/abnormal ears, asymmetric face, micrognatia, cleft lip, cardiac, renal,	Normal	Uncertain, chromosomal, AD, AR, multifactorial		-
Poland–Fokin syndrome	Variable	Oligodactyly, skin syndactyly	Normal	Dextrocardia, renal anomalies	Normal	Uncertain		-
Okihiro–Duane radial ray syndrome	Variable	Absent or hypoplastic thumbs	Absent or hypoplastic fibula	Cardiac, renal agenesis	Normal	AD	*SALL4*	-
Fetal valproate syndrome	Variable	Oligodactyly, polydactyly	Talipes	Cardiac, CNS, cleft lip, micrognathia	IUGR	Environment		Maternal drug history
Lower limb anomalies								
Campomelic dysplasia	Normal	Normal	Short bowed femora, tibiae and fibulae	Cardiac, micrognathia, ambiguous genitalia/sex reversal in males	Normal	AD	*SOX9*	NIPD for fetal sex
Osteogenesis imperfecta III	May be short +/- bowed, may be normal in early pregnancy	Normal	Bilateral short bowed femora/tibiae and fibulae	Rib fractures	Decrease in growth velocity of long bones	AD, germinal mosaic	*COL1A1, COL1A2*	
Osteogenesis imperfecta IV	Normal	Normal	Bilateral mild bowing of femora +/- tibiae	-	May have normal/slight decrease in velocity	AD, germinal mosaic	*COL1A1, COL1A2*	
Femoral hypoplasia – unusual facies syndrome	Normal	Normal	Asymmetrical hypoplasia/absence of the femora	Short humeri, micrognathia, spinal anomalies, cardiac, renal and CNS		Sporadic/familial form type		Maternal diabetes, GTT
Proximal femoral focal deficiency	Normal	Normal	Usually unilateral hypoplastic/bowed femur +/- tibia and fibular, talipes			Sporadic		
Caudal regression syndrome	Normal	Normal	Bilateral, often asymmetrical hypoplasia of femora, +/- abnormal tibiae and fibulae	Spinal anomalies with lumbar/sacral agenesis, abnormal pelvis, urogenital anomalies		Sporadic		Maternal diabetes, GTT

Adapted from reference 11. AD, autosomal dominant; AR, autosomal recessive; ASD, atrioseptal defect; CNS, central nervous system; GTT, glucose tolerance test; IUFGR, intrauterine fetal growth restriction; N/A, not applicable; NIPT, noninvasive prenatal testing; PAPP-A, pregnancy-associated plasma protein A; USS, ultrasound scan.

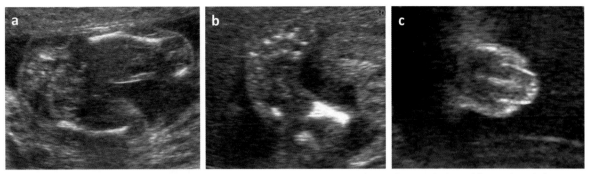

Figure 11.2 Ultrasound images of a fetus with campomelic dysplasia at 20 weeks' gestation, showing the bowed femurs: (a) with short lower leg bones and talipes; (b) this fetus had ambiguous genitalia but was confirmed to be male on cell-free DNA analysis (c).

obvious findings until the midtrimester, when they may be detected on a routine fetal anomaly scan[14], others present later[3], but many do not present until later in postnatal life. The challenge prenatally is to try and arrive at a definitive diagnosis in order to offer parents accurate information regarding prognosis. As this is frequently not possible, at a minimum we should aim to distinguish lethal from nonlethal[15] and provide some degree of differential diagnosis upon which parents can make decisions regarding further pregnancy management. Definitive diagnosis prenatally usually requires molecular genetic confirmation. This is increasingly possible since the molecular genetic defects underlying many of these conditions is now known (Table 11.4;[16]), further emphasizing the need to involve a clinical geneticist in the prenatal evaluation of these conditions. Furthermore, the advent of next-generation sequencing (NGS) and the development of NGS gene panels can further enhance the ability to screen affected pregnancies for multiple mutations in many genes. This increases the possibility of arriving at a definitive diagnosis in a timely fashion in pregnancy either following invasive testing by analysis of fetal amniocytes or chorionic villi[17] or using NIPD and analysis of cfDNA in maternal plasma[4].

Examination of long bones

The first indication of a generalized skeletal dysplasia is often the identification of a short femur at the time of a scan for another reason. Careful examination of the rest of the fetal anatomy can reveal further signs of a skeletal dysplasia (Table 11.3). If limb shortening appears to be isolated, then constitutional short stature may be the cause. Parents may be short or there may be a family history of short stature, and serial scanning should

demonstrate a normal long bone growth velocity, albeit along a line below the normal centiles. Intrauterine fetal growth restriction (IUFGR) must be considered as a possible etiology and review of maternal serum screening results for levels of pregnancy-associated plasma protein A, beta-human chorionic gonadotropin and maternal serum alpha-fetoprotein with assessment of fetal and maternal Dopplers may indicate placental insufficiency[18]. Personal experience is that around 30% of fetuses referred to our unit for evaluation of short limbs have early IUFGR.

The length of long bones should be checked against appropriate charts[8] and the gestational age at onset, degree and pattern of shortening determined (Table 11.3). In some conditions, the changes may be confined to the legs (e.g., campomelic dysplasia; Figure 11.2) or arms (e.g., Holt–Oram) or not be apparent until the third trimester (e.g., achondroplasia; Figure 11.3). Evidence of and the pattern of bowing or fracturing the long bones is a very useful diagnostic feature. Bones may appear short, thick and crumpled, indicating severe degrees of fracturing and undermodelling as in osteogenesis imperfecta (OI) IIA/C (Figure 11.4), whereas in other conditions, lesser degrees of deformity of the long bones may be present such as osteogenesis imperfecta III/IV (Figure 11.5) or campomelic dysplasia (Figure 11.2). Absence or hypoplasia of long bones should be assessed. The ends of the bones should be carefully examined to detect epiphyseal stippling, which is associated with chondrodysplasia punctata and some maternal conditions (Figure 11.6). If stippling is identified, various metabolic and cytogenetic investigations can be undertaken to aid definitive diagnosis (Table 11.3). Finally, the metaphyses may be flared in some of the collagen disorders, such as Kniest syndrome.

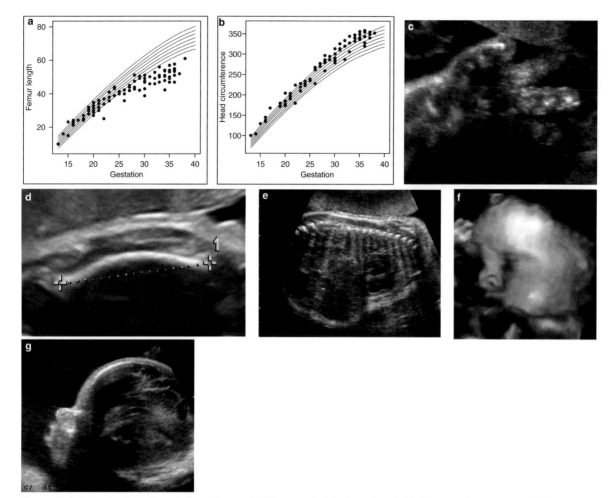

Figure 11.3. Achondroplasia. Growth charts showing the fall in growth of the femur length: (a) after 25 weeks' gestation and relative macrocephaly; (b) with sonographic images showing the short fingers; (c) slight bowing of the femora that can sometimes be observed; (d) the slight narrowing of the chest; (e) frontal bossing visible in three-dimensional view (f) but is often easier to recognize when visualizing the profile using two-dimensional ultrasound; and (g) the increased liquor volume can be seen. (a and b, courtesy of Chitty et al.[3])

Examination of the extremities

Polydactyly, either pre- or postaxial, can be a feature of a number of conditions (Figure 11.7; Table 11.3). Polysyndactyly, syndactyly and oligodactyly are less common findings but can be a very useful aid to diagnosis (Figure 11.7; Table 11.3). Hitchhiker thumbs and toes are pathognomonic of diastrophic dysplasia (Figure 11.7). Talipes can be seen in campomelic dysplasia, Kniest syndrome and oral-facial-digital (OFD) syndrome type IV.

Examination of the limb girdles

The limb girdles, shoulder and pelvis can be more difficult to examine. Hypoplastic clavicles may be seen in cleidocranial dysostosis and small scapulae in campomelic dysplasia.

Examination of the skull

The skull should be examined for shape, relative size and mineralization. In contrast to a normally mineralized skull, one which is hypomineralized will cast little or no acoustic shadow (Figure 11.4). Furthermore, the intracranial contents will be more clearly visualized than normal and, as the cerebral hemispheres appear relatively anechoic, the appearances are not infrequently mistaken for cerebral ventriculomegaly. In conditions associated with profound hypomineralization, in later pregnancy the skull shape can be distorted by pressure

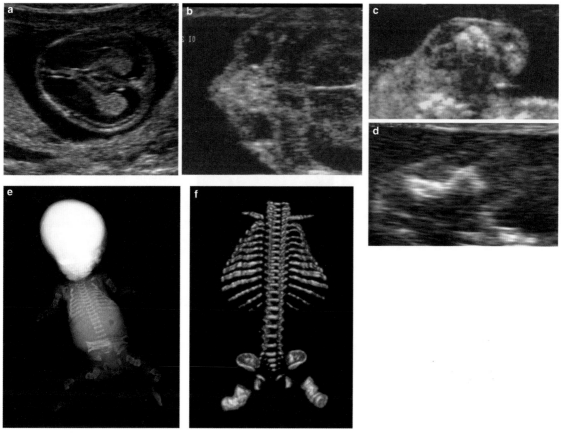

Figure 11.4 A fetus with osteogenesis imperfecta (OI) IIA, showing the profoundly hypomineralized skull, which casts no acoustic shadow (a) and facial bones (b), together with the very crumpled undermodelled humerus (c) and femur (d). A radiograph of a fetus with OI IIA also shows the beaded ribs (e) and reconstruction using computed tomography imaging shows these features in more detail (f). (e and f, courtesy of A Owens, Great Ormond Street NHS Foundation Trust)

from the ultrasound transducer. Abnormal skull shape can be seen as a result of associated craniosynostosis in a variety of conditions, including short-ribbed poly-dactyly syndrome, Apert syndrome and thanatophoric dysplasia type II (Figure 11.8), where a cloverleaf skull is a relatively common finding. Skull size can be a useful diagnostic aid. For example, in achondroplasia and thanatophoric dysplasia, there is frequently relative macrocephaly (Figures 11.3 and 11.8), whilst a small head circumference can aid diagnosis in conditions such as rhizomelic chondrodysplasia punctate and de Lange syndrome.

Examination of the face

The face should be carefully examined in the coronal, axial and sagittal planes using both two- and three-dimensional ultrasound as many skeletal dysplasias have associated facial anomalies. Examination in the coronal view can reveal a cleft lip, which can be very small and difficult to detect in some conditions, such as OFD syndrome type IV or Ellis–van Creveld. A sagittal view can reveal micrognathia (Figure 11.9), mid-face hypoplasia, frontal bossing (Figures 11.3 and 11.8) or a depressed nasal bridge (Figure 11.6). If possible, the mandible and orbital diameters should be measured, although acoustic shadowing from surrounding bony structures may impede accuracy later in pregnancy.

Examination of the thorax

The thorax should be examined in the axial, coronal and sagittal planes as most lethal dysplasias are associated with thoracic abnormalities; indeed, it is the small thorax and resultant pulmonary hypoplasia

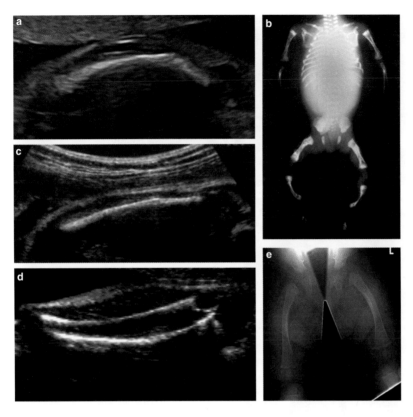

Figure 11.5 Types of osteogenesis imperfecta present with less obvious bowing. In (a) the femur is bowed proximally. There was also some mild bowing of the humeri and all long bones lay just below the 3rd centile at 21 weeks' gestation. A diagnosis of probable osteogenesis imperfecta (OI) III was made and confirmed radiologically after delivery shortly thereafter (b). OI IV can present with less obvious features, as in the fetus seen here, where scanning at 25 weeks' gestation detected minimal bowing of the femur (c) and tibia and fibula (d). The long bones remained within normal length for most of pregnancy, falling to the 3rd centile towards term. The baby was liveborn and the radiograph showed minor bowing of the femurs (e). The baby suffered further fractures in childhood.

that is usually the cause of death. The chest can be measured as there are various nomograms of thoracic size available, but a small chest can often be inferred by comparison of the chest and abdominal size in the axial plane. Usually, these structures are approximately the same size, but when there is a significant degree of thoracic hypoplasia, the size discrepancy is obvious (Figure 11.8). The heart should normally occupy one-third of the chest but, in the presence of short ribs, the heart will appear to occupy a greater proportion of the chest when viewed in the axial plane, and can, when the ribs are extremely short as in thanatophoric dysplasia[19], for example, appear to lie outside the thoracic cavity (Figure 11.8). Examination in the sagittal plane can show a narrow thorax with an apparently protuberant abdomen, the 'champagne-cork appearance' (Figure 11.8). The chest can also appear to be small secondary to a short spine, as in some of the spondylo-dysplasias, for example, spondylo-epiphyseal dysplasia congenita[20] (Figure 11.9). Here, the chest may appear small in a sagittal plane, but when viewed in the axial plane in comparison with the abdomen, the ribs are of normal length and the heart:thoracic ratio appears normal. Clearly, the importance of accurate assessment of chest size is for the prediction of pulmonary hypoplasia, which if significant can result in neonatal death. A further aid to the prediction of lethality is the use of a femur length:abdominal circumference (FL/AC) ratio which, if <0.16, distinguishes lethal from nonlethal skeletal dysplasias[21]. The ribs should be examined carefully as they may be short, thick, thin, beaded or irregular in organization or number. Short ribs can readily be identified in the axial plane (Figure 11.8), whilst beading or fracturing may be more easily seen in the sagittal or coronal planes (Figure 11.4) where three-dimensional (3D) ultrasound may prove a useful aid. Absent or disorganized ribs (usually seen in association with spinal anomalies) are also more readily visualized in the sagittal or coronal planes with 2D and 3D ultrasound (Figure 11.10). This is to be distinguished from the extra calcification that can give the appearance of a disorganized spine in some chondrodysplasia punctatas (Figure 11.10). Absence of mineralization of the vertebral bodies can also be a key clue to the diagnosis of achondrogenesis (Figure 11.11).

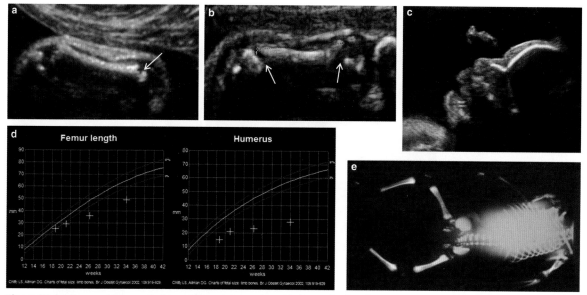

Figure 11.6 Ultrasound images of a fetus at 20 weeks' gestation with rhizomelic chondrodysplasia punctata showing (a) and (b) the short humerus with stippled epiphyses (arrows) and (c) the profile demonstrating the mid-face hypoplasia and slightly depressed nasal bridge. The charts (d) of humeral and femoral length demonstrate the relatively greater shortening of the humeri in a series of fetuses with rhizomelic chondrodysplasia punctata seen by the authors. The radiograph (e) shows the postnatal findings in an affected fetus.

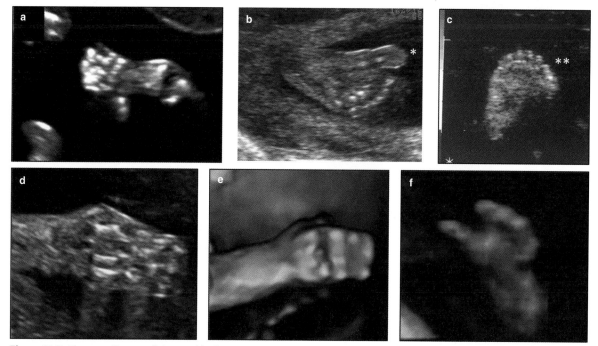

Figure 11.7 Ultrasound images of abnormal fetal extremities to demonstrate how this can aid sonographic diagnosis of skeletal dysplasia. In (a) the classic 'hitchhiker thumb' pathognomic of diastrophic dysplasia can be seen as early as 13 weeks. Pre-axial polydactyly of the toes is found in Ellis–van Creveld (b) as indicated by the large duplicated great toe (*) and the extra digits (**) in oral-facial-digital IV (c). A two-dimensional view (d) and three-dimensional image (e) of the syndactyly seen in Apert syndrome is shown, whilst oligodactyly (f) is found in conditions such as Cornelia de Lange.

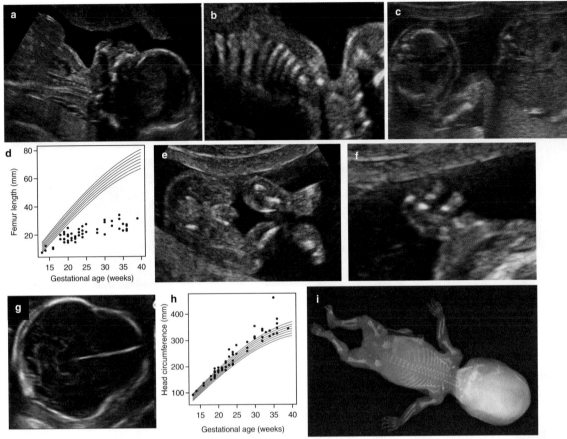

Figure 11.8 Some of the classical sonographic images seen in thanatophoric dysplasia with the very small 'champagne cork' appearance of the chest (a) with the bulging abdomen secondary to the very short ribs (b). When viewed in transverse section the chest is obviously smaller than the abdomen (c). Limb length is below the normal range from early pregnancy (d) and the legs are typically in the 'frog-like' position (e). Frontal bossing is always present (a) and the fingers are short (f). In thanatophoric dysplasia type II, there may be craniosynostosis, as indicated by an abnormal head shape (g). There is usually relative macrocephaly present (h). A postnatal radiograph is shown in (i).

Examination of the spine

The spine should be examined in all three planes. Hypomineralization of the vertebral bodies is a very useful aid to the diagnosis of achondrogenesis (Figure 11.11), but the sonographer should be wary of over-diagnosing this as ossification of the cervical and sacral vertebral bodies occurs late in pregnancy (Figure 11.1). The spine may appear to be disorganized secondary to hemivertebrae, which may or may not be associated with rib anomalies in conditions, such as VATER and Jarcot–Levin (Figure 11.10), but the ectopic calcification seen in some chondrodysplasia punctatas results in a disorganized appearance (Figure 11.10).

Examination of the skin for edema

One of the earliest signs of a fetal genetic problem is an increased nuchal translucency which, when seen in association with limb anomalies, can be indicative of an underlying skeletal dysplasia (Tables 11.3 and 11.4;[12]) as well as aneuploidy. Later in pregnancy, this can persist as an increased nuchal fold and generalized skin thickening as the skin appears to outgrow the bones, and thus long bones appear quite 'fat' (Figure 11.8). In conditions such as achondrogenesis and Greenberg dysplasia, frank hydrops can also occur.

Examination of the fetal viscera

Many skeletal dysplasias and other genetic syndromes associated with skeletal anomalies can have a variety of other

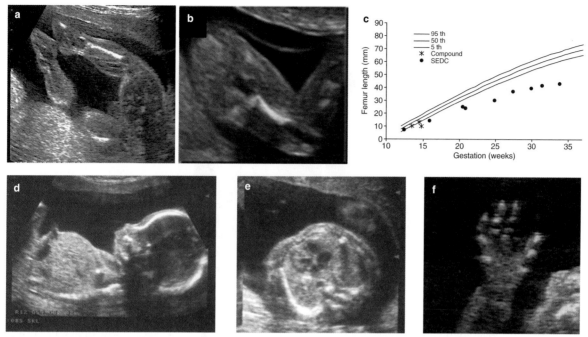

Figure 11.9 Ultrasound images of a fetus with spondylo-epiphyseal dysplasia congenita presenting with short straight legs (a), and short arms (b), falling below the 3rd centile from early in pregnancy (c, taken from Chitty et al.[20]). The chest is slightly small as seen in the sagittal view (d), which also shows the micrognathia. When viewed in transverse section (e) the ribs are of normal length. The heart is not protruding and only occupies one-third of the chest as normal (e).

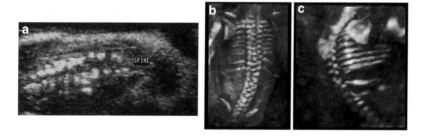

Figure 11.10 Abnormalities of the spine can be a useful aid to sonographic diagnosis of skeletal anomalies. In (a) the disorganized appearance of the spine in a fetus with chondrodysplasia punctata is very similar to that seen in the coronal view of the fetus with Jarcot Levin, but in this case (a) the disorganization seen is due to extra calcification. Disorganization of the spine is apparent in (b) secondary to multiple hemivertebrae in this fetus with Jarcot Levin syndrome. The associated rib gaps are clearly seen in the sagittal view (c).

abnormalities, some of which, if detected, can significantly aid the sonographic diagnosis (Table 11.3). For example, confirmation of a discrepancy between phenotypic sex and genetic sex determined by analysis of cell free DNA in maternal plasma in a fetus with bowed femora and female external or ambiguous genitalia can distinguish campomelic dysplasia from other cases of bilateral femoral bowing.

Assessment of amniotic fluid volume

The amniotic fluid may be increased as a result of a small chest in some dysplasias, but may also reflect the presence of esophageal atresia in VATER for example.

Conditions associated with more localized long bone anomalies

Fetal forearm anomalies

The etiology of fetal forearm defects is wide, and includes aneuploidy (particularly trisomy 18), teratogens, genetic syndromes or isolated findings. There are more than 200 syndromes associated with forearm anomalies such as radial club hand, transverse limb defects and digital anomalies. Table 11.5 gives a list of some of the more common associations, with

179

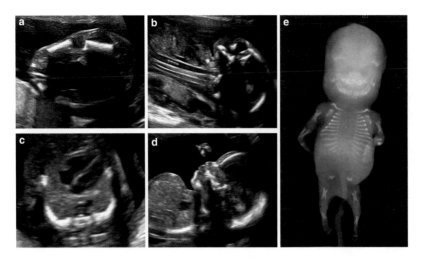

Figure 11.11 Ultrasound images of a fetus at 20 weeks' gestation with achondrogenesis type II. Note the very short, straight long bones (a), profoundly hypomineralized spine (b), short ribs seen in the axial view of the chest (c), and resulting in a very small chest seen in the parasagittal view (d). The postnatal radiograph with very short and straight long bones, and unmineralized vertebral bodies is shown in (e).

suggested aids to the prenatal diagnosis. As cardiac abnormalities are a relatively common association and can sometimes be very subtle, expert fetal echocardiography should be performed. The spine should also be carefully examined to exclude hemivertebrae. Experience suggests that if the forearm abnormality is isolated, the risk of an underlying genetic or chromosomal problem is very low, particularly where the growth is normal and the lesion is unilateral. Fetuses with associated abnormalities or bilateral forearm defects are much more likely to have an underlying genetic or chromosomal pathology[11].

Conditions associated with isolated lower limb defects

Femoral anomalies are rarely isolated, the majority being associated with other skeletal or visceral anomalies, which may give clues to the underlying diagnosis. Intrauterine fetal growth retardation and constitutional short stature should be considered if there appears to be isolated short but straight legs. When bowing or shortening is present and the lesion is unilateral or asymmetrical, the most likely diagnosis is one of proximal femoral focal hypoplasia, which is at the mild end of the caudal regression spectrum or femoral hypoplasia-unusual facies syndrome (Table 11.5). In the experience of the authors, the rate of growth for the affected long bone in several cases of femoral hypoplasia has continued at a relatively normal velocity, albeit below the normal centiles. This is useful information when discussing prognosis with the pediatric orthopedic team, as it narrows the postnatal management options. Again, in the authors' experience, where there was symmetrical bilateral bowing of the femora, all fetuses had an underlying skeletal dysplasia (Table 11.5).

Summary

The etiology of fetal skeletal abnormalities is broad, the prognosis highly varied and the prenatal diagnosis of cases arising unexpectedly in pregnancy is challenging. Nevertheless, by using a methodical and structured approach, a reasonably narrow differential diagnosis can often be reached and, with advances in molecular genetics, definitive diagnosis will increasingly be made in pregnancy. For some conditions, early drug or gene therapy may ameliorate the condition, for example, the use of bisphosphonates in osteogenesis imperfecta. However, a detailed description of the prognosis and management for all conditions is beyond the scope of this review. Given the high incidence of underlying genetic causes and the rapidly changing landscape, both for diagnosis and treatment, a multidisciplinary approach is essential and should involve an expert in clinical genetics, a radiologist familiar with skeletal dysplasias, and pediatric specialists. Referral to the relevant pediatric teams (orthopedic, hand specialists, skeletal dysplasia clinics, etc.) is useful for parents wanting to understand more about the long-term management, potential treatments and prognosis for the nonlethal conditions. Contact with relevant lay groups can also be very useful.

References

1. Sebire NJ, Weber MA, Thayyil S, et al. Minimally invasive perinatal autopsies using magnetic resonance imaging and endoscopic post-mortem examination ("keyhole autopsy"): feasibility and initial experience. *J Matern Fetal Neonatal Med* 2012; 25: 513–8.

2. Arthurs OJ, Thayyil S, Addison S, et al. Diagnostic accuracy of post-mortem MRI for musculoskeletal abnormalities in fetuses and children. *Prenat Diagn* 2014; 34: 1254–61.

3. Chitty LS, Griffin DR, Meaney C, et al. New aids for the non-invasive prenatal diagnosis of achondroplasia: dysmorphic features, charts of fetal size and molecular confirmation using cell free fetal DNA in maternal plasma. *Ultrasound Obstet Gynecol* 2011; 37: 283–9.

4. Chitty LS, Mason S, Barrett AN, et al. Non-invasive prenatal diagnosis of achondroplasia and thanatophoric dysplasia: next generation sequencing allows for a safer, more accurate and comprehensive approach. *Prenat Diagn* 2015; 35(7): 656–62.

5. Lench N, Barrett A, Fielding S, et al. The clinical implementation of non-invasive prenatal diagnosis for single gene disorders: challenges and progress made. *Prenat Diagn* 2013; 33: 555–62.

6. Calder AD, Offiah AC. Foetal radiography for suspected skeletal dysplasia: technique, normal appearances, diagnostic approach. *Pediatr Radiol* 2015; 45: 536–48.

7. Chitty LS, Campbell S, Altman DG. Measurement of the fetal mandible: feasibility and construction of a centile chart. *Prenat Diagn* 1993; 13: 749–56.

8. Chitty LS, Altman DG. Charts of fetal size: limb bones. *Br J Obstet Gynaecol* 2002; 109: 919–29.

9. Chitty LS, Altman DG. Charts of fetal size: kidney and renal pelvis measurements. *Prenat Diagn* 2003; 23: 891–7.

10. Chitty LS, Altman DG. Charts of fetal measurements. In: *Fetal Medicine: Basic Science and Clinical Practice*, CH Rodeck, M Whittle (eds). London: Churchill Livingstone, 2009: 721–66.

11. Pajkrt E, Cicero S, Griffin DR, et al. Fetal forearm anomalies: prenatal diagnosis, associations and management strategy. *Prenat Diagn* 2012; 32: 1084–93.

12. Khalil A, Pajkrt E, Chitty LS. Early prenatal diagnosis of skeletal anomalies. *Prenat Diagn* 2011; 31: 115–24.

13. Pajkrt E, Griffin DR, Chitty LS. Brachmann-de Lange syndrome: definition of prenatal sonographic features to facilitate prenatal diagnosis. *Prenat Diagn* 2010; 30: 865–72.

14. Schramm T, Gloning KP, Minderer S, et al. Prenatal sonographic diagnosis of skeletal dysplasias. *Ultrasound Obstet Gynecol* 2009; 34: 160–70.

15. Yeh P, Saeed F, Paramasivam G, et al. Accuracy of prenatal diagnosis and prediction of lethality for fetal skeletal dysplasias. *Prenat Diagn* 2011; 31: 515–8.

16. Krakow D, Rimoin DL. The skeletal dysplasias. *Genet Med* 2010; 12: 327–41.

17. Drury S, Williams H, Trump N, et al. Exome sequencing for prenatal diagnosis of fetuses with sonographic abnormalities. *Prenat Diagn* 2015; 35(10): 1010–7.

18. Vermeer N, Bekker MN. Association of isolated short fetal femur with intrauterine growth restriction. *Prenat Diagn* 2013; 33: 365–70.

19. Chitty LS, Khalil A, Barrett AN, et al. Safer, accurate prenatal diagnosis of thanatophoric dysplasia using ultrasound and cell free fetal DNA. *Prenat Diagn* 2013; 33: 416–23.

20. Chitty LS, Tan AW, Nesbit DL, et al. Sonographic diagnosis of SEDC and double heterozygote of SEDC and achondroplasia: a report of six pregnancies. *Prenat Diagn* 2006; 26: 861–5.

21. Nelson DB, Dashe JS, McIntire DD, et al. Fetal skeletal dysplasias: sonographic indices associated with adverse outcomes. *J Ultrasound Med* 2014; 33: 1085–90.

Chapter

12

Fetal genitourinary anomalies

Ashis Sau

Ultrasound detection of fetal urinary tract abnormality was first reported by Garrett et al. in 1970[1]. Since that time there have been significant improvements in the detection of fetal structural anomalies with the use of high resolution ultrasound machines. Currently, about 80% of all genitourinary malformations are detected by ultrasound in the second and third trimester[2]. These malformations contribute to about 20% of all major fetal structural abnormalities[3].

Embryology

The intermediate mesoderm differentiates into pro-nephros, mesonephros and metanephros around the 4th week of gestation. Later on, the pronephros and mesonephros regress and the metanephros gives rise to functional nephrons.

The ureteric bud grows out of the distal mesone-phic duct cranially and fuses with the metanephros. The ureteric bud forms the ureter, renal pelvis, papil-lae, and collecting system. The functional fetal kidney arises from the fusion of the ureteric bud and metane-phros, which is completed by 7 weeks of gestation. By the 9th week of gestation, the kidneys move up from its sacral position to the lumbar region.

Fetal renal function

Fetal urine production starts at 13 weeks of gestation. Initially there is no tubular reabsorption, so fetal urine consists of ultrafiltrate of serum containing high levels of sodium and chloride. Tubular reabsorption starts as the fetal kidneys become more mature from 15–16 weeks of gestation. The urinary sodium, chloride, amino acids level and urinary osmolality fall gradually. Urinary sodium levels of above 100 mmol/L, chloride above 90 mmol and osmolarity above 210 mosmol are considered to be associated with severe renal damage[4]. High concentrations of neutral amino acids in the fetal urine are also a predictor of poor renal function[5].

Sonographic appearances of the urinary tract

Fetal kidneys can be demonstrated by transvaginal scan as bilateral hyperechoic structures in about 92–99% cases around 13 weeks of gestation[6]. The bladder is visualized as a rounded sonolucent area at the center of the pelvis and a color flow will demonstrate two umbil-ical arteries around the bladder (Figure 12.1).

During the anomaly scan between 18–20 weeks, the kidneys are slightly hyperechoic in comparison with the surrounding bowels and paravertebral tissue. Two renal arteries can be easily demonstrated as originat-ing from the aorta by color flow Doppler (Figure 12.2). The ureters, which are not usually visualized during the anomaly scan, measure 1 mm or less in diameter.

A systematic assessment of fetal kidneys, bladder and liquor volume will help in the detection of renal tract abnormalities.

Renal agenesis

Failure of development and fusion of the ureteric bud with the metanephros is thought to be the result of renal agenesis. It can affect one or both kidneys. Unilateral renal agenesis is more common than bilateral with the incidence being 1 in 1,000 and 1 in 4,000 live births, respectively[7,8].

Diagnosis of unilateral renal agenesis is difficult unless a meticulous search is made of the renal fossa during the 18–20 weeks anomaly scan. In absence of renal tissue, fetal adrenal gland expands into the renal

Fetal Medicine, ed. Bidyut Kumar and Zarko Alfirevic. Published by Cambridge University Press. © Cambridge University Press 2016.

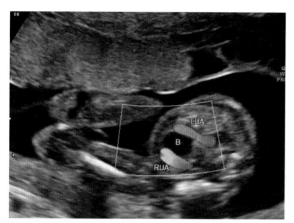

Figure 12.1 Transverse scan through fetal pelvis showing bladder (B) surrounded by right and left umbilical arteries (LUA and RUA).

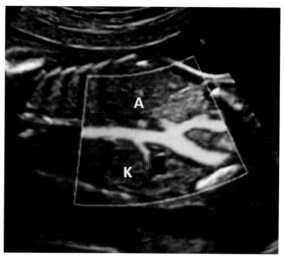

Figure 12.3 Unilateral renal agenesis. Kidney (K) and renal artery present in one side and the contralateral renal fossa is occupied by adrenal (A) with absence of renal artery.

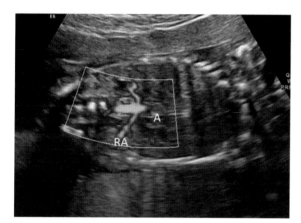

Figure 12.2 Coronal scan showing renal arteries (RA) originating from aorta (A) in color flow Doppler.

fossa mimicking the kidney. Furthermore, the liquor and bladder will also be normal. Demonstration of the unilateral absence of renal artery in color-flow Doppler will confirm the diagnosis of unilateral renal agenesis (Figure 12.3). The fetal pelvis should be checked carefully to rule out pelvic kidney. Similarly, normal size and shape of contralateral kidney will rule out crossed renal ectopi.

In contrast, there will be anhydramnios/severe oligohydramnios with absent bladder in bilateral renal agenesis. Lack of amniotic fluid and abnormal fetal position usually make the visualization of the renal fossa very difficult. Both renal arteries will be absent on color flow Doppler. Presence of normal liquor at 11–14 weeks scan does not preclude the diagnosis of bilateral renal agenesis as the kidneys do not become the major source of amniotic fluid until 14–16 weeks.

Bilateral renal agenesis should be differentiated from other renal diseases, particularly bilateral multicystic dyspalstic kidney or infantile polycystic kidney. Severe early onset intrauterine growth restriction and spontaneous rupture of membranes need to be excluded before confirming the diagnosis.

Renal agenesis may occur as an isolated anomaly or as a part of genetic syndrome. As a consequence of anhydramnios, a fetus with bilateral renal agenesis will be associated with Potter's facies, limb deformities and pulmonary hypoplasia. Major structural anomalies such as cardiac and VATER (vertebral, anal, tracheoesophageal, renal) abnormalities could be associated in about 1 in 4 cases[9].

Bilateral renal agenesis is a lethal abnormality and babies usually die soon after birth or in the early neonatal period due to pulmonary hypoplasia. Termination of pregnancy is an option that should be offered to the parents following a diagnosis. Unilateral renal agenesis is associated with normal prognosis, but babies will need a follow-up renal scan in the neonatal period to exclude any abnormality of contralateral kidney. Parents need to be aware that the recurrence risk of bilateral renal agenesis in future pregnancy is around 3–6%[10].

Pelvic kidney

This is the most common location of an ectopic kidney with an overall incidence of 1 in 700 live births[11], and is due to the failure in the ascension of the definitive

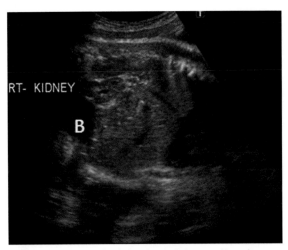

Figure 12.4 Right pelvic kidney located above and lateral to bladder (B).

kidney to the lumbar region in the first trimester of pregnancy.

A midtrimester scan will reveal that the renal fossa is occupied by the adrenal gland and absence of renal artery on the affected side, mimicking renal agenesis. Careful scanning of the fetal pelvis will show presence of the kidney lying above the bladder (Figure 12.4).

This condition is usually not associated with any other anomalies and has a very good prognosis if isolated.

Renal cystic disease

Cystic diseases of the kidney are of varied etiology. Based on etiological factors, they are classified into four different groups.

Two inheritable conditions are:

(1) infantile polycystic kidney (autosomal recessive or Potter type I)
(2) adult polycystic renal disease (autosomal dominant or Potter Type III).

Two developmental or acquired disorders are:

(3) multicystic dysplastic kidney (Potter type II)
(4) obstructive cystic disease (Potter type IV).

Infantile polycystic kidney: Potter type I

This is an autosomal recessive disease with an incidence of 1 in 40,000 to 50,000 live births[12]. Sonographic features of bilateral symmetrically enlarged hyper-echogenic kidney with small or absent bladder and oligohydramnios/anhydramnios are suggestive of Potter type I disease. This condition is also associated with hepatic fibrosis. The renal appearances are similar to adult polycystic kidney (Potter type III), but the presence of reduced/absent liquor will differentiate it from Potter type III disease.

Prognosis is very poor when diagnosed in utero. Although commonly diagnosed after 24 weeks of gestation, diagnosis as early as the end of the first trimester has also been reported[13]. In general, the earlier the prenatal manifestation of the disease, the poorer the prognosis. An option of termination of pregnancy can be offered to the parents, particularly if there is history of an affected sibling.

Multicystic dysplastic kidney: Potter type II

Multicystic dyspalstic kidney results from incomplete union of the metanephros to the branching ureteric bud leading to dilatation of the collecting tubules, which is a sporadic condition. The affected kidney appears enlarged with multiple noncommunicating cysts of different sizes. Usually, there is little or no renal parenchyma and the dyspalstic areas are echogenic (Figure 12.5). It is commonly seen in males with an overall incidence of 1 in 3,000 live births. In the majority of cases, it affects only one kidney, but bilateral disease can be seen in up to 23% of cases[14]. Contralateral kidney may have other abnormalities such as vesicoureteric reflux, renal hypoplasia and pelviureteric junction obstruction. Extra renal abnormalities including cardiac, gastrointestinal and central nervous system abnormalities may be seen.

Bilateral disease is associated with anhydramnios leading to pulmonary hypoplasia and neonatal death. Termination of pregnancy is an appropriate management option. The prognosis of unilateral disease is good provided the contralateral kidney maintains normal function and is managed conservatively. During the antenatal period, serial scans are performed to check the liquor volume, parenchyma of the normal kidney as well as the affected kidney. Renal scans are performed after delivery to confirm the diagnosis followed by micturating cystourethrogram (MCUG) and dimercaptosuccinic acid (DMSA) scans. The unilateral multicystic kidney usually atrophies in childhood and nephrectomy is rarely required.

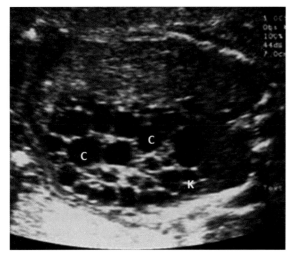

Figure 12.5 Multicystic dysplastic kidney. A sagittal scan showing kidney (K) with multiple cysts (C) with echogenic parenchyma.

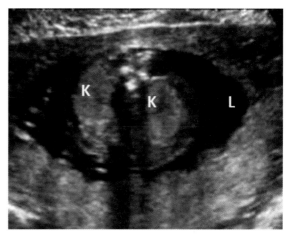

Figure 12.6 Adult polycystic kidney. A transverse scan showing bilateral enlarged echogenic kidneys (K) with normal liquor (L).

Adult polycystic renal disease: Potter type III

Adult polycystic renal disease is an autosomal dominant disease with an incidence of 1 in 1,000 live births. The condition is most commonly caused by a mutation in the chromosome 16 and manifests as cystic dilatation of the nephrons of both kidneys, which are rarely seen in utero[15].

Prenatally, a symmetrically enlarged and echogenic kidney with presence of a normal bladder, normal or reduced liquor and family history will help in diagnosing this condition (Figure 12.6). It is important to scan the kidneys of parents if there is no known family history. The presence of two or more cysts in each kidney of either of the parents will confirm the diagnosis. Kidneys may look normal at the 20 weeks' anomaly scan, so it is important to repeat the scan later in a pregnancy where there is a family history.

The most common associated abnormalities are cysts in the liver, spleen and pancreas, which are mainly seen in adults.

The prognosis of antenatally detected adult polycystic kidneys is difficult to determine. Presence or absence of a previously affected sibling and family history will help in counseling regarding the short- and long-term outlook of the baby. Around 43% of babies will die within first year of life in the absence of previous affected pregnancy [16]. Being an autosomal dominant condition, there is a 50% risk of recurrence in future pregnancy.

Obstructive cystic dysplasia: Potter type IV

Urinary tract obstruction in the first-trimester or early second-trimester pregnancy will lead to dysplastic lesion in the kidneys, which is a sporadic condition. It is very difficult to ascertain the actual incidence of this condition as only a minority of cases of urinary tract obstruction will progress to cystic dysplasia. An incidence of approximately 1 in 8,000 live births has been reported[17].

The condition can be unilateral or bilateral. Unilateral disease is most commonly due to pelviureteric or vesicoureteric junction obstruction. Presence of duplex kidneys with associated ureterocele can lead to unilateral obstructive disease. Bilateral disease is mainly caused by posterior urethral vale or urethral atresia.

Sonographic features of small echogenic kidney containing peripheral cortical cysts along with other evidence of obstruction are suggestive of obstructive cystic dysplasia. Bilateral diseases are associated with bilateral hydronephrosis, hydroureter, a large thick-walled bladder and oligo- or anhydramnios. In a duplex system, dysplasia can affect only the upper moiety of the kidney. Normal echogenicity of the renal cortex does not always exclude dyspepsia so a serial assessment of the renal cortex is essential.

This condition can be associated with other abnormalities, such as vertebral, anorectal atresia, cardiac abnormalities, tracheoesophageal fistula and limb abnormalities (VACTERL).

Prognosis is very poor in a bilateral disease and an option of termination pregnancy should be discussed with the parents. In the absence of other abnormalities and contralateral renal disease, the prognosis of unilateral disease is good and it can be managed conservatively.

Renal obstruction

Urinary tract obstruction in the midtrimester of pregnancy will manifest as renal pelvic dilatation or hydronephrosis. There are controversies regarding the cutoff value of anteroposterior (AP) diameter of the renal pelvis, above which it should be considered abnormal. An AP diameter of above 15mm (severe) at 20 weeks gestation is associated with about 50% reduction in the mean differential renal function and 30% reduction is seen when the diameter is between 10 and 15 mm (moderate)[18]. A mild renal pelvic dilatation (AP diameter of 5–8 mm) is not associated with significant reduction of renal function but can be associated with vesicoureteric reflux in up to 12% of cases. The UK National Health Service Fetal Anomaly Screening Programme (FASP) recommends a follow-up scan in third trimester for renal pelvic dilatation of more than 7 mm at 18–20 weeks.

The common causes of renal pelvic dilatation or hydronephrosis are pelviureteric junction (PUJ) obstruction, vesicoureteric junction (VUJ) obstruction, vesicoureteric reflux, posterior urethral valve and duplex renal system, with or without ureterocele.

Pelviureteric junction obstruction

PUJ obstruction is the most common urinary tract abnormality, which is unilateral in 90% of cases. This condition is seen commonly in males with an overall incidence of 1 in 2,000 live births.

The presence of unilateral dilatation of the renal pelvis without dilatation of the bladder and ureter in the midtrimester scan will lead to the suspicion of PUJ obstruction. Severe obstruction will cause calyceal dilatation with thinning of the renal cortex (Figure 12.7). Evidence of cortical dysplasia in the form of increased echogenicity or small cortical cyst can be seen in severe disease. Liquor volume is usually normal. It is essential to assess the contralateral kidney to rule out bilateral disease or other associated renal abnormality, such as renal agenesis, multicystic dysplastic kidney, which can be seen in about 25% cases[19]. Bilateral disease needs to be differentiated

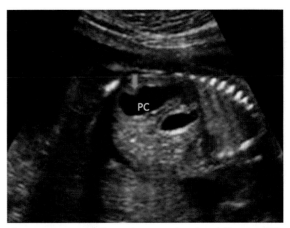

Figure 12.7 A sagittal scan showing pelvicalyceal dilatation (PC) with thin renal cortex (arrow).

from VUJ obstruction, vesicoureteric reflux and bladder neck obstruction. Bilateral renal pelvis dilatation in the absence of ureteric dilatation will make a strong case of PUJ obstruction.

It is very important to organize a follow-up scan in the third trimester following suspicion of PUJ obstruction at 20 weeks to assess the severity of the disease, liquor volume and contralateral kidney. A neonatologist should be informed and the baby will need prophylactic antibiotics. A follow-up renal scan during the neonatal period, an MCUG and DMSA scan will be helpful to confirm the antenatal diagnosis and severity of the disease. Although the majority of cases are managed conservatively, severe disease with poor differential renal function will need surgical correction to prevent further renal cortical damage.

Severity of renal pelvic dilatation during antenatal period correlates well with the degree of renal impairment. In general, the prognosis is good. Due to the sporadic nature of the condition, the risk of recurrence in any future pregnancy is low.

Vesicoureteric junction obstruction

VUJ obstruction constitutes about 10% of all antenatally detected significant renal tract abnormalities[20]. Similar to PUJ obstruction, this condition is more common in males. It is bilateral in about 25% of cases.

A diagnosis of VUJ obstruction should be considered when there is sonographic evidence of unilateral or bilateral renal pelvic dilatation along with dilated ureter (Figure 12.8). Dilated sonolucent ureter can be differentiated from the bowels, which show a low level

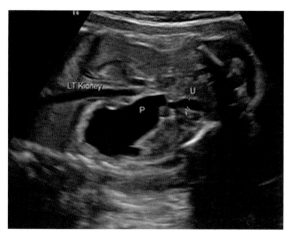

Figure 12.8 Coronal section through left kidney showing hydronephrosis (P) and dilated ureter (U).

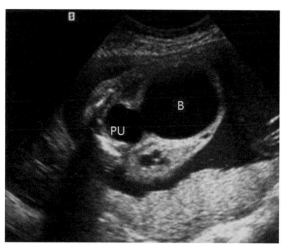

Figure 12.9 Transverse scan through fetal pelvis showing distended bladder (B) and dilated posterior urethra (PU). "Keyhole sign," PU valve.

of echos. In a unilateral disease, the bladder and liquor volume are usually normal but may be reduced in bilateral disease. Similar to any other renal tract abnormality, it is important to assess the contralateral kidney, which may be affected with VUJ obstruction, muticystic dysplatic kidney or renal agenesis. It is very difficult to differentiate a bilateral VUJ obstruction from vesicoureteric reflux antenatally. MCUG after delivery will differentiate between these two conditions. An obstruction caused by a ureterocele in a duplex kidney will have similar features as unilateral VUJ obstruction but the presence of a ureterocele within the bladder and dilatation of the upper moiety will differentiate it from a VUJ obstruction.

A follow-up scan in the third trimester should be arranged to assess liquor volume and severity of the condition. During the neonatal period, the baby will need prophylactic antibiotics until further investigations rule out vesicoureteric reflux. Renal function can be assessed by a DMSA scan. The majority of the babies are managed conservatively with a good outcome. In cases of severe disease with deteriorating renal function, ureteric reimplantation will be required.

The recurrence in any future pregnancy is very low.

Bladder outlet obstruction

Bladder outlet obstruction could be due to posterior urethral valve or urethral atresia.

Posterior urethral valve

This condition only affects males with an overall incidence of 1 in 5,000 to 8,000. The presence of a

membranous tissue within the posterior urethra leads to bladder neck obstruction.

A second-trimester scan will show evidence of a distended, thick-walled bladder with dilated posterior urethra (Figure 12.9). There will be oligohydramnios or anhydramnios along with hydroureter and hydronephrosis. In cases of incomplete obstruction, the liquor volume and bladder may look normal at the 20 weeks' scan. The condition should be differentiated from urethral atresia, severe bilateral vesicoureteric reflux and megacystis-microcolon syndrome.

It is important to rule out chromosomal anomaly in cases of posterior urethral valve, which is seen in about 8% of cases. Other associated structural anomalies are cardiac anomalies, anal atresia and VATER syndrome.

Prognosis depends on the severity of the disease and gestational age of diagnosis. Diagnosis before 24 weeks, oligohydramnios, hydroureter and hydronephrosis, along with echogenic/cystic renal cortex, indicate very poor prognosis[21]. About 44% of the babies who survive the early neonatal period will develop end-stage renal failure by the age of 4–5 years.

Antenatal management will depend upon the severity of the disease. Termination of pregnancy can be offered in the poor prognostic group; on the other hand, conservative management is appropriate where the liquor volume is normal and hydronephrosis remain stable. In utero insertion of the vesicoamniotic shunt to bypass the bladder obstruction is considered only in a few cases where there is progression of obstruction in the third trimester, and repeated

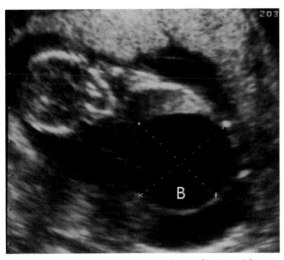

Figure 12.10 Urethral atresia. A sagittal scan of a 15-week fetus showing distended bladder (B) occupying the whole abdomen with no dilatation of posterior urethra.

vesicocentesis confirm preservation of renal function. There are controversies regarding the role of antenatal insertion of the shunt, and a multicenter randomized trial in the UK was closed early because of poor recruitment. It is important to discuss in a multidisciplinary team involving the fetal medicine consultant, neonatologist and pediatric urologist.

The recurrence risk in future pregnancy is low.

Urethral atresia

Urethral atresia results from incomplete canalization of distal urogenital sinus, which forms the proximal urethra. This is seen more commonly in males and may constitute up to 60% of all prenatal diagnosed bladder neck obstruction[22].

The presence of a distended bladder, severe oligohydramnios/anhydramnios, hydroureter and hydronephrosis are characteristics of urethral atresia. The condition is manifested early in the pregnancy (Figure 12.10). The absence of a dilated proximal urethra will differentiate this condition from posterior urethral valve.

Chromosomal and other structural anomalies are associated in about two-thirds of the cases. It may be difficult to rule out structural anomalies due to the presence of anhydramnios.

Termination of pregnancy is an appropriate management option due to poor prognosis of the baby. The majority of the babies will die in the early neonatal period due to pulmonary hypoplasia.

The condition is sporadic with a very low risk of recurrence in future pregnancy.

Vesicoureteric reflux

Vesicoureteric reflux accounts for about 10% of all fetal hydronephrosis and about 20% of all prenatally detected significant renal abnormality[20]. About 30–50% of children who present with recurrent urinary tract infection will show some evidence of vesicoureteric reflux. In-utero reflux is thought to be caused by the distortion of VUJ by the high-voiding pressure.

Bilateral or unilateral dilatation of the renal pelvis may be the only feature of vesicoureteric reflux. In severe cases there will be associated ureteric dilatation and thin-walled distended bladder. A high grade of bilateral reflux can cause renal scarring in utero. Liquor volume is usually normal even in bilateral disease. Unilateral disease needs to be differentiated from unilateral PUJ or VUJ obstruction. Bladder neck obstruction needs to be considered in cases of bilateral disease with distended bladder. Confirmation of diagnosis is possible only after delivery by MCUG. In a unilateral condition, contralateral kidney should be checked for associated anomalies, such as PUJ obstruction, muticystic kidney, duplex kidney and renal agenesis.

A follow-up scan at the third trimester is essential to assess the severity of the disease and liquor volume. After delivery, the baby should have prophylactic antibiotics followed by a renal scan in the first week of life, and MCUG depending on the renal scan findings. In some cases, MCUG is considered in all neonates with antenatal diagnosis of renal pelvic dilatation irrespective of postnatal renal scan findings[23].

Vesicoureteric reflux can lead to renal scarring and reflux nephropathy if not treated appropriately. The majority (70%) of mild reflux can resolve spontaneously in the first few months of life, but spontaneous resolution is seen in around 40% of severe refluxes by 15 months of age[24].

Reflux disease is thought to be genetically linked as there is high risk of recurrence. Two-thirds of babies will be affected if the mother suffers from reflux and one-third of siblings of an affected child will have reflux[25].

Megacystis-microcolon-intestinal-hypoperistalsis syndrome

Megacystis-microcolon-intestinal-hypoperistalsis syndrome is an autosomal recessive condition more

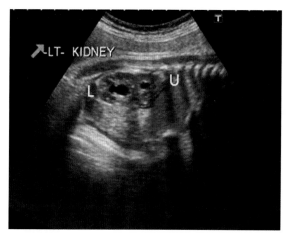

Figure 12.11 Duplex kidney. Sagittal scan showing upper and lower moiety (U and L) with two renal pelvis.

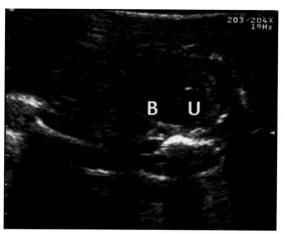

Figure 12.12 Scan through fetal pelvis showing ureterocele (U) within the bladder (B).

commonly seen in girls with a female-to-male ratio of 4 to1. Exact etiology is unknown but it manifests as a functional small bowel obstruction with nonobstructed distended urinary bladder.

The antenatal scan will show a distended thick-walled bladder with bilateral hydronephrosis. The presence of normal or excessive liquor will differentiate it from posterior urethral valve. The past history of an affected sibling and a female baby are two important factors in diagnosing this condition.

The prognosis is very poor. Termination of pregnancy is an appropriate option, particularly when there is a family history.

Risk of recurrence is 25%.

Ureterocele

Stenosis of distal ureteric orifice leads to dilatation of the intravesical part of the ureter, which is known as ureterocele. It is commonly associated with a duplex renal system (Figure 12.11) in females, but in males it may develop from a normal kidney[2]. This condition is bilateral in about 10–15% of cases.

Ureterocele is commonly associated with dilated ureter and renal pelvis. In a duplex system, it is the upper moiety that is commonly affected. Sometimes a large ureterocele can obstruct the contralateral ureteric orifice leading to hydroureter and hydronephrosis of the opposite kidney. Rarely, it can obstruct the bladder neck. Liquor volume is usually normal in unilateral cases. Detection of ureterocele within the bladder is the confirmatory sign but is not always possible to visualize on the scan (Figure 12.12).

Vesicoureteric reflux is commonly associated with this condition and can affect the lower pole moiety. Prognosis is usually good. A follow-up scan in the third trimester is essential to assess the liquor volume and renal parenchyma of the affected kidney. Diagnosis is confirmed and renal function is assessed by neonatal renal scan, DMSA scan and MCUG. Cystoscopic puncture of the ureterocele is the treatment of choice.

The risk of recurrence in future pregnancy is low.

Cloacal exstrophy

Cloacal exstrophy is a sporadic condition with an incidence of 1 in 250,000 live births[26]. Rupture of the cloacal membrane before the completion of caudal growth of the urorectal septum will lead to this abnormality. It is usually manifested as bladder exstrophy, herniation of small and large bowels through the lower part of anterior abdominal wall and bifid phallus. An exomphalus and lumbosacral spina bifida are usually associated with this abnormality.

An absent bladder and an anterior abdominal wall defect below the umbilicus on the antenatal scan will lead to a strong suspicion of cloacal exstrophy. Liquor volume is usually normal but sometimes the condition can be associated with polyhydramnios. Associated abnormality can be seen in up to 85% of cases. Renal anomalies, such as unilateral renal agenesis, pelvic kidney and multicystic kidney, are the most common association.

Absence of bladder and defect below the umbilicus will differentiate this condition from exomphalus and gastroschisis.

Major surgical correction after delivery is required and an option of termination of pregnancy should be discussed with the parents following antenatal detection of cloacal exstrophy.

Recurrence risk in future pregnancy is low.

Bladder exstrophy

Rupture of cloacal membrane after the completion of caudal growth of urorectal septum will cause bladder exstrophy. The condition is commonly seen in males with an overall incidence of 1 in 30,000 live births[27].

Ultrasonographic features of absent bladder, along with lower abdominal bulge, a small penis along with anteriorly displaced scrotum, normal liquor and kidneys, are suggestive of bladder exstrophy. Other anomalies are usually not associated with this condition, which differentiates it from cloacal exstrophy.

Long-term prognosis following surgical correction after delivery is generally good. The recurrence is less than 1%.

Ambiguous genitalia

It is a rare disorder caused either by chromosomal abnormality or by abnormal hormonal effect.

Female pseudohermaphroditism is due to either maternal ingestion of androgen or congenital adrenal hyperplasia. Excess androgen will cause clitoral enlargement of variable degree. The karyotype is 46,XX.

The abnormal response of external genitalia to testosterone or under production of testosterone in a genetically male fetus will lead to male pseudohermaphroditism. In this condition, a male fetus will have a blind vagina or micropenis with or without cryptorchidism.

Chromosomal defects such as mixed gonadal dysgenesis, pure gonadal dysgenesis and true hermaphroditism are the other causes of ambiguous genitalia.

It is hard to detect ambiguous genitalia during the antenatal period. A micropenis with undescended testes will have a similar ultrasound appearance to that of clitoromegaly with normal labia (Figure 12.13). Ultrasound features of male genitalia in a genetically female baby are suggestive of congenital adrenal hyperplasia. Diagnosis can be confirmed by estimating 17-hydroxyprogesterone levels in amniotic fluid. A follow-up scan in the latter half of pregnancy will be helpful to assess fetal genitalia but not accurate enough to assign a gender during the antenatal period. A final diagnosis should be made after a thorough neonatal assessment.

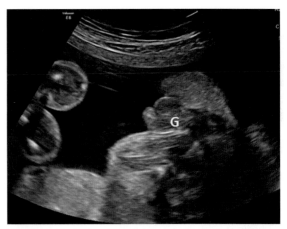

Figure 12.13 Section through the external genitalia (G) showing scrotum and micropenis in a genetically male fetus.

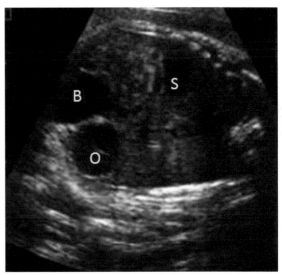

Figure 12.14 Coronal scan showing right ovarian cyst (O) located just above and lateral to bladder (B). Stomach (S) on the left side.

Ovarian cyst

Ovarian cysts are relatively common intra-abdominal cystic lesions in the female fetus. Ovarian cysts develop in response to high maternal hormones and resolve spontaneously after delivery. Sonographically, a unilocular/occasionally multilocular cystic structure below the kidney and beside the bladder in a female fetus will raise the suspicion of an ovarian cyst (Figure 12. 14). Absence of two umbilical arteries surrounding the cyst will differentiate it from the fetal bladder. Usually no intervention is required during antenatal period. Very rarely, a large ovarian cyst can cause pressure effects on other organs or obstructed labor. A transabdominal aspiration of the cyst is an appropriate option in those circumstances. A scan during the neonatal period will confirm the diagnosis and assess the size of the cyst.

References

1. Garrett WJ, Grunwald G, Robinson DE. Prenatal diagnosis of fetal polycystic kidney by ultrasound. *Aust N Z J Obstet Gynecol* 1970; 10: 7–9.

2. Wiesel A, Queisser-luft A, Clementi M, et al. Prenatal detection of congenital renal malformations by fetal ultrasonographic examination: An analysis of 709,030 births in 12 European countries. *Eur J Med Genet* 2005; 48: 131–44.

3. Elder JS. Antenatal hydronephrosis fetal and neonatal management. *Pediatr Clin North Am* 1997; 44: 1299–321.

4. Appleman Z, Globus MS. The management of fetal urinary tract obstruction. *Clin Obstet Gynaecol* 1986; 29: 483–9.

5. Lenz S, Lund-Hansen T, Bang J, et al. A possible prenatal evaluation of renal function by amnio acid analysis on fetal urine. *Prenat Diagn* 1985; 5: 259–67.

6. Rosati P, Guariglia L. Transvaginal sonographic assessment of the fetal urinary tract in early pregnancy. *Ultrasound Obstet Gynecol* 1996; 7: 95–100.

7. Hitchcock R, Burge DM. Renal agenesis: an acquired condition? *J Pediatr Surg* 1994; 29: 454–5.

8. Bronshtein M, Amil A, Achiron R, et al. The early prenatal diagnosis of renal agenesis: techniques and possible pitfalls. *Prenat Diagn* 1994; 14: 291–7.

9. Newbold MJ, Lendon M, Barson AJ. Oligohydramnios sequence: the spectrum of renal malformations. *Br J Obstet Gynaecol* 1994; 101: 598–604.

10. Bankier A, De Campo M, Newell R, et al. A pedigree study of prenatally lethal renal disease. *J Med Genet* 1985; 22: 104–11.

11. Hill L, Peterson CS. Antenatal diagnosis of fetal pelvic kidneys. *J Ultrasound Med* 1987; 6: 393–6.

12. Tsuda H, Matsumota M, Imanaka M, et al. Measurement of fetal urine production in mild infantile polycystic kidney disease-a case report. *Prenat Diagn* 1994; 14: 1083–5.

13. Bronshtein M, Yoffe N, Brandes JM, et al. First and second trimester diagnosis of fetal urinary tract anomalies using transvaginal ultrasound. *Prenat Diagn* 1990; 10: 653–6.

14. Gough DCS, Postlethwaite RJ, Lewis MA, et al. Muticystic renal dysplasia diagnosed in the antenatal period: a note of caution. *Br J Urol* 1995; 76: 244–8.

15. Reeders ST, Breuning MH, Davies KE, et al. A highly polymorphic DNA marker linked to adult type polycystic kidney disease on chromosome 16. *Nature* 1985; 317: 542–4.

16. MacDermot KD, Saggar-Malik AK, Economides SJ. Prenatal diagnosis of autosomal dominant polycystic kidney disease (PDK 1) presenting in utero and prognosis for very early onset disease. *J Med Genet* 1998; 35: 13–6.

17. Scott JE, Renwick M. Urological anomalies in the northern region fetal abnormality survey. *Arch Dis Child* 1993; 68: 22–6.

18. Barker AF, Cave MM, Thomas DFM, et al. Fetal pelvi-ureteric junction obstruction: predictions of outcome. *Br J Urol* 1995; 76: 649–52.

19. Drake DP, Stevens P, Eckstein HB. Hydronephrosis secondary to uretero-pelvic obstruction in children: a review of 14 years experience. *J Urol* 1978; 119: 649–51.

20. Thomas DFM. Prenatally detected uropathies: Epidemiological considerations. *Br J Urol* 1998; 81 (Suppl 2): 8–12.

21. Twining P. Urinary tract abnormalities. In: Twining P, McHugo JM, Pilling DW, eds. *Textbook of fetal abnormalities.* London: Churchill Livingstone, 2000.

22. Reuss A, Wladimiroff JW, Stewart PA, et al. Non-invasive management of fetal obstructive uropathy. *Lancet* 1988; 2: 949–50.

23. Tibballs JM, De Bruyn R. Primary vesico-ureteric reflux – how useful is postnatal ultrasound? *Arch Dis Child* 1996; 75: 444–7.

24. Yeung C, Godley M, Dhillon H, et al. The characteristics of primary vesico-ureteric reflux in male and female infants with prenatal hydronephrosis. *Br J Urol* 1997; 80: 319–27.

25. Noe N, Wyatt R, Peeden J, et al. The transmission of vesicoureteral reflux from parent to child. *J Urol* 1992; 148: 1869–71.

26. Chtril Y, Zorn B, Filidori M, et al. Cloacal exstrophy in monozygotic twins detected through antenatal ultrasound scanning. *J Clin Ultrasound* 1993; 21: 339–42.

27. Shapiro E, Lepor H, Jeffs R. The inheritance of exstrophy – epispadias complex. *J Urol* 1984; 132: 308–10.

Chapter

13

Fetal tumors

Andrew Sharp and Zarko Alfirevic

Fetal tumors are rare but are often detectable with antenatal ultrasound in the second or third trimester. Ultrasound is helpful to determine tumor location, content (solid, cystic, mixed or calcified), vascular involvement, compressive effects, as well as likely tissue of origin. Furthermore, serial ultrasound assessments allow monitoring of growth and cardiovascular effects. However, difficulties do exist, particularly with very large tumors, and the addition of fetal magnetic resonance imaging (MRI) can provide further information.

The range of fetal tumors is vast (Table 13.1) and includes those of benign and malignant potential, tumors that affect widely varying tissues and locations within the fetus and those that are isolated or associated with other conditions. It is important to remember that tumors may have significant effects on fetal prognosis either directly, due to pressure effects, or secondary to effects upon the fetal circulation.

The management of many fetal tumors requires a multidisciplinary approach. There may also be significant management plans that are required in fetuses with tumors, which may necessitate elective cesarean section or the involvement of other specialities, such as general or ear, nose and throat (ENT) surgeons.

Fetal tumors are commonly located in the heart (24%), face and neck (22%) and abdomen (19%), with rarer sites including the sacrococcygeal region (11%), extremities (11%), chest (10%) and central nervous system (CNS) (4%)[1]. On histological assessment, two-thirds of fetal tumors are lymphangiomas (25%), rhabdomyomas (23%), teratomas (17%) or hemangiomas (14%).

Central nervous system tumors

CNS tumors comprise 10% of all prenatally diagnosed tumors with most being supratentorial, in marked contrast to pediatric tumors, which are mostly infratentorial[2]. Generally the prognosis is poor and worse if the diagnosis is made prior to 30 weeks where mortality secondary to severe hydrocephalus can be up to 96%[3].

Most CNS tumors will be identified as an intracranial mass with associated hydrocephalus, macrocephaly or polyhydramnios. The mainstay of diagnosis should be to identify potentially curable CNS tumors, such as choroid plexus papillomas, from rapidly fatal ones, such as teratomas or neuroepithelial tumors. The use of fetal MRI may aid determination of tissue type.

Hydrocephalus and macrocephaly develop secondary to obstruction of the ventricular system and cerebrospinal fluid outflow. Rapid growth of a tumor may also lead to macrocephaly secondary to tumor size or the development of hydrops due to cardiovascular compromise. Twenty-one percent of fetuses with CNS tumors will be stillborn as a result of these complications[4]. Due to the high incidence of hemorrhage (18%) in CNS tumors, all diagnoses of intracranial hemorrhage should include assessment of the possibility of an underlying brain lesion. Pediatric neurosurgeons should be involved in the development of a multidisciplinary management plan. Delivery may be complicated by the presence of significant macrocephaly and cesarean section or predelivery decompression of the skull may be required to prevent labor dystocia.

Teratoma

Although rare in older children, intracranial teratoma is the most common CNS tumor in the fetus (>50%) [5]. Most will be located within the ventricles, hypothalamic, suprasellar or cerebral regions. As with all teratomas, they appear as an irregular solid and cystic

Fetal Medicine, ed. Bidyut Kumar and Zarko Alfirevic. Published by Cambridge University Press. © Cambridge University Press 2016.

Table 13.1 Ultrasound features of tumor by location and tumor type

Tumor location	Tumor type	Ultrasound features	Differential diagnoses
CNS	Teratoma	Mixed echogenicity, calcifications, distortion of anatomy	Arachnoid cyst; Choroid plexus cyst; Vein of Galen aneurysm
	Astrocytoma	Unilateral echogenic mass in cerebral hemisphere	
	Medulloblastoma	Infratentorial/cerebellar	
	Ependymoma	Usually fourth ventricle Mixed echos, may include cystic areas, hemorrhage or calcification	
	Choroid plexus tumor (papilloma)	Large lobulated echogenic mass, unilateral, lateral ventricle (rarely third ventricle)	
Head and neck	Lymphangioma/cystic hygroma	Large cystic mass with multiple septations commonly observed in the posterior triangle of the neck	
	Cervical teratoma	Large (5–12 cm) multiloculated, unilateral lesion with solid and cystic components. Calcifications	
Cardiac	Fibroma	Solid interventricular lesion	
	Rhabdomyoma	Single or multiple intramural hyperechoic masses	
	Teratoma	Solid and cystic components calcifications	
Abdomen	Adrenal neuroblastoma	Cystic, solid or mixed appearance. Well circumscribed Right sided	Ovarian cyst (follicular, lutein)
	Congenital mesoblastic nephroma	Unilateral solid, homogeneous mass may have cystic areas	
	Hemangioma	Single or multiple heterogeneous mass within the liver	
	Hamartoma	Homogeneous or mixed cystic lesions within the liver	
	Hepatoblastoma	Homogeneous liver lesion	
	Lymphangioma	Cystic mass with septations	
	Sacrococcygeal teratoma	Cystic and solid elements and may be significantly vascularized May be very large	
	Wilm's tumor	Unilateral solid, homogeneous mass may have cystic areas	
	Ovarian tumor	Unilateral cystic, solid or complex mass	

echogenic mass with calcifications that distort the normal appearance of the brain. Teratomas comprise tissue from all three germ cell layers with immature neuroglial elements. Prognosis is extremely poor and is related to the size of the tumor and presence of associated hydrocephalus. A third will die in utero with only 12% surviving the neonatal period and 7% reaching 1 year of age[5].

Astrocytomas

Astrocytomas are the second most common congenital CNS tumor and represent a wide range of pathologies from subependymal giant cell astrocytomas to glioblastoma multiforme[5]. The appearances on ultrasound are of a unilateral echogenic mass within the cerebral hemisphere, which may have internal hemorrhage and often causes midline shift. The prognosis is generally poor with 13% stillborn and 37% surviving the neonatal period. The situation is even worse in the more aggressive glioblastoma multiforme where only 13% will survive[4].

Ependymoma

Ependymomas are tumors of the ependymal cells lining the ventricles or spinal canal. Ultrasound appearances are of mixed echogenic masses arising from the ventricle, which may include cystic areas, hemorrhage or calcification. They commonly arise from the fourth ventricle. There can be extension into the subarachnoid space with resultant involvement of the spinal cord. Macrocephaly and hydrocephalus are common features, and stillbirth, intracerebral hemorrhage and labor dystocia are complications.

Neuroepithelial tumors/medulloblastoma

Tumors comprised of neuroepithelial tissue can be termed primitive neuroepithelial tumors or medulloblastoma, and whilst common in the pediatric population, this is a much less common finding in the perinatal period. Unlike most other perinatal CNS tumors they are often infratentorial, arising from the cerebellar vermis and extending into the fourth ventricle. Survival is very poor at 12%[6].

Choroid plexus tumor

Tumors of the choroid plexus are rare and mostly papillomas or occasionally carcinomas. They represent 20% of congenital brain tumors and are less common in older children. The hallmark of choroid plexus tumors is excessive cerebrospinal fluid (CSF) production with associated hydrocephalus and macrocephaly. The appearance on ultrasound is of a large lobulated highly echogenic (cauliflower-like) mass, usually unilateral and located in the atria of the lateral ventricle, or rarely in the third ventricle. Treatment is with surgical excision, with adjuvant chemotherapy and radiotherapy for carcinoma, and survival rates of >70% are common[5].

Craniopharyngioma

These tumors are rare in the perinatal period. When found, they present as large heterogeneous cystic lesions with calcifications. They arise in the suprasellar region from epithelial origin. The prognosis is worse when identified in the perinatal period.

Spinal cord tumors

Congenital tumors of the spinal cord are extremely rare and most commonly are actually saccrococcygeal teratomas. Occasionally astrocytomas can present in this location, and as with most CNS tumors the prognosis is poor.

Differential diagnoses: CNS cysts and vascular malformations

Whilst technically not tumors, these lesions are included as they are important differential diagnoses when investigating CNS lesions.

Choroid plexus cysts

These fluid-filled cystic areas are located within the choroid plexus and form during normal development. They can be found in up to 1% of fetuses on routine ultrasound scanning where they appear as well-circumscribed sonolucent, unilocular or septated cysts >3 mm diameter within the choroid plexus itself. They tend to resolve by the third trimester or soon after birth. They have historically been linked to chromosomal disorders such as trisomy 18, but this risk is low and if found in isolation, does not warrant invasive testing.

Particularly large cysts are usually unilateral and may lead to ventriculomegaly due to obstruction of the flow of cerebrospinal fluid, but in invariably the outcomes are good[7]. Treatment in the neonatal period may be required with removal or fenestration techniques.

Arachnoid cysts

These cysts are benign congenital collections of CSF and may account for 1% of all CNS masses in children. The cysts are lined with collagen arising from the arachnoid mater and there may be communication to the subarachnoid space. Ultrasound appearances are of peripherally placed discrete sonolucent lesion with thin, smooth walls. They are usually supratentorial with the majority located within the sylvian fissure, but they may be found in the posterior fossa[8].

The main effect of arachnoid cysts is as a space-occupying lesion, and therefore the size and location of the cysts can be critical to prognosis. Small cysts may be of no clinical importance, whereas large cysts may cause seizures and neurologic symptoms in the newborn period. Isolated cysts usually have a good prognosis, although regular follow-up is required as they may increase in size in the third trimester leading to the development of hydrocephaly, particularly if located in the posterior fossa. Intrauterine cyst drainage has been attempted for the rapidly enlarging cyst, but usually this can be deferred until after birth.

Arachnoid cysts are usually isolated lesions, but they may be associated with other CNS malformations, such as agenesis of the corpus callosum, absent septum pellucidum, Arnold–Chiari malformation type I, and a variety of chromosomal/genetic syndromes, such as distichiasis-lymphedema, Mohr syndrome, trisomy 18, triploidy and unbalanced translocations. Therefore, amniocentesis should be offered in all cases of arachnoid cysts due to the association with genetic anomalies.

Vein of Galen aneurysm

Aneurysm of the great cerebral vein (of Galen) is extremely rare but relatively easy to diagnose with approximately 50% being diagnosed before infancy. The vein of Galen is part of the network of deep cerebral veins and curves under the splenium of the corpus callosum joining with the inferior sagittal sinus to form the straight sinus. This aneurysmal defect occurs as a result of an arteriovenous malformation between the primitive choroidal vessels and the median prosencephalic vein of Markowski.

Ultrasound appearances are of a well-defined midline sonolucent mass above the corpus callosum and cerebellum extending to the cranium. The use of color Doppler shows a nonpulsatile turbulent flow within the dilated vessel. Additional features within the head include macrocephaly or hydrocephalus. Fetal MRI is important to detect other anomalies and to exclude other differential diagnoses, such as arachnoid, porencephalic or choroid plexus cysts. Common complications include hydrocephaly, high-output cardiac failure and stillbirth. Other sequelae of a vein of Galen aneurysm may occur within the rest of the fetus, and include cardiomegaly, pericardial effusion, dilated neck veins, hepatomegaly, ascites, polyhydramnios and hydrops fetalis. In addition, ballantyne (mirror) syndrome may also present due to a hydropic placenta.

The prognosis for antenatally diagnosed vein of Galen aneurysms is related to the presence of associated cardiac or cerebral anomalies. When other anomalies are present the outcome is invariably poor[9]. For those fetuses that survive to the neonatal period, surgical treatment options exist and some success has been reported with the use of postnatal vein embolization, although the mortality for this procedure is around 30%.

Head and neck tumors

The range of head and neck tumors is significant and includes teratoma, lymphangioma, congenital goitre, thyroid or parathyroid tumors, thyroid cysts, neuroblasmtoma or hamartomas. Tumors of the fetal face usually present early with a persistently open fetal mouth even before the development of associated polyhydramnios. Head and neck tumors may grow large enough to cause obstruction of the fetal airway. If inadequately prepared for, this can be both fatal for the fetus and extremely distressing for the attending clinical team. Other potential complications include polyhydramnios and preterm birth secondary to esophageal obstruction, labor dystocia secondary to tumor size, or spontaneous rupture of the tumor leading to fetal death from exsanguination.

Lymphangioma

Cystic hygroma, otherwise called lymphangioma, is a benign malformation of the lymphatic drainage. They can develop anywhere within the body but commonly affect the neck and thorax. Normally, the lymphatic system begins to form at 5 weeks of gestation. Failure of the jugular lymph sacs to join with the lymphatic system leads to the development of progressively enlarging cystic structures on the lateral and posterior aspects of the neck.

Identification of a cystic hygroma in the first or second trimester carries the risk of fetal demise in utero, and also requires discussion of invasive testing as >50% will have an underlying chromosomal disorder and may also have other anomalies. The common associations include Turner syndrome, Down's syndrome (trisomy 21), Edward's syndrome (trisomy 18) and Noonan syndrome. Even with a normal karyotype, the risk of major structural anomalies in these fetuses remains high (34%), predominantly cardiac or skeletal[10]. Overall, a normal outcome can be expected in 17% of fetuses diagnosed with a first-trimester cystic hygroma.

Lymphangioma can also present later in the third trimester after normal routine ultrasound examination. These later onset lymphangiomas are usually located on the anterior neck and the prognosis is generally better. They do not appear to have the same association with aneuploidy or coexistent anomalies.

Appearances on ultrasound are of a large cystic mass with multiple septations commonly observed in the posterior triangle of the neck (Figure 13.1). It may be difficult to differentiate increased nuchal translucency from cystic hygroma at early gestations as both may contains septations[11]. Other differential diagnoses need to be excluded by confirming integrity of the skull (posterior encephalocele) and lack of solid or calcified components (teratoma), ascites or pleural effusions (nonimmune hydrops). If there is doubt, fetal MRI may be beneficial to distinguish between cystic hygroma and cervical teratoma (Figure 13.2).

Prognosis depends greatly upon gestation at presentation and associated chromosomal or structural anomalies. The majority of early cystic hygromas have a very poor prognosis due to the high incidence of chromosomal abnormalities and hydrops. In the presence of a normal karyotype, no hydrops and no other structural anomalies, the prognosis is excellent.

Management relies upon invasive testing, detailed cardiac assessment, serial scans for progression or compression. Occasionally, amnioreduction will be required due to polyhydramnios secondary to esophageal compression. Vascular compression can lead to nonimmune hydrops, and if the tumor is large elective cesarean section or ex utero intrapartum treatment (EXIT) procedure may be required (Figure 13.3). There is limited data on the use of sclerosing agents for in utero treatment of cystic hygroma but not enough evidence to offer this treatment outside of research protocols.

Postnatal management of cystic hygroma relies upon imaging with computed tomography or MRI, followed by surgery or use of sclerosing agents, such as bleomycin. Complete resection is possible in only 77% of cases, with recurrence in 11–52%[12].

Cervical teratoma

These tumors are rare and, in common with other teratomas, consist of tissue from all three germ layers. Due to their location within the neck, the predominant tissue is neural, although 40% may also have thyroid tissue.

Ultrasound commonly demonstrates a large (5–12 cm) multiloculated, unilateral lesion with solid and cystic components. Calcifications may be present in 50% of cases[13]. Extension is commonly to the mandible, mastoid process, suprasternal notch and mediastinum. Involvement of the floor or the oropharynx can lead to mandibular hypoplasia and polyhydramnios.

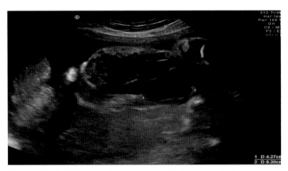

Figure 13.1 Ultrasound appearance of a large cervical lymphangioma.

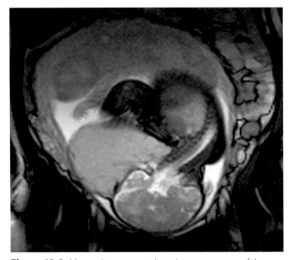

Figure 13.2 Magnetic resonance imaging appearance of the same cervical lymphangioma shown in Figure 13.1.

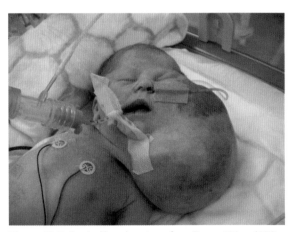

Figure 13.3 Cervical lymphangioma from Figures 13.1 and 13.2 following an ex utero intrapartum treatment procedure.

Management requires repeated ultrasound assessments to monitor tumor growth and liquor volume. Amnioreduction may be required if there is significant polyhydramnios to reduce the likelihood of preterm birth. Stillbirth remains a concern secondary to high-output cardiac failure. Delivery is almost always by cesarean section due to tumor size, hyperextension of the fetal neck and risk of tumor rupture at delivery. Elective intubation at delivery is mandatory and EXIT procedures have been advocated[14] due to the high risk of airway obstruction and respiratory compromise. Even with adequate ventilation, mortality is high at 45% and up to 80–100% in untreated cases. Fetal MRI may help to define the extent of the tumor and allow preparation for an EXIT procedure and postnatal surgery.

Postnatal surgery can be extremely complex and multiple operations may be required to give a good functional and cosmetic result. Endocrine disorders due to loss of thyroid and parathyroid tissue are common but malignant transformation is rare. Recurrence in future pregnancies is extremely rare.

Ex utero intrapartum treatment (EXIT)

In the fetus with a large neck mass, there is a high risk of airway compromise at birth secondary to laryngeal obstruction or laryngomalacia. If the mass is unrecognized or inadequately planned for, the risk of anoxic brain injury and death is substantial[14].

In cases where a giant neck mass has been identified in the antenatal period appropriate planning of delivery can occur in collaboration with neonatal physicians and ENT surgeons. In these cases it may be appropriate to perform an elective cesarean section with an EXIT procedure (Figure 13.3 and supplementary video).

The EXIT procedure involves delivery of the fetal head and neck at cesarean and establishing a secure airway whilst the fetus is still attached to the placenta. This technique can provide a window of up to 2 h of adequate placental oxygenation in order to secure the airway or even resect the tumor[15]. Once an airway is secured, the rest of the fetus is delivered and separated from the placenta. The main maternal risk from an EXIT procedure is hemorrhage due to the prolonged use of inhalational agents, which relax the uterus.

Cardiac tumors

Fetal cardiac tumors are rare and almost always benign. Most of the cardiac tumors identified in the fetus will

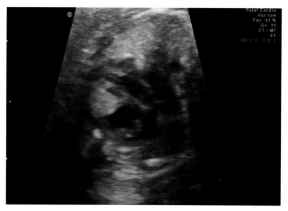

Figure 13.4 Ultrasound appearance of a large septal rhabdomyoma.

be rhabdomyomas, although teratomas and fibromas can also be identified[16]. Due to the location of cardiac tumors, they may have significant effects upon cardiac function or conduction (arrhythmias).

Rhabdomyoma

Rhabdomyoma is by far the most common cardiac tumor and is often identified as single or multiple intramural hyperechoic masses (Figure 13.4). Technically, these are hamartomas, an overgrowth of normal tissues, rather than neoplasms. Occasionally, due to the location or size of these masses, they may predispose to cardiac arrythmyias or hydrops due to intracardiac flow disruption. Arrhythmia or cardiac dysfunction are poor prognostic factors and are associated with stillbirth and neonatal death.

The most significant feature of the identification of cardiac rhabdomyomas is their association with tuberous sclerosis, which is present in 50–80% of cases[16]. The presence of multiple cardiac rhabdomyomas is sufficient to give a diagnosis of tuberous sclerosus.

Tuberous sclerosus is an autosomal dominant condition with an incidence of 1 in 6,000, with two-thirds occurring as sporadic mutations. Mutations occur within the tumor suppressor TSC1 or TSC2 genes, located on chromosome 9q34 and 16p13.3, respectively. The resulting hamartoma formation can be lethal. Characteristic features of the condition include mental retardation, epilepsy and facial angiofibromas. Neonatal seizures are common due to cortical and subependymal tubers (gliomas). The use of fetal MRI can significantly aid prognosis as the presence of CNS tubers may provide valuable prognostic evidence that may help decision making regarding continuance of the pregnancy[17]. Antenatal diagnosis of cardiac rhabdomyomas should prompt a careful history and examination of parents and siblings to elucidate family mutations.

Teratoma

The second most commont fetal cardiac tumor is a teratoma but they are far more commonly located elsewhere. Teratomas can originate from the pericardium or less commonly from the myocardium. The most common presentation will be with a mass with a resultant pericardial effusion, or rarely nonimmune hydrops. Stillbirth or neonatal death is an uncommon possibility.

Cardiac fibroma

These are a rare benign tumor of fibroblast or myofibroblast origin often arising from the interventricular septum. Main features relate to left ventricular dysfunction or arrhythmia (ventricular tachycardia or ventricular fibrillation). Occasionally, cardiac fibromas may be associated with cleft lip and palate or syndromes such as Beckwith–Wiedeman syndrome or nevoid basal cell carcinoma syndrome (Gorlin's syndrome). Cardiac fibromas should be removed surgically after birth to ensure unimpaired cardiac function, although survival can be low (23%) if surgery is performed in the neonatal period[16].

Cardiac myxoma

Myxoma is a common benign neoplasm in adults but is extremely rare in the fetus. Most commonly located within the atrium they can cause valvular dysfunction and cardiac failure. Case reports have suggested its involvement in stillbirth.

Abdominal and pelvic tumors

The abdomen and pelvis is the most common site for fetal tumors and the tissue of origin is usually readily identified.

Hepatic tumors

The most common cause of a hepatic lesion is not a tumor but actually a hepatic, biliary or choledochal cyst, which require observation and postnatal review.

Hepatic tumors constitute only 5% of fetal tumors[2]. The most common hepatic tumor is a hemangioma. This benign vascular tumor can be singular or multiple and appear heterogeneous when compared with normal liver. Growth can be rapid and lead to cardiovascular compromise, but spontaneous postnatal resolution can occur.

Hamartomas can also occur and are of hepatic, biliary tree or fibrous origin. They appear as solid or mixed cystic lesions on ultrasound and may be associated with Beckwith–Weidemann syndrome[18]. Hepatoblastoma is a malignant tumor of the liver that appears as a solid nodule and is associated with Beckwith–Wiedemann syndrome and other malformations.

Neuroblastoma

Neuroblastoma is the most common fetal malignancy and arises from cells of the sympathetic nervous system. Generally these tumors are sporadic but there can be associations with neural crest malformations or a rare familial form (1–2%), which can be screened for[19]. In the nonfamilial form, recurrence is low. The use of folic acid may reduce incidence.

Ninety percent of neuroblastomas are located within the adrenal gland with a right-sided predominance. Ultrasound demonstrates a cystic, solid or mixed appearance. They are normally well circumscribed and cause caudal displacement of the kidney. Fetal MRI may be of assistance in confirming the origin. In utero metastasis to the liver, umbilical cord or placenta has been reported and may lead to hydrops due to compressive effects. Serial ultrasound assessments are required to look for metastases and monitor the size and development of hydrops. Preterm delivery and in utero therapy are not indicated. Maternal complications include pre-eclampsia secondary to secretion of fetal catecholamines, which may be more common in metastatic disease.

Postnatal management usually consists of biopsy to confirm diagnosis and surgery when appropriate. A small number may regress and overall outcome is good with a >90% survival[18].

Renal mass

Tumors of the kidney are rare, with most renal anomalies being due to renal function or cystic lesions. The most common solid renal tumor identified prenatally is a mesoblastic nephroma, which is indistinguishable from Wilm's tumor (nephroblastoma) on imaging[2]. Appearances are of a unilateral solid homogeneous mass, which may have cystic areas within, representing hemorrhage or necrosis. Polyhydramnios is a common finding, although the exact mechanism of its development is unclear. Tumors are rarely large enough to preclude vaginal delivery.

Assessment for associated anomalies is important as Wilm's tumor may exist as part of Perlman's syndrome (ascites, hepatomegaly, macrosomia and polyhydramnios). If Wilm's tumor is a possibility, a clear history from the mother is required as 20% are associated with mutations of the *WT1* gene on chromosome 11.

Ovarian mass

The female fetus may have a tumor arising from the ovary. These are usually cystic follicular or lutein cysts, which regress postnatally. Solid or complex lesions are more likely to represent immature teratomas, which require postnatal resection. Very large lesions >5 cm are at risk of prenatal torsion with resulting ovarian necrosis. Cystectomy with conservation of ovarian tissue should be performed postnatally for persistently large cysts.

Sacrococcygeal teratoma

Teratomas are tumors that have tissue from all three germ cell layers (ectoderm, mesoderm and endoderm). Mature teratomas are benign, whereas immature teratomas have malignant potential. They are mostly located within the midline. Over 60% arise from the sacrococcygeal area, with other sites including the gonads (20%), neck, mediastinum, pericardium, retroperitoneum, brain, heart, pharynx and pleura[20].

Sacrococcygeal teratomas (SCT) represent the most common congenital neoplasm with a high perinatal morbidity and mortality. The tumor is often large and can be classified in relation to its intra-abdominal contents (Table 13.2)[21]; however, this classification does not give useful information regarding prognosis. SCTs often contain both cystic and solid elements and may be significantly vascularized. Despite these characteristic features antenatal detection is only 50%[22] (Figure 13.5).

Ultrasound forms the mainstay of management and 3D imaging may aid physicians' and parents' understanding of the tumor anatomy. Ultrasound may be less good at determining the extent of pelvic masses due to the "drop out" generated by the bony pelvis, and in these circumstances fetal MRI may have a role to determine the extent of the tumor and its interactions with other tissues.

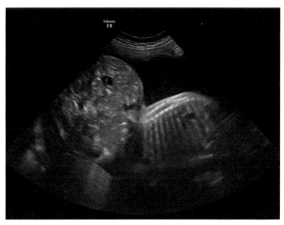

Figure 13.5 Ultrasound of a large sacrococcygeal teratoma at 26 weeks showing the cystic appearance. In this example, the tumor is actually larger than the abdominal circumference.
Supplementary video: video of an ex utero intrapartum treatment (EXIT) procedure performed for massive cervical lymphangioma.

Table 13.2 Classification of SCT tumors

Type of sacrococcygeal teratoma tumor as per American Academy of Pediatrics Surgical Section (AAPS)[21]	
Type I	Predominantly external, with minimal intrapelvic extension
Type II	Mainly external, with significant intrapelvic extension
Type III	Visible external, but predominantly internal
Type IV	Internal, although external parts may be visible

Isolated SCT is not associated with an abnormal karyotype and amniocentesis is not indicated.

Regular assessment with ultrasound and MRI is required as tumors can grow rapidly and may lead to development of hydrops. Fetal MRI may be superior to ultrasound for the assessment of tumor extension within the abdomen/pelvis.

Congenital teratomas themselves are virtually always benign but should be removed after birth as there is a significant potential for malignant change in the infant period.

Management of fetal tumors

Initial diagnosis and management is likely to be via the fetal medicine unit. It is important to remember that in most cases the management of fetal tumors will involve a multidisciplinary approach, involving fetal medicine specialists, neonatologists, pediatric surgeons or neurosurgeons and midwifes. Pregnancy support groups (www.Bliss.org.uk; www.uk-sands.org) and parent groups may also be useful in providing personalized advice and support to the mother and family of the affected fetus.

The good safety profile and ready availability of ultrasound, supports the use of ultrasound as the primary modality for the detection and follow-up of fetal tumors, especially as repeated assessments are needed.

The use of fetal MRI may be beneficial, particularly when there is uncertainty over tissue of origin or involvement of other organs[2]. The main advantage of fetal MRI is excellent tissue resolution[2].

Summary

Fetal tumors are rare but ultrasound detection is increasingly common in the antenatal period with standard ultrasound based screening modalities. A careful assessment of the tumor location and ultrasound features may aid the determination of tissue type, which could have a significant impact on counseling and request for termination of pregnancy. The use of fetal MRI is beneficial where the tissue of origin or extent of tumor is unclear.

Overall, fetal tumors have a poor prognosis and are associated with high stillbirth rates, labor dystocia and postnatal surgery. However, determination of the underlying tissue type is vitally important as it can drastically alter the prognosis.

References

1. Kamil D, Tepelmann J, Berg C, et al. Spectrum and outcome of prenatally diagnosed fetal tumors. *Ultrasound Obstet Gynecol* 2008; 31(3): 296–302.

2. Lee C, Olutoye O. Evaluation of the prenatally diagnosed mass. *Semin Fetal Neonatal Med* 2012; 17(4): 185–91.

3. Isaacs H. Fetal brain tumors: a review of 154 cases. *Am J Perinatol* 2009; 26(6): 453–66.

4. Isaacs HI. Perinatal brain tumours: a review of 250 cases. *Pediatr Neurol* 2002; 27(4): 249–61.

5. Hwang S, Su J, Jea A. Diagnosis and management of brain and spinal cord tumors in the neonate. *Semin Fetal Neonatal Med*, 2012; 17(4): 202–6.

6. Parmar HA, et al. Imaging of congenital brain tumors. *Semin Ultrasound CT MR* 2011; 32(6): 578–89.

7. Fong K, Chong K, Toi A, et al. Fetal ventriculomegaly secondary to isolated large choroid plexuscysts: prenatal findings and postnatal outcome. *Prenat Diagn* 2011; 31(4): 395–400.

8. Chen C. Prenatal diagnosis of arachnoid cysts. *Taiwan J Obstet Gynecol*, 2007; 46(3): 187–98.

9. Deloison B, Chalouhi GE, Sonigo P, et al. Hidden mortality of prenatally diagnosed vein of Galen aneurysmal malformation: retrospective study and review of the literature. *Ultrasound Obstet Gynecol* 2012; 40(6): 652–8.

10. Malone F, Ball RH, Nyberg DA, et al. First-trimester septated cystic hygroma: prevalence, natural history, and pediatric outcome. *Obstet Gynecol* 2005; 106(2): 288–94.

11. Molina F, Avgidou K, Kagan KO, et al. Cystic hygroma, nuchal edema, and nuchal translucency at 11–14 weeks of gestation. *Obstet Gynecol* 2006; 107(3): 678–83.

12. Hancock B, St-Vil D, Luks FI, et al. Complications of lymphangiomas in children. *J Pediatr Surg* 1992; 27(2): 220–4.

13. Tonni G, De Felice C, Centini G, et al. Cervical and oral teratoma in the fetus: a systematic review of etiology, pathology, diagnosis, treatment and prognosis. *Arch Gynecol Obstet* 2010; 282(4): 355–61.

14. Ogamo M, Sugiyama T, Maeda Y, et al. The ex utero intrapartum treatment (EXIT) procedure in giant fetal neck masses. *Fetal Diagn Ther* 2005; 20(3): 214–8.

15. Lazar D, Olutoye OO, Moise KJ Jr, et al. Ex-utero intrapartum treatment procedure for giant neck masses-fetal and maternal outcomes. *J Pediatr Surg* 2011; 46(5): 817–22.

16. Isaacs H. Fetal and neonatal cardiac tumors. *Pediatr Cardiol* 2004; 25(3): 252–73.

17. Muhler M, Rake A, Schwabe M, et al. Value of fetal cerebral MRI in sonographically proven cardiac rhabdomyoma. *Pediatr Radiol*, 2007; 37(5): 467–74.

18. Avni F, Massez A, Cassart M. Tumours of the fetal body: a review. *Pediatr Radiol* 2009; 39(11): 1147–57.

19. Fisher J, Tweddle D. Neonatal neuroblastoma. *Semin Fetal Neonatal Med* 2012; 17(4): 207–15.

20. Gucciardo L, Uyttebroek A, De Wever I, et al. Prenatal assessment and management of sacrococcygeal teratoma. *Prenat Diagn* 2011; 31(7): 678–88.

21. Altman R, Randolph J, Lilly J. Sacrococcygeal teratoma: American Academy of Pediatrics Surgical Section Survey 1973. *J Pediatr Surg* 1974; 9(3): 389–98.

22. Swamy R, Embleton N, Hale J. Sacrococcygeal teratoma over two decades: birth prevalence, prenatal diagnosis and clinical outcomes. *Prenat Diagn* 2008; 28(11): 1048–51.

Fetal infections

Amarnath Bhide

The contents of this chapter will be limited to those infections that are transmitted to the fetus in the prenatal period, and where there may be evidence of fetal effects identified on prenatal imaging. The following infections will be discussed:

- cytomegalovirus (CMV)
- toxoplasma
- parvovirus B19
- varicella
- syphilis
- rubella.

Infections cannot be transmitted to the fetus without maternal infection. The first time a susceptible individual contacts an infectious agent is termed "primary" infection. Following exposure to an infectious agent, the body develops antibodies. Initial antibodies are of immunoglobulin M (IgM) variety, followed by specific IgG class antibodies. The interval between entry of the pathogen into the maternal body and the development of protective antibodies is the time window in which the pathogen is circulating in maternal systems, and can reach the fetus. The IgG class of antibodies can cross the placenta and are protective for the fetus. The pathogen may attempt to enter the host again in the future. This is not possible (due to the presence of protective antibodies) unless the antigen has undergone a slight change (a different strain of the same virus as in the case of CMV). The antibodies still provide partial protection, and the risk to the fetus is much smaller. Antibodies against syphilis are not protective, and therefore reinfections can take place.

The fetus is particularly susceptible during a primary maternal infection when there are no protective maternal antibodies. With the exception of syphilis and CMV, infection with all other agents listed above leads to long-standing maternal immunity, and reinfections

do not occur. Although maternal re-infection and subsequent fetal infection can take place with CMV, fetal infection is much less common as compared with primary maternal infection. Primary maternal infection must occur during pregnancy for fetal infection to take place. For many infectious agents, the first half of pregnancy is particularly vulnerable for the fetus due to immaturity of the fetal immune system. In this case, the resultant damage can be substantial.

Immunization is available against certain pathogens. Active immunization is achieved by the use of live but nonpathogenic organisms (rubella, measles). Passive immunization is achieved with the use of inactivated (killed) organisms (pertussis, some varieties of polio vaccine). Both approaches lead to development of antibodies in the recipients, although response to active immunization is longer lasting.

Rubella immunization is offered routinely in the UK to all adolescent girls. Immunization leads to lifelong immunity. Antibodies against syphilis are not protective. Reinfection can occur, and the fetus is at risk. Seropositivity following infection may remain for several years.

Table 14.1 shows the burden of these infections in pregnancy in the UK.

Clinical presentations

There are essentially two ways in which fetal infection can present as a possibility to fetal medicine specialists.

1. Identification of primary maternal infection in pregnancy or a positive screening test

Screening for rubella and syphilis antibodies is part of booking investigations. The presence of rubella antibodies is evidence of maternal immunity and that the mother is protected. The absence of rubella antibodies implies that the mother is susceptible to the infection.

Fetal Medicine, ed. Bidyut Kumar and Zarko Alfirevic. Published by Cambridge University Press. © Cambridge University Press 2016.

Table 14.1 Burden of disease in the UK

Infectious agent	Prevalence of maternal seropositivity (past infection) (%)	Annual number of infections in pregnancy in UK	Reference
Cytomegalovirus	77[a]	2240[b]	Townsend et al., 2013[2]
Toxoplasma	17	47[c]	Flatt & Shetty 2013[5]; Halsby et al., 2014[6]
Parvovirus	60–70	944[c]	Vyse et al., 2007[7]
Varicella	90–95	2100[c]	Pembrey et al., 2013[4]; RCOG Green-Top Guideline No. 13, 2007[9]
Syphilis	0.47 (antibodies not protective)	4.7/1,000[c]	Giraudon et al., 2009[3]
Rubella	95.9	1–2[b]	Wise, 2013[8]

[a] Significant ethnic variation (49% in white British, 98% in South Asians born abroad).
[b] Number of fetal infections.
[c] Number of maternal infections.

Immunization is recommended after delivery. Syphilis screening tests need to be followed by further diagnostic tests to confirm infection and assess its stage as well as any potential infectivity and risk to the unborn child. Maternal treatment of syphilis is effective in preventing congenital syphilis and its fetal sequels.

Sometimes, maternal infection can be diagnosed following signs and symptoms. Varicella and parvovirus infection in the mother are commonly diagnosed due to the presence of a skin rash. Varicella skin lesions are characteristic. Both varicella and parvovirus infections can be confirmed by maternal serology showing a positive IgM, and negative IgG specific antibodies. Both these infections are generally self-limiting in the mother. Rarely, maternal varicella can be complicated by varicella pneumonia or encephalitis, which are serious conditions. Maternal CMV or toxoplasma infections are uncommonly diagnosed because of nonspecific signs and symptoms. Primary maternal infection is confirmed by evidence of maternal seroconversion, and the presence of positive IgM and negative IgG specific antibodies in maternal serum. Testing of booking blood showing negative results for both IgG and IgM antibodies with later positivity for these antibodies is a reliable evidence of seroconversion.

Performing a TORCH (toxoplasma, rubella, CMV and herpes) test without a clear indication is generally not recommended. The test detects antibodies but is unable to distinguish between a recent and a past infection. The majority of positive test results are as a result of past infection.

Table 14.2 Ultrasound features of fetal infection

Ultrasound feature	Possible infection
Hydrops fetalis	Parvovirus, rubella, varicella, CMV, toxoplasmosis
Ventriculomegaly	CMV, toxoplasmosis
Microcephaly	CMV, toxoplasmosis, syphilis, rubella
Intrauterine growth restriction	CMV, rubella, syphilis, toxoplasmosis
Placentomegaly	Parvovirus, syphilis, toxoplasmosis
Cardiomegaly and hyperdynamic circulation	Parvovirus
Calcifications	CMV, syphilis, toxoplasmosis
Limb deformities	Varicella, syphilis
CMV: cytomegalovirus.	

2. Ultrasound features that raise the possibility of fetal infection as the underlying cause

Some ultrasound features raise the suspicion of fetal infection as the underlying cause[15]. Table 14.2 shows suspicious ultrasound features and possible responsible agents.

Identification of a positive TORCH test

A common practice is to perform a TORCH test, this being testing without a clear reason. These tests are not carried out as part of routine antenatal investigations. Serology for rubella and syphilis is tested at booking.

Table 14.3 Serology and its interpretation

IgG	IgM	Interpretation	Action
Negative	Negative	Mother susceptible but not infected	Reassure Suggest precautions to prevent infection
Negative	Positive	Possible acute infection (primary)	Test booking blood Repeat serology in a few days
Positive	Negative	Mother immune, infection unlikely	Reassure[a]
Positive	Positive	Likely primary infection	Test booking blood Perform IgG avidity

[a] Test booking blood. Perform IgG avidity if the clinical suspicion is strong or test is performed several weeks after booking.

Serologic investigations

In general, the first step in cases of suspected fetal infection is to explore if the mother shows evidence of recent infection (Table 14.3). Fetal infection is not possible without maternal infection, but all maternal infections are not passed on to the fetus. The first response after contacting an infection is the production of IgM antibodies. This is followed by production of IgG antibodies. Both these antibody types are specific to the infecting organism. Newly formed IgG antibodies are less 'sticky' to the antigen, and show a low (<30%) avidity. Low-avidity antibodies are suggestive of a recent seroconversion. Over time, the IgG antibodies mature and the avidity is high (>70%). High-avidity antibodies are suggestive of seroconversion >6 months prior.

If the mother showed primary infection in the pregnancy, fetal infection is a possibility. At this stage, the probability of fetal infection and its implications should be explained to the parents. Fetal infection can be tested by amniocentesis/fetal blood sampling after some time (making allowance for the time it takes to reach the fetus) if the parents request it. Fetal infection can be detected by looking for the specific antigen of the infecting agent. Implications of fetal infection can be a wide spectrum from being asymptomatic to severe damage.

Cytomegalovirus

CMV is the most common cause of fetal infection occurring in 3–4 per 1,000 live births with significant racial variation. Pregnant women usually acquire CMV infection by exposure to children in their home or from occupational exposure to children. Infection can potentially occur from close contact with body fluids, such as saliva, blood, semen, urine and cervical secretion. Maternal infection is usually asymptomatic and the mother is generally unaware of being infected with CMV. A small proportion of patients may experience symptoms such as malaise, fever, generalized lymphadenopathy and hepatosplenomegaly.

Routine screening for maternal CMV seroconversion during pregnancy is not recommended in the UK. In some countries, such as Italy and France, serologic screening is performed in the first half of pregnancy. The main argument for not offering routine screening is lack of an effective treatment for reducing the rate of fetal transmission.

Fetal infection with CMV is a result of a transplacental passage of the virus during primary maternal CMV infection. Reinfection is uncommon and can be the result of a reactivation of the virus in the host or reinfection with a different CMV strain. The outcome of the fetus/newborn is directly correlated to the type and timing of infection. The most severe forms occur as the result of a primary infection contracted in the first 2 months of pregnancy.

The risk of transmission from mother to fetus is 30–50% during a primary infection. Of those infected, 90% of the fetuses are usually asymptomatic at birth, while 10% may manifest signs or symptoms related to CMV infection. Of the 10% of fetuses showing signs of infection, a third experience a fetal or neonatal demise. Among the survivors, half present major sequelae. Among asymptomatic fetuses, 10% may experience sensorineural hearing loss. Transmission from mother to fetus is considerably lower in a nonprimary infection and occurs in around 1% of the cases. The course of fetal disease is no different in primary or secondary maternal infection once infection has established.

The following diagram shows a mathematical modeling of a hypothetical cohort of 1,000 pregnant women with primary CMV infection (Figure 14.1).

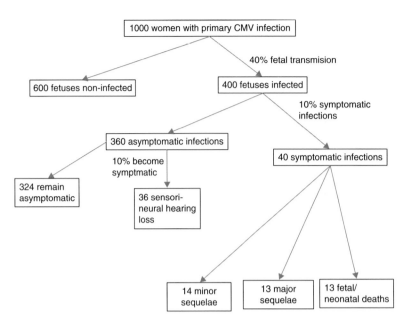

Figure 14.1 Laboratory investigations. CMV: cytomegalovirus.

The gold standard of serologic diagnosis of CMV infection is maternal seroconversion or the presence of anti-CMV IgM antibodies combined with anti-CMV IgG antibodies of low avidity. When a serum sample from early pregnancy is available, the diagnosis of CMV is facilitated by the documentation of seroconversion to CMV-specific antibodies in a previously seronegative woman.

A rise in IgM antibody titer may indicate a reactivation or reinfection with CMV. The rate of vertical transmission during a nonprimary infection is significantly lower compared with a primary infection. Moreover, IgM antibodies can be produced for months after the acute phase of infection. An increase in IgG antibody titre with or without the presence of IgM antibodies and high avidity is suggestive of a nonprimary CMV infection.

Ultrasound features of CMV infection

- CNS (ventriculomegaly, microcephaly, intraventricular hemorrhage, intraventricular adhesions, periventricular echogenicities, lissencephaly, porecephaly, cerebellar agenesis/hypoplasia, microphthalmia)
- Intrauterine growth restriction (IUGR)
- Placental enlargement
- Gastrointestinal tract (hepatomegaly, splenomegaly, echogenic bowel, intra-abdominal and liver calcification, ascites)
- Heart (cardiomegaly, pericardial effusions and calcifications)
- Hydrops fetalis

A serologic assessment of the mother is warranted when dealing with a fetus presenting with apparently isolated ventriculomegaly at the scan, particularly if a recent history of flu-like symptoms is reported. Periventricular intracranial calcifications are also relatively commonly associated with congenital CMV infection. Although in the presence of CMV infection fetal brain malformations are common, isolated extracerebral abnormalities can be detected in around 30% of the cases. Echogenic bowel and bowel dilation are the most common extracerebral findings detected at the scan in an infected fetus and are the result of viral enterocolitis. Hepatosplenomegaly and multiple liver calcifications can also be seen.

Although ultrasound has a low sensitivity in detecting congenital CMV infection even in patients at risk, the presence of ultrasound signs is an independent, poor prognostic factor. Therefore, a detailed ultrasonographic assessment in centers of excellence is warranted. It is important to state that a negative ultrasound scan in the second trimester does not exclude fetal infection. Magnetic resonance imaging (MRI) has a better spatial resolution compared with ultrasound, and may be helpful in detecting additional brain abnormalities, especially late in gestation.

Congenital CMV infection may cause a wide range of neurologic disabilities, including mental retardation, cerebral palsy, autism, epilepsy, blindness or visual deficits and learning disabilities. CMV is also the main cause of sensorineural hearing loss during childhood, which is present in about 10–15% of all infected babies, with the risk being greater if the infection was symptomatic in the neonatal period. See also Table 14.2.

Management

Confirmation of fetal infection through an invasive test (amniocentesis or fetal blood sampling) should be offered to the parents. Fetal infection is very unlikely if CMV is not detected in a fetal sample obtained at least 6–8 weeks after maternal infection or after 20 weeks of gestation. Isolation of CMV in the amniotic fluid by polymerase chain reaction (PCR) confirms the diagnosis of fetal infection, but does not predict the outcome of these babies at birth. In this case, viral load assessment through the use of quantitative PCR may be useful. A high viral load in the amniotic fluid (defined as the presence of $>10^3$ copies/mL) is likely to indicate a symptomatic infection. Recently, several authors have tried to correlate antenatal virologic, biochemical, hematologic and imaging parameters with the likelihood of an adverse outcome following confirmed fetal infection using fetal blood biochemistry. Fetal thrombocytopenia, elevated liver enzymes and abnormal findings at ultrasound correlate with poor neonatal outcome.

There is currently no proven prenatal treatment for congenital CMV infection. The use of CMV hyperimmune globulin or antiviral drugs given to the mother has been proposed to reduce the course of infection and the rate of vertical transmission. In a non-randomized prospective study, it was reported that maternal treatment with hyperimmune globulin was associated with a lower chance (3%) of symptomatic babies compared to 50% of the control group[11]. In another study it was proposed that antenatal valaciclovir given to the mother reduces the viral load in fetal blood. Randomized clinical trials are needed in order to clarify the role of antenatal treatment with immunoglobulins or antiviral drugs in congenital CMV infection. Postnatal diagnosis of congenital CMV infection relies on the isolation of the virus in the urine or saliva of the baby in the first 2 weeks of life. Symptoms of congenital CMV infection include hepatosplenomegaly, jaundice and petechiae. Neurologic symptoms include hypotonia, lethargy and seizure. Not all newborns presenting with symptoms related to congenital infection have a poor neurologic outcome and one-third of these babies have been reported not to have severe neurologic impairment. Microcephaly and abnormal brain findings at postnatal imaging are highly correlated with adverse neurodevelopmental outcome. Babies with a confirmed congenital CMV infection should be assessed sequentially during childhood by a multidisciplinary team including a pediatric neurologist, ophthalmologist and ENT surgeon. Figures 14.2 and 14.3 show the above discussion diagrammatically.

Key counseling points

- Maternal infection with CMV is often asymptomatic.
- The greatest risk to the fetus is with a primary CMV infection in early pregnancy (first trimester).
- The risk of fetal infection following maternal infection is 30–40%.
- Fetal infection can be tested by an invasive test (amniocentesis/fetal blood sampling). Amniotic fluid sample is more reliable for the detection of CMV antigen.
- A majority (90%) of congenitally infected fetuses are asymptomatic at birth.
- There are no reliable tests to exclude symptomatic fetal infection. However, abnormal ultrasound features (particularly microcephaly, ventriculomegaly) or abnormal fetal brain MRI are highly suggestive of developmental delay.
- Abnormal fetal liver function tests or presence of anemia or thrombocytopenia in the fetal blood are also suggestive of a guarded prognosis.
- No drug has a proven effectiveness to prevent or limit fetal damage.

Toxoplasmosis

Toxoplasma gondii is an obligate intracellular protozoan, whose lifecycle is characterized by a sexual phase occurring only in cats and an asexual phase taking place within virtually all warm-blooded animals, including humans. The mother acquires infection by ingestion of uncooked or raw meat containing *Toxoplasma* cysts. Water or food contaminated by oocysts excreted in the feces of infected cats represents another source of infection. After ingestion, *Toxoplasma* acquires its

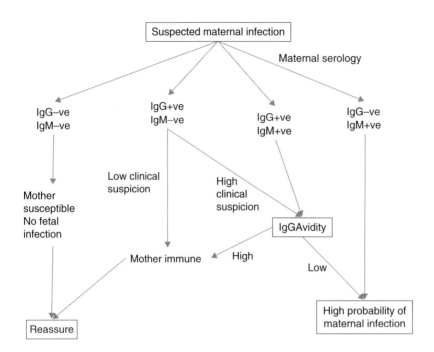

Figure 14.2 Management of women with suspected cytomegalovirus infection. IgG: immunoglobulin G IgM: immunoglobulin M..

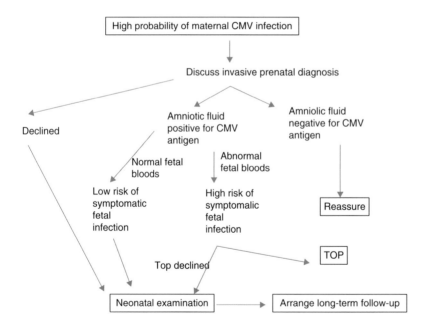

Figure 14.3 Management of women with serology suggesting a high probability of cytomegalovirus (CMV) infection. TOP: termination of pregnancy.

active form and invades intestinal epithelial cells, thus spreading in the circulation.

Maternal infection is usually asymptomatic and only a small proportion of women develop low-grade fever, malaise or lymphadenopathy. Rarely, *Toxoplasma* infection manifests primarily as chorio-retinitis.

Transmission from the mother to fetus occurs almost exclusively during a primary maternal infection. The frequency of vertical transmission increases with the gestational age and is around 70% in the third trimester, while being as low as 5–6% in the first trimester of pregnancy. Risk of fetal infection with toxoplasmosis

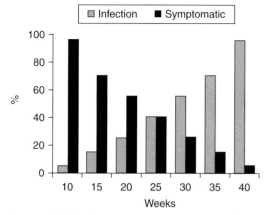

Figure 14.4 Risk of vertical transmission (gray bars) with toxoplasmosis and the risk of being symptomatic if infected (dark bars).

and the risk of being symptomatic if infected is shown in Figure 14.4 [13]. At no point is the overall risk of a symptomatic infection less than 5–8%.

Laboratory investigation

Detection of specific anti-*Toxoplasma* IgM and IgG in the maternal serum is the most commonly adopted technique for diagnosing maternal infection (see Table 14.3). Any positive test needs confirmation in the reference laboratory. *Toxoplasma* IgG avidity test is usually performed as a confirmatory test in the case of positive results at serology. High-avidity IgG results in the first trimester of pregnancy are reassuring as they indicate past infection.

Ultrasound features of fetal *Toxoplasma* infection

- CNS abnormalities (ventriculomegaly, calcifications in the brain parenchyma, periventricular zone and caudothalamic zone, periventricular echogenicity or cysts)
- Ocular abnormalities (cataracts)
- GI abnormalities (hepatomegaly, liver calcifications, ascites)
- Placental enlargement/thickening

The outcome of fetuses with congenital toxoplasmosis is worse when signs of infection are detected at the scan. When mothers acquired the infection during the first trimester of pregnancy and where a prenatal scan showed no structural abnormalities suggestive of infection, the outcome of fetuses at 2 years of age was

not significantly different from that of fetuses whose mothers were infected later in pregnancy. See also Table 14.2.

Management

Once serologic tests have confirmed that a recent maternal infection has occurred, particularly in the first 18 weeks of gestation, antenatal administration of spiramycin to the mother should be considered. Isolation of *Toxoplasma* in the amniotic fluid by PCR is the gold standard for the diagnosis of fetal infection. Invasive prenatal tests should be performed after 18 weeks of gestation when sensitivity and specificity for the diagnosis of infection are significantly higher than in earlier gestations.

Spiramycin is reported to reduce the rate of vertical transmission by 60%, particularly if administered in the first trimester of pregnancy. Spiramicin should be started at the dose of 1 g (3 million units) every 8 h. It should be continued even in the presence of negative PCR results on amniotic fluid and/or normal findings at the scan. However, a recent systematic review has failed to find a strong association between maternal administration of spiramycin and prevention of fetal infection.

In women in whom fetal infection is confirmed by positive PCR on amniotic fluid, in fetuses presenting abnormalities suggestive of fetal infection at the scan or in mothers acquiring infection after 18 weeks of gestation, a combination of pyrimethamine (50 mg every 12 h for 48 h followed by 50 mg daily), Sulfadiazine (75 mg/kg, followed by 50 mg/kg every 12 h) and folinic acid (10–20 mg daily) is indicated. Spiramycin is intended for prophylactic use (prevention of fetal transmission), whereas the intended use for pyrimethamine is therapeutic (used in proven fetal infection). Pyrimethamine crosses the placenta and should not be used in the first trimester of pregnancy due to the possibility of teratogenicity. The rational of this multidrug therapy is mainly to cure rather than prevent fetal infection. However, the rate of serious neurologic sequel or death in treated cases is no better than those without treatment.

The majority of newborns with congenital toxoplasmosis do not show any clinical signs of the disease at birth. When present, clinical manifestations include epilepsy, psychomotor or mental retardation, blindness, strabismus, petechiae due to thrombocytopenia and anemia. Babies should be carefully examined at

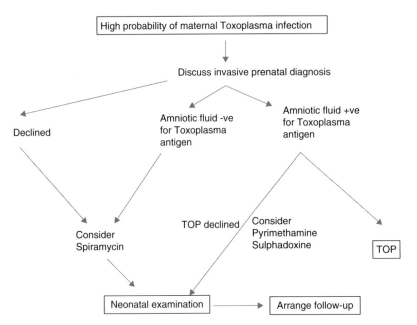

High probability of maternal Toxoplasma infection

Discuss invasive prenatal diagnosis

Declined

Amniotic fluid -ve for Toxoplasma antigen

Amniotic fluid +ve for Toxoplasma antigen

Consider Spiramycin

TOP declined

Consider Pyrimethamine Sulphadoxine

TOP

Neonatal examination → Arrange follow-up

Figure 14.5 Management of women with high probability of *Toxoplasma* infection. TOP: termination of pregnancy.

birth by a multidisciplinary team involving a pediatric neurologist and ophthalmologist. MRI or computed tomography imaging is useful to assess normality of neonatal brain. Babies that are asymptomatic at birth need a prolonged follow-up.

Key counseling points

- Congenital toxoplasmosis is a relatively uncommon occurrence.
- The fetus is at risk if the mother contracts *Toxoplasma* infection in pregnancy. Presence of IgG antibodies usually indicates past infection and maternal immunity.
- The risk of fetal infection increases with advancing gestation.
- The risk of resultant fetal damage reduces with advancing gestation, but at no time is the risk less than 5–8%.
- Fetal infection can be tested by *Toxoplasma* antigen in the amniotic fluid/fetal blood.
- The intended purpose of the use of spiramycin is to prevent mother-to-fetus transmission of *Toxoplasma*. However, this has not been proven in prospective studies.
- The intended purpose of the use of pyrimethamine + sulfadiazine is treatment of established fetal infection. Evidence for the

efficacy in improving fetal outcome is not very robust.

Parvovirus B19

Parvovirus B19 (PB19) epidemics tend to occur every 4 years with a yearly peak of incidence in spring. Risk of PB19 infection is higher in day-care personnel and among women of child-bearing age with young children. Maternal infection usually occurs through respiratory droplets. Maternal viremia reaches its peak approximately 7 days after the infection, and IgM antibodies are detected in maternal blood between 7 and 14 days, while IgG antibodies are produced between 14 and 21 days. Maternal infection is usually asymptomatic, although symptoms such as mild fever, headache, arthralgia and erythema infectiosum may occur. Vertical transmission from mother to fetus by transplacental passage of the virus is related to maternal viremia, and occurs in 30–50% of the cases. For maternal infection before 24 weeks, the risk of adverse fetal outcome is 10%. Fetal infection with PB19 infection is linked with miscarriage, intrauterine fetal death, fetal anemia and nonimmune hydrops fetalis. PB19 cell-related damage is due to the destruction of erythroid precursors leading to fetal anemia, high-output cardiac failure, hydrops fetalis and eventually death. PB19 can also

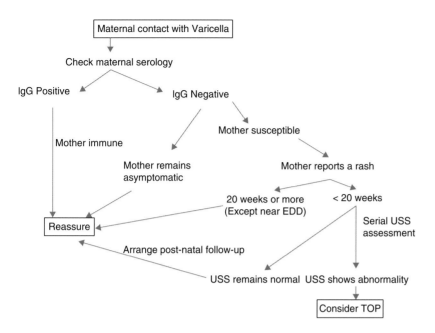

Figure 14.6 Management of women with a contact with varicella. EDD: estimated date of delivery; Ig: immunoglobulin; TOP: termination of pregnancy; USS, ultrasound scan.

lead to myocarditis, which can cause arrhythmias or even cardiac arrest.

Laboratory investigations

Maternal serology is the first step for the confirmation of PB19 infection in patients at risk. Following maternal infection, PB19 IgM is detectable in maternal blood between 7 and 14 days, reaching a peak at 10–14 days, and then rapidly decreasing within 2 or 3 months. It is very informative to test maternal booking blood samples if available. Presence of IgG antibodies at booking is reassuring and excludes the possibility of acute infection later in pregnancy. IgG antibodies are produced between 14 and 21 days. A positive maternal IgM titer has a high sensitivity and specificity for the diagnosis of a recent PB19 infection. After the contact between the mother and the virus, there is a window of 7 days during which both IgM and IgG remain negative. This can lead to a false-negative result if the mother is tested at that time. The interval between maternal infection and occurrence of hydrops is usually between 2 and 6 weeks. PCR for PB19 DNA should be performed when analyzing fetal or neonatal samples.

Ultrasound features of PB19 infection

In a woman with confirmed parvovirus infection, increased nuchal translucency and abnormal flow in the ductus venosus may be the only signs linked to PB19 infection in the first trimester. Later in pregnancy, parvovirus infection presents as fetal anemia with or without fetal hydrops. Fetal anemia due to PB19 infection should always be suspected in the presence of an increased peak systolic velocity (PSV) in the fetal middle cerebral artery (MCA) when the mother is known to be negative for atypical red-cell antibodies. Fetal anemia leads to progressive high-output cardiac failure and fetal hydops. The peak incidence of fetal hydrops is between 17 and 24 weeks of gestations. The interval between maternal infection and appearance of fetal hydrops is between 2 and 6 weeks. See also Table 14.2.

Management

Pregnant women presenting with a rash should be tested for PB19 IgG and IgM. A positive IgM antibody test or a negative IgM/IgG ratio indicates a recent PB19 infection, and an appropriate fetal follow-up should be arranged. No specific antiviral therapy or vaccine is available for PB19 infection.

The fetus should be checked for the occurrence of anemia or signs of hydrops within 4 weeks from confirmed maternal infection. In the case of negative ultrasound examination, follow-up scans should be arranged every 1 or 2 weeks up to 10 weeks after exposure. After that the risk of fetal disease is minimal. If there is no fetal abnormality at or later than 30 weeks gestation, the mother can be reassured that adverse sequelae from the PB19 infection are unlikely. If ultrasound shows signs of anemia or overt hydrops fetalis, the patient should be referred to centers with a high level of expertise for an intrauterine transfusion. Fetal blood transfusion is warranted in hydropic fetusus as it leads to an improved fetal outcome compared with expectant management. Overall prognosis is very good, although there is some evidence suggesting a higher rate of adverse neuro-developmental outcome for the baby if hydrops develops, even with prenatal treatment. Viral isolation by PCR is used to diagnose infection. A full blood count should be requested at birth in order to assess the degree of anemia and thrombocytopenia in the newborn.

Key counseling points

- Parvovirus infection is often seasonal, and is usually clinically apparent, with the mother reporting exanthematous skin rash and fever.
- The infection is particularly dangerous for the fetus in the first half of the pregnancy as a result of immaturity of the fetal immune system.
- Women with confirmed parvovirus infection in pregnancy should be followed-up with serial scans. MCA-PSV is used for noninvasive detection of fetal anemia.
- Weekly scans are necessary for 10 weeks following maternal infection.
- Fetal blood sampling and intrauterine transfusion are indicated if significant fetal anemia is suspected.
- The outcome of infected fetuses is excellent with appropriate treatment.

Varicella-zoster infection (chickenpox)

While chickenpox is the consequence of a primary infection with varicella-zoster virus (VZV), herpes zoster is caused by the reactivation of the virus from its latency in the nucleus of the para-spinal cells. VZV is a highly contagious and readily transmissible infective agent with more than 90% of household contacts becoming infected after exposure. The first contact between the virus and the host is usually through the conjunctivae and the mucous membranes of the nasopharynx. After an incubation period of 15 days (range, 10–21 days), nonspecific prodromal symptoms, such as fever, headache and malaise, usually precede a maculopapular rash. This becomes vesicular before

crusting usually after 5 days. The host can potentially transmit the infection from 2 days before to 5 days after the onset of the rash until the vesicles crust over (7–10 days). Pneumonia represents the most serious complication of maternal infection, occurring in about 5–10% of cases, with even a possibility of mortality (<1%). Although primary infection provides lifelong immunity, the virus persists in a latent form in the nucleus of the paraspinal cells and can potentially reactivate, particularly if immunosuppression coexists.

Although contraindicated in pregnancy, varicella vaccine does not seem to be harmful for the fetus if accidentally administered. The most likely mechanism of fetal infection is a reactivation of the VZV in utero as a consequence of the immature fetal cell-mediated immunity. The fetus can be infected only during a primary maternal infection. The risk of transmission following herpes zoster (reactivation) is negligible.

The rate of vertical transmission before 20 weeks has been reported to be at around 8–9% and congenital varicella syndrome occurs in about 10% of the fetuses developing infection (0.4–2% of all infected mothers), particularly if maternal infection is acquired before 20 weeks of gestation. The risk of congenital varicella syndrome is negligible if maternal infection occurs after 20 weeks, with only sporadic cases reported in the literature.

Congenital varicella syndrome is characterized by CNS abnormalities (microcephaly and cortical atrophy), limb hypoplasia, skin scarring and ocular abnormalities (cataracts, chorioretinitis).

Neonatal varicella can occur if delivery takes place between 5 days before and 2 days after the onset of the rash. In this scenario, the lack of an adequate immune response from the mother results in low levels of IgG in fetal blood, thus predisposing the fetus to neonatal varicella that occurs in up to 30% of the cases. Neonatal varicella is characterized by the presence of neurologic, ocular, muscular, cutaneous, gastrointestinal and genitourinary abnormalities, and leads to neonatal death in approximately 7% of the cases. Herpes zoster does not pose a risk of fetal infection.

Laboratory investigations

Maternal varicella is usually diagnosed based on clinical findings. Detection either of specific IgM or isolation of varicella virus by PCR in maternal blood confirms the diagnosis. Isolation of the virus by PCR in the amniotic fluid confirms the presence of fetal infection. An interval of at least 5 weeks between maternal onset of the rash and prenatal invasive tests is required in order to avoid a false-negative test.

Ultrasound features of congenital varicella syndrome

- Cutaneous scarring causing limb contractures
- Anomalies of the CNS (ventriculomegaly, microcephaly, intracranial calcifications, cerebral hypoplasia, porencephaly)
- Ocular abnormalities (microphthalmia, cataract)
- IUGR
- Placental anomalies
- Hydrops fetalis

Some abnormalities associated with congenital varicella syndrome, such as cutaneous and neuronal lesions, are not usually diagnosed with ultrasound, thus highlighting the importance of a detailed postnatal assessment.

Management

Women exposed to varicella zoster virus who are found to be seronegative should receive VZV IgG within 72–96 h of exposure in order to attenuate maternal symptoms. VZV IgG has no effect once infection has established.

Severe complications, such as pneumonia, can occur in up to 10% of pregnant women infected with varicella. Therefore, all pregnant women with confirmed infection should receive oral aciclovir (15 mg/kg every 8 h) within 24 h of the onset of the rash in order to treat the disease and to reduce the rate of severe complications. If the maternal infection develops before 20 weeks of gestation, the parents should be counseled about the presence of a small (0.4–2%) risk of developing congenital varicella syndrome. Abnormal ultrasound suggests the presence of congenital varicella syndrome and carries a poor prognosis for the fetus. In such cases, an offer of pregnancy termination is reasonable.

Serial antenatal scans should be arranged. In the presence of a normal scan, parents should be reassured about the positive outcome of the pregnancy. A complete detailed postnatal examination is required in order to rule out those abnormalities, such as cataracts, chorioretinitis and skin scarring, not detected at ultrasound. If maternal varicella occurs in the third trimester of pregnancy close to the expected date of delivery, an attempt

to delay the delivery until 2 days after the onset of rash should be made in order to prevent neonatal varicella.

Newborns with a confirmed diagnosis of varicella infection in the amniotic fluid should undergo a detailed anatomic examination. Abnormalities such as cataracts, skin scarring or chorioretinitis may be present even if the prenatal scan was negative. VZV IgG should be given to the baby if maternal varicella occurs in the third trimester of pregnancy and the delivery takes place between 5 days before and 2 days after the onset of the rash. Aciclovir should also be used if neonatal infection is confirmed.

Key counseling points

- Varicella infection is usually clinically apparent. The mother reports a vesicular skin rash with constitutional symptoms.
- If the mother develops varicella infection in pregnancy, the risk to the fetus is small in the first half and negligible in the second half of pregnancy.
- Maternal shingles has minimal fetal risk because of the presence of antibodies in the maternal blood.
- Onset of maternal varicella rash within 5 days prior to 2 days after delivery can lead to severe neonatal disease.
- Aciclovir is recommended to shorten the maternal disease course.
- The risk of congenital varicella syndrome is small (0.4–2.0%). Detailed ultrasound examination at a referral center is indicated.
- All fetuses born to mothers suffering from varicella in the first half of the pregnancy should be assessed at birth by a neonatologist.

Syphilis

Syphilis is the result of the infection of *Treponema pallidum*, a Gram-negative bacterium. Syphilis is transmitted by sexual contact. The *Treponema* organism enters the body through small abrasions of the skin or the genital mucosa. A primary lesion known as chancre appears after an incubation period of approximately 3 weeks. The chancre is a painless, red, round ulceration with an indurated base and well-formed border. Regional painless lymphadenopathy is always present.

The chancre disappears spontaneously in 3–8 weeks even if untreated. If the immune response is unable to eradicate the infection, secondary syphilis

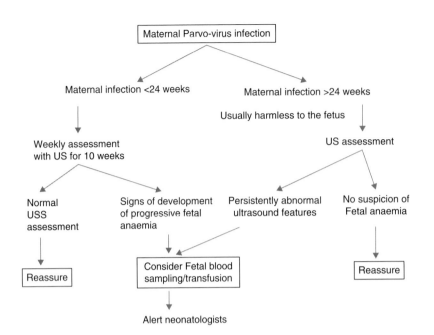

Figure 14.7 Management of women with parvovirus infection. US, USS, ultrasound scan.

follows. The *Treponema* organisms multiply locally and spread through the perivascular lymphatic system to the systemic circulation causing lesions in ectodermal tissues, such as the skin and mucous membranes. The clinical picture of secondary syphilis resolves even if untreated, and most of the infected patients remain asymptomatic (latent phase). This stage is characterized by serologic evidence of syphilis without signs or symptoms of primary or secondary disease. After several years of latent syphilis, approximately 30% of affected individuals develop tertiary syphilitic lesions that predominantly affect the CNS and cardiovascular systems, the bones and other viscera. *T. pallidum* can cross the placenta and may cause congenital fetal infection at any time during pregnancy. The degree of fetal involvement is more severe if infection is acquired during the early stages of pregnancy. *T. pallidum* is responsible for a multiorgan disease in the fetus. Congenital syphilis may cause stillbirth, preterm labor, growth retardation, fetal hydrops and neonatal infection. Fetal hepatosplenomegaly is frequent and can lead to hypoalbuminemia and ascites. Anemia and thrombocytopenia are frequent. Hydrops is usually the result of high-output congestive heart failure induced by severe anemia. Skeletal involvement, such as osteomyelitis, osteochondritis or periostitis, is also observed.

In liveborn infants, early signs of congenital syphilis usually appear within 2 years of life, and include respiratory symptoms, generalized lymphadenopathy, hepatosplenomegaly, abnormal liver function, jaundice, hepatitis, anemia, thrombocytopenia, osteochondritis or periostitis, and maculopapular rash involving hands and feet. CNS involvement is also frequent and may manifest with meningitis-like symptoms.

Laboratory investigations

The most common tests using non-specific antibodies are the rapid plasma reagin (RPR) and the venereal disease research laboratory (VDRL) tests.

Approximately 1–5% of positive RPR and VDRL results are false positives. False-positive results usually have low titers and suggest the possibility of autoimmune disease, particularly antiphospholipid antibody syndrome. The VDRL and RPR tests are used for rapid screening. Their false-positive and false-negative rates are comparable to the nonpregnant status. Specific serologic reactions for syphilis are the fluorescent treponemal antibody adsorption test (FTA-ABS) and the microhemagglutination assay for antibodies against *T. pallidum* (MHA-TP).

The FTA-ABS test and the MHA-TP tests are used to verify a positive screening test.

Ultrasound features of congenital syphilis

- IUGR
- Hydrops, ascites, pleural and pericardial effusion, generalized skin edema

- Placental thickening
- Hyperechogenic bowel, hepatic calcifications
- Hepatosplenomegaly
- Shortening of the long bone
- Bone deformity (bowing, curvature and thickening)

Management

Parental penicillin G is the drug of choice for all the stages of syphilis. Maternal treatment should be started soon after serologic confirmation of infection according to the stage of the disease. Women treated in the first two trimesters of pregnancy are more likely to have a healthy infant. Penicillin is effective in preventing the transplacental transmission of the *Treponema* organism from the mother to the fetus, and to treat fetal infection once established.

Antibiotic treatment in patients with confirmed syphilis infection is as follows[14]:

- primary and secondary syphilis, or early latent syphilis (less than 1 year duration): benzathine penicillin G, 2.4 million units intramuscularly in a single dose
- late latent syphilis (more than 1-year duration) or latent syphilis of unknown duration: benzathine penicillin G, 7.2 million units total, administered as three doses of 2.4 million units IM each at one-week intervals
- neurosyphilis: procaine penicillin G, 2.4 million units IM once daily plus probenecid, 500 mg orally four times daily, both for 10–14 days *or* aqueous crystalline penicillin G, 18–24 million units per day, administered as 3–4 million units intravenously every 4 hours or by continuous infusion for 10–14 days.

The penicillin-allergic pregnant woman poses a major management dilemma. At present, there is no effective drug that can be substituted in pregnant women allergic to penicillin. The best approach is to perform skin testing to document serious allergy followed by desensitization.

Serologic evidence of adequately treated syphilis in patients with early syphilis is demonstrated by at least a four-fold decrease in VDRL or RPR titers. If the disease has entered the latent phase before treatment, a large percentage of patients may never attain a completely negative VDRL result. In these cases, the evidence of adequate treatment will be a stable or declining RPR or VDRL titers of ≤1:4. Babies of mothers with syphilis infection should be considered at high risk of congenital infection, irrespective of maternal antibiotic treatment during pregnancy.

Maternal treatment commenced before 20 weeks is nearly uniformly successful. The risk of treatment failure increases if the ultrasound features of congenital syphilis are observed. No fetus with ultrasound signs suggestive of syphilis was successfully treated, and all liveborn infants required treatment for congenital syphilis.

The presence of anti-treponemal IgM antibodies in neonates is diagnostic of congenital syphilis. IgG antibodies are the result of transplacental transmission from a mother. An RPR or VDRL titer in the neonate four times greater than the maternal titer is also consistent with congenital syphilis. Penicillin treatment should be started only after serologic confirmation of neonatal syphilis, and these babies should be closely followed-up over a long term. In a study reporting eight children with congenital syphilis[17], four infants had long-term sequelae (vision impairment due to keratitis, deafness and abnormal dentition (Hutchinson's teeth)).

Key counseling points

- Offer of screening is recommended in all pregnancies.
- Treatment is relatively simple, cheap and highly effective. Reinfection can occur.
- False-positive serologic tests are known to occur, particularly with autoimmune diseases.
- Despite effective screening and treatment, the disease has not been eradicated.
- Treatment with penicillin is highly effective.
- Presence of antenatal ultrasound features suggestive of congenital syphilis increases the risk of treatment failure.

Rubella (German measles)

Before the introduction of vaccination programs, rubella used to be an endemic infection. The contact between the virus and the host occurs through respiratory droplets. After an incubation period of 14 (range, 12–23) days, a maculopapular rash appears on the face and then rapidly spreads to the trunk and limbs. The rash is usually associated with lymphadenopathy of the cervical region. Nonspecific symptoms, such as headache, sore throat, low-grade fever and conjunctivitis, may also be present. Up to 50% of infections are asymptomatic. Primary infection confers life-long immunity. The risk of transmission from the mother to the fetus and the rate of congenital defects have been reported to be 80% and 85%, respectively, with a high risk of birth defects if the infection occurs in the first 8 weeks of pregnancy. The rate of miscarriage in the first trimester of pregnancy is around 20%. The risk of fetal infection progressively reduces after the first trimester of pregnancy. The risk of fetal compromise is negligible if infection occurs after the second trimester of pregnancy.

Rubella induces a characteristic pattern of multiorgan disease in the fetus, known as congenital rubella syndrome (CRS). It is characterized by heart defects (pulmonary stenosis, patent ductus arteriosus), neurologic deficits (neurodevelopmental delay, speech defect, psychomotor retardation), eye defects (cataracts, microphthalmia, retinopathy), sensorineural or central deafness, hematological abnormalities (thrombocytopenia, purpura), hepatosplenomegaly and diabetes. After the second trimester of pregnancy, the developing fetal immune system is able to induce an immune response against the virus, leading to a low rate of congenital abnormalities and adverse outcomes.

In countries where rubella immunization is routinely offered, such as in the UK, the occurrence of CRS is exceedingly rare.

Laboratory investigations

Clinical diagnosis of rubella infection is unreliable. Therefore, it is important that mothers undergo serologic examination if they are nonimmune to rubella and present with rubella-like symptoms or exposed to individuals with rubella infection in the first 16 weeks of pregnancy. Negative rubella IgG and positive IgM in sera in the presence of rubella-like symptoms or a history of contact with patients showing a macopapular rash are indicative of primary maternal infection. Fetal compromise occurs almost exclusively in mothers with a primary rubella infection. In this author's experience, all rubella infections in pregnancy were acquired during foreign travel.

Ultrasound features of rubella

- CNS abnormalities (ventriculomegaly, microcephaly, intracranial calcifications, intraventricular adhesions, subependymal cysts)
- Ocular abnormalities (microphtalmia, cataract)

- Heart defects (pulmonary artery stenosis and hypoplasia, atrial septal defect, ventricular septal defect, cardiomegaly)
- IUGR
- Hepatomegaly
- Hydrops
- Polyhydramnios
- Ascites
- Hyperechogenic bowel
- Placental enlargement

Because the risk of congenital abnormalities is higher during the first trimester of pregnancy, early ultrasound examination is warranted in women with a confirmed rubella infection on the basis of a serologic diagnosis. See also Table 14.2.

Management

Women with a serologic diagnosis of rubella infection in the first trimester should be counseled about the likely occurrence of an adverse outcome of the pregnancy. If the infection has occurred after the first trimester of pregnancy, it may be explained to the parents that fetal infection is unlikely between 13 and 18 weeks, and negligible after 18 weeks of gestation.

PCR is the technique of choice in confirming fetal infection. An invasive test (amniocentesis) should be delayed until at least 7–8 weeks after infection. A positive PCR test, particularly if associated with the presence of structural abnormalities at the scan, indicates a poor outcome. An offer of pregnancy termination is reasonable. A negative PCR result indicates no infection, although false negatives are possible.

A detailed ultrasound assessment in centers with high skills in fetal medicine should be carried out in order to detect structural abnormalities associated with congenital rubella syndrome. An early fetal echocardiography is also warranted. Currently, there is no evidence that giving rubella hyperimmune globulins to the mother reduces the rate of transmission or alters the course of fetal infection, although it may modify maternal disease. After birth, the baby should be examined carefully in order to rule out the presence of congenital rubella syndrome. Blood and urine should be obtained and tested for the presence of the virus if a prenatal work-up was not available. A longer follow-up is needed.

On the basis of the high morbidity and mortality associated with rubella infection in pregnancy, and of the lack of a cure if infection has been established, it is important that women of child-bearing age are confirmed to be immune and that rubella vaccine should be offered to all who are susceptible. A pregnancy should be avoided for at least one month after vaccination. Pregnancy represents a contraindication to rubella vaccination. However, the rate of congenital abnormalities does not appear to increase if vaccination had been inadvertently administered during pregnancy.

Key counseling points

- Clinical diagnosis of rubella (a maculopapular rash) is unreliable.
- Congenital rubella syndrome is exceedingly rare due to the universal offer of rubella immunization.
- The disease may make a comeback because many parents are choosing not to get their babies vaccinated against rubella infection due to fears of adverse effects.
- The virus is highly infective. Maternal infection in the first trimester often leads to devastating consequences. Fetal risk is negligible after 18 weeks.
- Rubella vaccine should be offered to all susceptible women after delivery.

References

1. MacLean A, Regan L, Carrington D (eds). *Infection in Pregnancy*. London: RCOG Press, 2001.

2. Townsend CL, Forsgren M, Ahlfors K, et al. Long-term outcomes of congenital cytomegalovirus infection in Sweden and the United Kingdom. *Clin Infect Dis* 2013; 56: 1232–9.

3. Giraudon I, Forde J, Maguire H, et al. Antenatal screening and prevalence of infection: surveillance in London, 2000–2007. *Euro Surveill* 2009; 14(9): 8–12.

4. Pembrey L, Raynor P, Griffiths P, et al. Seroprevalence of cytomegalovirus, Epstein Barr virus and varicella zoster virus among pregnant women in Bradford: a cohort study. *PLoS One* 2013; 8(11): e81881.

5. Flatt A, Shetty N. Seroprevalence and risk factors for toxoplasmosis among antenatal women in London: a re-examination of risk in an ethnically diverse population. *Eur J Public Health* 2013; 23: 648–52.

6. Halsby K, Guy E, Said B, et al. Enhanced surveillance of toxoplasmosis in England and Wales, 2008–2012. *Epidemiol Infect* 2014; 142(8): 1653–60.

7. Vyse AJ, Andrews NJ, Hesketh LM, et al. The burden of parvovirus B19 infection in women of childbearing age in England and Wales. *Epidemiol Infect* 2007; 135: 1354–62.

8. Wise J. Small rise in rubella cases triggers warning. *BMJ* 2013; 346: f2935.

9. Royal College of Obstetricians and Gynaecologists (RCOG). Chickenpox in pregnancy. RCOG Green-top Guideline No. 13. London: RCOG, September 2007.

10. Jacquemard F, Yamamoto M, Costa JM, et al. Maternal administration of valaciclovir in symptomatic intrauterine cytomegalovirus infection. *BJOG* 2007; 114: 1113–21.

11. Nigro G, Adler SP, La Torre R, et al; Congenital Cytomegalovirus Collaborating Group. Passive immunization during pregnancy for congenital cytomegalovirus infection. *N Engl J Med* 2005; 353: 1350–62.

12. Bhide A, Papageorghiou AT. Managing primary CMV infection in pregnancy. *BJOG* 2008; 115: 805–7.

13. Dunn D, Wallon M, Peyron F, et al. Mother-to-child transmission of toxoplasmosis: risk estimates for clinical counseling. *Lancet* 1999; 353(9167): 1829–33.

14. Center for disease Prevention and Control (CDC). Treatment guidelines: Sexually transmitted diseases. Atlanta: CDC, 2010.

15. Crino JP. Ultrasound and fetal diagnosis of perinatal infection. *Clin Obstet Gynecol* 1999; 42: 71–80.

16. Wendel GD Jr, Sheffield JS, Hollier LM, et al. Treatment of syphilis in pregnancy and prevention of congenital syphilis. *Clin Infect Dis* 2002; 35: S200–9.

17. Caddy SC, Lee BE, Sutherland K, et al. Pregnancy and neonatal outcomes of women with reactive syphilis serology in Alberta, 2002 to 2006. *J Obstet Gynaecol Can* 2011; 33: 453–9.

Chapter 15

Red blood cell alloimmunization

Bidyut Kumar and Zarko Alfirevic

Rhesus antigens

Hemolytic disease of the fetus and newborn (HDFN) is caused by maternal alloantibodies directed against fetal red cell surface antigens that the mother herself lacks. Erythrocytes or red blood cells contain multiple surface antigens of which the rhesus (Rh) blood group has the most clinical importance in obstetrics. The Rh antigens are a family of small integral proteins associated with the lipid component of the red blood cell membrane. The most frequently involved antigen in HDFN is the D antigen of the Rh blood group and it remains so despite the widespread use of prophylactic antenatal and postpartum anti-D immunoglobulin (Ig). In addition, alloimmunization to "c", "C" and "E" antigens of the Rh system and the "K" antigen of the Kell blood group system, although rare, can lead to HDFN. The commonly implicated antigen pairs are Dd, Cc and Ee, and the genes which determine these antigens are inherited from the parents.

Of the approximately 45 Rh antigens, D is the major cause of Rh incompatibility. It is estimated that 15–17% of whites, 5–7% of blacks and about 2% of Indo-Eurasians do not express the D antigen and so are called "Rh-negative." The D antigen and anti-D has never been isolated but for ease of explanation it is included in any description.

The Kell blood group comprises 24 antigens. At least eight of the antigens have been associated with HDFN, of which Kell (K or KEL1) and Cellano (k or KEL2) appear to be the most common and the strongest immunogens. Ninety-one percent of the population are Kell negative (i.e., kk). The rest are Kell positive having the genotype KK or Kk. The development of anti-K antibodies is primarily a result of prior maternal

transfusion, and only a few cases occur following a previous pregnancy or are present naturally[1,2].

Generally, blood group antigens are biallelic codominant systems, and if the father is heterozygously positive for a particular blood group antigen, then there will be a 50% chance that the fetus will be carrying the risky antigen. If the blood group antigen is not present, then such a fetus will have no risk of HDFN and no further follow-up will be necessary. If, however, the fetus does inherit the implicated antigen, careful monitoring for fetal anemia with Doppler ultrasound and serial assessment of maternal antibody titers may be indicated.

Pathophysiology of hemolytic disease of the newborn

Red blood cell alloimmunization secondary to pregnancy involves three key stages. First, a paternally derived red blood cell antigen foreign to the mother must be inherited by the fetus. Second, the volume of fetal red cells that gain access to the maternal circulation must be sufficient to stimulate an immune response in the particular individual. Finally, maternal antibodies to fetal red cells must gain transplacental access and cause immune destruction of sensitized red cells by Fc receptor-bearing effector cells in the fetus and neonate.

Although alloimmunization can occur at a lesser amount of fetomaternal hemorrhage (FMH), most women who become alloimmunized do so as a result of FMH of >0.1 mL. Several first- and second-trimester clinical events may cause alloimmunization. Therapeutic and spontaneous abortions are associated with a 4–5% and a 1.5–2% risk, respectively, of alloimmunization in susceptible women[3]. Ectopic pregnancy is also associated with alloimmunization

Fetal Medicine, ed. Bidyut Kumar and Zarko Alfirevic. Published by Cambridge University Press. © Cambridge University Press 2016.

in susceptible women. Although threatened abortion is an infrequent cause, 10% of women with threatened abortion show evidence of FMH[4]. Clinical procedures that may breach the integrity of the choriodecidual space, may also cause Rh alloimmunization. Chorionic villus sampling (CVS) is associated with a 14% risk of FMH of more than 0.6 mL[5], and amniocentesis is associated with a 7–15% risk of FMH, even if the placenta is not traversed[6]. Likewise, cordocentesis and other percutaneous fetal procedures pose a risk for FMH. External cephalic version whether or not it is successful, results in FMH in 2–6% cases[7].

When an Rh-negative individual is first exposed to an adequate volume of Rh-positive red blood cells, a primary immune response is mounted following a latent period of several weeks. It is believed to take between 5 and 15 weeks for such antibodies to appear in the maternal circulation following such an event. This is called sensitization or immunization. IgM is the primary Ig produced, increasing in exponential fashion to a plateau, then decreasing over a period of months. Because IgM antibodies are unable to cross the placenta, there is no fetal effect of a primary response, and hence, HDFN does not usually take place in a first pregnancy. However, IgM (and IgG if present) can be detected on screening tests on maternal blood samples. The primary response also involves expansion of a population of memory B cells with high affinity for binding the Rh antigen, primed to produce IgG antibody earlier and in much greater quantity on subsequent exposure to antigen. With later exposure to Rh-positive red cells, often a much smaller antigenic dose, a secondary response occurs, resulting in the production of mainly IgG antibodies. IgG production has a shorter lag phase, a much longer plateau and a titer of perhaps 10 times that of the primary response. IgG actively crosses the placenta by Fc binding to specific receptors on trophoblastic cells and produces the clinical manifestations of Rh isoimmunization.

Incidence and epidemiology

Only four antibodies seem to be associated with severe fetal disease: anti-RhD, anti-Rhc, anti-Kell (K1) and anti-E. In most cases, non-D antibodies are of low titer and of no clinical significance, and when HDFN does occur, it is usually less severe than with anti-D. However, fetal death has been reported due to anti-c[8] and anti-Kell[9]. Isolated cases of HDFN due to anti-E, anti-C, anti-k (Kell system) and anti-Fy^a (Duffy

system) and rare cases of severe fetal anemia due to Kidd (JkA, JkB), MNS system (M, N, S, s), Lutheran (Lu^a, Lu^b), Diego (Di^a, Di^b) have been reported. Anti-c, anti-Kell and anti-E may cause hemolytic disease of the newborn as severe as that seen in anti-D hemolytic disease of the newborn[10]. Often, the D antibody is found in conjunction with other Rh antibodies (c, C, E, e) of weaker titer.

D disease

The presence of D antigen on maternal erythrocytes confers Rh-positive status to the mother. About 10% of all pregnancies involve an Rh-negative mother with a Rh-positive fetus and in a first pregnancy, about 60% of Rh-negative women will have an Rh-positive baby[11]. Although sensitization to the C, E, D and e antigens can cause fetal anemia, sensitization to D is the most common and clinically important. As no antibody to a 'D' antigen has been identified, the designation 'D' actually describes the absence of the D antigen.

Kell alloimmunization (anti-K antibody)

Kell hemolytic disease accounts for 10% of the cases of antibody-mediated severe fetal anemia[12]. The reason that Kell sensitization is uncommon is that, while 9% of the population has at least one Kell (K) antigen allele, only 5% of the 91% who are Kell-negative will develop anti-Kell antibodies after incompatible transfusion. This is because partners of Kell-negative women are likely to be Kell-positive in 10% of pregnancies and only half of these pregnancies are likely to be incompatible because of paternal heterozygosity. Published results on the outcome of maternal Kell alloimmunization indicate that between 2.5% and 10% of Kell-immunized pregnancies end in the delivery of affected infants[13 –15], with about half the infants requiring intervention.

Fetal disease caused by anti-Kell anitbodies tends to be more aggressive compared with other antibodies. Maternal Kell antibody levels do not correlate well with the risk of fetal anemia and fetal erythropoietic suppression[11–14,16] Severe HDFN in Kell alloimmunization may occur earlier and at lower maternal antibody titers than with anti-D disease.

Anti-k antibody (Cellano or K$_2$)

Several authors have reported a small number of cases of anti-k alloimmunisation. Most of these have been mild, involving single neonatal transfusion, neonatal exchange transfusion and neonatal phototherapy alone. Hydropic fetal loss and need for intrauterine transfusion (IUT) has been reported but is very rare. The maternal antibody titer bears no relation to the severity of disease and it has been suggested that anti-k antibody might produce fetal erythropoietic suppression at lower maternal titers in the same way as anti-Kell.

Rhc, RhC, RhE and Rhe antibodies

Rhc has been associated with severe HDFN. In more than half of women with anti-Rhc, there is a history of previous blood transfusion. The hemolytic effect of anti-Rhc is very similar to that of anti-RhD. Cases of neonatal death, hydrops, hydropic stillbirth and perinatal deaths have been reported. In the most recent series reported by Hackney et al. in 2004, 25% of Rhc antigen-positive fetuses exhibited severe HDFN, 7% of the total group were hydropic and 17% required IUTs[17].

Anti-RhC, anti-RhE and anti-Rhe usually occur in low titers in conjunction with anti-RhD antibody, and their presence can be additive to the hemolytic effect of the anti-RhD. IUTs are reported only rarely when these antibodies occur as the sole finding.

MNS antigen system

The MNS antigen system consists of 40 red cell antigens; the M, N, S, s, and the U antigens are constituents of this group that have been associated with HDFN. In the great majority of cases, the paternal phenotype will be positive for the antigen with the majority of individuals being heterozygous. Anti-M is a naturally occurring IgM that typically presents as a cold agglutinin. Conversion to IgG occurs rarely and has been associated with HDFN.

Multiple maternal antibodies

The management of these cases has typically been equivalent to that of Rh D-isoimmunisation[18,19]. Although some studies have reported that the presence of multiple maternal antibodies (anti-C + anti-D[20]; anti-E + anti-c[21]) appear to have more severe disease than those with only anti-D red blood cell antibody.

ABO hemolytic disease

ABO hemolytic disease is estimated to occur in about 2–3% of all births, but only in 1 in 3,000 births does severe hemolytic disease of newborn (HDN) occur. Mild cases not requiring exchange transfusion are identified as 1 in 150 births. Less than 5% of affected newborns require phototherapy and only in very rare cases is exchange transfusion required.

ABO hemolytic disease of the newborn is limited to mothers with blood group type O whose babies are group A or B. One of the most important reasons for low incidence and severity of ABO HDN, despite considerable fetomaternal ABO incompatibility, is that most anti-A and anti-B antibodies are of the IgM type and do not cross the placenta. Unlike Rh disease, ABO hemolytic disease of the newborn occurs with the same frequency in the first as in subsequent pregnancies, since maternal anti-A and anti-B antibodies are present normally, probably secondary to sensitization against A or B substances in food or bacteria.

Prevention of red cell (RhD) alloimmunization

There are about 105,000 births to RhD negative women each year in England and Wales. This constitutes some 17% of all births. Of these babies, about 59% or 62,000 are RhD positive. This represents about 10% of all births each year in England and Wales. Before immunoprophylaxis became available, the frequency of HDFN was 1% of all births, and HDFN was responsible for the death of one baby in every 2200 births. Anti-D prophylaxis (mostly administered postnatally) and advances in neonatal care have reduced the frequency of HDN by a factor of 10, to 1 in 21,000 births. In England and Wales, about 500 fetuses develop hemolytic disease each year, resulting in the loss of 20 fetuses before 28 weeks' gestation, death of 25–30 babies due to HDFN and a further 45 fetuses being affected with developmental problems[22].

The correct administration of anti-D immune globulin dramatically reduces the rate of alloimmunization. In the UK, the National Institute of Clinical Excellence[23] now recommends antenatal prophylaxis at 28 and 34 weeks of gestation, and the dose for each antenatal administration as well as the dose given after delivery is 500 IU.

It has also been shown experimentally that one prophylactic dose of 300 mcg (1,500 IU) of anti-D immune globulin can prevent RhD alloimmunization after an exposure to up to 30 mL of RhD-positive blood or 15 mL of fetal cells[24]. In its guidance, NICE indicate that one dose of 1,500 international units (IU) at 28 weeks appears to be as effective as two doses as mentioned above. Considering cost, manpower resource factors and patient convenience, there has been some debate on the optimum dosage regimen to be used for routine antenatal anti-D prophylaxis and many trust hospitals now prefer to use the single prophylactic dose between 28–30 weeks.

Initial studies proved that the postpartum administration of a single dose of anti-D immune globulin to susceptible RhD-negative women within 72 h of delivery reduced the alloimmunization rate by 90%[25].

The British Committee for Standards in Haematology recommend that RhD-negative mothers delivering RhD-positive infants or following a potentially sensitizing event in pregnancy, undergo a test to screen for FMH in excess of the amount covered by the standard dose of anti-D immune globulin. This test, the Kleihauer–Betke test, will determine if additional anti-D immune globulin is necessary[26].

The Kleihauer–Betke test is a test on maternal blood to quantify the amount of FMH. The amount of fetal blood transfused into the mother's circulation can vary, ranging from 0.1 mL to 30 mL. Knowing the amount can help better determine how much anti-D Ig will be needed to prevent the formation of antibodies in the maternal blood. It is estimated that more than 50% of women will have amounts of 0.1 mL or less in their blood, but it is possible for the amount to reach up to 30 mL (in 0.6% of cases). The basis of the test is that, hemoglobin (Hb) A is readily eluted from adult red cells at a low pH, whilst red cells, which contain Hb F, are more resistant. A suitable reagent will fully elute the adult Hb A from a thin blood film without eluting the red cells containing Hb F. The resistant Hb can then be stained red with an appropriate counter stain, which will make them stand out clearly against the ghost-like appearance of the eluted adult cells when viewed under a microscope.

Where applicable, a Kleihauer–Betke test should be undertaken, and if FMH is found to be more than 4 mL, then follow-up samples are required at 48 h following an intravenous (IV) dose of anti-D or 72 h following an intramuscular (IM) dose to check for clearance of fetal cells. Additional doses of anti-D should be administered as necessary.

Potentially sensitizing events requiring anti-D prophylaxis are as follows[26]:

- amniocentesis, CVS, cordocentesis
- antepartum hemorrhage/uterine or vaginal bleeding in pregnancy
- external cephalic version
- abdominal trauma (sharp/blunt, open/closed)

- ectopic pregnancy
- evacuation of molar regnancy
- intrauterine death and stillbirth
- in utero therapeutic interventions (transfusion, surgery, insertion of shunts, laser)
- miscarriage, threatened miscarriage
- therapeutic termination of pregnancy
- delivery – normal, instrumental or cesarean section.
- intra-operative cell salvage.

If anti-D is identified in an Rh-negative pregnant woman, further history should be obtained and investigation undertaken to determine whether this is immune or passive, as a result of previous injection of anti-D Ig. If no clear conclusion can be reached about the origin of the anti-D detected, then in the case of a potentially sensitizing event at less than or more than 20 weeks, the woman should continue to be offered anti-D prophylaxis on the assumption that the detectable anti-D may be passive. Women with indeterminate RhD typing results should be treated as D-negative until confirmatory testing is completed[26].

Preventable RhD alloimmunization occurs in susceptible RhD-negative women for the following reasons:

- failure to administer antenatal doses of anti-D Ig at 28 and 34 weeks' gestation
- failure to recognize antenatal clinical events that place patients at risk for alloimmunization and failure to administer the adequate dose of anti-D Ig appropriately
- failure to administer anti-D Ig postnatally.

Safety, availability, dosage and administration of anti-D Ig

Anti-D Ig used in the UK is polyclonal and is prepared from pooled plasma from non-UK blood donors who have high levels of anti-D Ig, either due to previous sensitization or intentional immunization. In addition to screening for hepatitis B surface antigen, anti-human immunodeficiency virus infection and hepatitis C virus RNA, the plasma also undergoes viral inactivation steps in order to reduce risk of viral transmission. The theoretical transmission of Creutzfeldt–Jakob disease remains unquantifiable, though is likely to be extremely small. The incidence of possible adverse events from an injection of anti-D is estimated to be less than one event per 80,000 doses of anti-D Ig, the majority of which are not considered serious.

Table 15.1 Indication and dose of anti-D in previously non-sensitized RhD-negative women[26]

Event/procedure	Recommended dose of anti-D	Comments or conditions that must apply
Spontaneous complete miscarriage <12 week	Anti-D not necessary	Where uterus is not instrumented and mild painless bleeding. Test for FMH not required.
Therapeutic termination of pregnancy	250 IU within 72 h of the event	Irrespective of gestational age. Test for FMH not required.
Ectopic pregnancy	250 IU within 72 h	Regardless of method of management. Test for FMH not required.
Molar pregnancy	250 IU within 72 h of evacuation	
Threatened miscarriage	Anti-D not necessary	Where viable fetus and bleeding stops before 12 weeks. Test for FMH not required.
Amnniocentesis/CVS/ cordocentesis	250 IU within 72 h 500 IU within 72 h	At any gestation up to 20 weeks. Test for FMH not required. After 20 weeks of gestation.
Persistent uterine bleeding	250 IU to be given at a minimum interval of 6-weekly interval	Between 12 and 20 weeks. Test for FMH not required.
ECV	500 IU within 72 h	Test for FMH required.
All other potential sensitising events after 20 weeks as mentioned above	500 IU within 72 h	Test for FMH required.

CVS: chorionic villus sampling; ECV: external cephalic version; FMH: fetomaternal hemorrhage; IU: international units; h: hours.

Although very rare, severe hypersensitivity, including anaphylaxis, may occur. Medications to treat anaphylaxis, such as adrenaline and steroids, should be readily available in case of such severe reactions. The probable mechanism by which anti-D works includes rapid clearance of anti-D coated D-positive red cells by macrophages and downregulation of antigen-specific B cells.

The minimum recommended dose of anti-D is mentioned above. The actual dose depends on the quantity of FMH and type of anti-D Ig preparations available in individual centers, and thus may be higher than is clinically necessary. The dose of anti-D is specified in IU and 1 mcg of anti-D Ig is equivalent to 5 IU. A dose of 500 IU, IM is considered sufficient to treat a FMH of up to 4 mL fetal red cells. Where it is necessary to give additional doses of anti-D Ig, as guided by tests for FMH, the dose calculation is traditionally based on 125 IU anti-D Ig/mL fetal or inadvertently transfused D-positive red cells for IM administration.

Management of red cell alloimmunization

In current clinical practice, obstetricians will encounter two clinical scenarios where knowledge of Rh disease becomes important:

(1) positive Rh antibody screening report, indicating presence of antibodies that may cause HDN
(2) raised Rh antibodies and affected fetus or newborn in a previous pregnancy.

As with most other areas of fetal medicine, the key elements of appropriate management strategy include careful history taking, maternal and fetal diagnostic tests, antenatal surveillance and treatment when necessary.

Obstetric history

An attempt should be made to establish the sensitizing event. Faced with a parous patient with no previous history of Rh sensitization, the following questions are helpful.

(1) Did you have any pregnancy losses, ectopic pregnancy or invasive tests in previous pregnancies? If yes, did you receive an (anti-D) injection?
(2) Did you receive antenatal/postnatal anti-D prophylaxis in previous pregnancies?
(3) Did you receive any blood transfusions in the past? (This is particularly relevant in the presence of non-D antibodies.)

The following questions are helpful when faced with a patient with history of Rh sensitization in previous pregnancy, particularly when full obstetric records are not available.

(1) Were you refered to a fetal medicine unit for monitoring in your last pregnancy?

(2) Did you have any invasive tests/fetal blood transfusions in your last pregnancy?

(3) Was your labor induced because of antibodies? If yes, at which gestation?

(4) Did any of your babies need a transfusion after birth?

(5) Did your baby need phototherapy ("under blue light") after birth?

As a rule, the HDN tends to worsen in subsequent affected pregnancies. History of early fetal death or hydrops is particularly ominous, as hydrops recurs in 90% of affected pregnancies, often at an earlier gestation. Neonatal jaundice due to hemolysis is also likely to recur to the same degree of severity in subsequent affected pregnancies.

Paternal testing

Testing for paternal genotype should be considered routine in the presence of maternal Rh antibodies. If the father is homozygous then all his children will be at risk of Rh disease, whereas if he is heterozygous there is a 50:50 chance of his fathering a baby who will not be affected.

However, this counseling should not be trivialized because in certain scenarios this is effectively a test of paternity. For example, if presumed father is shown to be RhD homozygous, but the baby is found to be RhD negative, this may cause a considerable distress to the family in question. In the authors' practice, a frank discussion is often held with a pregnant woman without the partner's presence. If there is even a remote possibility that the current partner may not be the father of the child, then fetal genotyping should be considered (see below) without checking paternal blood group.

Prenatal diagnosis of fetal RhD status

One of the most important advances in recent years in the antenatal management of red cell alloimmunization has been the introduction of fetal blood grouping using cell-free fetal DNA (cffDNA) from maternal blood. Several studies have shown that detection of fetal RhD, RhC, RhE, Rhc and Kell antigens in maternal blood in alloimmunized pregnancies is highly accurate and can eliminate unnecessary fetal monitoring[27–30]. For antigens other than those mentioned above, invasive

testing (CVS or amniocentesis) may be considered if fetal anemia is a concern or if invasive testing is performed for another reason, e.g., karyotyping.

In the UK, the Bristol International Blood Group Reference Laboratory (http://ibgrl.blood.co.uk/) perform prenatal diagnosis for the blood group antigen RhD, Kell, Rhc and RhE. When a test is negative, either the fetus is antigen negative or there was no fetal DNA in the maternal blood sample. In such circumstances, testing for the presence of the sex-determining region Y (SRY) gene in the fetal cells in maternal plasma can confirm the presence of a male fetus, and hence the presence of fetal DNA in the sample. The presence of a female fetus can potentially complicate the test result, but one useful option is to repeat the test after a few weeks. The last option would be to do the genetic testing of amniocytes obtained from amniocentesis, but this option is rarely needed. As diagnostic accuracy of cffDNA testing is not quite 100%, blood levels of antibody should be tested every 4 weeks to detect any false-negative results[31].

Routine testing of cffDNA for fetal RhD genotyping for all D-negative pregnant women can potentially limit the administration of prophylactic anti-D only to those women in whom it is needed. This could result in a significant saving of anti-D Ig, as women with D-negative fetuses (about one-third) will not require routine immunoprophylaxis or prenatal anti-D following sensitizing events (e.g., invasive procedures). It may also negate the need for testing the serologic status of the newborn at delivery, as DNA testing is more accurate than serology.

Maternal serology

The aims of antenatal serologic testing are to identify Rh-negative women who will benefit from anti-D Ig prophylaxis, to detect maternal alloimmunization and to ascertain risk to the fetus from alloimmune hemolytic disease. All pregnant women should be tested for ABO, RhD typing and for irregular serum antibodies at the initial antenatal visit, preferably in the first trimester and repeated at 28 weeks' gestation (prior to administration of prophylactic anti-D).

Conventionally, an indirect antiglobulin test (IAT) is performed with untreated red cells in order to detect clinically important IgG antibodies, which may cross the placenta. Often an additional test is carried out using enzyme modified red cells, which facilitates early detection of low levels of antibodies, some of which may be clinically important.

When clinically significant alloantibodies are detected, quantification is usually performed by an autoanalyser technique (for anti-D and anti-c) or by IAT titration, usually reported as a titer score. Anti-D and anti-c values are expressed as IU/mL.

By convention, the quantification of other other antibodies is reported as the integer of the greatest tube dilution with a positive agglutination reaction (i.e., a titer of 16 is equivalent to a dilution of 1:16).

It is important to note that an increase in titer from 1 in 32 to 1 in 64 or from 1 in 64 and to 1 in 128 is not considered clinically significant. The increase should be more than double, i.e., from 1 in 32 to 1 in 128. This is the reason why old samples should be stored frozen and tested in parallel with the current sample using the same techniques.

The absolute level of antibody is not as important as the trend, with a rising level requiring more frequent monitoring, particularly if there is a history of previous HDFN. Significant HDFN due to anti-D is highly unlikely below a concentration of 4 IU/mL. Where quantification is not routine, antibody titration is performed using the IAT, with different laboratories establishing critical titers for RhD antibody, varying from 1:8 to 1:32. Close monitoring is usually indicated if the titre is >1/8[32–35] .

Ultrasound monitoring

A variety of ultrasonographic parameters have been used in an attempt to determine when fetal anemia is present. These have included placental thickness, umbilical vein diameter, hepatic length, splenic perimeter and polyhydramnios[36]. However, most of these features have not proven reliable in clinical practice. Late ultrasound findings include abdominal ascites, pleural and pericardial effusion and scalp edema.

The major breakthrough in the monitoring of Rh disease came with the introduction of the use of Doppler ultrasound to measure peak systolic velocity (PSV) of blood flow in the fetal middle cerebral artery (MCA) of the fetus[37].

The technique for obtaining fetal MCA Doppler waveforms is as follows[38].

- An axial section of the brain, including the thalami and the sphenoid bone wings, should be obtained and magnified.
- Color flow mapping should be used to identify the circle of Willis and the proximal MCA.
- The pulsed-wave Doppler gate should then be placed at the proximal third of the MCA, close to its origin in the internal carotid artery (the systolic velocity decreases with distance from the point of origin of this vessel).
- The angle between the ultrasound beam and the direction of blood flow should be kept as close as possible to zero degrees.
- Care should be taken to avoid any unnecessary pressure on the fetal head.
- At least three and fewer than 10 consecutive waveforms should be recorded. The highest point of the waveform is considered as the PSV (cm/s).

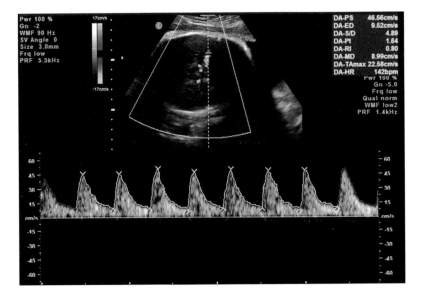

Figure 15.1 Doppler ultrasound examination of middle cerebral artery.

Table 15.2 Values for peak systolic velocity in the middle cerebral artery at different gestational ages[a]

Week of gestation	Multiples of the median (MoM)			
	1.00 MoM	1.29 MoM	1.50 MoM	1.55 MoM
18	23.2	29.9	34.8	36.0
20	25.5	32.8	38.2	39.5
22	27.9	36.0	41.9	43.3
24	30.7	39.5	46.0	47.5
26	33.6	43.3	50.4	52.1
28	36.9	47.6	55.4	57.2
30	40.5	52.2	60.7	62.8
32	44.4	57.3	66.6	68.9
34	48.7	62.9	73.1	75.6
36	53.5	69.0	80.2	82.9
38	58.7	75.7	88.0	91.0
40	64.4	83.0	96.6	99.8

[a] Reproduced with permission from the Massachusetts Medical Society[37].

- The PSV can be measured using manual calipers or autotrace. The latter yields significantly lower medians than does the former, but more closely approximates published medians used in clinical practice.

The threshold values for PSV in the MCA at different gestational ages are shown in Table 15.2. All of the fetuses with moderate or severe anemia had PSV values above 1.50 times the median.

Amniotic fluid spectrophotometry

In most developed countries and many developing countries, amniotic fluid spectrophotometry (AFS) has now been superseded by antenatal fetal Doppler ultrasound examination for assessment and monitoring. Briefly, AFS was first introduced by Liley[39] in 1961 when he obtained amniotic fluid from 101 Rh-sensitized pregnant women between 27 and 41 weeks' gestation, and spectrophotometrically analyzed it for bilirubin at an optical density of 450 nm. Liley used his data to delineate three zones related to gestational age. The optical density difference (ΔOD450) values in the lower zone (zone 1) indicated a fetus with mild or no hemolytic disease, whilst those in the upper zone (zone 3) indicated severe hemolytic disease with fetal death probable within 7–10 days.

In order to decide the optimum time of intervention (delivery or in utero transfusion), Whitfield et al.

[40] introduced the concept of an action line based on the presence, severity and likely further trend of hemolysis in the fetus as indicated by the trend of amniotic fluid bilirubin concentration.

Fetal blood sampling and intrauterine transfusion

Fetal blood sampling (FBS) is ultrasound-directed, which allows for the direct measurement of fetal blood indices as early as 17–18 weeks' gestation.

Traditionally, fetal blood is obtained from placental cord insertion or intrahepatic umbilical vein. In certain circumstances when access is a problem, it may be necessary to puncture a loop of cord that floats freely in the amniotic fluid. Specimens of fetal blood can be used for direct measurement of complete blood count, reticulocyte, and red cell antigen phenotyping. Full blood count is done in the local hematology laboratory and may take 5–10 min. Most fetal medicine units also use preliminary bedside testing (e.g., Hamecue) to decide whether to start fetal transfusion whilst waiting for the confirmatory result from the laboratory.

There is no universal agreement on a critical Hb level that indicates the need for transfusion. In modern practice, FBS is only performed in sensitized pregnancies with fetal hydrops or significantly raised PSVs in the fetal MCA. It is therefore extremely rare to perform FBS and find fetal Hb >10 g/L. When indicated, fetal transfusion is perfomed with O, Rh-negative, cytomegalovirus-negative, washed irradiated packed cells crossmatched against maternal blood. It is important to have the blood ready.

Transfusion volume depends on estimated fetoplacental blood volume for a particular gestation, fetal hematocrit and donor hematocrit.

In order to calculate exact transfusion, volume nomograms have been created by Nicolaides's group from the Harris Birthright Fetal Medicine Unit at King's College Hospital, London. Total fetoplacental blood volume increases from around 26 mL at 18 weeks to 241 mL at 36 weeks of gestation (Table 15.3)[41]. Based on pretransfusion fetal hematocrit and donor blood hematocrit, they derived a multiplication factor (F) in order to achieve a post-transfusion fetal hematocrit of around 40% (Table 15.4)[42]. The amount of blood to be transfused is calculated by multiplying the fetopalcental volume with this factor F. In current practice, these calculations are used to determine the initial volume of transfused blood. Post-transfusion

Table 15.3 Estimated fetoplacental blood volume in fetuses with erythroblastosis fetalis

Gestational age (weeks)	Estimated fetoplacental blood volume in fetuses with erythroblastosis fetalis (mL)
18	26
20	34
22	50
24	69
26	86
28	112
30	136
32	166
34	203
36	241

Table 15.4 Multiplication factor to be used to calculate volume of donor blood to be transfused to achieve a post-transfusion fetal hematocrit of approximately 40%

Donor hematocrit (%) ▶ Fetal hematocrit (%) ▼	50	60	70	80
10	3	1.5	1	0.75
20	2	1	0.7	0.5
30	1.125	0.55	0.35	0.3

fetal Hb is checked using a bedside test for full blood count. Additional volume is transfused, if necessary, aiming for a post-transfusion fetal Hb of around 130–150 g/L. In certain circumstances, particularly in a hydropic baby, the risk of volume overload is high, and it may be necessary to 'under-transfuse' in the first instance before a further top-up transfusion a week later. This will allow the fetal cardiovascular system to compensate for the acute change in viscosity. In the past, the follow-up transfusion was scheduled based on an anticipated decline in hematocrit of approximately 1% per day. Increasingly, MCA Doppler measurements are used to determine the timing of subsequent transfusions.

Intraperitoneal transfusion

Intraperitoneal transfusion (IPT) is a technique in which donor red cells are placed in the fetal peritoneal cavity and are absorbed via subdiaphragmatic lymphatics and thoracic duct into the fetal circulation. This

was superseded by intravascular intrauterine transfusion because of several disadvantages such as being less effective in hydropic fetus, a lack of information on pre- and post- transfusion blood indices, and possibly, increased intraperitoneal pressure compromising the venous return. However, IPT may be the only choice when treatment becomes essential at very early gestations (<18 weeks) because intravascular access is technically difficult[43]. Some have suggested that combined intravascular and intraperitoneal transfusion may be useful in prolonging the interval between the transfusion, but most centers use intravascular transfusion alone to avoid the need for two procedures and shorten the procedure time[44].

Management protocol

Stable antibodies <4 IU/mL or <1:64

Confirm that the partner is homozygous for the relevant antigen. If in doubt, organize fetal gentotyping. Serial antibody measurement is performed every 4 weeks before 28 weeks and 2 weeks after 28 weeks. Some minor antibodies can be repeated every 4 weeks. Multiple antibodies should be repeated every fortnight.

In such cases, timing, mode and place of delivery is dependent on standard obstetric grounds. Good quality evidence is not available to influence decision making. Usually, delivery is undertaken around 38–39 weeks' gestation.

Antibodies >4 IU/mL or >1:64 and/or previously affected child

All such cases should be referred/discussed with tertiary fetal medicine units. Women with hydrops in previous pregnancy should be seen as early as 14–16 weeks. As a rule, MCA Doppler to estimate PSV should start around 18 weeks and usually continued fortnightly. If antibody levels rise, then Doppler studies may be needed weekly or even twice per week. Timing of repeat Doppler studies depends on the history, antibody levels and MCA values. Stable MCA below 1.29 multiples of the median (MoM) is reassuring.

When MCA-PSV exceeds 1.5 MoM before 32 weeks, most centers are likely to opt for FBS to detect fetal Hb levels. The authors' view is that each FBS procedure has to be organized and planned meticulously, with blood for transfusion being readily available and an operating theatre on stand-by (after 24 weeks' gestation).

As a rule, this group of women will be delivered between 36 and 38 weeks and the timing of invasive procedures often reflect that. In the past, the last in-utero transfusion used to be scheduled around 32 weeks, but with more experience and better results the upper cut-off point seems to be shifting towards later gestations, particularly when access is thought to be easier (e.g., anterior placenta).

Some units have attempted to modify the disease using high-dose IV gammaglobulins, plasmapheresis or steroids as an adjunct to intravascular transfusion in severe hemolytic disease where treatment is required prior to 20 weeks[44], or even before pregnancy. The mechanism of action could be downregulation of the maternal immune system or antagonistic action in the fetal reticular endothelial system[46].

Indications for referral to a fetal medicine specialist for a fetus at risk of HDFN[47]

- Anti-D level of >4 IU/mL. At antibody levels >4 IU/mL but <15 IU/mL the fetus carries a moderate risk of HDFN and levels above 15 IU/mL can cause severe HDFN.
- Anti-c level of >7.5 IU/mL. At antibody levels >7.5 IU/mL but < 20 IU/mL the fetus carries a moderate risk of HDFN, whereas antibody levels >20 IU/mL correlate with a high risk of HDFN.
- Anti-K antibodies can lead to severe anemia even at low titres, and therefore referral should take place once anti-K antibody is detected.
- Anti-E potentiates the severity of HDFN due to anti-c antibodies, and hence referral is indicated at lower titers or levels when both these antibodies are present simultaneously.

References

1. Vaughan JI, Warwick R, Welch CR, et al. Anti-Kell in pregnancy (letter). *Br J Obstet Gynaecol* 1991; 98: 944–5.

2. Anonymous. Dangers of anti-Kell in pregnancy (editorial). *Lancet* 1991; 3376: 1319–20.

3. Society of Obstetricians and Gynaecologists of Canada (SOGC). Prevention of RH Alloimmunization. RCOG Clinical Practice Guidelines No. 133. London: RCOG, September 2003.

4. Von Stein GA, Munsick RA, Stiver K, et al. Fetomaternal haemorrhage in threatened abortion. *Obstet Gynaecol* 1992; 79: 383–6.

5. Blakemore KJ, Baumgarten A, Schoenfeld-Dimaio M, et al. Rise in maternal serum alpha-fetoprotein concentration after chorionic villus sampling and the possibility of isoimmunisation. *Am J Obstet Gynecol* 1986; 155: 988–93.

6. Bowman JM. Controversies in Rh prophylaxis. Who needs Rh immune globulin and when should it be given? *Am J Obstet Gynecol* 1985; 151: 289–94.

7. Lau TK, Stock A, Rogers M. Fetomaternal haemorrhage after external cephalic version at term. *Aust NZ J Obstet Gynaecol* 1995; 35: 173–4.

8. Tovey LAD. Haemolytic disease of the newborn-the changing scene. *Br J Obstet Gynaecol* 1986; 93: 960–6.

9. Mayne KM, Bowell PJ, Pratt GA. The significance of anti-Kell sensitisation in pregnancy. *Clin Lab Haematol* 1990a; 12: 379–85.

10. Bowman JM. Maternal blood group immunisation: Haemolytic disease (erythroblastosis fetalis). In: Creasy RK, Resnik R (eds). *Maternal-Fetal Medicine: Principles and Practice*, 4th edn. Philadelphia: Saunders, 1994; 711.

11. Chilcott J, Lloyd Jones M, Wight J, et al. A review of the clinical effectiveness and cost effectiveness of routine anti-D prophylaxis for pregnant women who are Rhesus (RhD) negative. London: National Institute of Clinical Excellence, 2002.

12. Vaughan JI, Warwick R, Letsky E, et al. Erythropoietic suppression in fetal anemia because of Kell alloimmunization. *Am J Obstet Gynecol* 1994; 171: 247–52.

13. Caine ME, Mueller-Heubach E. Kell sensitisation in pregnancy. *Am J Obstet Gynecol* 1986; 154: 85–90.

14. Leggat HM, Gibson JM, Barron SL, et al. Anti-Kell in pregnancy. *Br J Obstet Gynaecol* 1991; 98: 162–5.

15. Bowman JM, Pollack JM, Manning FA, et al. Maternal Kell blood group alloimmunization. *Obstet Gynecol* 1992: 79: 239–44.

16. Vaughan J, Manning M, Warwick R, et al. Inhibition of erythroid progenitor cells by anti-Kell antibodies in fetal alloimmune anemia. *N Engl J Med* 1998; 338: 798–803.

17. Hackney DN, Knudtson EJ, Rossi KQ, et al. Management of pregnancies complicated by anti-c isoimmunization. *Obstet Gynecol* 2004; 103: 24–30.

18. American College of Obstetricians and Gynecologists (ACOG). Technical Bulletin. Management of isoimmunisation in pregnancy. *Int J Obstet Gynecol* 1996; 55: 183–90.

19. Queenan JT, ed. Rh and other blood group immunizations. In: *Management of High-Risk Pregnancies*, 4th edn. Maldan (MA): Blackwell Science, 1999; 399–412.

20. Sponge CY, Porter AE, Queenan JT. Management of isoimmunization in the presence of multiple maternal antibodies. *Am J Obstet Gynecol* 2001; 185: 481–4.

21. Babinszki A, Berkowitz RL. Haemolytic disease of the newborn caused by anti-c, anti-E and anti-Fya

antibodies: report of five cases. *Prenat Diagn* 1999; 19: 533–6.

22. National Institute for Health and Care Excellence (NICE). Guidance on the use of routine antenatal anti-D prophylaxis for RhD-negative women. Technology Appraisal Guidance No. 41, May 2002.

23. National Institute of Clinical Excellence (NICE). Routine antenatal anti-D prophylaxis for women who are rhesus D negative. NICE Technology Appraisal Guidance (TA156), August 27, 2008 (nice.org.uk/guidance/ta156).

24. Pollack W, Ascari WQ, Kochesky RJ, et al. Studies on Rh prophylaxis. 1. Relationship between doses of anti-Rh and size of antigenic stimulus. *Transfusion* 1971; 11: 333–9.

25. Freda VJ, Gorman JG, Pollack W, et al. Prevention of Rh haemolytic disease-ten years' clinical experience with Rh immune globulin. *N Engl J Med* 1975; 292: 1014–6.

26. Qureshi H, Massey E, Kirwan D, et al. BCSH guideline for the use of anti-D immunoglobulin for the prevention of haemolytic disease of the fetus and newborn. *Transfus Med* 2014; 24: 8–20.

27. Schefferr PG, van der Schoot CE, Page-Christiaens GC, et al. Noninvasive fetal blood group genotyping of rhesus D, c, E and of K in alloimmunised pregnant women: evaluation of a 7-year clinical experience. *BJOG* 2011; 118(11): 1340–8.

28. Hromandnikova I, Vesela K, Benesova B, et al. Non-invasive fetal RHD and RHCE genotyping from maternal plasma in alloimmunized pregnancies. *Prenat Diagn* 2005; 25: 1079–83.

29. Geifman-Holtzman O, Grotegut CA, Gaughan CA, et al. Non-invasive fetal RhCE genotyping from maternal blood. *BJOG* 2009; 116(2): 144–51.

30. Gutensohn K, Muller SP, Thomann K, et al. Diagnostic accuracy of non-invasive polymerase chain reaction testing for the determination of fetal rhesus C, c and E status in early pregnancy. *BJOG* 2010; 117(6): 722–9.

31. Illanes S, Soothill P. Management of red cell alloimmunisation in pregnancy: the non-invasive monitoring of the disease. *Prenat Diagn* 2010; 30: 668–73.

32. Voak D, Mitchell R, Bowell P, et al. Guidelines for blood grouping and red cell antibody testing during pregnancy. *Transfus Med* 1996; 6: 71–4.

33. Urbaniak SJ, Greiss MA. RhD haemolytic disease of the fetus and the newborn. 2000; 14: 44–61.

34. Bruce M, Chapman JF, Duguid J, et al. Addendum for guidelines for blood grouping and red cell antibody testing during pregnancy. *Transfus Med* 1999; 9: 99.

35. Clark AC. Red cell antibodies in pregnancy: evidence overturned. *Lancet* 1996; 347: 485–6.

36. Whitecar PW, Moise KJ Jr. Sonographic methods to detect fetal anaemia in red blood cell alloimmunization. *Obstet Gynecol Surv* 2000; 55: 240–50.

37. Mari G, Deter RL, Carpenter RL, et al. Non-invasive diagnosis by Doppler ultrasonography of fetal anaemia due to maternal red-cell alloimmunization. *N Engl J Med* 2000; 342(1): 9–14.

38. ISUOG Practice Guidelines: use of Doppler ultrasonography in Obstetrics. *Ultrasound Obstet Gynecol* 2013; 41: 233–9.

39. Liley AW. Liquor amnii analysis in the management of the pregnancy complicated by Rhesus sensitisation. *Am J Obstet Gynecol* 1961; 82: 1359–70.

40. Whitfield, CR, Lappin, TRJ, Carson, M. Further development and experience in an action line method for the management of Rhesus isoimmunisation. *J Obstet Gynaec Brit Cwlth* 1970; 77: 791–5.

41. Nicolaides KH, Clewell WH, Rodeck CH. Measurement of human fetoplacental blood volume in erythroblastosis fetalis. *Am J Obstet Gynecol* 1987; 157: 50–3.

42. Nicolaides KH, Soothill PW, Rodeck CH, et al. Rh disease: Intravascular fetal blood transfusion by cordocentesis. *Fetal Therapy* 1986; 1: 185–92.

43. Rodeck CH, Deans A. Red cell alloimmunisation. In: Charles H Rodeck, Martin J Whittle (eds). *Fetal Medicine: Basic Science and Clinical Practice*. Churchill Livingstone, 2001; 785–802.

44. Moise KJ Jr. Haemolytic Disease of the fetus and newborn. In: RK Creasy, R Resnik (eds). *Maternal-Fetal medicine*. Pennsylvania: Saunders, 2004; 537–61.

45. Ruma MS, Moise KJ Jr, Kim E, et al. Combined plasmapheresis and intravenous immune globulin for the treatment of severe maternal red cell alloimmunization. *AJOG* 2007; 196(2): 138.e1–6.

46. Voto LS, Mathet ER, Zapaterio JL, et al. High-dose gammaglobulin (IVIG) followed by intrauterine transfusions (IUTs): a new alternative for the treatment of severe fetal hemolytic disease. *J Perinat Med* 1997; 25(1): 85–8.

47. Royal College of Obstetricians and Gynaecologists (RCOG). The management of women with red cell antibodies during pregnancy. Green-Top Guideline No. 65, May 2014.

Chapter 16

Fetal and neonatal alloimmune thrombocytopenia

Bidyut Kumar and Zarko Alfirevic

Fetal and neonatal thrombocytopenia is defined as a platelet count below 150×10^9/L and can be classified into mild ($100–149 \times 10^9$/L), moderate ($50–99 \times 10^9$/L), severe ($20–49 \times 10^9$/L) and very severe ($<20 \times 10^9$/L). Mild and moderate thrombocytopenias do not require treatment but may lead to investigative tests. Very severe thrombocytopenia is associated with a high risk of intracranial hemorrhage (ICH) and requires immediate steps towards a diagnosis, followed by urgent treatment.

The most common cause of severe and very severe fetal and neonatal thrombocytopenia (FNAIT) is fetomaternal platelet incompatibility resulting in alloimmunization.

Nomenclature and prevalence

An alloimmune etiology for neonatal thrombocytopenia was first suggested in the early 1950s (Harrington et al.). Since 1990, the human platelet antigen (HPA) nomenclature has been adopted and the polymorphic biallelic platelet alloantigen systems have been numbered chronologically in order of their discovery. The letter "a" or "b" is assigned to the high- and low-frequency alleles, respectively. "W" marks an HPA system antigen for which only one allele is identified so far. Apart from HPA 1a and HPA 1b, many lower frequency HPAs (polymorphisms of glycoprotein IIIa) have been identified.

Of all Caucasians, 97% are HPA-1a positive, 69% are homozygous HPA-1a and 28% are heterozygous. Those who are HPA-1a negative account for about 85% of FNAIT. The other antigens most commonly involved in fetal and neonatal alloimmune thrombocytopenia (FNAIT) among whites are HPA-1b, HPA-5b, HPA-3a and HPA-3b. In Asians, sensitization against HPA-4 is the most common cause of FNAIT.

Anti-HPA-1a antibodies are produced in approximately 11% of the HPA-1a-negative mothers.

The development of anti-HPA-1a antibodies is strongly associated with the presence of the HLA class type II DRB3*0101. About one-third of HPA-1a-negative women who are DRB3*0101-positive develop antibodies. The absence of DRB3*0101 in an HPA-1a-negative women virtually precludes the development of antibodies. These alloantibodies are of IgG type and can cross the placental barrier early in pregnancy, causing destruction of fetal platelets even before 20 weeks' gestation.

Incidence of clinically affected infants is about 1 in 15,000 births in European populations[1,2]. A UK national study involving the UK Obstetric Surveillance System recently reported a UK-wide incidence of clinically detected FNAIT of 12.4 cases per 100,000 total births, following a survey spanning 2 years[3]. Eighty-one percent of cases were due to anti-HPA-1a, 7% due to anti-HPA-5b, 5% were associated with both anti-HPA-1a and anti- HPA-5b.

Clinical features and differential diagnosis

FNAIT ranges from subclinical, mild-to-moderate thrombocytopenia to life-threatening bleeding in the fetal and early neonatal period. After birth, the duration of thrombocytopenia depends on the rate of removal of the maternal antibody from the neonatal circulation. The platelet count usually reaches normal levels in 1–3 weeks. In contrast to hemolytic disease of the fetus and newborn, first pregnancies are often severely affected and the diagnosis is usually made with the birth of a first affected infant.

Accurate diagnosis of FNAIT is essential for management of any subsequent pregnancy. Therefore, FNAIT should be part of the differential diagnosis in all cases of neonatal thrombocytopenia (with platelet

Fetal Medicine, ed. Bidyut Kumar and Zarko Alfirevic. Published by Cambridge University Press. © Cambridge University Press 2016.

count of $<100 \times 10^9$/L). The laboratory investigations should include[4]:

- confirming the presence of anti-HPA antibodies in maternal serum
- crossmatching of maternal serum with paternal platelets, both untreated and chloroquine-treated (to remove HLA antigens that may cause a "false-positive" test)
- HPA pheno- or genotyping of mother and father
- exclusion of maternal thrombocytopenia.

Neonatal presentation

The most common clinical presentation of FNAIT includes petechiae, purpura or cephalohematoma at birth. ICH can result in neurologic sequelae or demise. Visceral hemorrhages, such as gastrointestinal bleeding or hematuria, occur less frequently.

Careful examination of the infant and consideration of the maternal history should exclude most of the other causes. These include the following:

- infection – bacterial, viral or parasitic infections that may occur in intensive care units
- disseminated intravascular coagulation, most often secondary to acute fetal distress or sepsis
- immune-mediated – autoimmune thrombocytopenic purpura, lupus erythematosus, maternal use of drugs
- platelet consumption – hemangioma, extensive thrombosis
- megakaryocytopoiesis impairment – chromosomal abnormalities, bone marrow metastases, congenital leukemia, downregualtion as part of rhesus hemolytic disease or chronic hypoxia
- inherited causes, e.g., thrombocytopenia associated with absent radii syndrome, congenital amegakaryocytopenia, von Willebrand 2B disease or thrombotic thrombocytopenic purpura.

Fetal presentation

Most commonly, fetal medicine specialists will encounter FNAIT in two clinical scenarios.

(1) Prepregnancy or antenatal referral of woman with a previously affected child.
(2) Antenatal diagnosis of ICH by ultrasound and/or fetal magnetic resonance imaging (MRI) associated with maternal antiplatelet antibodies.

ICH occurs in 7–26% of untreated pregnancies with FNAIT and 25–50% of such hemorrhages occur in utero. This diagnosis should always be considered when porenecephalic cysts, hydrocephalus or ICH is discovered antenatally. MRI is particularly helpful in identifying ICH.

The risk of ICH in untreated pregnancy that follows the birth of a thrombocytopenic sibling without ICH is around 7%[5]. In a UK national study, 24 out of 173 (15%) infants clinically identified as cases of FNAIT had an ICH(3).

Routine screening programme is currently not available for HPA antibodies. Therefore, presentation of FNAIT in a first pregnancy or without any previous history is invariably unexpected.

Management

The fetus of an HPA-1a mother is always considered at risk if the father is HPA-1a homozygous. If the father is heterozygous, amniocentesis can be performed to identify fetal HPA type. Recently, determination of fetal platelet antigen from cell-free fetal DNA (cffDNA) in maternal plasma has been reported and this technique is now used in many centers on a regular basis[6]. A fetus who is positive for the offending antigen should be managed in a specialized fetal medicine center.

Current antenatal antibody screening techniques are not always able to distinguish between clinically significant cases of FNAIT and cases with no or minor clinical consequences, and thus have the potential to overdiagnose clinically significant FNAIT. High maternal alloantibody concentration (28 IU/mL or more) measured before 28 weeks' gestation is associated with a high sensitivity (81%) and specificity (83%) for detection of severe thrombocytopenia (platelet count less than 50×10^9/L)[7]. In the UK, the antibody levels are rarely used to determine the management plan. Once the fetus is identified as high risk based on previous history and fetal genotype, the treatment is instituted.

In the last decade, there has been an important shift from an invasive management involving serial fetal platelet transfusion to a completely noninvasive management policy based on intravenous immunoglobulin (IVIG) therapy. A group in Leiden have been the main advocates of this much safer approach[7].

Intravenous immunoglobulin

In an analysis of prospectively collected data from Netherlands, 52 FNAIT pregnancies (53 babies) were treated with IVIG alone (without fetal blood sampling (FBS)). Weekly IVIG at a dose of 1 g/kg of maternal body weight was started at 16 weeks of gestation if the sibling had a history of ICH and at 32 weeks if there was no such history. Women were allowed to labor if there was no history ICH, and of these 65% (n = 31) achieved a vaginal birth. Following this management plan, only 10 out of 53 neonates had severe thrombocytopenia with ICH or signs of internal or external bleeding[7].

IVIG is expensive, but is well tolerated and known to be safe. Because of its source from human blood donors, risk of microbial infection exists but is very low. Although the mechanism of action is unclear, it seems to involve depression of antiplatelet antibody production, interference with antibody attachment to platelets, inhibition of macrophage receptor-mediated immune complex clearance and blockage of Fc receptors in the reticuloendothelial system.

The latest guideline on Ig use assigns FNAIT to the "red" category. "Red" indicates conditions for which treatment is considered the highest priority because of a risk to life without treatment. The guideline also states that this condition is an appropriate indication for treatment of long duration, which implies treatment of equal to or more than 3 months' duration[8]

Corticosteroids

In the UK national study, 45 fetuses were known to be affected at the outset of pregnancy. IVIG alone and a combination of IVIG, maternal steroids and intrauterine transfusion were the most common management strategies[3].

A systematic review was undertaken to determine the optimal antenatal treatment of fetomaternal alloimmune thrombocytopenia to prevent fetal and neonatal hemorrhage and death[9]. Only one trial of 54 women met the selection criteria for this review. This trial had adequate methodologic quality, but the method used to calculate sample size was inappropriate, and therefore the power calculation was not sufficient to determine any significance in differences between the treatment groups. The trial compared IVIGs plus corticosteroid (dexamethasone) with IVIGs alone. No significant differences were reported between the treatment and control groups in any of the outcomes measured. The authors concluded that there were insufficient data from randomized controlled trials to determine the optimal antenatal management of fetomaternal alloimmune thrombocytopenia. Future trials should consider the dose of IVIGs, the timing of initial treatment, monitoring of response to treatment by FBS, laboratory measures to define pregnancies with a high risk of intercranial

hemorrhage, management of nonresponders and long-term follow-up of children.

FBS to test directly for the presence of fetal thrombocytopenia has theoretical advantages; normal fetal platelet count would avoid unnecessary treatment with IVIG and may provide information about response to treatment. However, it is associated with the clinically important risk of fetal hemorrhage and pregnancy loss. If FBS is planned, fetal platelet transfusion must be immediately available in case severe fetal thombocytopenia is detected. Most UK fetal medicine units have completely abandoned serial FBS and platelet transfusions as a therapeutic option for FNAIT.

Antenatal surveillance

Ultrasound remains the mainstay of antenatal surveillance for all potentially affected pregnancies. The focus is on presence/absence of ICH. If ultrasound assessment is difficult or inconclusive, MRI in the third trimester is very helpful as it readily distinguishes ICH from other pathology.

Labor and delivery

In a recent prospective study from Leiden, out of 32 women who had a child with thrombocytopenia without ICH, 23 were delivered vaginally and nine underwent cesarean section, all for obstetric indications. All women received weekly 1 g/kg bodyweight of IVIG from 32 to 38 weeks followed by induction of labor. No diagnostic FBS was performed. Assisted vaginal delivery was considered contraindicated. Nine neonates needed treatment for thrombocytopenia, six from the vaginal birth group and three from the cesarean section group. None of the neonates had signs of ICH at ultrasound examination[10]. For women with a history of FNAIT-related ICH, most specialists recommend cesarean delivery.

A suggested management plan is shown in the following flow chart (Figure 16.1).

Key learning points

- FNAIT is rare but a potentially disastrous condition.
- Management should focus on prevention of ICH.
- The majority of ICH occurs during intrauterine life.
- There is a lack of good quality evidence to guide management.

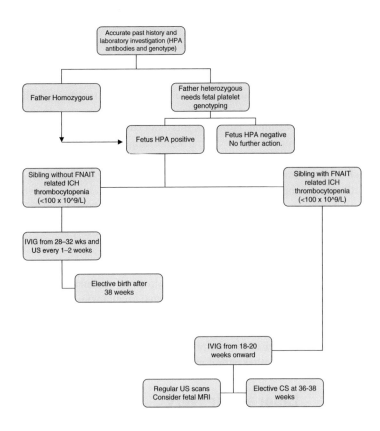

Figure 16.1 Suggested management plan.

CS: cesarean section;
FNAIT: fetal and neonatal alloimmune thrombocytopenia;
HPA: human platelet antigen;
ICH: intracranial hemorrhage;
IVIG: intravenous immunoglobulin;
MRI: magnetic resonance imaging;
US, USS: ultrasound scan;
FBS: fetal blood sampling;
IUPT: intrauterine platelet transfusion.

- The index pregnancy is the most important factor for risk estimation of ICH.
- Maternal IVIG administration appears to reduce risk of ICH even when the platelet count shows no response.

References

1. Williamson LM, Hackett G, Rennie J, et al. The natural history of fetomaternal alloimmunization to the paltelet-specific antigen PA-1a (PIA1, Zwa) as determined by antenatal screening. *Blood* 1998; 92: 2280–7.

2. Serrarens-Janssen v M, Steegers EA, van den Bos A, et al. Experiences with fetomaternal alloimmune thrombocytopenia in the Netherlands over a 2-year period. *Acta Obstetrica et Gynecologica Scandinavica* 2005; 84: 203.

3. Knight M, Pierce M, Allen D, et al. The incidence and outcome of fetomaternal alloimmune thrombocytopenia: a UK national study using three data sources. *Br J Haematol* 2011; 152: 460–8.

4. Vandenbussche FPHA, Brand A, Kanhai HHH. Fetal thrombocytopenia. In: *High Risk Pregnancy – Management Options.* James D, Steer P, Weiner C, et al. (eds). Elsevier Saunders, 2011; 229–37.

5. Radder CM, Brand A, Kanhai HHH. Will it ever be possible to balance the risk of intrasranial haemorrhage in fetal or neonatal alloimmune thrombocytopenia against the risk of treatment strategies to prevent it? *Vox Sang* 2003; 84; 318–25.

6. Scheffer P, Ait Soussan A, Verhagen O, et al. Noninvasive fetal genotyping of human platelet antigen-1a. *BJOG*, 2011; 118: 1392–5.

7. van den Akker E, Oepkes D, Lopriore E, et al. Noninvasive antenatal management of fetal and neonatal alloimmune thrombocytopenia: safe and effective. *BJOG* 2007; 114: 469–73.

8. UK Department of Health. *Clinical Guidelines for Immunoglobulin Use*, 2nd edn, July 2011.

9. Rayment R, Brunskill SJ, Stanworth S, et al. Antenatal interventions for fetomaternal alloimmune thrombocytopenia. *Cochrane Database Syst Rev* 2005; (1): CD004226. Update in *Cochrane Database Syst Rev* 2011; (5): CD004226.

10. van den Akker E, Oepkes D, Brand A, et al. Vaginal delivery for fetuses at risk of alloimmune thrombocytopenia? *BJOG* 2006; 113: 781–3.

Prescribing and teratogenesis in pregnancy

Geeta Kumar

Pregnancy is one of the most challenging situations for clinicians to prescribe medications. Fear of potential harm to the fetus is widespread among women as well as prescribers, leading to reluctance in both prescribing and compliance. It is therefore vital for the clinician to provide an informed estimate of the perceived teratogenic risks of medications and the risks of untreated medical condition endangering maternal and fetal health.

Approximately 2% of all pregnancies in the UK are associated with congenital anomalies. While the majority of these are attributed to unknown causes, it is estimated that nearly 1% of congenital anomalies are caused by prescribed drugs and other exogenous agents (Figure 17.1)[1].

The susceptibility of an embryo or fetus for a teratogenic response is related to various factors, including the stage of development at the time of exposure, the amount of drug exposure, the chemical composition of the drug, the genetic make-up of the mother and other concurrent exposures. Exposure to a toxin during the pre-embryonic phase (up to 17 days postconception) when the cells are rapidly multiplying, either results in a miscarriage owing to death of the embryo or survival of a fetus without any harmful consequences: the 'all or nothing' effect[2]. Exposure to a drug during the embryonic phase from 18 days to 8 weeks postconception can result in permanent organ damage (teratogenicity). Beyond 8 weeks, if the fetus is exposed to drugs, it is unlikely to result in significant organ damage, although certain subtle changes in the growing organs, such as the brain, kidneys or gut, may go undetected until late in life. As the gestational age of exposure to a drug is the single most important determinant of the teratogenic potential, it becomes crucial to determine the correct gestational age of the fetus to be able to counsel about the potential risks involved (Figure 17.2)[1].

Counseling and management in pregnancy

Good knowledge of basic embryology, as well as the physiologic changes encountered in pregnancy, is vital to aid appropriate counseling. As most women attend for an antenatal booking visit around 8–10 weeks of gestation, the majority of the vital organogenesis will have already occurred, and thus it is ideal for women to have preconception counseling about the potential benefits versus risks of medication. Clinical condition permitting, nonessential drugs should be discontinued and appropriate medication with the least teratogenic potential should be selected for treatment. Counseling for exposure to drugs or exogenous agents during pregnancy should be based on the principles discussed above, and patients should be made aware of the background risk of congenital anomalies to enable them to understand that even if a particular drug is considered to be safe based on animal or human studies, one can never guarantee that the fetus will not have any congenital abnormality. The flow diagram (Figure 17.3) below serves as a simplistic guide for counseling a drug-exposed pregnant woman[3].

In cases where drugs are thought to be linked with congenital anomalies, a detailed ultrasound scan should be offered to check normality of the fetus. The woman must be informed beforehand of the limitations of scanning and that functional abnormalities, such as mental restriction, are not detectable on ultrasound scan.

In the UK, a clinician is immune from civil liability for the adverse effects on the fetus of a drug appropriately

Fetal Medicine, ed. Bidyut Kumar and Zarko Alfirevic. Published by Cambridge University Press. © Cambridge University Press 2016.

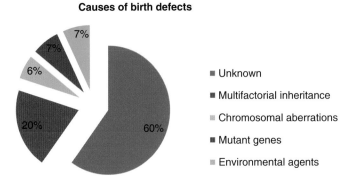

Causes of birth defects

- Unknown
- Multifactorial inheritance
- Chromosomal aberrations
- Mutant genes
- Environmental agents

Figure 17.1 Causes of congenital abnormalities, the majority being of unknown etiology.

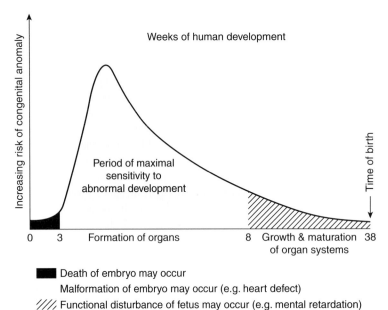

Weeks of human development

Increasing risk of congenital anomaly

Period of maximal sensitivity to abnormal development

Time of birth

0   3   Formation of organs   8   Growth & maturation   38
of organ systems

Death of embryo may occur
Malformation of embryo may occur (e.g. heart defect)
Functional disturbance of fetus may occur (e.g. mental retardation)

Figure 17.2 Schematic illustration showing the increasing risk of birth defects developed during organogenesis.
Adapted from Moore KL, Persaud TVN. *The Developing Human: Clinically Orientated Embryology*, 8th edn. Philadelphia: Elsevier 2008, with permission.

prescribed in pregnancy if it is in-line with established medical practice (Congenital Disabilities [Civil Liability] Act 1976). In situations where the clinician is confronted with having to offer advice to women who have inadvertently taken drugs for minor illnesses in pregnancy, it is best to base the advice on current information attained from the UK Teratology Information Service (UKTIS)[4].

Specific medications and pregnancy

Analgesics in pregnancy

Analgesics are one of the most commonly used class of medications in pregnancy, either prescribed or bought over the counter. Although there are no clinical trials to recommend its applicability and safety,

if used with caution, the World Health Organization analgesic ladder (Figure 17.4) may serve as a simplistic model for control of pain during first two trimesters of pregnancy[2].

In-utero exposure to paracetamol has not been known to be associated with an increased risk of congenital abnormalities. Paracetamol usage in therapeutic dosages or paracetamol poisoning in pregnancy per se is not an indication for termination of pregnancy or any additional fetal investigations[4].

Aspirin, a commonly used nonselective nonsteroidal anti-inflammatory drug (NSAID), has been shown to be teratogenic in animal studies when taken in high doses (>300 mg/day) and when consumed in analgesic doses, particularly in late gestation, may have adverse effects including increased risk of maternal and

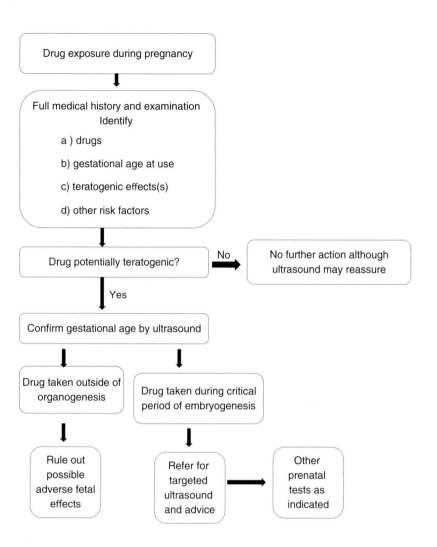

Figure 17.3 Flow diagram for counseling a drug-exposed pregnant woman.

Adapted from Little BB. Introduction to Drugs in Pregnancy. In: *Drugs and Pregnancy: A Handbook*. CRC Press 2006, with permission.

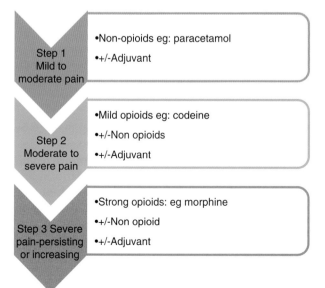

Figure 17.4 The World Health Organization analgesic pain relief ladder.

neonatal bleeding due to its antiplatelet effects, premature closure of ductus arteriosus (DA) in utero, and thus is best avoided, particularly in the third trimester. However, aspirin exposure at any stage of pregnancy is not in itself a ground for termination of pregnancy or for any further diagnostic tests. Low-dose aspirin, commonly used for its antiplatelet effect in pregnancy is not known to cause any adverse fetal or maternal effects.

NSAIDs should generally be avoided during the third trimester due to their association with an increased risk of premature closure of DA and oligohydramnios. It is advised that any NSAID exposure after 30 weeks of pregnancy should be monitored by fetal echocardiogram and serial scans for early detection of ologohydramnios. However, inadvertent exposure to NSAIDs at any stage in pregnancy is not an indication for termination of pregnancy in the absence of other indications. Ibuprofen is the preferred NSAID if clinically indicated in the first two trimesters of pregnancy[4].

Opioids are considered reasonably safe for use during pregnancy and are commonly prescribed for pain relief as second-line treatment. If used regularly in the third trimester close to delivery, one should ensure close monitoring of the newborn to detect opioid withdrawal symptoms.

Anticonvulsant drugs in pregnancy

Evidence suggests that congenital malformations linked with epilepsy are perhaps a combination of exposure of anticonvulsants in an individual who may be genetically susceptible. Polytherapy in contrast to monotherapy is known to increase the risk of anomalies. Kaneko et al. reported a 6.5% malformation rate with multiple drugs compared to 15.6% amongst women on a single drug[5]. The most common congenital malformations associated with the intake of antiepileptics, particularly first-generation drugs such as phenytoin and phenobarbitone, are neural tube defects (spina bifida and hydrocephalus), cardiac and skeletal malformations and cleft lip and palate. Fetal anticonvulsant syndrome, characterized by midfacial abnormalities such as wide-spaced eyes, depressed nasal bridge, low-set ears and hypoplasia of distal digits, has been associated with the use of these antiepileptic drugs. Second-generation drugs, such as sodium valproate and carbamazepine, have also been associated with neural tube defects, with a quoted risk of about 2% for spina bifida with valproate and 1% with carbamazepine[2]. A statistically significant association has been noted with cleft lip and/or palate and use of valproate and carbamazepine in pregnancy, the risk being more from valproate usage.

Lamotrigine, increasingly used for monotherapy, has been found to have a major malformation rate of 2.9% in the UK Registry, with a clear dose–response effect similar to valproate exposure[2]. The available published data on levetiracetam administration during pregnancy suggests an overall risk (2.2%) of major congenital malformations, which is well within the background risk (1–3%), the risk being lower (1.3%) with monotherapy compared to polytherapy (4%)[6]. There is no known effect on long-term developmental outcome, and further study results are awaited before labeling it as one of the safest antiepileptic in pregnancy.

Supplementation with high-dose folic acid (5 mg/day) is recommended for patients on anticonvulsants in the preconception period and throughout pregnancy.

Anticoagulants in pregnancy

Low molecular weight heparins (LMWH), such as enoxaparin, dalteparin and tinzaparin, are much more commonly used in pregnancy in UK and are overall known to be as efficacious and safe as unfractionated heparin. Danaparoid sodium is a LMWH with very little cross-reactivity with other heparins, and thus may be used as an alternative in pregnant women allergic to heparins or who develop heparin induced thrombocytopenia, an antibody-mediated reaction, which usually develops 5–10 days after initiation of heparin treatment. Any further treatment with heparin is contraindicated as there is a potential risk of life-threatening thrombus formation in this condition[7]. Heparins, however, do not cross the placenta due to their large molecular size, and thus there are no known risks to the fetus with their usage.

Warfarin is a coumarin anticoagulant that acts by blocking the activation of vitamin K-dependent clotting factors across the placenta and is a known teratogen. Studies looking at exposure to warfarin in first trimester of pregnancy have reported a risk as high as 30% of warfarin embryopathy or fetal warfarin syndrome (FWS), whilst more recent reports suggest a risk of 6–10%. FWS is characterized by nasal hypoplasia, stippled chondral calcification (chondrodysplasiapunctata) and scoliosis and fetal bleeding complications. This risk may be dose-dependent with doses higher than 5 mg/day carrying a higher risk. Exposure in later gestations may still be associated with central nervous system (CNS) and eye anomalies[4]. Warfarin exposure should be avoided in pregnancy and the anticoagulant should be changed to a LMWH prepregnancy or as soon as pregnancy is suspected.

The only exceptions are women with prosthetic heart valves in whom thromboembolic prophylaxis may need to be achieved with warfarin even in early pregnancy. Use of LMWH is not considered adequate in this situation[8]. While inadvertent warfarin exposure would not be regarded as medical grounds for termination of pregnancy, detailed ultrasound scans to screen the exposed fetus for any major structural malformations should be requested from the fetal medicine department[4].

Antiasthmatics in pregnancy

Treatment of asthma during pregnancy is no different from that in nonpregnant woman and the majority of the antiasthmatic drugs are considered safe during pregnancy. There is conflicting evidence about the safety of systemic steroids such as prednisolone in the first trimester as these may be associated with an increased risk of oral clefts[9]. Topical and inhaled or nebulized exposure is not known to carry any increased risks. It is, however, recommended that steroids in any form – inhaled, nebulized, oral or parenteral – should not be withheld in pregnancy as inadequate treatment is likely to lead to exacerbation of asthma, putting the mother and fetus both at increased risks. Maternal folate supplementation during early pregnancy may reduce the risk of oral clefts according to some studies[4].

Beta-agonists, such as salbutamol and terbutaline, are also considered safe in pregnancy and no adverse fetal or neonatal effects have been reported with their usage in pregnancy.

Antibiotics in pregnancy

It is advisable to treat pregnant women with the standard adult doses of antibiotics whenever clinically indicated as inadequate treatment is more likely to cause maternal and fetal harm by its inability to control infectious illness during pregnancy (Table 17.1). Penicillins or cephalosporins may be commenced when urgent treatment is indicated for maternal infections while awaiting results of culture and sensitivity. In cases of preterm premature rupture of membranes, the prophylactic antibiotic of choice is erythromycin,

while co-amoxiclav is best avoided due to increased risk of necrotizing enterocolitis[10]. A single dose of intravenous antibiotic in the form of cefuroxime with or without metronidazole is recommended as prophylaxis during cesarean sections and should be administered early enough for the antibiotic to be present in the blood circulation at the time of surgical incision[11]. This has not demonstrated any harmful effects on the baby.

Anti-HIV medications in pregnancy

Highly active antiretroviral therapy (HAART) usage in pregnancy has been reported to be associated with increased risk of gestational diabetes and preterm delivery. There are case reports of increased risk of congenital malformations following in-utero exposure to didanosine and efavirez. However, no other antiretrovirals have been known to be teratogenic[12].

Antiemetics in pregnancy

If nausea and vomiting in pregnancy are not controlled with conservative measures, drug treatment may be required. There is no evidence of teratogenesis with the use of commonly used antiemetics such as antihistamines, phenothiazines and pyridoxine[13,14] Dopamine antagonists like metoclopramide[15] and 5-hydroxytryptamine (5-HT3) antagonists such as ondansetron, although considered safe[16] and effective, are recommended as second-line therapy due to limited data.

Antihypertensive drugs during pregnancy

Labetolol, a combined alpha-beta adrenergic blocker, is offered as first-line treatment for hypertension in pregnancy[17]. Labetolol crosses the placenta and maternal serum and amniotic fluid levels are approximately similar nearly 1–3 h after a single intravenous dose[18]. Labetolol usage is not known to alter uteroplacental blood flow despite a reduction in maternal blood pressure, and although there are occasional observations of neonatal bradycardia and hypotension following treatment with labetolol of maternal hypertension near delivery, overall there is no evidence of clinically significant beta-blocker effect in mature infants. While there is limited evidence to prove its safety in the first trimester, there are no published reports of fetal malformations attributable to labetolol specifically in the available literature. Although fetal growth restriction

Table 17.1 An overview of safety data for antibiotics in pregnancy[4]

Antibiotic	Effects in pregnancy
Penicillins: amoxicillin, ampicillin, benzylpenicillin, co-amoxiclav, flucloxacillin	No evidence of any increase in risk of congenital anomalies with therapeutic doses.
Cephalosporins: cephalexin, cefaclor, cefadroxil, cefixime, cefuroxime, ceftriaxone	Majority of studies do not suggest increased risk of congenital malformations. Two small studies found an increases risk of cardiovascular defects and oral clefts but causal link with cephalosporins is unproven.
Tetracyclines: tetracycline, doxycycline, minocycline, oxytetracycline	Discoloration of teeth and bones as well as impaired bone growth is observed following second- or third-trimester exposure. Hence, should be generally avoided after the first trimester.
Aminoglycosides: gentamicin, neomycin	Based on limited data, there is no increased teratogenic risk, but theoretical concerns about fetal ototoxicity and nephrotoxicity exist.
Macrolides: erythromycin, clarithromycin, azithromycin	No established causal link with congenital anomalies.
Quinolones: ciprofloxacin, nalidixic acid, norfloxacin, ofloxacin	Based on limited data and theoretical risk of arthropathy, these are not generally recommended except for life-threatening conditions not responding to other antibiotics. If indicated, ciprofloxacin is the preferred agent.
Chloramphenicol	Based on limited data there is no increased risk. Near-term use may be associated with Grey baby syndrome, although supporting evidence for this is lacking.
Triemethoprim	Increased risk of neural tube defects, or-facial clefts and cardiac defects have been reported[4]. Theoretical concerns about folic acid deficiency also exist.
Nitrofurantoin	Not associated with increase in congenital malformations based on limited studies. Associated with hemolysis in patients with glucose-6-phosphate dehydrogenase deficiency.
Metronidazole	Available data do not show any increase in risk of congenital malformations.

is a potential side effect of all beta-blockers, benefits of controlling maternal hypertension with labetolol outweighs any potential small risks.

Methyldopa, a centrally acting antiadrenergic medication, has been the most frequently used medication for treatment of hypertension in pregnancy. Methyldopa crosses the placenta to achieve fetal concentrations similar to maternal serum levels, but there is no evidence of any risks to the fetus known with its usage in pregnancy.

Nifedipine, a calcium-channel blocker, is used for treatment of hypertension and increasingly for tocolysis in pregnancy. No increase in the risk of major congenital malformations is reported with its usage.

Exposure to angiotensin-converting enzyme inhibitors (ACE-I) and angiotensin–ll receptor blockers in the first trimester of pregnancy has been associated with an increased risk of congenital abnormalities, including cardiovascular, renal and CNS malformations, and therefore it is advisable to substitute these with an alternative antihypertensive treatment for managing hypertension prepregnancy[4]. ACE-I fetopathy, characterized by oligohydramnios, renal tubular dysgenesis, lung hypoplasia, persistent ductus arteriosus, mild-to-moderate growth restriction and fetal/neonatal death, has been observed following exposure to ACE-I in the second and third trimesters of pregnancy[4]. Exposure to ACE-I in pregnancy should be considered an indication for a detailed structural anomaly fetal scan, and careful monitoring of the pregnancy with advice from maternal and/or fetal medicine specialist, as well as UKTIS, is recommended[4].

There may be an increased risk of congenital abnormality and neonatal complications if thiazide diuretics are taken during pregnancy. Hence, alternative antihypertensive treatment should be considered for women in the reproductive age group on these medications if contemplating pregnancy.

Antineoplastic drugs during pregnancy

Methotrexate is a folic acid antagonist and its use during organogenesis is associated with a spectrum of congenital anomalies termed "methotrexate embryopathy" or the fetal aminopterin–methotrexate syndrome. The critical period of exposure is 6–8 weeks postconception and the critical dose is thought to be ≥10 mg/week[19]. The drug is known to cause fetal growth restriction, hypoplastic supraorbital ridges, low-set ears, micrognathia, limb anomalies and possibly mental retardation. Second- and third-trimester exposures may cause *fetal toxicity* and death. While it is advisable to avoid pregnancy for at least 12 weeks after medical treatment of ectopic pregnancy with methotrexate, there is not enough data related to any toxic after-effects, and thus there is no indication for recommending termination of pregnancy. Referral to a fetal medicine unit and a detailed fetal anomaly scan, as well as fetal echocardiography, should be considered[4]. In one study, pregnancies occurring even within the first 6 months of treatment with methotrexate – single or repeated injections for ectopic pregnancy – did not appear to cause any excessive risk when compared with unexposed pregnancies[20].

Anthracycline regimens are considered relatively safe for treatment of breast cancer in pregnancy, particularly during the second and third trimesters, while data on the use of taxanes is limited, thus reserving its use for high-risk node positive or metastatic disease. Tamoxifen and trastuzumab (Herceptin), a monoclonal antibody that blocks the epidermal growth factor receptor 2 protein, are contraindicated in pregnancy and should not be used due to reported adverse fetal outcomes, such as miscarriage and oligohydramnios[21]. However, inadvertent exposure is not an indication per se for termination of pregnancy or any further invasive testing.

Drugs used for treatment of diabetes in pregnancy

Use of metformin, a biguanide used in the treatment of type 2 diabetes, is not known to be associated with an increased risk of congenital abnormalities or any other adverse pregnancy outcomes. Women with pre-existing diabetes on metformin may be advised to continue use of metformin, either as an adjunct or alternative to insulin or both, prepregnancy and during pregnancy[22]. Glibenclamide, an oral suplhonylurea, although not generally recommended in pregnancy, is not known to have any teratogenic effects when used after the first trimester of pregnancy.

Insulin does not cross the placenta and there is no evidence from clinical trials to suggest any adverse fetal or neonatal effects with any type of insulin analogues during pregnancy.

Drugs used for thyroid disorders in pregnancy

Levothyroxine (T4) is considered effective and safe as replacement therapy during pregnancy and not known to have any teratogenic effects. Propylthiouracil (PTU), a thioamide, is considered the medication of choice for treatment of hyperthyroidism in pregnancy, and carbimazole is an acceptable alternative if PTU is not effective. PTU prevents synthesis of thyroid hormones as well as inhibiting peripheral deiodination of T4 to T3. PTU crosses the placenta but is not known to be associated with an increased risk of congenital anomalies. Long-term follow-up amongst children exposed to PTU in utero did not reveal any difference in their intellectual or physical development apart from a very small risk of fetal goiter formation (5% or less), particularly when administered close to term[23]. Exposure to carbimazole in pregnancy is known to be associated with a small risk of aplasia cutis (fetal scalp lesions) and esophageal or choanal atresia, particularly when used in the first trimester. The lowest possible dose of antithyroid medications for the shortest possible duration should be used when managing hyperthyroidism in pregnancy, and regular thyroid function tests are advisable as these drugs cross the placenta and can cause fetal hypothyroidism. It is advisable to maintain maternal thyroid-stimulating hormone towards the lower range of normal and T4 towards upper reference range.

Psychotropic medications during pregnancy

The absolute risk of fetal anomalies following use of psychotropic medication in pregnancy is very low and the clinician should always weigh up the benefits of treatment versus risks of relapse following discontinuation of these medications. Tricyclic antidepressants are not known to increase the risk of congenital malformations when used in pregnancy. Limited human studies have not indicated any relationship between fluoxetine exposure in utero and any teratogenic effects[24]. If used towards the end of pregnancy, newborns may show some neurologic signs, which are self-resolving.

Steroids in pregnancy

Although in animal studies corticosteroids have been shown to have some adverse effects on fetuses, such as cleft palate and sex organ defects, they are generally considered safe for use in pregnancy. Prednisolone is the oral steroid used for treatment of asthma in pregnancy and the benefits are known to outweigh the potential risks to mother and baby.

Topical corticosteroids are used commonly for treatment of autoimmune or inflammatory skin conditions, although little is known about the potential effects on the fetus. A Cochrane review concluded that, based on the limited data available, there is no linkage between use of topical steroids and birth defects, preterm delivery or stillbirth. However, use of very potent topical steroids has been related to low birthweight babies[25].

Substance misuse during pregnancy

Heroin usage in pregnancy is associated with fetal growth restriction, increased perinatal morbidity and mortality and sudden infant death syndrome. It is postulated that the adverse effects of heroin are as a result of repeated minor degrees of withdrawal related to its short half-life causing smooth muscle spasm, which results in premature uterine contractions leading to preterm delivery or spasm of fetal gut leading to antenatal passage of meconium. There is no good evidence to link usage of illicit drugs in pregnancy to teratogenicity apart from some inconsistent case reports of increased risk of congenital abnormalities such as cleft palate with benzodiazepine consumption in early pregnancy[2].

Isotretinoin (Accutane), a vitamin A analogue used for treatment of severe acne, is a known potent human teratogen. It is associated with increased rate of spontaneous miscarriage and fetal malformations if taken during pregnancy. There are strict guidelines for prescription of isotretinoin to help avoid the embryopathy. Common anomalies include craniofacial conditions, such as microtic ears, stenosis or agenesis of external ear canal, micrognathia, flattened nose bridge and hyperteorism, and cardiac conditions such as transposition of the great arteries, Fallot's tetralogy and ventricular septal defects. Concerns have also been raised about significant functional impairment in exposed infants who seemingly have no visible abnormalities on imaging studies and appear normal at birth. However, there appears to be no increased risk if the drug is discontinued prior to conception.

Miscellaneous drugs and pregnancy

Oral contraceptives If taken inadvertently in pregnancy, these do not per se constitute an indication for termination of pregnancy but additional fetal monitoring for fetal growth may be warranted[4].

Ergotamine An ergot alkaloid – usage should be avoided during pregnancy. Genitourinary abnormalities, such as unilateral renal agenesis, urethral atresia and pulmonary hypoplasia, have been reported with its usage for treatment of migraine during early pregnancy[26].

Misoprostol A synthetic prostaglandin E1 analogue – used increasingly for inducing medical termination of pregnancy as well as in treatment of gastric and duodenal ulcers. While the majority of animal studies do not report any teratogenicity, fetal malformations, including cranial nerve defects (Mobius syndrome affecting cranial nerves 6 and 7) and limb abnormalities as a result of possible vascular disruption, have been reported in literature with misoprostol usage. If a woman wishes to continue her pregnancy after a failed attempt at misoprostol-induced termination, she should be counseled appropriately about the potential marginally increased risk to the fetus and one needs to be aware of the fact that cranial nerve damage, if any, is rarely detectable using ultrasound[27].

Statins These are generally contraindicated in pregnancy and close monitoring of pregnancy is advisable following inadvertent exposure during pregnancy. Although rare, there are reports of CNS and limb defects in newborns exposed to statins in utero. Hence, until availability of additional data, it is advisable to discontinue statins before pregnancy or as soon as pregnancy is confirmed.

Drugs used in inflammatory bowel disease during pregnancy Aminosalicylates and thiopurines are considered relatively safe for use in pregnancy when indicated. Infliximab and adalimumab are relatively safe during the first and second trimesters of pregnancy and should be used with caution in the third trimester as they cross the placenta. Methotrexate is contraindicated as stated earlier.

Deferoxamine An iron chelator – used for treating iron overload in women with thalassemia and can be considered if required for pregnant women as there is no definitive evidence to prove its teratogenicity.

Table 17.2 Estimated fetal absorbed dose range from common diagnostic radiation procedures[28]

Maternal imaging procedure	Estimated fetal absorbed dose range (mGy)
Dental, skull, chest, thoracic spine and breast X-ray Head and/or neck X-ray CT	0.001–0.01
Pulmonary angiogram X-ray CT 99mTc lung ventilation scan	0.01–0.1
Abdomen, barium meal, pelvis and hip X-ray Pelvimetry and chest and liver X-ray CT 99mTc lung perfusions, thyroid, lung ventilation (DTPA), renal (MAG3 and DMSA) and white cell scans	0.1–1.0
Barium enema, IV urography and lumbar spine X-ray Lumbar spine and abdomen X-ray CT 18F PET tumor scan	1.0–10
Pelvis, pelvis abdomen and chest X-ray CT 18F PET/CT whole body scan	10–50

CT, computed tomography; DMSA, dimercaptosuccinic acid; DTPA, diethylenetriamine pentaacetate; IV, intravenous; MAG3, mercaptoacetyltriglycine; PET, positron emission tomography.

Herbal products usage in pregnancy

There is limited good quality evidence to prove safety of herbal products in pregnancy. In one prospective controlled study looking at safety of the herb echinacea (used for upper respiratory tract conditions) during pregnancy, no statistically significant difference in the rate of major malformations between the study group and disease-matched control group was observed[28]. However, women must be informed that the evidence is very limited, if any, on the safety of these medications during pregnancy.

Ionizing radiation and pregnancy

Exposure to ionizing radiation in pregnancy can be a cause for extreme concern about the potential risks to the fetus. Ionizing radiation can cause damage directly or by secondary reaction, and this includes physical, physiochemical, chemical, biologic damage to DNA and RNA structures. The effects depend upon the total dose of radiation, amount of body area exposed, dose distribution within the body, patient's size, source-to-skin and patient-to-image intensifier distances.

Overall, the risks following ionizing radiation exposure during pregnancy are limited but adverse "deterministic effects" include miscarriage, congenital anomalies such as microcephaly, microphthalmia and cataracts, fetal growth restriction, neurobehavioral abnormalities and stillbirth, which are increased above a threshold dose, and "stochastic effects" such as childhood cancers or germ cell mutations, which are

not associated with a threshold dose[4]. An exposure of more than 100 mGy equivalent to 10 rad (>1,000 chest X-rays) is considered a threshold dose above which the adverse deterministic outcomes listed above is increased. Hence, applying a safety margin, pregnant women are advised to avoid exposed to radiation doses in excess of 50 mGy[4]. Estimated average fetal absorbed dose for different maternal imaging procedures listed in Table 17.2 provides a guideline, and actual fetal dose may vary depending on, e.g., maternal body mass index and the type of imaging equipment used. National guidance on the use of diagnostic radiology and nuclear medicine should be consulted if in doubt[29].

Radiation dose to the fetus from any diagnostic procedure in current use in the UK should not present any risk of adverse fetal outcomes. Hence, all the diagnostic procedures can be carried out when clinically indicated, and radiation dose is kept to a minimum required. Exposure to total absorbed dose of radiation <50 mGy at any stage of pregnancy would not be regarded as medical grounds for offering additional fetal monitoring or termination of pregnancy in the absence of other additional risk factors[30]. Magnetic resonance imaging does not use ionizing radiation and is considered ideal for fetal imaging.

Vaccinations in pregnancy

Immunization is only advisable in pregnancy in the presence of a clear indication and where the benefits of immunization clearly outweigh the potential risks (Table 17.3). None of the vaccines or immunoglobulins

Table 17.3 Vaccines and recommendations in pregnant women

Disease	Type of vaccine	Recommendation in pregnancy
Polio (oral) Polio (injection)	Live attenuated virus Killed virus	Generally contraindicated in pregnancy as fetal/neonatal risks are largely unknown. Recommended only to unimmunized women travelling to endemic areas. Injectable vaccine is considered safer in pregnancy when indicated
Yellow fever	Live attenuated virus	Generally contraindicated in pregnancy as fetal/neonatal risks are largely unknown. However important to weigh the risk of maternal infection against the potential risks following immunization
Measles	Live attenuated virus	Contraindicated
Mumps	Live attenuated virus	Contraindicated
Rubella	Live attenuated virus	Contraindicated. Inadvertent exposure to MMR does not constitute an indication for termination of pregnancy
BCG	Live bacteria	Not recommended in pregnancy although no harmful effects have been observed
Hepatitis B	Killed virus	For high-risk individuals, pre- and post-exposure prophylaxis advisable. Considered safe
Influenza	Killed virus	Follow seasonal guidance from Department of Health/RCOG
Rabies	Killed virus	Consider if benefits outweigh risks in individual cases. No evidence of harm
Cholera	Killed bacteria	Recommended for pregnant woman only if it is unavoidable. Risks not known
Meningococcus	Killed bacteria	Consider if benefits outweigh risks
Typhoid	Killed bacteria	Consider only where benefits clearly outweigh the potential risks. Avoid unless high risk of exposure
Diphtheria	Toxoid: modified or inactivated bacterial toxin	Recommended prior to travel to high-risk areas or in case of close contact with a suspected case if the woman has not had diphtheria immunization or booster toxoid within last ten years. Considered safe
Tetanus	Killed bacteria	No reported adverse outcomes following post-exposure prophylaxis to tetanus toxoid administration in pregnancy
Hepatitis A	Immunoglobulin	Offers protection for up to four months and not known to have any adverse risks in pregnancy. It is advisable for prophylaxis to those travelling to high risk regions. HAV is, however, only recommended for frequent travellers and HNIG is generally preferred to HAV during pregnancy
Varicella-zoster	Immunoglobulin	Post-exposure prophylaxis recommended
Hepatitis B	Killed virus	Active immunization with HBsAg offers up to five years of protection and immunization of pregnant women at high risk of contracting this infection should be considered. Babies born to mothers who suffer from hepatitis B or carriers of this condition should be offered a full course of immunization in addition to hepatitis B immunoglobulin administration
Human papilloma virus	Virus-like particles	Not recommended for use in pregnancy. If pregnancy detected after initiating the vaccination course, the remainder of the doses should be delayed until completion of pregnancy and no further intervention is advised

BCG, Bacillus Calmette–Guérin; HAV, hepatitis A vaccine; HBsAg, hepatitis B surface antigen; HNIG, human normal immunoglobulin; MMR, measles, mumps and rubella; RCOG, Royal College of Obstetricians and Gynaecologists.

are categorized as completely safe in pregnancy and the risk of contracting the disease and its harmful effects on the mother and fetus have to be balanced against the beneficial effects of the vaccine. There can be situations where travel to endemic areas is unavoidable or an epidemic sets in. Some women may have vaccination inadvertently in the early pregnancy before a pregnancy is recognized. It is advisable to undertake an individualized risk assessment before recommending any vaccination during pregnancy. Potential risks of

vaccination include preterm labor and risk of in-utero infection. As a rule of thumb, live vaccines like Bacillus Calmette–Guérin (BCG), measles, mumps and rubella (MMR), yellow fever and oral polio preparations should be avoided in pregnancy.

The UK Teratology Information Centre provides up-to-date information on drugs and chemicals in pregnancy via telephone information service and online through Toxbase. The types of enquiries answered include:

Table 17.4 Sources of drug and toxicology information

Information source	Contact details
British National Formulary	www.bnf.org BNF app
Toxbase	www.toxbase.org
UK Teratology Information Centre (UKTIS)	www.uktis.org
Manufacturer's information	Summary of product characteristics
Cochrane Database of Systematic Reviews	www.cochrane.org
Medicines information pharmacists	
Textbooks	
Electronic medicines compendium	www.medicines.org.uk/emc
Prescribing support	Email: rdtc.rxsupp@nuth.nhs.uk
Medicines information service	Email: rdtc.mi@nuth.nhs.uk

- the effect of inadvertent early exposure to a drug, in advance of knowledge of the pregnancy
- the therapeutic options available to a patient who needs to continue treatment for a particular indication, such as epilepsy
- the therapeutic options available to treat an acute condition that occurs during pregnancy, such as threadworm
- the effect of an acute or chronic exposure to a particular drug during pregnancy, such as an antibiotic
- advice to support prepregnancy counseling.

Key learning points

- Pregnancy status must be checked in all women of childbearing age before prescribing any medication/exogenous agent.
- Drugs should be prescribed only when necessary. Where applicable, nondrug measures should be tried first, e.g., changes in diet for constipation.
- Appropriate counseling should be undertaken wherever feasible before conception.
- Majority of congenital abnormalities are unrelated to drug use in pregnancy.
- Women may refrain from using medications during pregnancy and it is vital for them to be informed about the risks of not taking the drug

on both maternal and fetal wellbeing against the potential risks of the medication, if any.
- The lowest effective dose of the most suitable drug for the shortest possible duration must be recommended.
- Wherever possible, a drug with the best safety record should be chosen.
- Appropriate sources must be referred to for additional information.

References

1. Moore KL, Persaud TVN. *The Developing Human: Clinically Orientated Embryology*, 8th edn. Elsevier, 2008.

2. Rubin P, Ramsay M. *Prescribing in Pregnancy*, 4th ed. Oxford: Blackwell Publishing, 2008.

3. Little BB. Introduction to drugs in pregnancy. Chapter 1: *Drugs and Pregnancy: A Handbook*. CRC Press, 2006.

4. UK National Teratology Information Service (UKTIS). www.toxbase.org

5. Kaneko S, Otani k, Fukushima Y, et al. Teratogenicity of antiepileptic drugs: Analysis of possible risk factors. *Epilepsia* 1988; 29: 459–67.

6. Safety of levatiracetam in pregnancy. *Birth Defects Res A Clin Mol Teratol 2012*; 94(5): 407.

7. Myers B, Westby J, Strong J. Prophylactic use of danaparoid in high-risk pregnancy with heparin-induced thrombocytopenia positive skin reaction. *Blood Coagul Fibrinolysis* 2003; 14; 485–7.

8. Chan WS, Anand S, Ginsberg JS. Anticoagulation of pregnant women with mechanical heart valves. *Arch Intern Med* 2000; 160: 191–6.

9. Park-Wyllie L, Mazzotta P, Pastuszak A, et al. Birth defects after maternal exposure to corticosteroids: prospective cohort study and meta-analysis of epidemiological studies. *Teratology* 2000; 62: 385–92.

10. Royal College of Obstetricians and Gynaecologists (RCOG). Preterm prelabor rupture of membranes. RCOG Green Top Guideline No, 44. London: ROCG, 2010.

11. National Institute for Health and Care Excellence (NICE). Caesarean section. NICE Clinical Guideline CG132, November 2011 (last modified August 2012).

12. Royal College of Obstetricians and Gynaecologists (RCOG). Management of HIV in pregnancy. RCOG Green top Guideline No. 39. London: ROCG, 2010.

13. Jewell D, Young G. Interventions for nausea and vomiting in early pregnancy. *Cochrane Database Syst Rev* 2010; (9): CD000145.

14. Magee LA, Mazzotta P, Koren G. Evidence-based view of safety and effectiveness of pharmacologic therapy for nausea and vomiting of pregnancy (NVP). *Am J Obstet Gynecol* 2002: 186 (5 Suppl. Understanding); S256–61.

15. Tan PC. Metoclopramide during pregnancy did not increase risk for major congenital malformations or fetal death. *Ann Intern Med* 2014; 160(94): JC 13.

16. Pasternak B, Svanstrom H, Hviid A. Ondansetron in pregnancy and risk of adverse fetal outcomes. *N Engl J Med* 2013; 368(9): 814–23.

17. National Institute for Health and Care Excellence (NICE). Hypertension in pregnancy. NICE Clinical Guideline CG107, August 2010 (last modified January 2011).

18. Lunell NO, Hjemdahl P, Fredholm BB, et al. Acute effects of labetolol on maternal metabolism and uteroplacental circulation in hypertension of pregnancy. In: Riley A, Symonds EM (eds). *The Investigation of Labetolol in the Management of Hypertension in Pregnancy*. Amsterdam, Netherlands: Excerpta Medica, 1982; 34–45.

19. Briggs GG, freeman RK, Yaffe SJ. *A Reference Guide to Fetal and Neonatal Risk: Drugs in pregnancy and lactation*, 9th edn. Lippincot Williams and Wilkins; 2011: 928.

20. Svirsky R, et al. The safety of conception occurring shortly after methotrexate treatment of an ectopic pregnancy. *Reprod Toxicol* 2009; 27(91): 85–7.

21. Royal College of Obstetricians and Gynaecologists (RCOG). Pregnancy and breast cancer. RCOG Green Top Guideline No. 12. London: ROCG, 2011.

22. National Institute for Health and Care Excellence (NICE). Diabetes in pregnancy. NICE Clinical Guideline CG63, March 2008.

23. Burrow GN, Bartsocas C, Klatskin EH, et al. Children exposed in utero to propylthiouracil. *Am J Dis Child* 1968; 116: 161–5.

24. Baum AL, Misri S. Selective serotonin-reuptake inhibitors in pregnancy and lactation. *Harv Rev Psychiatry* 1996; 4(3): 117–25.

25. Chi CC, Lee CW, Wojnarowska F, et al. Safety of topical corticosteroids in pregnancy. *Cochrane Database Syst Rev* 2009; (3): CD007346.

26. Demirel G, et al. Unilateral renal agenesis and urethral atresia associated with ergotamine intake during pregnancy. *Renal fail* 2012; 34(5): 643–4.

27. Anonymous. Misoprostol and pregnancy: risk of malformations. *Prescrire Int* 2008; 17(94): 64–6.

28. Gallo M, Sarkar M, Au W, et al. Pregnancy outcome following gestational exposure to echinacea: a prospective controlled study. *Arch Intern Med* 2000; 160(20): 3141–3.

29. Public Health England. Protection of Pregnant Patients during Diagnostic Medical Exposures to Ionising Radiation (RCE-9). Radiation: HPA-RCE report series, March 2009.

30. Koch D, Drugan A. Exposure to ionizing radiation during pregnancy. In: Evans MI, et al. (eds) *Prenatal Diagnosis*. McGraw Hill, 2006.

Chapter 18

The law and epidemiology of induced abortion

Kristina Naidoo

Abortion and the law in the UK

The Abortion Act 1967[1] and Human Fertilisation and Embryology Act 1990[2] govern induced abortion in England, Scotland and Wales (UK). Compliance with the provisions of the Abortion Act 1967 creates a series of defences to the Offences against the Person Act 1861, Section 58, which prohibited the unlawful induction of a miscarriage and the Infant Life (Preservation Act) 1929, which prohibited abortion except where it was done in good faith for the purpose only of preserving the life of the woman.

The Human Fertilisation and Embryology Act 1990 introduced a time limit on most abortions of 24 weeks of gestation, but permitted termination at any gestation on the grounds of serious fetal abnormality, Ground E (Section 1(1)(d) of the Abortion Act.

Statutory grounds for induced abortion

The grounds for abortion (A–G) are set out in Sections 1(1)(a)–(d) of the Abortion Act.

(A) The continuance of the pregnancy would involve risk to the life of the pregnant woman greater than if the pregnancy were terminated: Abortion Act 1967 as amended, Section 1(1)(c).

(B) The termination is necessary to prevent grave permanent injury to the physical or mental health of the pregnant woman: Section 1(1)(b).

(C) The pregnancy has not exceeded its 24th week and the continuance of the pregnancy would involve risk, greater than if the pregnancy were terminated, of injury to the physical or mental health of the pregnant woman: Section 1(1)(a).

(D) The pregnancy has not exceeded its 24th week and the continuance of the pregnancy would involve risk, greater than if the pregnancy were terminated, of injury to the physical or mental health of any existing child(ren) of the family of the pregnant woman: Section 1(1)(a).

(E) There is a substantial risk that if the child were born it would suffer from such physical or mental abnormalities as to be seriously handicapped: Section 1(1)(d).

Abortion is legal in the UK if two registered doctors are of the opinion, formed in good faith (except in an emergency), that one of the stipulated grounds are met.

The Act also permits abortion to be performed in an emergency if one doctor is of the opinion, formed in good faith, that termination is immediately necessary:

(F) to save the life of the pregnant woman: Section 1(4)

(G) to prevent grave permanent injury to the physical or mental health of the pregnant woman: Section 1(4).

In pregnancies under 24 weeks where there is a fetal abnormality and which the woman wishes to terminate, doctors who believe in good faith that the continuation of the pregnancy involves a greater risk to her physical and mental health than its termination have the option of choosing either Ground C or Ground E.

What constitutes substantial risk and serious handicap becomes a particular issue for doctors when abortion is likely to take place after 24 weeks of gestation, when abortion is no longer lawful under Ground C of the Abortion Act. There is no legal definition of substantial risk or severe handicap.

Fetal Medicine, ed. Bidyut Kumar and Zarko Alfirevic. Published by Cambridge University Press. © Cambridge University Press 2016.

As the law is not specific, practice regarding which fetal abnormalities meet the legal criteria for the offer of termination after 24 weeks appears to be governed largely by consensus between colleagues within a fetal medicine unit or with other units, and in discussion with other specialists, particularly pediatricians and neonatologists[3].

Abortion forms

Doctors are under a legal obligation to complete the following forms:

HSA1 (Certificate A in Scotland) Two doctors are required to sign the HSA1 form, which is the certificate of opinion before an abortion is performed under Section 1(1) of the Abortion Act[4]. The HSA1 form must be kept for 3 years.

HSA2 (Certificate B in Scotland) To be completed by the doctor within 24 h of an emergency abortion and kept for 3 years. In cases such as these, the requirement for the opinion of two doctors does not apply.

HSA4 Must be completed by the doctor taking responsibility for the abortion and sent to the Chief Medical Officer (CMO), either manually or electronically, within 14 days of the abortion taking place. As is the case with the manual form, only doctors terminating the pregnancy are able to authorize the electronic form. In Scotland, the equivalent Notification Form must be sent to the CMO in Scotland within 7 days of the abortion taking place. There are as yet no electronic means of notification.

Doctors are legally required under the Abortion Act 1967 (as amended) (1) to complete abortion forms for every abortion performed, whether carried out in the National Health Service (NHS) or an approved independent sector place, and whether or not the woman is a UK resident[5].

The EPICure2 study collected data for all deliveries between 22+0 and 26+6 from all maternity units in England in 2006 using methods ensuring comprehensive data collection[6]. It found that there was a substantial under-reporting of abortions over 22 weeks to the Department of Health. Misclassification of late abortion as a miscarriage or stillbirth and inconsistencies between hospitals as to whether induction of labor for a fetus judged to be nonviable is classified correctly as an induced abortion were found. Education of staff regarding documentation and notification of abortion was recommended with internal audit to ensure continued compliance.

Two doctors in good faith

The Abortion Act 1967 requires that for an abortion to take place it has to be agreed by two doctors in good faith, and if challenged they could persuade a court that their belief is honestly held. There has been only one successful prosecution, R v Smith [1974][7]] "for unlawful procurement of miscarriage," where a doctor had neither examined internally nor enquired about the medical history of the woman, before agreeing to perform the operation. It was held that the doctor had no defence under the Act as he had allowed himself no opportunity to form a bona fide opinion regarding the balance of risks between termination and continuation of the pregnancy.

To quote Lord Scarman:

> "The question of good faith is essentially one for the jury to determine on the totality of the evidence. A medical view put forward in evidence by one or more doctors is no substitute for the verdict of the jury. An opinion may be absurd professionally and yet formed in good faith; conversely, an opinion may be one which a doctor could have entertained and yet in the particular circumstances of the case may be found either to have been formed in bad faith or not to have been formed at all."

In 2012, the Care Quality Commission (CQC) found evidence during an inspection of a private clinic that HSA1 forms were being pre-signed by one doctor. This is in breach of the Abortion Act and allows the second doctor to take a solo decision to allow an abortion. The Secretary of State for Health then asked the CQC to undertake an unannounced inspection of all providers of abortion services, which looked specifically for evidence of pre-signed HSA1 forms. CQC identified clear evidence of pre-signing at 14 locations, all of which were NHS Trusts. They were asked to stop this practice in order to comply with the Abortion Act, and to take steps including internal audits and staff training to ensure continued compliance[8]. No prosecutions have been brought in relation to this matter.

Although there is no legal requirement for at least one of the certifying doctors to have seen the pregnant woman before reaching a decision about an abortion, the UK Department of Health's view is that it is good practice for this to be the case. This does not necessarily mean a doctor has to physically meet the woman and may include discussion over the phone or by webcam. In order to form an opinion in good faith, doctors signing the HSA1 form must be aware of the woman's history through standard record keeping. They can rely on advice given by other members of the multidisciplinary team involved in her care but must personally review such information before forming an opinion[9].

Professionals' rights: conscientious objection to abortion

The Abortion Act 1967 contains a conscientious objection, clause s4, which states that "no person shall be under any duty, whether by contract or by any statutory or other legal requirement, to participate in any treatment authorised by this Act to which he has a conscientious objection." This clause applies equally to both signatories of the HSA1 form. It does not apply where an abortion is immediately necessary to save the life of or prevent grave permanent injury to the woman's physical or mental health, which is certified by one practitioner.

The leading case concerning the conscientious objection clause is Janaway v Salford HA 1988[10], where a doctor's secretary refused to type a referral letter for a woman to have an abortion and was unsuccessful when she claimed that she was protected by the clause. The House of Lords, in interpreting the word "participate" decided to give the word its *ordinary and natural meaning,* which meant that the clause only applied to those who were being required to take part in the treatment, that is to say, the doctors, nurses or midwives. Administration or routine care not directly connected with the abortion procedures lies outside the terms of the conscientious objection clause.

Since then there have been three important legal developments affecting the religious freedom of doctors, nurses and midwives, namely the Human Rights Act 1998, the Employment Equality (Religion or Belief) Regulations 2003 and Part 2 of the Equality Act 2006 (Discrimination on Grounds of Religion or Belief). In 2013, a case involving two midwives, the judgement gave a wider meaning to "participate in terminations of pregnancy" than the determination in the Janaway case in 1989. The appeal judges ruled the midwives' right to conscientious objection as meaning they can refuse to delegate, supervize or support staff involved in abortions[11].

The General Medical Council's guidance covering personal beliefs and medical practice (2013) states that "patients have a right to information about their condition and the options open to them. If you have a conscientious objection to a treatment or procedure that may be clinically appropriate for the patient, you must do the following. Tell the patient that you do not provide the particular treatment or procedure, being careful not to cause distress. You may wish to mention the reason for your objection, but you must be careful not to imply any judgment of the patient. Tell the patient that they have a right to discuss their condition and the options for treatment (including the option that you object to) with another practitioner who does not hold the same objection as you and can advise them about the treatment or procedure you object to. If it's not practical for a patient to arrange to see another doctor, you must make sure that arrangements are made – without delay – for another suitably qualified colleague to advise, treat or refer the patient. You must bear in mind the patient's vulnerability and act promptly to make sure they are not denied appropriate treatment or services"[12].

In the UK, the Royal College of Nursing has produced guidance on the rights of nurses and midwives to refuse to take part in abortion care[13].

Rights of the spouse or partner

The decision to have an abortion lies with the woman and her doctors. The woman's spouse and/or the putative father of the child has no right to demand or refuse an abortion in law. In individual cases, men have brought unsuccessful legal actions in an attempt to prevent their female partner obtaining an abortion (Kelly 1997[14]; Hansell 2001[15]). In Paton vs BPAS[16], a husband applied unsuccessfully for an injunction to prevent a clinic from carrying out an abortion of his wife's pregnancy. The request for a hearing before the European Commission of Human Rights was also denied[17].

Application of the Abortion Act in Northern Ireland and Crown dependencies

The Abortion Act 1967 does not apply in Northern Ireland. The relevant legislation in Northern Ireland is the Offences Against the Person Act 1861 and the Criminal Justice Act (Northern Ireland) 1945. It is lawful to perform an abortion in Northern Ireland only where it is necessary to preserve the life of the woman or there is a risk of real and serious adverse effect on the woman's physical or mental health, which is either long term or permanent. There is no limit set on the gestational age at which the abortion may be carried out. In any other circumstance it would be unlawful to perform such a procedure[18]. Fetal abnormality is not recognized as a ground in itself for abortion. There have been 35–57 terminations of pregnancy carried out in Northern Ireland between 2006 and 2012[19]. The background birth rate during this time was between 23,300–25,269 per year[20].

Whilst all maternity units in Northern Ireland offer anomaly scanning in the second trimester, the provision of screening tests for Down's syndrome is inconsistent. Between 2002 and 2005, there was a fall in the number of units offering serum screening for Down's syndrome, and in 2005 none of the units provided nuchal translucency scanning. As abortion for fetal abnormality cannot be offered in Northern Ireland, this may create a conflict for health professionals when offering screening and may have led to maternity units not having developed screening programmes in line with UK guidance[21].

The Abortion Act does not apply in the Crown dependencies Isle of Man, Jersey or Guernsey, and women from these countries are not considered to be residents of the UK.

Feticide

The Royal College of Obstetricians and Gynaecologists (RCOG) in the UK recommends that feticide for abortions over 21+6 weeks is routinely offered to ensure that the fetus is not born alive[22]. In 2012, of the 1312 abortions performed at 22 weeks of gestation and over, 71% were reported as preceded by feticide and a further 26% were performed by a method whereby fetal demise occurs as part of the procedure. Of the remaining 3%, all but eight cases were confirmed as having no feticide.

The EPICure2 study found evidence of under-reporting of feticide prior to abortion, with only 65% of cases it recorded in 2006 in England notified to the Department of Health. In some cases this may have arisen where feticide was performed at a specialist unit and the woman then returned to her local hospital to undergo the abortion procedure[6].

Selective feticide

The Human Fertilisation and Embryology Act 1990 also clarifies that selective reduction of a multiple pregnancy is covered by abortion legislation. Most specialists in this area believe that the continuation of multiple pregnancies could involve a greater risk to the woman than the termination of one of the fetuses, and Ground C is usually relied upon in pregnancies of under 24 weeks of gestation.

There were 82 abortions in 2012 in England and Wales that involved selective feticide. In 38 cases, a twin pregnancy was reduced to a singleton. In 28 cases, triplets were reduced to twins and in 11 cases triplets were reduced to one fetus. Over three-quarters (76%) of these selective abortions were performed under Ground E[23].

A fetus born alive after induced abortion

Feticide after 21+6 weeks is not a legal or statutory requirement but 'strongly recommended practice' as per RCOG guidance. Legal issues would arise if the fetus is born with signs of life when s/he must be managed (and registered) as a live birth, and if not given appropriate care, doctors could be accused of manslaughter or even murder.

The possible outcomes if feticide is not performed after 21+6 weeks should be fully explained to the woman. If the fetal abnormality is certain to be incompatible with survival, insisting on feticide may not be in her best interest and induced abortion followed by terminal care of the child may be the most favorable outcome for a woman and her partner. Care should be individualized and compassionate. It is for the woman to decide how to proceed based on the information she is given.

If feticide is not to be performed, then a care plan must be drawn up and agreed before the abortion takes place following discussion with the woman and her partner, with input from the obstetric, midwifery and neonatal staff. If the fetus is born alive, it becomes entitled to legal protection as would any other child, although the decisions concerning the type of care that is offered should be made on the basis of what the best interests of the fetus/child and the family would be[24]. If the prognosis based on the gestational age is considered to be very poor, active support would be inappropriate and palliative care should be given until the child dies. If the fetus is born alive and has a condition that is known to be incompatible with life, there is no requirement for neonatal staff to initiate resuscitation and intensive care[25]. In a situation where a child is born alive as a result of an induced abortion for a condition that is not immediately life-threatening at a gestational

Table 18.1 Legal abortions: grounds by gestation weeks, residents of England and Wales in 2012[23]

England and Wales, residents	Number of cases				
		Gestation weeks			
Ground	Total	3–9	10–12	13–19	20 and over
A (alone, or with B, C, D) or F or G	61	14	9	21	17
B (alone, or with C or D)	130	81	21	18	10
C (alone)	180,117	141,644	24,257	12,259	1,957
D (alone, or with C)	2,122	1,605	431	85	1
E (alone, or with A, B, C or D)	2,692	20	366	1,431	875
Total	185,122	143,364	25,084	13,814	2,860

age when such care would normally be given, then resuscitation and intensive care must be initiated. Once established in neonatal care, a decision regarding palliative care can be made depending on the situation of the child[26]. Failure to follow this guidance could result in a prosecution for murder or manslaughter.

Where feticide could not be performed for whatever reason, the patient should be counseled about the possibility of a live birth, and sympathetic explanation given that no attempts at resuscitation would be undertaken but that the fetus would be dealt with respectfully and sensitively.

Live birth before 22 weeks is uncommon. However, women should be counseled about this possibility and delivery unit staff trained to deal appropriately with this eventuality. After an induced abortion under 22 weeks of gestation, resuscitation should not be attempted even if a fetus is delivered showing signs of life as it would be considered as below the limit of viability. The child should receive comfort and be treated with dignity until its demise.

To certify a live birth below 22 weeks of gestation, the attending delivery unit staff must be certain that signs of life are present. Regular respiratory effort and a regular heartbeat or pulsation of the cord should be observed. Sporadic gasps, transient heart beats or reflex movements should not be considered as signs of life[27].

If an induced abortion results in a live birth and subsequent neonatal death, there are consequences for the mother and her partner and the doctors involved in her care. The parents are responsible for registering the birth and death, although they can delegate this to a health professional. Unless the fetus has a lethal abnormality, the cause of the neonatal death would be primarily extreme prematurity as a result of induced abortion. This would be required to be stated on the death certificate and it

may be considered necessary to inform the coroner. In the UK, no doctor has faced legal proceedings in these circumstances and it would be very unlikely if the abortion has been carried out lawfully; that is to say, two registered practitioners are of the opinion, formed in good faith, that the grounds for the abortion are met.

Epidemiology

The Abortion Notification forms (HSA4) sent to the Department of Health are used to collate statistics on legal abortions performed in England and Wales and are published annually[22]. The most recent report refers to abortions performed in 2012 when there were 195,296 abortions to residents in England and Wales.

In Scotland, the equivalent notification forms sent to the CMO are used to collate statistics. In 2012, 12,447 abortions were carried out in Scotland representing 8% of the total carried out in the UK[28]. This is a rate of 12/1,000 women aged 15–44 years compared with 16.5/1,000 in England and Wales[23].

The overall proportion of abortions of pregnancies with a fetal abnormality is unknown since, before 24 weeks, this might not be the prime indication for the abortion. Of the total number of abortions, 1.4% (2,692) were performed under Ground E of the Abortion Act, namely that there was a substantial risk that, if the child were born, it would suffer physical or mental abnormalities that would result in serious handicap (Table 18.1).

The HSA4 form allows the recording of all medical conditions and other details associated with the ground, such as the method used to make the diagnosis. In previous years, only the principal medical condition was published. Table 18.2 shows totals for the number of mentions of a medical condition in 2012. For example,

Table 18.2 Legal abortions: principal medical condition and total mentions of medical conditions for abortions performed under Ground E, residents of England and Wales in 2012[23]

England and Wales, residents		Numbers and percentages[b]					
ICD-10 code	Condition[a]	Number of abortions by principal medical condition		Number of mentions by principal medical condition		Over 24 weeks' gestation	
		Number	%	Number	%	Number	%
Total ground	E alone or with any other[c]	2,692	100			160	100
Q00–Q89	Congenital malformations total	1,197	44	1,676	49	106	66
Q00–Q07	Nervous system total	607	23	755	22	69	43
Q00	Anencephaly	208	8	216	6	5	3
Q01	Encephalocele	33	1	39	1	1	1
Q02	Microcephaly	6	0	13	0	4	3
Q03	Hydrocephalus	26	1	36	1	3	2
Q04	Other malformations of the brain	109	4	156	5	30	19
Q05	Spina bifida	149	6	167	5	5	3
Q06–O07	Other	76	3	128	4	21	13
Q10–Q18	Eye, ear, face and neck	2	0	2	0	0	0
Q20–Q28	Cardiovascular system	191	7	305	9	12	8
G30–Q34	Respiratory system	16	1	26	1	1	1
Q35–Q37	Cleft lip and cleft palate	4	0	12	0	0	0
Q38–Q45	Other malformations of the digestive system	6	0	16	0	1	1
Q60–Q64	Urinary system	104	4	162	5	7	4
Q65–Q79	Musculoskeletal system	174	6	287	8	11	7
G80–G85	Skin, breast integument phakomatoses	7	0	11	0	1	1
Q86–Q89	Other	86	3	100	3	4	3
Q90–Q99	Chromosomal abnormalities total	1,012	38	1,088	32	32	20
Q90	Down's syndrome	544	20	570	17	3	2
0910–Q913	Edwards' syndrome	211	8	226	7	8	5
Q914–Q917	Patau's syndrome	79	3	93	3	7	4
Q92–Q99	Other	178	7	199	6	14	9
	Other conditions total	483	18	663	19	22	14
P00–P04	Fetus affected by maternal factors	165	6	235	7	1	1
P05–P08	Fetal disorders related to gestation and growth	27	1	38	1	11	7
P35–P39	Fetus affected by congenital infectious disease	0	0	0	0	0	0
P529	Intercranial nontraumatic hemorrhage of fetus	7	0	7	0	4	3
P832–P833	Hydrop fetalis not due to hemolytic disease	39	1	81	2	1	1
O30	Multiple gestation	39	1	45	1	0	0
O41	Disorder of the amniotic fluids	4	0	8	0	0	0
Z20–Z22	Exposure to communicable disease	6	0	7	0	5	3

Table 18.2 (*cont.*)

England and Wales, residents		Numbers and percentages[b]				
Z80–Z84	Family history of heritable disorder	154	6	191	6	0	0
E84	Cystic fibrosis	15	1	17	0	0	0
G71	Disorder of the muscles	11	0	18	1	0	0
	Other	11	0	11	0	0	0
	Not known[d]	5	0	5	0	0	0

[a] 'Other' conditions may be available by ICD-10 code on request.
[b] Percentages are rounded and may not add up to 100.
[c] ICD-10 codes are taken from the International Statistical Classification of Diseases and Related Health Problems (10th revision), published by the World Health Organization.
[d] 'Not known' includes one case that on further investigation was found to be performed under Ground C and not Ground E, and it was too late to amend the tables.
[2] The all mentions totals show abortions where more than one medical condition is reported. Totals therefore do not equal the number of abortions performed under Ground E.

congenital malformations were mentioned 1,676 times within the 2,692 Ground E cases, although they were cited as the principal condition in 1,197 cases[23].

In 2012 in England and Wales, congenital malformations were reported as the principal medical condition in nearly half (44%) of the 2,692 abortions undertaken under Ground E. The most commonly reported malformations were of the nervous system (23%), cardiovascular system (7%) and musculoskeletal system abnormalities (6%). About one-third (38%) of pregnancies terminated under Ground E were reported to be for chromosomal abnormalities. Down's syndrome was the most commonly reported and accounted for 20% of all Ground E cases[23] (Table 18.2).

Major structural abnormalities still constitute a major cause of perinatal mortality, accounting for 9.6% of stillbirths and 21.5% of neonatal deaths in 2009 in the UK[29].

In 2012 in Scotland, 159 (1.3%) abortions were carried out under Ground E of the Abortion Act. Of these, 30 were for Down's syndrome, 26 for other chromosomal anomalies, 15 for anencephaly and 13 for musculoskeletal conditions[23] (Table 18.3).

Between 2006 and 2009 the number of abortions performed per year under Ground E in England and Wales was static. Between 2009 and 2012 there was an increase of 29%, whilst overall there was a slight fall in the total number of abortions. The percentage of the total number performed under Ground E has increased from 0.98% to 1.45% over 5 years from 2007. These figures may be a reflection of improved antenatal screening programmes (Table 18.4).

Abortions over 24 weeks of gestation accounted for less than 0.1% of the total. Although there were 160 abortions at or over 24 weeks in 2012 in England and Wales compared with 135 in 2007, they represent 5.9% of the total number of abortions carried out under Ground E compared with 7% in 2007. Whilst the proportion of abortions at 24 weeks and over has fallen slightly since 2007 there has been no change in the proportion at 20–23 weeks of gestation, which has remained at around 27% of the total under Ground E (Table 18.4).

Current national guidelines recommend that routine screening for Down's syndrome should be performed before 14 completed weeks of pregnancy to allow early decisions to be made, including whether to have an invasive diagnostic test and, if fetal aneuploidy is confirmed, whether to undergo induced abortion[30]. This would allow women to have an abortion at an earlier gestation with a reduced complication rate and avoid the necessity of feticide.

There were no abortions associated with rubella under Ground E in 2012. In the past 10 years, there have been seven abortions associated with rubella in England and Wales: two in 2003, three in 2005, and one in each 2006 and 2007[23].

In 2012, 75% of abortions under Ground E overall were performed medically compared with 48% of all abortions. Under 15 weeks of gestation, approximately half of the abortions under Ground E were medical. At 15–16 weeks, the ratio of medical to surgical abortions under Ground E was 4:1 and at 17–19 weeks it was 9:1. At 20–21 weeks, 99% were performed medically and at 22 weeks and over it was 97%[23] (Table 18.5).

The National Down's Syndrome Cytogenetic Register (NDSCR) began collecting data for England and Wales in 1989[31]. Screening tests for Down's syndrome were introduced at that time, and since 2003

Table 18.3 Legal abortions: countries of the UK by principal medical condition for abortions performed under Ground E in 2012 [23]

Country of abortion	Numbers and percentages					
	England and Wales		Scotland		UK	
All legal abortions	190,972	100%	12,447	100%	203,419	100%
Total under Ground E	2,692	100%	159	100%	2,851	100%
Nervous system (Q00–Q007)	607	23	41	26	648	23
Other congenital malformations (Q10–Q89)	590	22	40	25	630	22
Chromosomal abnormalities	1,012	38	56	35	1,068	37
Other	483	18	22	14	505	18

Table 18.4 Legal abortions performed under ground E, by gestation weeks, England and Wales in 2006–2012 [23]

Year	Total number abortions	Total abortions under Ground E (% of total number abortions)	Abortions under Ground E under13 weeks (% of abortions under Ground E)	Abortions under Ground E 13–19 weeks (% of abortions under Ground E)	Abortions under Ground E 20–23 weeks (% of abortions under Ground E)	Abortions under Ground E ≥24 weeks (% of abortions under Ground E)
2006	193,700	2,036 (1.05)	315 (15.5)	1,018 (50.0)	567 (27.8)	136 (6.7)
2007	198,500	1,939 (0.98)	291 (15.0)	1,000 (51.6)	513 (26.5)	135 (7.0)
2008	195,296	1,988 (1.02)	309 (15.5)	999 (50.3)	556 (28.0)	124 (6.2)
2009	189,100	2,085 (1.10)	329 (15.8)	1,020 (48.9)	600 (28.8)	136 (6.5)
2010	189,574	2,290 (1.21)	382 (16.7)	1,116 (48.7)	645 (28.2)	147 (6.4)
2011	189,931	2,307 (1.21)	338 (14.7)	1,191 (51.6)	631 (27.4)	147 (6.4)
2012	185,122	2,692 (1.45)	386 (14.3)	1,431 (53.2)	715 (26.6)	160 (5.9)

Table 18.5 Legal abortions performed under ground E by gestation weeks, residents of England and Wales numbers in 2012[23]

England and Wales, residents	Number of cases						
		Gestation weeks for abortions performed under Ground E					
Procedure	Total	Under 13	13 & 14	15 & 16	17 to 19	20 & 21	22 and over
Total abortions	2,692	386	795	353	283	482	393
Surgical	676	213	344	72	28	6	13
Vacuum aspiration	452	175	261	16	0	0	0
Dilatation and evacuation	154	16	64	52	19	3	0
Feticide with a surgical evacuation[a]	70	22	19	4	9	3	13
Medical	2,016	173	451	281	255	476	380
Antiprogesterone with or without prostaglandin	1,463	165	420	256	221	372	29
Other medical agent	127	8	31	25	29	24	10
Feticide with a medical evacuation[b]	426	0	0	0	5	80	341

[a] Includes feticide with no method of evacuation and surgical 'other'.
[b] Includes eight cases where use of feticide was not confirmed at time of publication.

Table 18.6 Legal abortions: complication[a] rates by procedure and gestation weeks, residents of England and Wales in 2012[23]

England and Wales, residents	Complication rates per 1,000 abortions		
Gestation weeks	Total all procedures	Procedure	
		Surgical	Medical
Total complications (number of cases)	278	91	187
All gestations	2	1	2
3–9 weeks	1	1	1
10–12 weeks	2	2	3
13–19 weeks	5	1	16
20 weeks and over	12	3	29

[a] Complications include hemorrhage, uterine perforation and/or sepsis, and are those reported up to the time of discharge from the place of termination.

when the UK National Screening Programme was introduced, first-trimester screening has become gradually available to all women in England and Wales. This has resulted in an increase in the number of antenatal diagnoses of Down's syndrome. An increase in maternal age has contributed to this rise. The prevalence of Down's syndrome has also increased as pregnancies that would previously have resulted in miscarriage are being diagnosed.

In 1989, the NDSCR reported a total of 1066 Down's syndrome diagnoses, 318 (30%) of which were made antenatally. In 2012, the total number of diagnoses had risen to 1982, of which 1259 (64%) were antenatal. Around 90% of women with an antenatal diagnosis of Down's syndrome undergo termination of pregnancy. There has been a slight decrease in this proportion, from 92% between 1989–2010 to 90% in 2011–2012. However, the NDSCR data show that overall the number of terminations of pregnancy that were performed after a diagnosis of Down's syndrome has increased more than fourfold from 302 in 1989 to 1331 in 2012.

First-trimester screening has resulted in the diagnosis of Down's syndrome being made earlier in pregnancy, thereby allowing termination of pregnancy to be carried out at lower gestations. In women under 35 years of age in 1989, only 2% of abortions after a diagnosis of Down's syndrome were performed under 15 weeks of gestation, which increased to 46% in 2012. In women over 35 years old, the increase was from 18%–50%. The proportion of terminations of pregnancy performed at 21 weeks of gestation and over reduced from 52% in 1989 to 12% in 2012 in women under 35, and from 19% to 6% in women over 35 years old[26].

These figures reflect those of the UK Department of Health statistics but are considerably higher, possibly as in some cases the abortion if under 24 weeks of gestation, will have been legally performed under clause C of the Abortion Act or due to under-reporting to the Department of Health.

The number and prevalence of live births affected by Down's syndrome have not changed significantly, there being 750 cases in 1989 and 775 in 2012.

Complications

Complications of abortion increase with gestational age. This is especially the case with medical abortion. Complications were reported in 278 cases in 2012, a rate of about one in every 700 abortions, which was the same as in 2011 and 41% less than in 2002[22] (Table 18.6).

There were no maternal deaths following abortion notified to the Department of Health in 2012. In the triennium 2006–2008, there were 107 direct maternal deaths in the UK. Two were associated with abortion and both of these were from genital tract sepsis. There were a total of 628,342 abortions in the triennium 2006–2008, making the mortality rate of induced abortion 0.32/100,000[32].

References

1. Abortion Act 1967. London: HMSO; 1967. http://www.legislation.gov.uk/ukpga/1967/87/contents.

2. Human Fertilisation and Embryology Act 1990. London: HMSO; 1990. http://www.legislation.gov.uk/ukpga/1990/37/contents.

3. Statham H, Solomou W, Green J. Late termination of pregnancy: law, policy and decision making in four English fetal medicine units. *BJOG* 2006; 113: 1402–11.

4. Abortion Act 1967. London: HMSO; 1967. https://www.gov.uk/government/publications/abortion-notification-forms-for-england-and-wales.

5. Abortion Act 1967. Section 3. London: HMSO; 1967. http://www.legislation.gov.uk/ukpga/1967/87/section/3.

6. Draper E, Alfirevic Z, Stacey F, et al. for the EPICure Study Group. An investigation into the reporting and management of late terminations of pregnancy (between 22+0 and 26+6 weeks of gestation) within NHS Hospitals in England in 2006: the EPICure preterm cohort study. *BJOG* 2012; 119: 710–5.

7. R v Smith [1974]. 1 All ER 376, 1 WLR 1510, 58 Cr App Rep 106.

8. Care Quality Commission (CQC). Findings of termination of pregnancy inspections 2012. http://www.cqc.org.uk/media/findings-termination-pregnancy-inspections-published.

9. Department of Health. Guidance in relation to requirements of the Abortion Act 1967, May 2014. https://www.gov.uk/government/uploads/system/uploads/attachment_data/file/313459/20140509_-_Abortion_Guidance_Document.pdf.

10. Janaway v Salford Health Authority: All England Law Rep 1988 Dec1; [1988] 3: 1079–84.

11. Doogan and Wood v. NHS Greater Glasgow and Clyde Health Board [2013] CSIH 36 P876/11. http://www.bailii.org/scot/cases/ScotCS/2013/2013CSIH36.html.

12. General Medical Council. Personal beliefs and medical practice, 2013. http://www.gmc-uk.org/Personal_beliefs_and_medical_practice.pdf_51462245.pdf.

13. Royal College of Nursing. Termination of pregnancy, an RCN nursing framework, 2013. http://www.rcn.org.uk/__data/assets/pdf_file/0004/529654/Terminationofpregnancy_WEB.pdf.

14. Kelly v Kelly [1997]. ScotCS CSIH_2 (24 May 1997). http://www.bailii.org/scot/cases/ScotCS/1997/1997_SC_285.html.

15. Hone v Hansell [unrep, March 2001].

16. Paton v BPAS [1979] QB 276.

17. Paton v UK [1981] 3 EHRR 408.

18. Northern Ireland Department of Health, Social Services and Public Safety. The limited circumstances for a lawful termination of pregnancy in Northern Ireland. A guidance document, 2013. http://www.dhsspsni.gov.uk/guidance-limited-circumstances-termination-pregnancy-april-2013.pdf.

19. Northern Ireland Department of Health, Social Services and Public Safety. Written statement to the Assembly, 2012. http://www.dhsspsni.gov.uk/termination-statement.

20. Northern Ireland Statistics and Research Agency. Birth and Deaths Reports. www.nisra.gov.uk/demography/default.asp23.htm.

21. Lynn F, McNeill J, Alderdice F. Current trends in antenatal screening services: results from a regional survey. *Ulster Med J* 2010; 79(1): 12–5.

22. Royal College of Obstetricians and Gynaecologists (RCOG). Termination of Pregnancy for Fetal Abnormality in England, Wales and Scotland. Working Party Report. London: RCOG, 1996.

23. Department of Health. Report on abortion statistics in England and Wales for 2012, July 2013. https://www.gov.uk/government/publications/report-on-abortion-statistics-in-england-and-wales-for-2012.

24. Nuffield Council on Bioethics. Critical Care Decisions in Fetal and Neonatal Medicine: Ethical Issues. London: Nuffield Council on Bioethics, 2006. www.nuffieldbioethics.org/go/ourwork/neonatal/publication_406.html.

25. British Association of Perinatal Medicine. Palliative care (supportive and end of life care). A framework for clinical practice in perinatal medicine, 2010. http://www.bapm.org/publications/documents/guidelines/Palliative_Care_Report_final_%20Aug10.pdf.

26. Royal College of Paediatrics and Child Health (RCPCH). Withholding or Withdrawing Life Sustaining Treatment in Children: A Framework for Practice, 2nd edn. London: RCPCH, 2004. [www.library.nhs.uk/GUIDELINESFINDER/ViewResource.aspx?resID=298393].

27. Royal College of Obstetricians and Gynaecologists (RCOG). Additional report from the RCOG Ethics Committee. Further issues relating to late abortion, fetal viability and registration of births and deaths. London. RCOG, 2001.

28. National Health Service Scotland. Information Services Division (ISD) Scotland Abortion Statistics 2012, May 2013. http://www.isdscotland.org/Health-Topics/Sexual-Health/Publications/2013-05-28/2013-05-28-Abortions-Summary.pdf?58079165221.

29. Healthcare Quality Improvement Partnership UK. Confidential Enquiry into Maternal and Child Health: Perinatal Mortality, 2009. www.hqip.org.uk/assets/NCAPOP-Library/CMACE-Reports/35.-March-2011-Perinatal-Mortality-2009.pdf.

30. National Institute for Clinical Excellence (NICE). Antenatal Care: Routine Care for the Healthy

Pregnant Woman. NICE Clinical Guideline CG62. London: NICE, 2008 http://guidance.nice.org.uk/CG62.

31. Public Health England. The National Down Syndrome Cytogenetic Register for England and Wales. 2012 Annual Report, 2013. http://www.wolfson.qmul.ac.uk/current-projects/downs-syndrome-register#annual-report

32. Centre for Maternal and Child Enquiries (CMACE). Saving mothers' lives. Reviewing maternal deaths to make motherhood safer: 2006–2008. *BJOG* 2011; 118 (Suppl. 1): 1–203.

Chapter

19

Methods of abortion

Kristina Naidoo

Once a woman has made the decision to undergo an abortion, treatment should be arranged without delay. This will reduce the anxiety of waiting and allows an abortion to be performed at an earlier gestation. However, there is no evidence that this lessens the emotional impact of the pregnancy loss. Although doctors working in fetal medicine are reconciled to offering women induced abortion in certain circumstances, those who are ethically opposed to abortion have a duty of care to refer women who choose to undergo an abortion in a timely manner[1].

If a woman remains uncertain, she must be given sufficient time to make her decision as far as is practicable. It must not be assumed that a woman will choose to have an abortion even if the fetus has a lethal condition such as anencephaly. If she wishes to continue with the pregnancy, the likely outcomes should be clearly explained to her and an individualized care plan agreed. Whatever her decision, it must be respected and fully supported[2].

A multidisciplinary approach is required to provide optimal care to women after a diagnosis of fetal abnormality. Those involved should be clear as to their role and ensure that the woman and her partner are carefully guided along a planned pathway of care by fully briefed and supportive staff. When care is divided between local and specialist units, clear lines of communication must be in place. It is also essential that the woman's general practitioner and community midwife are informed of the diagnosis and management plan so that ongoing support can be offered to her when she returns home.

Pre-abortion care

Once a woman has decided to undergo an abortion she must be given accurate evidence-guided information about the methods of abortion appropriate to the gestational age and their potential adverse effects and complications. Written information should be available in a variety of languages. Where possible a woman should be given the abortion method of her choice. Women value the ability to choose the method, and their preferences are based on their individual emotional coping styles[3].

A woman should be able to choose to have a surgical abortion in the second trimester. If required, she should be given the option of referral to a provider with expertise in this method, such as an independent clinic under contract to the National Health Service (NHS). There must be no undue delay in referral.

Wherever the place of treatment, health professionals should be sensitive and responsive to a woman's needs and should respect her privacy and dignity. For instance, a private room with facilities for her partner to stay should be provided if she undergoes a medical abortion.

The options available for pain relief, whether she wants to see the baby and have any momentoes should be discussed. The woman should be informed about the care plan after the process of abortion is completed, including potential complications and the benefit of further investigations such as a postmortem examination. The options for sensitive disposal of the fetal remains should also be offered.

It is essential that all the staff involved in the woman's care are well informed, appropriately trained and with the requisite skills. The most important factors associated with satisfaction regarding induced abortion due to a fetal abnormality are the human aspects of care[4].

Feticide

The Royal College of Obstetricians and Gynaecologists (RCOG) in the UK, recommends that feticide should

Fetal Medicine, ed. Bidyut Kumar and Zarko Alfirevic. Published by Cambridge University Press. © Cambridge University Press 2016.

be offered to all women undergoing abortion after 21+6 weeks of gestation to ensure that the fetus is not born alive[5].

Data were reported on live birth rates in medical abortions for fetal abnormality in the West Midlands between 1995 and 2004[6]. Overall, 102 of the 3189 (3.2%) fetuses were born alive, of which 36% survived 1 h or less and 6% for 6 or more hours. Between 1995 and 2003, the proportion of live births at 22–23 weeks gestation decreased from 6.5% to 3%. This was likely to be due to the impact of the UK RCOG guidelines recommending feticide above 21+6 weeks. The data also showed that there was a significant chance of a live birth at 20 and 21 weeks, at 3.5% and 5.4% respectively.

In a prospective study (EPICure2), data were collected for the late abortions performed in all maternity units in England in 2006[7]. There were 3782 deliveries between 22+0 and 26+6 weeks of gestation, which were the result of induced abortion; 90.3% for fetal abnormality and 9.7% for maternal or fetal compromise. Feticide was carried out prior to 83.7% of abortions for fetal abnormality and 60.3% of abortions for maternal or fetal compromise. Live births resulted from 2.2% abortions for fetal abnormality and 4.8% abortions for maternal or fetal compromise. All liveborn infants died within a short time. Median time to death was 1 h (interquartile range 42 min to 2 h 15 min). They received terminal care, and resuscitation was not attempted. Fetal compromise was mainly due to severe fetal growth restriction, with or without premature rupture of membranes.

With regard to feticide for prevention of fetal pain and awareness, the UK RCOG's published guidance concluded: "In reviewing the neuroanatomical and physiological evidence in the fetus, it was apparent that connections from the periphery to the cortex are not intact before 24 weeks of gestation and, as most neuroscientists believe that the cortex is necessary for pain perception, it can be concluded that the fetus cannot experience pain in any sense prior to this gestation"[8].

Whilst many health professionals will find the procedure stressful, most agree that feticide will prevent a woman or couple and delivery unit staff from facing the difficult situation of a live birth after induced abortion. A woman and her partner should receive support before, during and after feticide. The decision and their experience of the procedure itself are likely to have had a significant psychologic impact[9].

Feticide should be performed by an appropriately trained practitioner using aseptic conditions and continuous ultrasound guidance. An intracardiac injection of potassium chloride is the method recommended to ensure fetal asystole[1]. The needle should be placed into a cardiac ventricle and after aspiration of fetal blood to ensure correct placement, 2–5 ml of 15% potassium chloride is injected. A further injection may be required if asystole has not occurred after 30–60 s. Asystole should be documented for at least 5 min. It is a good practice to repeat a scan 10–20 min later to confirm fetal demise.

There were no live births in a series of 239 cases of feticide using this technique between 20+5 and 37+5 weeks of gestation. Asystole was confirmed in all cases within 2 min of the first injection, with no woman requiring a second needle insertion and no maternal complications[11]. Potassium chloride can be administered by the umbilical route after cordocentesis but failures have been recorded[12].

Fetal demise may also be induced by intra-amniotic or intrathoracic injection of digoxin (up to 1 mg) and by umbilical venous or intracardiac injection of 1% lignocaine (up to 30 mL). Neither technique consistently results in cardiac asystole[1]. A large retrospective review concluded that the overall failure rate with intrafetal or intra-amniotic digoxin at various doses was 7%, although there were no failures with a 1 mg intrafetal dose[13]. The review found there were no adverse effects at any of the doses of digoxin used.

Intracardiac injection of either potassium chloride or intrathoracic injection of digoxin require considerably more skill than intra-amniotic injection of digoxin. Whilst the latter may be slightly less effective in inducing fetal demise, it may be an option for units where the practitioners do not have the necessary skill to administer intracardiac injections.

Methods of abortion

Whenever possible, women should be given a choice of abortion method appropriate for them. Medical and surgical abortion methods are possible at all gestations (Table 19.1).

Whilst the majority of induced abortions are performed in the first trimester, most abortions for fetal abnormality are not undertaken until the second trimester. The optimal method of second trimester abortion continues to be debated[14]. Surgical abortion by dilatation and evacuation preceded by cervical preparation is safe, effective and preferred by women in the second trimester, yet it is offered in relatively few cases in the UK for abortion under Ground E [15]. In

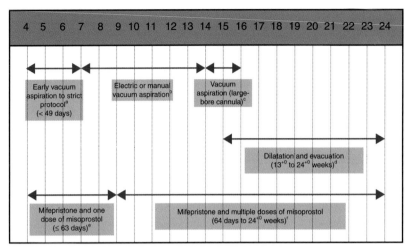

Table 19.1 Summary of abortion methods appropriate for use in abortion services in the UK by gestational age in weeks[1]

a. Surgical abortion by means of vacuum aspiration at gestations below 7 weeks. To increase confidence that the gestation sac has been removed, protocols should include safeguards such as examination of the aspirate for the presence of the gestational sac and follow-up serum human chorionic gonadotrophin estimation if needed.
b. Surgical abortion using electric or manual vaccum aspiration. The uterus is emptied using a suction cannula, sharp curettage is not recommended.
c. Surgical abortion using vaccum aspiration which may require large bore suction cannula and tubing.
d. Surgical abortion using a combination of vaccum aspiration and specialised forceps.
e. Medical abortion using a single oral dose of the anaprogesterone mifepristone, followed by a single dose of a prostaglandin analogue.
f. Medical abortion using a single oral dose of the antiprogesterone mifepristone, followed by multiple doses of a prostaglandin analogue.

a UK randomized controlled trial of abortion methods for fetal abnormality, 100% of women in the surgical group stated that they would prefer that treatment again against 53% in the medical induction group (P < 0.001)[16].

In the USA, dilatation and evacuation (D&E) is the primary method of second trimester abortion for any indication and one-third of fetal medicine specialists provide D&E. Whilst D&E is the most commonly used method at gestations over 14 weeks by independent sector providers in England, very few gynecologists in the NHS in the UK perform D&E. Women value choice and the RCOG endorses surgical abortion in the second trimester[2]. However, surgical abortion in the second trimester is not a core surgical skill for trainees in obstetrics and gynecology in the UK, and it is only an optional requirement for the small proportion of trainees who undertake the advanced training skills module in Abortion Care. Addressing these training issues and developing services within the NHS should be a priority.

Medical methods of abortion

The recommended method for medical abortion is mifepristone, a progesterone receptor antagonist,

followed 1–2 days later by misoprostol, a synthetic prostaglandin analogue. This regimen is effective and appropriate at any gestation[17].

Mifepristone is administered orally and the recommended dose is 200 mg. Level 1B evidence from a randomized trial showed that a dose of 200 mg of mifepristone is as effective as 400 mg or 600 mg[18]. This study used vaginal gemeprost rather than misoprostol, but level III evidence from large case series using oral misoprostol following 200 mg or 600 mg of mifepristone confirmed that there was no difference in efficacy between the two doses of mifepristone, with a reduced cost of the lower dose. This applies at all gestational ages[19].

Gemeprost is a prostaglandin E1 analogue, which was used routinely for a number of years. It is much more expensive than misoprostol, requires refrigeration and can only be administered vaginally. A series of studies reviewed in a UK RCOG guideline[2] demonstrated that misoprostol is equally, if not more effective than gemeprost in early medical abortion, cervical priming and medical abortion from 13 to 24 weeks of gestation[2]. Misoprostol is therefore the prostaglandin analogue of choice for abortion care. A number of other prostaglandins, such as sulprostone and prostaglandin F2α, are no longer used because of their adverse side effects and relative lack of efficacy.

Several of the recommended regimens and routes of administration of mifepristone and misoprostol are outside their product licenses. However, the European Economic Community Council Directive 65/65/EEC specifically permits doctors to use "licensed medicines for indications or in doses or by routes of administration outside the recommendations given in the licence"[20].

Women should be informed before a drug is prescribed for an unlicenced indication. Mifepristone and misoprostol can be dispensed by pharmacists and administered by nurses and midwives, provided a medical practitioner has prepared and signed an individual prescription.

Early medical abortion for pregnancies up to 9 weeks (63 days) of gestation

Mifepristone with misoprostol is highly effective, safe and acceptable up to 9 weeks of gestation. Efficacy rates up to 98% are reported[21]. Mifepristone 200 mg orally followed 24–48 h later by misoprostol 800 mcg administered by the vaginal, buccal or sublingual routes is recommended. Women should be advised of the greater risk of adverse effects with nonvaginal routes. Side effects include nausea, vomiting, diarrhea and fever.

At 7–9 weeks of gestation, if abortion has not occurred 4 h after administration of misoprostol, a second dose of misoprostol 400 mcg may be administered vaginally or orally depending on the woman's preference and amount of bleeding[2].

Very few abortions under Ground E in the UK are performed under 9 weeks of gestation. There were only 20 such cases in England and Wales in 2012[15].

Medical abortion at 9–13 weeks of gestation

The recommended method for medical abortion between 9 and 13 weeks of gestation is mifepristone 200 mg administered orally followed 36–48 h later by misoprostol 800 mcg administered vaginally. A maximum of four further doses of misoprostol 400 mcg may be administered at 3-hourly intervals, orally or vaginally until expulsion of the products of conception occurs[2].

In a consecutive series of 483 women at 9–13 weeks of gestation, managed with mifepristone 200 mg

followed 36–48 h later by repeated doses of misoprostol, the complete abortion rate was 95% and was gestation dependent[22]. In this series, up to five doses of misoprostol were permitted.

In a randomized trial involving 368 women at 10–13 weeks of gestation, participants were randomly allocated to medical or surgical abortion[23]. Complete abortion rates were 95% in the medical group and 98% in the surgical group, which was not significant. There were more adverse events in the medical group, but 70% of the women in this group indicated that they would opt for the same method in the future compared to 79% in the surgical group.

Medical abortion at 13–24 weeks of gestation

For medical abortion between 13 and 24 weeks of gestation, the following regimen is recommended. Mifepristone 200 mg administered orally followed 36–48 h later by misoprostol 800 mcg administered vaginally (or 400 mcg orally), then misoprostol 400 mcg orally, sublingually or vaginally at 3-hourly intervals, up to a maximum of four further doses[2].

Second-trimester medical abortion with mifepristone followed by a prostaglandin analogue is effective and is associated with shorter induction-to-abortion intervals than methods using a prostaglandin analogue alone. Evidence from a randomized trial of second trimester medical abortion showed that as for the first trimester, mifepristone at a dose of 200 mg is effective[24].

In a study of 386 consecutive cases between 12 and 20 weeks of gestation, an abortion rate of 97.9% was reported. If abortion was not completed by 15 h, a second dose of 200 mg mifepristone was given and the course of prostaglandin analogue repeated starting 24 h later. Treatment was completed within 36 h in over 99% of women.

A randomized trial comparing gemeprost and vaginal misoprostol 36–48 h after 200 mg mifepristone at 12–20 weeks' gestation found no significant difference in complete abortion rates. Surgical evacuation rates and adverse effect profiles were similar in the two groups[25].

A systematic review, which included 40 randomized controlled trials (RCTs) addressing various agents and methods of administration for medical abortion between 12 and 28 weeks of gestation, concluded that the combination of mifepristone and misoprostol appeared to have the highest efficacy and shortest abortion time interval. The optimal route for administering misoprostol was vaginally, preferably using tablets at 3-hourly intervals. Further conclusions from this review were limited by the variable gestational age ranges and medical regimens of the included trials[17].

In countries where mifepristone is unavailable, misoprostol alone is a reasonable alternative. A higher total dose is needed and the induction to abortion interval is longer than with the combined regime, resulting in a higher incidence of side effects. However, the abortion will be completed within 24–36 h in 80–90% of women[26].

A meta-analysis of randomized trials comparing gemeprost with misoprostol showed that vaginal misoprostol compared to gemeprost was associated with a reduced need for opiate analgesia and surgical evacuation of the uterus[26].

Over 24 weeks of gestation

Over 24 weeks of gestation, the regimens used for medical abortion will generally be the same as for induction of labor. The dose of misoprostol should be reduced due to the greater sensitivity of the uterus to prostaglandins at higher gestational age. There is a lack of clinical studies to recommend specific doses. The International Federation of Gynecology and Obstetrics recommendations are misoprostol 25 mcg vaginally 6-hourly or orally at 2-hourly intervals based on the World Health Organization (WHO) guidance for induction of labor[27].

Regimens for delayed expulsion

There are few studies that report regimens for women who do not complete the abortion within 24 h. According to some protocols, if abortion does not occur, a further dose of mifepristone is given, followed by repeated vaginal misoprostol 12 h later[28]. A woman who fails to expel the fetus during the second day would receive a third dose of mifepristone followed by gemeprost 1 mg every 3 h. There is insufficient consensus to set a guideline for women who have a failed or delayed medical abortion. For women going on to a second or third day, D&E would be an appropriate option[28]. If possible, the woman should be given a preference of which way to proceed.

The Society of Obstetricians and Gynaecologists of Canada have advocated the use of intramuscular 15-methyl prostaglandin F2α (Hemabate) in women not responding to conventional therapy. It is successful

in 95% cases within 10–20 h. The recommended dose for failed late second trimester abortion is 250 mcg by deep intramuscular injection repeated every 2 h as required. The total dose ranges from 1250–2500 mcg[29]. Hysterotomy is essentially a classical cesarean section that is rarely indicated as a method of abortion. It has a much greater morbidity and mortality than any other technique and should only be considered as a last resort after all medical therapies have failed.

Surgical evacuation of placenta

The placenta is usually expelled within a short time of the fetus. An injection of oxytocin may be given to help expulsion of the placenta. If the placenta is not delivered within 1–2 h, an infusion of 10 units oxytocin in 500 mL of normal saline at a rate of 2 mL per min or other uterotonic drugs may be given[30]. After expulsion, the placenta should be examined to ensure it is complete, and the woman observed in hospital to monitor vital signs and vaginal blood loss. If the uterus is not contracting well and bleeding persists, the uterine cavity should be explored to see whether there are any retained products of conception. Routine surgical evacuation of the uterus is not required following medical abortion. It should only be undertaken if there is clinical evidence that the abortion is incomplete or the woman starts bleeding excessively[2].

Medical abortion and prior cesarean section

The cesarean section rate is increasing worldwide. Although many studies have described the risk of complications with subsequent vaginal birth after a cesarean section, experience with second trimester abortion is limited. Uterine rupture, hemorrhage, hysterotomy and hysterectomy are possible complications of a second-trimester medical abortion in women with a uterine scar.

A systematic review concluded that although the use of misoprostol for second-trimester medical abortion was safe for women with one prior cesarean section, it was associated with incidence rates of 0.4% for uterine rupture and 0.2% for need for transfusion; the hysterectomy rate was 0%[31]. In another review, the reported risk of uterine rupture was less than 0.3%[32].

There are little data on the risk of uterine rupture for women with two or more cesarean deliveries. In a retrospective review of 279 women between 14–26 weeks of gestation, the overall rate of uterine rupture was 1.1%[33]. No uterine ruptures occurred among the 60 women with one prior cesarean, even though they received multiple low doses of misoprostol vaginally. However, 3 of 26 (11.5%) women with two or more prior cesarean sections had a scar rupture. One woman with three previous cesarean sections was at 24 weeks of gestation and underwent hysterectomy. Two women each with two prior cesarean sections were at 16 and 20 weeks, respectively, and both had a laparotomy and repair of the scar. In this study, half of the routine misoprostol dose was used in the women with a uterine scar resulting in a longer time from induction to abortion and higher total doses of misoprostol.

A study evaluating the safety and efficacy of vaginal misoprostol for midtrimester medical abortion in 31 women with three or more prior cesarean deliveries concluded that it was safe and acceptably effective[34]. Owing to the lack of randomized trials, there are no conclusions about the safety and effectiveness of the administration routes or misoprostol dosage used in women with a prior uterine scar, or the time allowed between doses. Until then, management of women in this situation should be made on a case-by-case basis, after consideration of the number of cesarean sections and gestational age. Careful monitoring is required during the abortion procedure and awareness of the risk of uterine rupture by all staff.

Pain relief for medical abortion

Abdominal pain is one of the most common adverse effects of medical abortion and is most likely to be felt in the first few hours after prostaglandin analogue administration[35]. Analgesia should therefore be offered to all women with a range of options available to meet their needs.

There is a lack of research evidence to inform the choice of analgesic regimen. In a systematic review of pain control in medical abortion, only 10 of 361 articles identified met the inclusion criteria[7]. Oral paracetamol has been shown not to reduce pain more than placebo during medical abortion and is therefore not recommended. Nonsteroidal anti-inflammatory drugs (NSAIDs) are a possible first-line treatment. They inhibit the production of endogenous prostaglandins, which are important messengers responsible for uterine contractions, cramps and pain sensation. The main positive finding of a systematic review was that ibuprofen given after the onset of pain reduced further analgesic use[36].

In a randomized study examining the effect of paracetamol and codeine or diclofenac given with the first dose of misoprostol to women undergoing medical abortion between 13 and 22 weeks of gestation, women using diclofenac had a reduced need for opiate injections[37]. NSAIDs do not interfere with the action of misoprostol or mifepristone on inducing cervical ripening, uterine contractility or the time to abortion and expulsion of the products of conception[36].

Studies have shown that analgesic requirements and the perception of pain are significantly higher in younger women, those at a higher gestational age, with a longer induction-to-abortion interval and with a greater number of misoprostol doses. Conversely it is less in older, parous women and those at lower gestations. However, none of these factors is sufficiently predictive to be useful in the management of individual cases[38]. The role of advanced or prophylactic analgesia, conscious sedation and paracervical block and their effectiveness, as well as women's satisfaction and acceptability need further research.

Side effects

Side effects, including nausea, vomiting and diarrhea are characteristics of prostaglandin administration and are caused by a stimulatory effect on the gastrointestinal tract. Fever and chills can also occur and are more common with misoprostol than gemeprost. They are self-limiting and not indicative of infection and antipyrexial therapy is appropriate for symptomatic relief.

Surgical methods

Vacuum aspiration

Vacuum aspiration is the recommended technique of surgical abortion up to 14 weeks of gestation[2]. Either electric or manual vacuum aspiration may be used, as both are effective and acceptable to women and clinicians. Vacuum aspiration is preferable to sharp curettage for surgical abortion. Comparative trials of evacuation methods for miscarriage management found that vacuum aspiration is associated with less blood loss, less pain and shorter procedure times than sharp curettage[39]. Comparing flexible and rigid cannulae, one randomized trial found no statistically significant differences in cervical injury, febrile morbidity, blood transfusion, antibiotic use or incomplete evacuations between them[40].

During vacuum aspiration, the uterus should be emptied using the suction cannula and blunt forceps if required. The UK RCOG guideline[2] does not recommend routine sharp curettage to ensure the cavity is empty. The "gritty" sensation experienced when the uterus clamps down on the cannula should provide sufficient reassurance that all the products of conception have been removed. The risks of sharp curettage include Asherman's syndrome. Access to ultrasound may be useful in some cases but routine use is not a requirement[2].

Vacuum aspiration may also be performed between 14 to 16 weeks of gestation. Large-bore cannulae and suction tubing are required for the procedure [41]. Cannulae over 12 mm in diameter may not be readily available in the UK, in which case forceps are used to remove larger fetal parts.

The method of choice at gestations above 13 weeks will depend on the available resources and the skills and experience of local clinicians.

Dilatation and evacuation

D&E preceded by cervical priming is a safe and effective method of surgical abortion for pregnancies above 14 weeks of gestation. Specialized training is required. Adequate prior cervical dilatation is particularly important (see "Cervical priming" below).

A 14–16 mm cannula is inserted into the uterine cavity and the amniotic fluid aspirated. When nothing further can be suctioned, usually after 1–2 min, Bierer or Sopher ovum forceps are introduced into the uterine cavity to remove fetal parts and other pregnancy tissue. Ultrasound guidance during D&E is helpful to locate fetal parts and reduce the risk of complications. Whenever possible, the evacuation should be completed from the lower uterine cavity and reaching high into the uterus avoided. After evacuation, the pregnancy tissue should be examined to ensure complete abortion.

Cervical priming

Cervical priming should be considered in all cases prior to surgical abortion as it may be beneficial, in particular if risk factors for cervical injury or uterine perforation exist. These risk factors include less than 18 years of age, advanced gestational age, particularly in multiparae, cervical anomalies or previous surgery, or when a less experienced surgeon is operating. It is unclear at what gestation cervical priming should be routine, but the risk of complications tends to increase after 9 weeks. The current WHO recommendation is that cervical preparation may be considered at any gestational age but is recommended at 12 weeks of gestation and above[21].

The following regimens are recommended for cervical preparation up to 14 weeks of gestation. Misoprostol 400 mcg administered vaginally 3 h prior to surgery or sublingually 2–3 h prior to surgery. Sublingual administration is superior to vaginal administration but is associated with more side effects. Gemeprost 1 mg vaginally 3 h or mifepristone 200 mg orally 36–48 h before surgery are effective and licenced for this indication. Gemeprost is expensive compared to misoprostol. The length of time that mifepristone has to be administered before the procedure makes it less practical[42].

Up to 18 weeks' gestation, misoprostol 800 mcg vaginally or 400 mcg sublingually or mifepristone 200mg are also acceptable for cervical preparation[42]. Few randomized controlled trials (RCTs) exist from which to determine the optimal regimen for cervical dilatation before D&E, particularly after 20 weeks of gestation.

A recent systematic review found that osmotic dilators were superior to prostaglandins throughout the second trimester with respect to cervical dilatation and in reducing the procedure time in the early second trimester[43].

All methods are generally safe, although their efficacy and adverse effects vary. No published study has investigated whether pharmacologic methods of cervical priming reduce uncommon complications, such as uterine perforation and cervical laceration. However, they do reduce the duration of the abortion procedure, which is important with increasing gestational age when mechanical cervical dilatation becomes more difficult. The adverse effects experienced with cervical priming, such as pain, need to be considered against the reduced time taken to complete the procedure.

Based on randomized trials, the routine use of uterotonic medication at the time of vacuum aspiration is of no benefit. However, the use of oxytocin is likely to be effective in reducing excessive blood loss[2]. Ergometrine is not recommended because of the high risk of postoperative vomiting.

The use of NSAIDs for analgesia does not reduce the efficacy of cervical priming with misoprostol[44].

Complications of abortion

Incomplete abortion

Incomplete abortion can occur following either medical or surgical abortion. The incidence is higher in women undergoing medical abortion[45].

Symptoms include vaginal bleeding and abdominal pain and signs of infection may be present. Diagnosis should be based on clinical criteria as ultrasound scanning is unreliable because of its low specificity.

Management of incomplete abortion may be surgical or medical. Rates of surgical evacuation vary according to diagnostic criteria, intervention thresholds and the woman's preference. Vacuum aspiration is recommended over dilatation and curettage for uterine evacuation, as it is associated with less blood loss, less pain and shorter procedure times[46].

Comparing the rate of surgical intervention after medical and surgical abortion up to 9 weeks in a partially randomized study, significantly more women undergoing medical abortion required surgical intervention, 6% compared to 2% of women undergoing surgical abortion. The results were similar at 10–13 weeks of gestation (5% versus 2%) [47]. In a registry-based study of more than 42,000 women undergoing induced abortion up to 9 weeks of gestation, 6% of women having medical abortions needed surgical intervention for retained products of conception compared to fewer than 1% having surgical abortion[45].

Incomplete abortion may be treated medically using misoprostol. The recommended dose and route of administration for this indication is either 600 mcg orally or 400 mcg sublingually[21]. The presence of bleeding may decrease misoprostol absorption when administered vaginally; thus, a nonvaginal route is generally preferable, although vaginal administration of 400–800 mcg has been used effectively. In a systematic review of women with incomplete miscarriage, there were no differences in the rates of complete abortion or of adverse events between vacuum aspiration and misoprostol, although there were more unplanned surgical interventions with the use of misoprostol[48].

Hemorrhage

The incidence of hemorrhage after surgical abortion is low, ranging from 0.7 to 1.5 in 1,000 with vacuum aspiration up to 14 weeks and increases in the midtrimester to 5.6–8.6 in 1,000. It has been reported as high as 21 per 1,000 with late second trimester D&E. The

risk of hemorrhage requiring transfusion in early medical abortion is 1.3 per 1000 and 6 per 1,000 in second trimester abortion[2].

Hemorrhage associated with induced abortion can result from retained products of conception, trauma to the cervix, bleeding disorders or rarely, uterine perforation. Depending on the cause, appropriate treatment may include evacuation of the uterus and administration of uterotonic drugs to stop the bleeding, intravenous fluid replacement, and, in severe cases, blood transfusion, replacement of clotting factors, laparoscopy or exploratory laparotomy. Because of the low incidence of hemorrhage using vacuum aspiration, oxytocic drugs are not routinely needed, although they may be indicated with D&E at gestations above 14 weeks.

Prolonged menstrual-like bleeding is an expected effect of medical methods of abortion. On average, vaginal bleeding gradually diminishes over about 2 weeks after expulsion of products of conception but in individual cases, bleeding and spotting may persist for up to 45 days. Such bleeding is rarely heavy enough to constitute an emergency. Surgical evacuation may be performed in cases where the bleeding is heavy or prolonged, is causing anemia, or when there is evidence of infection. Major hemorrhage is rare and is usually associated with prolonged retention of the placenta.

Infection

Infection of varying severity may occur after induced abortion when the genital tract is more susceptible to ascending organisms. It is usually caused by existing infection; screening and prophylactic antibiotics reduces the risk.

All women should be offered screening for *Chlamydia trachomatis* and undergo a risk assessment for other sexually transmitted infections (for example, human immunodeficiency virus, gonorrhea, syphilis), and be screened for them if appropriate[2].

A systematic review has shown that antibiotic prophylaxis at the time of first-trimester surgical abortion is effective in preventing pelvic inflammatory disease[49]. The antibiotic of choice is determined by the local epidemiology of genital tract infections, including sexually transmitted infections.

The UK RCOG guideline[2] recommends offering antibiotic prophylaxis effective against anerobes and *C. trachomatis* for surgical abortion (grade A recommendation) and for medical abortion (Grade C recommendation). The following regimens are suitable for use in the UK: metronidazole 1 g rectally or 800 mg orally prior to or at the time of abortion. Unless a woman has tested negative for *C. trachomatis* then either azithromycin 1 g orally or doxycycline 100 mg orally twice daily for 7 days, starting on the day of the abortion should be given.

There are few data on the incidence of clinically significant pelvic infection after medical abortion, but it occurs possibly less frequently than after vacuum aspiration. Whilst the WHO recommends universal prophylaxis for surgical abortion, it does not do so for medical abortion[21].

Post-abortion infection causes short-term morbidity and may result in tubal damage, leading to subfertility and increased risk of ectopic pregnancy. Many of the symptoms of pelvic infection are nonspecific and precise diagnosis is difficult; therefore, women with pelvic pain, abdominal or adnexal tenderness, vaginal discharge and fever should be treated with broad-spectrum antibiotics.

Rare cases of anerobic infection with little or no fever have been reported from North America following medical abortion where the women had *Clostridium*-related toxic shock, and cases have been reported during the postpartum period following a normal delivery[50]. There is no evidence that prophylactic antibiotic treatment during medical abortion would eliminate these rare fatal cases of serious infection[21].

Uterine perforation

Uterine perforation usually goes undetected and resolves without the need for intervention. A study of more than 700 women undergoing laparoscopic sterilization at the time of a first-trimester abortion found a rate of uterine perforation of 2%. However, 12 out of the 14 perforations were small and would not have been recognized had laparoscopy not been performed[51]. When uterine perforation is suspected, observation and antibiotic treatment is required. Laparoscopy is the investigation of choice if available and deemed necessary. If the laparoscopic findings and/or clinical condition of the woman suggest damage to the bowel, blood vessels or other structures, laparotomy may be necessary.

Serious complications, such as uterine rupture, major hemorrhage and cervical tear, are rare. The vast majority of women who have a properly performed induced abortion will not suffer any long-term effects on their general or reproductive health. Studies have shown that there is no association between safely induced first-trimester abortion and adverse outcomes in subsequent pregnancies[52]. Although second-trimester abortions have not been studied as extensively, there is no evidence of an increased risk of adverse outcomes in subsequent pregnancies[21].

References

1. Royal College of Obstetricians and Gynaecologists (RCOG). The Care of Women Requesting Induced Abortion. Evidence-based Clinical guideline No. 7. London: RCOG Press, 2011.

2. Royal College of Obstetricians and Gynaecologists (RCOG). Termination of Pregnancy for Fetal Abnormality in England, Scotland and Wales. Report of a Working Party. London: RCOG Press, 2010.

3. Kerns J, Vanjani R, Freedman L, et al. Women's decision making regarding choice of second trimester termination method for pregnancy complications. *Int J Gynaecol Obst* 2012; 116(3): 244–8.

4. Asplin N, Wessel H, Marions L, et al. Pregnancy termination due to fetal anomaly: Women's reactions, satisfaction and experiences of care. *Midwifery* 2014; 30(6): 620–7.

5. Royal College of Obstetricians and Gynaecologists (RCOG). Termination of Pregnancy for Fetal Abnormality in England, Wales and Scotland. Working Party Report. London: RCOG Press, 1996.

6. Wyldes MP, Tonks AM. Termination of pregnancy for fetal anomaly: a population-based study 1995 to 2004. *BJOG* 2007; 114: 639–42.

7. Draper E, Alfirevic Z, Stacey F, et al. for the EPICure Study Group. An investigation into the reporting and management of late terminations of pregnancy (between 22^{+0} and 26^{+6} weeks of gestation) within NHS Hospitals in England in 2006: the EPICure preterm cohort study. *BJOG* 2012; 119: 710–5.

8. Royal College of Obstetricians and Gynaecologists (RCOG). Fetal Awareness: Review of Research and Recommendations for Practice. Report of a Working Party. London: RCOG Press, 2010. http://www.rcog.org.uk/files/rcogcorp/RCOGFetalAwarenessWPR0610.pdf.

9. Graham RH, Mason K, Rankin J, et al. The role of feticide in the context of late termination of pregnancy: a qualitative study of health professionals' and parents' views. *Prenat Diagn* 2009; 29: 875–81.

10. Royal College of Obstetricians and Gynaecologists (RCOG). Further issues relating to late abortion, fetal

viability and registration of births and deaths. RCOG Statement. London: RCOG Press; 2001.

11. Pasquini L, Pontello V, Kumar S. Intracardiac injection of potassium chloride as a method for feticide: experience from a single UK tertiary centre. *BJOG* 2008; 115: 528–31.

12. Bhide A, Sairam S, Hollis B, et al. Comparison of feticide carried out by cordocentesis versus cardiac puncture. *Ultrasound Obstet Gynecol* 2002; 20: 230–2.

13. Molaei M, Jones HE, Weiselberg T, et al. Effectiveness and safety of digoxin to induce fetal demise prior to second-trimester abortion. *Contraception* 2008; 77: 223–5.

14. Lyus R, Robson S, Parsons J, et al. Second trimester abortion for fetal abnormality. *BMJ* 2013; 347: f4165.

15. Department of Health. Report on abortion statistics in England and Wales for 2012, July 2013. https://www.gov.uk/government/publications/report-on-abortion-statistics-in-england-and-wales-for-2012.

16. Kelly T, Suddes J, Howel D, et al. Comparing medical versus surgical termination of pregnancy at 13–20 weeks of gestation: a randomised controlled trial. *BJOG* 2010; 117: 1512–20.

17. Wildschut H, Both MI, Medema S, et al. Medical methods for mid-trimester termination of pregnancy. *Cochrane Database Syst Rev* 2011; (1): CD005216.

18. World Health Organization (WHO). WHO Task Force on Post-ovulatory Methods of Fertility Regulation. Termination of pregnancy with reduced doses of mifepristone. *BMJ* 1993; 307: 532–7.

19. World Health Organization (WHO). WHO Task Force on Post-ovulatory Methods of Fertility Regulation. Comparison of two doses of mifepristone in combination with misoprostol for early medical abortion: a randomised trial. *BJOG* 2000; 107: 524–30.

20. European Commission. Council Directive 65/65/EC on the approximation of provisions laid down by law, regulation or administrative action relating to medicinal products. *Official Journal* 1965; 22: 369–73. http://www.echamp.eu/fileadmin/user_upload/Regulation/Directive_65-65-EEC-Consolidated_Version.pdf.

21. World Health Organization. Safe Abortion: technical and policy guidance for health systems, 2nd edn, 2012.

22. Hamoda H, Ashok PW, Flett GM, et al. Medical abortion at 64 to 91 days of gestation: a review of 483 consecutive cases. *Am J Obstet Gynecol* 2003; 188: 1315–9.

23. Ashok PW, Kidd A, Flett GM, et al. A randomized comparison of medical abortion and surgical vacuum aspiration at 10–13 weeks gestation. *Hum Reprod* 2002; 17: 92–8.

24. Webster D, Penney GC, Templeton A. A comparison of 600 and 200 mg mifepristone prior to second trimester abortion with the prostaglandin misoprostol. *Br J Obstet Gynaecol* 1996; 103: 706–9.

25. Bartley J, Baird DT. A randomised study of misoprostol and gemeprost in combination with mifepristone for induction of abortion in the second trimester of pregnancy. *BJOG* 2002; 109: 1290–4.

26. Gemzell-Danielsson K, Lalitkumar S. Second trimester medical abortion with mifepristone-misprostol and misoprostol alone: a review of methods and management. *Reprod Health Matters* 2008; 16(31): 162–72.

27. World Health Organization (WHO). WHO recommendations for Induction of Labour. Geneva: WHO, 2011.

28. Ashok PW, Templeton A, Wagaarachchi PT, et al. Midtrimester medical termination of pregnancy: a review of 1002 consecutive cases. *Contraception* 2004; 69(1): 51–8.

29. Davis VJ. Induced abortion guidelines, Society of Obstetricians and Gynaecologists of Canada clinical practice guidelines No. 184. *J Obstet Gynaecol Can* 2008; 30(11): 1014–27.

30. Hammond C. Recent advances in second-trimester abortion: an evidence-based review. *Am J Obstet Gynecol* 2009; 200(4): 347–56.

31. Berghella V, Airoldi J, O'Neill AM, et al. Misoprostol for second trimester pregnancy termination in women with prior caesarean: a systematic review. *BJOG* 2009; 116(9): 1151–7.

32. Dodd JM, Crowther CA. Misoprostol versus cervagem for the induction of labour to terminate pregnancy in the second and third trimester: a systematic review. *Eur J Obstet Gynecol Reprod Biol* 2006; 125(1): 3–8.

33. Güleç UK, Urunsak IF, Eser E, et al. Misoprostol for midtrimester termination of pregnancy in women with 1 or more prior cesarean deliveries. *Int J of Gynecol Obstet* 2013; 120(1): 85–87.

34. Fawzy M, Abdel-Hady el-S. Midtrimester abortion using vaginal misoprostol for women with three or more prior cesarean deliveries. *Int J Gynecol Obstet* 2010; 110(1): 50–2.

35. Gemzell-Danielsson K, Ostlund E. Termination of second trimester pregnancy with mifepristone and gemeprost. The clinical experience of 197 consecutive cases. *Acta Obstet Gynecol Scand* 2000; 79(8): 702–6.

36. Jackson E, Kapp N. Pain control in first-trimester and second-trimester medical termination of pregnancy: a systematic review. *Contraception* 2011; 83: 116–26.

37. Fiala C, Swahn ML, Stephansson O, et al. The effect of non-steroidal anti-inflammatory drugs on medical

abortion with mifepristone and misoprostol at 13–22 weeks gestation. *Hum Reprod* 2005; 20: 3072–7.

38. Hamoda H, Ashok PW, Flett GM, et al. Analgesia requirements and predictors of analgesia use for women undergoing medical abortion up to 22 weeks of gestation. *BJOG* 2004; 111(9): 996–1000.

39. Tuncalp O, Gülmezoglu AM, Souza JP. Surgical procedures for evacuating incomplete miscarriage. *Cochrane Database Syst Rev* 2010; 9: CD001993.

40. Kulier R, Cheng L, Fekih A, et al. Surgical methods for first trimester termination of pregnancy. *Cochrane Database Syst Rev* 2001; 4: CD002900.

41. Stubblefield PG, Albrecht BH, Koos B, et al. A randomized study of 12 mm and 15.9 mm cannulas in midtrimester abortion by laminaria and vacuum curettage. *Fertil Steril* 1978; 29: 512–7.

42. Kapp N, Lohr PA, Ngo TD, et al. Cervical preparation for first trimester surgical abortion. *Cochrane Database Syst Rev* 2010; 2: CD007207.

43. Newmann SJ, Dalve-Endres A, Diedrich JT, et al. Cervical preparation for second trimester dilation and evacuation. *Cochrane Database Syst Rev* 2010; 8: CD007310.

44. Li CF, Wong CY, Chan CP, et al. A study of co-treatment of nonsteroidal anti-inflammatory drugs (NSAIDs) with misoprostol for cervical priming before suction termination of first trimester pregnancy. *Contraception* 2003; 67: 101–5.

45. Niinimäki M, Pouta A, Bloigu A, et al. Immediate complications after medical compared with surgical termination of pregnancy. *Obstet Gynecol* 2009; 114: 795–804.

46. Grimes DA, Schulz KF. Morbidity and mortality from second-trimester abortions. *J Reprod Med* 1985; 30: 505–14.

47. Ashok PW, Kidd A, Flett GM, et al. A randomized comparison of medical abortion and surgical vacuum aspiration at 10–13 weeks gestation. *Hum Reprod* 2002; 17: 92–8.

48. Neilson JP, Gyte GM, Hickey M, et al. Medical treatments for incomplete miscarriage (less than 24 weeks). *Cochrane Database Syst Rev* 2010; 1: CD007223.

49. Low N, Mueller M, Van Viet HAAM, et al. Perioperative antibiotics to prevent infection after first-trimester abortion. *Cochrane Database Syst Rev* 2012; 3: CD005217.

50. Ho CS, Bhatnagar J, Cohen AL, et al. Undiagnosed cases of fatal Clostridium-associated toxic shock in Californian women of childbearing age. *Am J Obstet Gynecol* 2009; 201: 459–7.

51. Kale SG, Szigetvari IA, Bartfai GS. The frequency and management of uterine perforations during 1st-trimester abortions. *Am J Obstet Gynecol* 1989; 161: 406–8.

52. Rowland Hogue CJ, Terry MPH, Boardman LA, et al. Answering questions about long-term outcomes. In: Paul M, Lichtenberg ES, Borgatta L, et al., (eds). *Management of Unintended and Abnormal Pregnancy: Comprehensive Abortion Care*. Hoboken, NJ: Wiley-Blackwell, 2009: 252–63.

Chapter

20

Post-abortion care

Kristina Naidoo

After undergoing induced abortion for fetal abnormality, a woman's ongoing physical, psychologic and practical needs should be addressed[1].

Post-abortion investigations

If further tests are required to confirm a diagnosis of fetal abnormality, they should be discussed and verbal consent obtained. These may include fetal chromosome analysis. If a postmortem is considered necessary, informed consent from the woman must be obtained. The options of a limited or external examination by a perinatal pathologist or geneticist can be offered if a full postmortem examination is declined. Once consent for a postmortem has been given, there should be a "cooling off" period to allow the woman to change her mind within a specified time[2].

Rhesus antibody prophylaxis

The UK Royal College of Obstetricians and Gynaecologists (RCOG) recommends that anti-D immunoglobulin G (IgG) immunoprophylaxis should be given within 72 h of an induced abortion to all Rhesus (Rh)-negative women regardless of gestation unless they are already sensitized[3]. Whilst there is little evidence to support anti-D prophylaxis in the first trimester, some studies indicate that the volume of a fetomaternal hemorrhage is potentially sufficient to cause sensitization[4]. The UK RCOG therefore recommends anti-D prophylaxis as routine in the first trimester[3].

The recommended dose of anti-D IgG is 250 international units (IU) before 20 weeks' gestation and 500 IU thereafter. For abortions undertaken after 20 weeks gestation, the volume of fetomaternal hemorrhage should be assessed. If the test indicates a fetomaternal

hemorrhage of >4 mL, an additional 125 IU of anti-D IgG per mL should be administered[3].

Lactation suppression

Women undergoing an abortion from the second trimester onwards should be informed about the possibility that lactation may be initiated. Treatments such as the use of a support brassiere, application of ice packs to engorged breasts and simple analgesia may be effective, but some women will experience severe discomfort[5]. Dopamine agonists have been shown to suppress lactation. Carbegoline appears superior to bromocriptene as it has fewer side effects and is a once daily dosage[6]. Dopamine agonists are contraindicated in women with hypertension or pre-eclampsia. Estrogen is of unproven benefit and increases the risk of thromboembolism. A recent Cochrane review found that there is weak evidence that pharmacologic treatments are better than no treatment in the 1st week and no evidence that nonpharmacologic approaches are more effective than no treatment[7].

Fertility and contraception

Information about fertility and contraception should be offered to women. Ovulation may occur as early as 2 weeks after an abortion so they should be advised about the possibility they could conceive before their next period[8].

Contraceptive supplies should be provided if required. Intrauterine contraceptives can be inserted immediately following medical and surgical abortion at all gestations. A systematic review of the literature concluded that the provision of combined oral contraceptives immediately following surgical or medical abortion was safe[9]. Use of the combined

Fetal Medicine, ed. Bidyut Kumar and Zarko Alfirevic. Published by Cambridge University Press. © Cambridge University Press 2016.

oral contraceptive pill does not affect either duration or amount of vaginal bleeding or the complete abortion rate.

The World Health Organization recommends that progestogen-only contraceptive pills, implants and injectables can all be started immediately following induced abortion; if started on the day of the abortion, contraceptive protection is immediate[10].

Psychologic sequelae

A woman or couple's emotional needs should be addressed immediately following an abortion for fetal abnormality.

Staff caring for women undergoing medical abortion for fetal abnormality must be sensitive to the fact that some women or couples may express a wish to see or hold the fetus. They should be made aware of the possible appearance of the fetus with respect to the gestational age and any structural abnormalities. They may wish to have mementoes, such as hand and footprints and photographs, and if not, staff should offer to store them securely in the case records for future access. Keeping such mementoes has not been associated with adverse outcomes and qualitative studies have shown that many couples value them highly[11].

Induced abortion for fetal abnormality can have significant psychologic consequences. In a longitudinal study, 4 months after abortion, 46% of 147 women showed pathologic levels of post-traumatic stress symptoms, decreasing to 20% after 16 months. Depression scores were 28% and 13% at 4 and 16 months, respectively. The most important predictor of persistent impaired psychologic outcome was outcome at 4 months; other predictors were low self-efficacy, high levels of doubt during decision making, lack of partner support, being religious and advanced gestational age. Strong feelings of regret for the decision were mentioned by only 2.7% of women[12].

It is also associated with long-lasting consequences for a substantial number of women. A cross-sectional study of 254 women, 2–7 years after induced abortion for fetal abnormality under 24 weeks of gestation, showed that women generally adapted well to grief. However, a substantial number of the participants (17.3%) had high scores for post-traumatic stress. Women who experienced little support from their partners and were low educated had the most unfavorable psychologic outcome. Advanced gestational age at the time of

abortion was associated with higher levels of grief, and post-traumatic stress symptoms and long-term psychologic morbidity were rare with abortions before 14 weeks of gestation[13].

Women's emotional and psychologic needs must therefore be addressed both immediately after the abortion and in the longer term. Referral should be available to any woman who may require additional support, including the possibility of self-referral.

There should also be an awareness that partners may experience adverse psychologic sequelae, such as extreme grief reactions and post-traumatic stress disorder[11].

Sensitive disposal of fetal tissue

All fetal tissue under 24 weeks of gestation, whether resulting from miscarriage or induced abortion, must be treated with dignity and respect[14]. Local policies should reflect the Human Tissue Authorities Code of Practice 5, "Disposal of human tissue for fetuses born dead at or before 24 weeks of gestation"[15]. Whilst fetal tissue from a pregnancy under 24 weeks may be incinerated, by the year 2000 this practice was felt to be unacceptable by health professionals working within this area[14]. Most UK National Health Service hospital trusts therefore developed policies and practices for the sensitive disposal of fetal tissue under 24 weeks of gestation[16].

A woman or couple should be informed about the options for disposal. This information must be freely available, taking into account any particular needs of the woman or couple, such as literacy skills and language. Verbal and written information should be provided by trained health professionals. The information should specify who a woman or couple should contact if they would like to request a particular option and in what timescale[17]. Many hospitals have specific staff, such as bereavement support officers, to fulfill this role.

Staff should be sensitive to the values and beliefs of a wide range of cultures and religions, particularly those of their local community. However, they should be aware that each decision is one for the individual concerned. A hospital should ensure that the necessary training and support is given so that staff are equipped to identify and meet the widest possible range of needs and wishes[14].

Some women or couples may not wish to receive information about, or take part in, the disposal of the fetal tissue. Provided that they have been made aware that the information is available, these wishes should be respected. It should be clearly documented in the woman's medical notes whether information has been requested or not and, if so, whether it has been given[17].

It is acknowledged that sometimes parents do not recognize their loss at the time, but may return months or even years later to enquire about disposal arrangements. It is therefore important that there is a well-documented audit trail to provide those details if needed at a later date[14]. Confidentiality must be ensured and it should not be possible to identify any individual from the information held by a crematorium or place of burial.

The hospital is responsible for the disposal of fetal remains. Both burial and cremation should be available to allow for cultural and religious differences. Hospital disposal usually involves communal cremation and burial. The hospital provides funding and makes the arrangements. The woman or couple should be informed and involved as appropriate and they and their family can choose whether to attend or not. In Scotland, there is an issue of whether multiple cremation and burial is allowed. Local policies may preclude it and if problems are encountered, advice can be sought from the Institute of Cemetery and Crematorium Management [14].

The woman or couple should be made aware that they can arrange a private burial or cremation themselves if they wish but that they may have to incur some or all of the costs. The UK Royal College of Nursing guidance for nurses and midwives on *Sensitive Disposal of All Fetal Remains* (2007) looks at the options[14]. The hospital should facilitate the arrangements and provide the necessary documentation. The woman or couple may wish to involve members of their religious community. There is no legal prohibition to burial outside a cemetery but certain requirements must be met. For instance, it must not cause a danger to the public, risk contamination of water supplies and must be buried to a depth of at least 45 cm.

Many hospitals provide a book of remembrance that is kept in a significant place, usually the hospital chapel. Parents should be informed of this and be aware that they can arrange for an entry to be placed in the book at any time. It is becoming commonplace to offer a regular service of remembrance to which couples are invited to attend. The format of this service should reflect the cultural, spiritual and diverse needs of the community the hospital serves.

Some units have developed a checklist to ensure that all the necessary information has been discussed. Timing is important in discussing issues about disposal arrangements. Guidance should be taken from experienced staff as to the most appropriate time. Many hospitals are looking at the issue of consent for disposal; some are including it on the consent form for the procedure or on a consent form for histologic examination[14].

Discharge

When a woman is ready to be discharged, there must be a clear well-organized plan for her follow-up and ongoing care. Women have reported inadequacies in aftercare that have tested their psychologic resources[18].

Verbal and written information should be provided about symptoms that a woman may experience after an induced abortion and how to recognize complications, particularly those that require urgent medical consultation. The medication required should be prescribed before the woman leaves the hospital.

The woman should be provided with contact details for clinical advice to contact hospital staff responsible for disposal arrangements, such as the bereavement support officer and relevant administration staff.

All key staff responsible for the care of the woman during pregnancy and afterwards should be informed about the outcome. Timely and appropriate communication between the hospital and primary care team is essential. The general practitioner must be informed when the woman is to be discharged and a home visit by the community midwife should be offered[19]. There should be a reliable system for ensuring that all existing hospital and community appointments are cancelled[1].

Follow-up appointment

The follow-up appointment needs careful management. Many women find it difficult to return to the hospital and this will be exacerbated if they are asked to wait in a busy antenatal clinic with expectant mothers[1].

An appointment to discuss postmortem results, if applicable, should be arranged as soon as possible. Any unavoidable delays must be explained to the woman or couple and the stress this may cause acknowledged. Many women will be anxious about this appointment because of the potential implications for future pregnancies. At the appointment with the obstetrician, the postmortem findings should be discussed and the risk of recurrence of a fetal abnormality clarified. It may be necessary to obtain additional genetic advice. If there are options for interventions to reduce the risk of a recurrence, such as high-dose folic acid therapy, these should be discussed. A provisional plan for antenatal diagnosis in a subsequent pregnancy should be drawn up. The next pregnancy is likely to cause anxiety for most women and will require sensitive management, with a care plan agreed as early in the pregnancy as possible[1].

References

1. Royal College of Obstetricians and Gynaecologists (RCOG). Termination of Pregnancy for Fetal Abnormality in England, Scotland and Wales. Report of a Working Party. London: RCOG Press, 2010.

2. Human Tissue Authority. The Sands perinatal post-mortem consent package, 2013. www.hta.gov.uk/licensingandinspections/sectorspecificinformation/postmortem/perinatalpostmortem/thesandsperinatalpostmortemconsentpackage.

3. Royal College of Obstetricians and Gynaecologists (RCOG). The Use of Anti-D Immunoglobulin for Rhesus D Prophylaxis. London: RCOG Press, 2011. http://www.rcog.org.uk/womens-health/clinical-guidance/ use-anti-d-immunoglobulin-rh-prophylaxis-green-top-22.

4. Jabara S, Barnhart KT. Is Rh immune globulin needed in early first-trimester abortion? A review. *Am J Obstet Gynecol* 2003; 188: 623–7.

5. Spitz AM, Lee NC, Peterson HB. Treatment for lactation suppression: little progress in one hundred years. *Am J Obstet Gynecol* 1998; 179: 1485–90.

6. European Multicentre Study Group for Cabergoline in Lactation Inhibition. Single dose cabergoline versus bromocriptine in inhibition of puerperal lactation: randomised, double blind, multicentre study. *BMJ* 1991; 302: 1367–71.

7. Oladapo OT, Fawole B. Treatment for suppression of lactation. *Cochrane Database Syst Rev* 2012; (9): CD005937.

8. Kremer JA, van der Heijden PF, Schellekens LA, et al. Postpartum return of pituitary and ovarian activity during lactation inhibition with the new dopamine agonist CV 205–502 and during normal lactation. *Acta Endocrinol (Copenh)* 1990; 122: 759–65.

9. Gaffield ME, Kapp N, Ravi A. Use of combined oral contraceptives post abortion. *Contraception* 2009; 80: 355–62.

10. World Health Organization (WHO). Selected practice recommendations for contraceptive use, 2nd edn. Geneva: WHO, 2004. http://whqlibdoc.who.int/publications/2004/9241562846.pdf.

11. Royal College of Obstetricians and Gynaecologists (RCOG). Late Intrauterine Fetal Death and Stillbirth. Green-Top Guideline No. 55. London: RCOG Press, 2010.

12. Korenromp MJ, Page-Christiaens GC, van den Bout J, et al. Adjustment to termination of pregnancy for fetal anomaly: a longitudinal study in women at 4, 8, and 16 months. *Am J Obstet Gynecol* 2009; 201(2): 160 e1–7.

13. Korenromp MJ, Page-Christiaens GC, van den Bout J, et al. Long-term psychological consequences of pregnancy termination for fetal abnormality: a cross-sectional study. *Prenat Diagn.* 2005; 25(3): 253–60.

14. Royal College of Nursing (RCN). Sensitive disposal of fetal remains. London: RCN, 2007. http://www.rcn.org.uk/__data/assets/pdf_file/0020/78500/001248.pdf.

15. Human Tissue Authority (HTA). Code of Practice 5 – Disposal of human tissue: Disposal following pregnancy loss. London: HTA, 2009.

16. Royal College of Obstetricians and Gynaecologists (RCOG). Disposal following pregnancy loss before 24 weeks of gestation. Good Practice No. 5. London: RCOG Press, 2005. http://www.rcog.org.uk/womens-health/clinical-guidance/disposal-following-pregnancy-loss-24-weeks-gestation.

17. Stillbirth and Neonatal Death Society. Pregnancy Loss and the Death of a Baby: Guidelines for Professionals, 2007. http://www.uk-sands.org/professionals/resources-for-health-professionals/the-sands-guidelines.

18. Lafarge C, Mitchell K, Fox P. Women's experiences of coping with pregnancy termination for fetal abnormality. *Qual Health Res* 2013; 23(7): 924–36.

19. Statham H, Solomou W, Green JM. *When the Baby has an Abnormality: A Study of Parents' Experiences.* Cambridge: Centre for Family Research, University of Cambridge, 2001.

Fetal growth disorders

Ai-Wei Tang and Umber Agarwal

Growth is a complex, dynamic process that starts from conception. A fertilized egg goes through multiple cycles of duplication and differentiation, followed by cell hyperplasia and hypertrophy in the uterus, to form a baby that is ready to be born. The growth pattern is commonly divided into three stages.

(1) The first stage occurs throughout the first trimester up to 20 weeks gestation and involves rapid cell division and hyperplasia, with cell differentiation and period of organogenesis. Thus, there is not much fetal weight gain with an average growth rate of about 5 g/day.

(2) In the second stage from 20–28 weeks, there is a mixture of cell hyperplasia and hypertrophy, with an average growth rate of 15–20 g/day.

(3) In the third stage from 28 weeks until term, the pattern of growth is cell hypertrophy that is associated with accumulation of fat, muscle and connective tissue in the fetus. This is a period of greatest weight gain, expected to be about 30–35 g/day.

This intricate process is controlled by a wide range of factors including genetic potential for growth, maternal health and nutrition, placental perfusion and function, fetal condition, and environmental factors. Changes to any of these factors can result in fetal growth disorders. About 20% of all babies are born at the extremes of birthweight, either small for gestational age (SGA) or large for dates (LFD). However, many of these are not diagnosed antenatally due to failure in identifying at risk pregnancies and lack of a robust screening strategy. Furthermore, studies are hampered from the inconsistencies in the definition of growth disorders. Yet, accurate prenatal assessment of fetal growth is essential to identify these fetuses for appropriate monitoring and intervention, which can result in improved pregnancy outcomes.

Definition of fetal growth disorders

Small for gestational age

The World Health Organization (WHO) defines SGA as a birthweight of less than 2500 g at term. Another common definition is the failure of the fetus to achieve a weight threshold, usually defined as the 10th centile. An estimated fetal weight (EFW) or abdominal circumference (AC) of <10th centile with no other abnormal parameters, will categorize a fetus as SGA. Commonly, severe SGA is defined as an EFW or AC of <3rd centile. However, these definitions do not take into account growth velocity and include a proportion of babies who are constitutionally small, thus normal and healthy. Although as a group, all SGA fetuses are at increased risk of perinatal morbidity and mortality, most adverse outcomes occur in fetuses that are growth restricted.

Fetal growth restriction

Fetal growth restriction (FGR) is defined as a failure to reach their genetic growth potential due to some pathologic reason. It is difficult to diagnose whether a fetus is constitutionally SGA or FGR from a single assessment. The use of customized growth charts (discussed below) would reduce the incidence of physiologically small fetuses being labeled as FGR. The common definition of FGR is a SGA fetus that has shown signs of compromise, either with decreased growth velocity, reduced liquor volume or abnormal Doppler studies. Although most FGR are SGA, a small proportion is of appropriate size for gestational age. However, FGR that is of appropriate

Fetal Medicine, ed. Bidyut Kumar and Zarko Alfirevic. Published by CAMBRIDGE UNIVERSITY PRESS. © Cambridge University Press 2016.

Table 21.1 Comparison between early onset and late onset FGR[1]

	Early onset FGR	Late onset FGR
FGR onset	<34 weeks' gestation	From about 33 weeks' gestation
Pathology	Placental bed pathology Inadequate vascular modeling leading to infarcts and insufficiency	Placental development pathology – placental villous immaturity and villous hypoplasia
Clinical association	Associated with hypertensive disorders and PET	Not associated with hypertensive disorders
Monitoring	UA Dopplers	UA Dopplers not useful for monitoring - possibility of using MCA Dopplers
Challenge	Difficulty in management	Difficulty in diagnosis

FGR, fetal growth restriction; MCA, middle cerebral artery; PET, pre-eclampsia; UA, umbilical artery.

gestational weight appear not to have as many adverse outcomes as those that are both FGR and SGA. FGR is currently classified into early onset (<34 weeks gestation) and late onset (>34 weeks gestation). They are two distinct entities of different etiology, pathology, and management strategies (Table 21.1)[1]. Accurate diagnosis of FGR is important as increased surveillance and timely intervention may improve the outcome.

Large for dates

At the other extreme are 10% of fetuses born as LFD, which is commonly defined as a birthweight of more than 4,000 g and termed "macrosomic." Prenatal diagnosis of macrosomic babies remains challenging despite the availability of modern ultrasound machines. It was previously thought that macrosomic babies only pose a problem of maternal or fetal injury at delivery, but evidence is emerging that being LFD is also associated with increased morbidity and mortality, and has implications for future health risks. Although risk factors exist for macrosomia, no combination can predict macrosomia adequately for it to be used clinically. Moreover, many LFD infants have no risk factors.

Etiology of fetal growth disorders

The determination of fetal size is multifactorial and can be divided into maternal, fetal or environmental factors. Failure of one or combination of any of these factors results in abnormal fetal growth (Table 21.2).

Maternal factors

The development of a healthy placenta, vital in maintaining adequate fetal growth, involves invasion and remodeling of the maternal spiral arteries by fetal trophoblast cells. Ideally, this results in a low-resistance circulation, promoting increased blood supply to the placental bed. Any chronic maternal vascular conditions that contribute to abnormal placentation or reduced blood supply to the placental bed can cause FGR. The most common of these are hypertensive disorders, including pre-eclampsia. However, antiphospholipid syndrome appears to carry the highest risk of FGR[2]. Diabetes is more commonly associated with fetal overgrowth, but there is risk of FGR if it is complicated by microvascular disease such as nephropathy. Some examples of other chronic diseases that are associated with FGR are listed in Table 21.2. Placental mosaicism, commonly associated with chromosome 16 and 22 is related to a reduced placental bulk and function, resulting in FGR.

Maternal conditions such as obesity and its associated metabolic changes, including type 2 and gestational diabetes, can result in a baby who is LFD. A macrosomic baby is a sign of poorly controlled diabetes, due to hyperglycemia in the fetus. This stimulates insulin, insulin-like growth factor, growth hormone and other growth factors, which results in stimulation of fetal growth and deposition of fat and glycogen. This theory also holds true for risk of LFD if there is excessive weight gain in pregnancy.

Fetal factors

Fetal chromosomal abnormalities or genetic syndromes are other causes of SGA. The earlier the SGA is detected, the higher the association with chromosomal problems. Congenital anomalies, such as omphalocoele, may increase the risk of chromosomal defects further or may be an independent reason for SGA. Most fetuses of higher order pregnancies are smaller, but may not be FGR.

Table 21.2 Causes of fetal growth disorders

	Small for gestational age	Large for dates (macrosomia)
Maternal	Hypertensive disorders (including pre-eclampsia)	Diabetes
	Thrombophilic disease (e.g., APS or thrombophilia)	Obesity
	Renal disease	Excessive weight gain in pregnancy
	Diabetes	
	Chronic diseases (e.g., anemia, sickle cell disease, SLE, IBD)	
	Placental mosaicism	
Fetal	Chromosomal or genetic abnormalities (e.g., trisomies, Silver–Russell syndrome)	Genetic abnormalities (e.g., Beckwith–Wiedermann syndrome)
	Structural abnormalities (e.g., omphalocoele, gastroshisis)	Post-dates pregnancy
	Multiple pregnancy	
Environmental	Congenital infections (e.g., CMV, toxoplasmosis, rubella, syphillis)	
	Smoking	
	Alcohol	
	Cocaine	
	Poor nutrition	

APS, antiphospholipid syndrome; CMV, cytomegalovirus; IBD, inflammatory bowel disease; SLE, systemic lupus erythematosus.

Although most genetic syndromes are associated with SGA fetus, Beckwith–Wiedermann syndrome is associated with fetal overgrowth. There are usually other features on ultrasound findings, such as macroglossia, organomegaly and abnormal digits, that raise the suspicion of this syndrome in a macrosomic fetus. A fetus that is of advanced gestational age may be large as fetal growth continues in utero.

Environmental factors

Reduced fetal growth is commonly seen in congenital infections, such as cytomegalovirus (CMV), syphilis or rubella. The most common of these is primary CMV infection, which occurs in 1% of the population. There is extensive evidence that both maternal smoking and passive smoking is associated with SGA fetuses. Similarly, alcohol and cocaine use are also linked to being SGA. The National Institute for Health and Clinical Excellence (NICE) in the UK has recommended that women should limit alcohol intake to 1–2 units (1 unit = ½ pint of ordinary strength beer or 25 ml of spirit) once or twice a week.

Screening and diagnosis

Accurate prenatal assessment to identify pregnancies, which may result in abnormal fetal growth, is important to allow for increased fetal monitoring and timely intervention if necessary. Prior to making any diagnosis, it is of upmost importance that the pregnancy has been accurately dated, and the fetus is of the right gestational age. The best method to date a pregnancy is by ultrasound measurements of the crown–rump length in the first trimester.

History

Many risk factors for growth disorders such as advanced maternal age, nulliparity, extremes of body mass index, smoking and poor diet, can be identified at the booking appointment. It is also important to enquire about maternal health status, in particular, chronic diseases and details of previous pregnancies and complications such as SGA or stillbirths.

Customized charts

Growth and birthweights vary with maternal characteristics such as weight at first antenatal-clinic visit, height, parity, and ethnic origin, and other factors, including birthweight of previous babies and fetal sex. However, antenatal population growth charts do not take into account these variables. A growth chart should be computer-generated and "customized" for each individual during pregnancy, taking into consideration the factors stated above[3]. An example is the gestation related optimal weight (GROW) customized

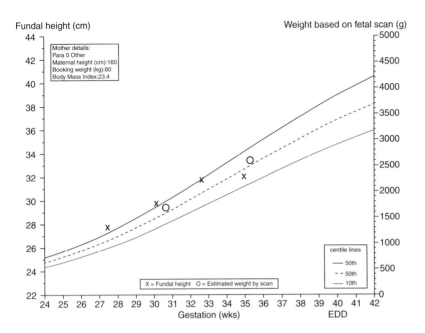

Figure 21.1 Example of a completed customized growth chart.

charts developed by the Perinatal Institute (www.gestation-net.com) for charting symphyseal fundal height (SFH) and EFW (Figure 21.1).

SFH measurements from abdominal palpation involve measuring the distance from the fundus of the uterus to the symphisis pubis, and the distance in centimeters plotted on a customized chart. Unfortunately, SFH measurements have a low sensitivity (27–83%), high intraobserver variability and high false-positive rates for detection of SGA or LFD fetuses, potentially due to inaccuracies from factors such as obesity, lie of fetus, hydramnios, large fibroids and measurements by different practitioners[4]. A single measurement that plots <10th centile, serial measurements that show static growth or cross centiles, or serial measurements that show accelerated growth, should be referred for an ultrasound assessment for EFW and hydramnios, and charted.

On normal population charts, up to 50% of fetuses in the <10th centile category would be normal and constitutionally small. Customized growth charts have reduced the incidence of the normally small fetus, and doubled the detection of FGR from 20–50%. Identification of these FGR pregnancies for appropriate intervention is starting to impact on an improvement in perinatal outcomes, especially reduction in stillbirth rates[5]. The same principle also applies in macrosomia where the baby has exceeded its growth

potential if growth plots above the 90th centile on the customized chart. The ultrasound assessment will address the issue of fetal size and polyhydramnios, and should prompt a re-evaluation of the fetus for structural anomalies.

The International Fetal and Newborn Growth Consortium for the 21st Century Project has recently published international growth and size standards for fetuses in a multicenter, population-based setting in eight countries where health and nutritional needs for mothers were met and adequate antenatal care was provided[6]. Named the Fetal Longitudinal Growth Study (FLGS), five ultrasound-based fetal anthropometric measurements were prospectively measured from 14 weeks until birth. The 3rd, 5th, 10th, 50th, 90th, 95th and 97th centile curves were generated for these ultrasound measures, representing the international standards for fetal growth. The researchers found that fetal growth and newborn size at birth were very similar across countries, if the mothers were healthy and well educated. The findings of the study challenge the widely held belief that race and ethnicity are primary factors for weight at birth.

Since publication of the study, there has been widespread debate on the need to customize fetal growth charts based on maternal variables and whether "one size fits all." More research is currently needed to address this issue.

Maternal serum screening

In view of the placental origin, several biochemical markers, such as alpha-fetoprotein (AFP), human chorionic gonadotropin (hCG), inhibin A, unconjugated estriol (uE3), and pregnancy associated plasma protein-A (PAPP-A), were investigated for screening tests for SGA. Abnormal AFP (>2.5 multiples of the median (MoM) or <0.25 MoM), raised hCG (>3 MoM), and inhibin A (≥2 MoM), low uE3 (<0.5 MoM) and triple test are found to be associated with increased adverse obstetric outcomes, but are of low predictive value for SGA fetuses in systematic reviews[7].

In the first trimester, there is evidence that low PAPP-A (<0.4 MoM) and/or low hCG (<0.5 MoM) are associated with SGA. In view of this, the UK RCOG have included low PAPP-A as a major risk factor for SGA where serial growth and assessment scans are needed throughout pregnancy[2].

There are no serum markers that have been investigated for associations with the fetus that are LFD.

Fetal echogenic bowel

Bright or echogenic fetal bowel at the 20-week anomaly scan is an independent risk factor for SGA and intrauterine death (IUD)[8]. In view of this, serial growth scans and close monitoring is recommended if this is found[2].

Ultrasound assessments

Serial fetal biometry

Ultrasound biometry measurements commonly include head circumference, biparietal diameter, AC and femur length, which will allow an EFW to be calculated from a formula. Of all parameters, fetal AC (<10th centile) has the highest sensitivity for identifying SGA fetuses. However, not all of these fetuses will have low birthweight, and may have unnecessary intervention if AC <10th centile alone were used to identify SGA fetuses. The accuracy of diagnosing SGA increases when both the AC and calculated EFW are <10th centile, and this group of fetuses are at higher risk of perinatal morbidity[9]. There are currently more than 30 published formulas for calculating EFW, taking into account different biometric parameters. Although there are considerable variations in the accuracy, they are generally acceptable for birthweights up to 3500 g. Most formulas overestimate SGA fetuses and underestimate LFD fetuses. In a population

at high risk of SGA, the sensitivity for detection ranged from 72–100%, while specificity was 41–88%. In this high-risk population, the Hadlock formula appears to have the optimal sensitivity/specificity trade-off in the detection for SGA[10].

A single set of fetal biometry <10th centile will not distinguish between a constitutionally SGA fetus and FGR. Thus, assessment should include repeated fetal biometry measurements and EFW, charted at each scan to assess for the pattern of fetal growth. There is no consensus on the frequency or optimal time interval between scans. If the aim of two different scans is to measure growth velocity, the interval should be at least 3 weeks to minimize false-positives diagnosis of FGR from scan error.

Liquor volume assessment

The liquor volume can be reported as maximum pool depth (MPD), a single measurement of the deepest vertical pocket of liquor, or amniotic fluid index (AFI), the sum of vertical measurement of liquor in four quadrants of the uterus. A Cochrane review has shown that when AFI was used, there were more diagnoses of oligohydramnios, leading to intervention of induction of labor and cesarean delivery for fetal distress without evidence of improvements in adverse peripartum outcomes, such as admission to neonatal intensive care unit, umbilical artery pH <7.1, and Apgar score <7 at 5 min. Thus, it is recommended that MPD is used as the tool to assess liquor volume[11]. An abnormality that requires further investigation would be MPD of <2 cm or >10 cm.

Uterine artery Doppler

An abnormal uterine artery (UtA) Doppler velocimetry (pulsatility index (PI) >95th centile, mean PI >1.45, and/or notching) correlates with high resistance in the maternal arterial blood supply to the placental bed, secondary to poor trophoblast invasion and remodeling of the maternal spiral arteries (Figures 21.2 and 21.3). A systematic review of 61 studies reported good predictive value of FGR if the UtA Doppler was abnormal with or without notching at 20–24 weeks[12]. In the majority of cases of abnormal UtA Doppler at 20–24 weeks, the PI remains raised when the test is repeated at 26–28 weeks gestation. Even if the PI normalizes, there is still an increased risk of FGR, and thus repeating UtA Dopplers at a later gestation is of limited value. Instead, a surveillance strategy should be in place to identify when FGR occurs.

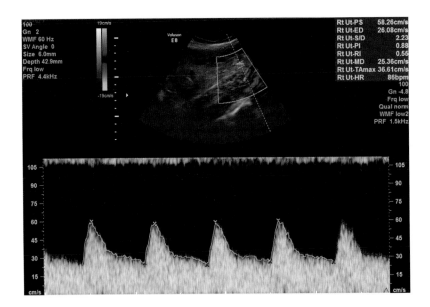

Figure 21.2 Normal uterine artery Doppler waveform.

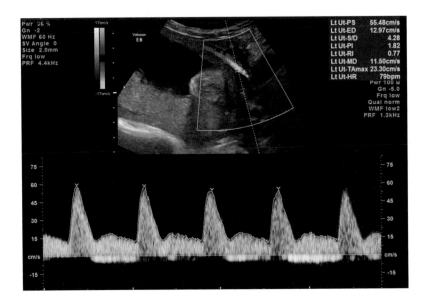

Figure 21.3 Abnormal uterine artery Doppler waveform with notching.

Fetal Dopplers

Referral for further assessment of detailed Doppler studies depends on the customized growth chart pattern where consecutive measurements show either tapering of growth, static growth or exponential growth. Doppler studies could include umbilical artery (UA), middle cerebral artery (MCA), aortic isthmus, and venous circulation such as ductus venosus (DV), umbilical vein or inferior vena cava to allow for an assessment of the fetal and maternal circulation. Arterial Dopplers assess the placental function and

fetal vasoregulation, while venous Dopplers provide information about fetal cardiac function. The commonly used Dopplers in the surveillance of high-risk pregnancies are UA, MCA and DV Dopplers[13].

There should be a low-resistance system with forward flow throughout the cardiac cycle in a normal pregnancy. The UA Doppler evaluates placental function and advancing severity of fetoplacental impairment leads to the progressive increase in the PI and resistence index of the UA Dopplers from a normal waveform to absent end-diastolic flow (EDF), to reversed EDF

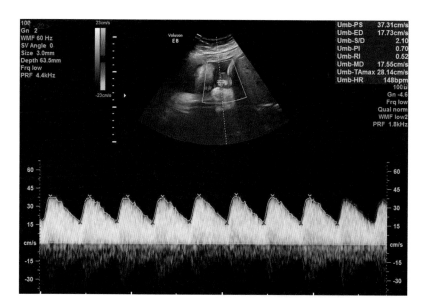

Figure 21.4 Normal umbilical artery waveform.

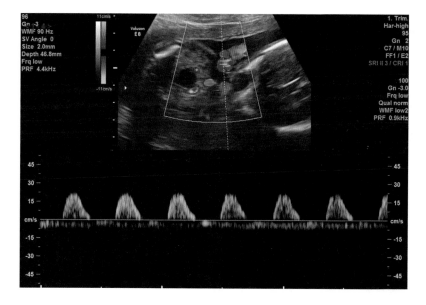

Figure 21.5 Absent end-diastolic flow in the umbilical artery waveform.

(Figures 21.4– 21.6). A systematic review of 18 studies on more than 10,000 women showed that use of UA Doppler in monitoring high-risk pregnancies, including SGA, was associated with a reduction in perinatal death from 1.7–1.2% (relative risk 0.71, 95% confidence interval 0.52–0.98), with fewer inductions of labor and cesarean sections[14]. Therefore, as a minimum, UA Doppler should be performed with all serial growth scans.

An abnormal flow pattern in the UA Doppler may lead to redistribution of blood flow to allow better oxygenation to vital organs, such as the brain and heart, leading to the "brain-sparing" effect. This is demonstrated by a reduced resistance to blood flow in the MCA (Figures 21.7 and 21.8). Another screening parameter is the cerebroplacental ratio (CPR), which is a measure of two Doppler indices, MCA PI/UA PI, and has been demonstrated to be more sensitive to fetal hypoxia[15]. A decreasing CPR suggests fetal compromise and correlates better with adverse outcome compared to its individual measurements.

Blood flow velocity patterns across the aortic isthmus is another modality of assessing fetal circulation.

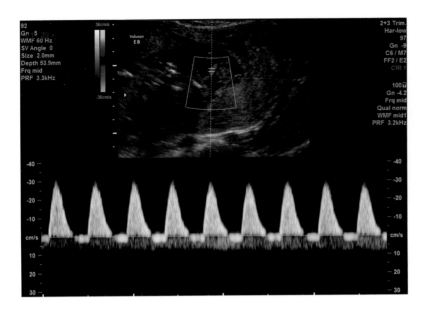

Figure 21.6 Reversed end-diastolic flow in the umbilical artery waveform.

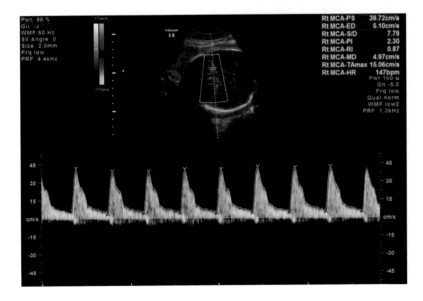

Figure 21.7 Normal middle cerebral artery waveform.

Aortic Doppler reflects the balance between the fetal right and left ventricle outputs, influenced by resistance to flow in the placenta and cerebral vascular systems. There should be forward flow in diastole as placental resistance should be lower than the cerebral circulation. However, in FGR, there is redistribution of cardiac output due to increased placental resistance and failure of the fetus to compensate, leading to retrograde flow in diastole. Unfortunately, it is technically difficult to sample this Doppler waveform reliably and consistently, which has led to a limitation in its clinical application.

Fetal vein Dopplers provide a direct reflection of the fetal heart function, and changes in waveforms are consistent with fetal cardiovascular adaptation mechanisms. The most commonly used venous Doppler is the DV, which is a four-phase waveform that is important in regulating distribution of oxygen and nutrition. The "a" wave, synonymous with atrial contraction of the fetal heart, is the common parameter used for monitoring in FGR. As FGR progresses, the rising cardiac afterload reduces forward venous flow during right atrial contraction, causing the a-wave to become progressively

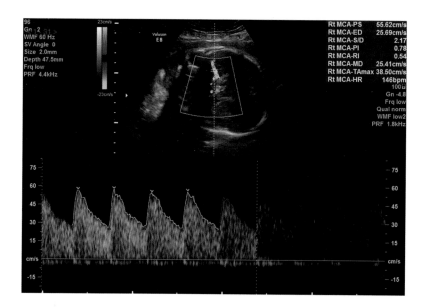

Figure 21.8 Middle cerebral artery with reduced pulsatility index consistent with the brain-sparing effect.

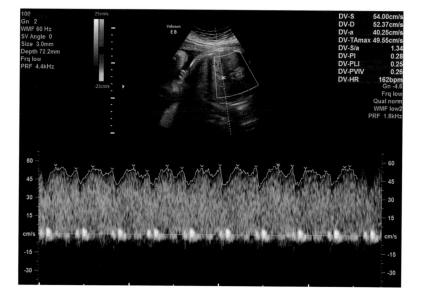

Figure 21.9 Normal ductus venosus waveform.

deeper (Figures 21.9 and 21.10). A reversed a-wave signifies heart failure and cardiac decompensation. The umbilical vein (UV) should be of constant velocity of flow to the fetus. In a compromised fetus, there may be retrograde pulsatility in the UV, which is commonly seen at the same degree of compromise when there is reversed a-wave in the DV. These findings are preterminal, indicating a need for immediate delivery, and associated with fetal acidosis and mortality[16]. The inferior vena cava Doppler waveform has also been investigated in monitoring compromised

fetuses. However, there is a wide variation in the indices measured, including retrograde flow in a normal fetus, which makes interpretation difficult, and thus is not commonly used.

Cardiotocography

Another means of antenatal monitoring is cardiotocography (CTG). Interpretation of conventional CTG can be subjective, but development of computerized fetal heart rate analysis systems has allowed automated

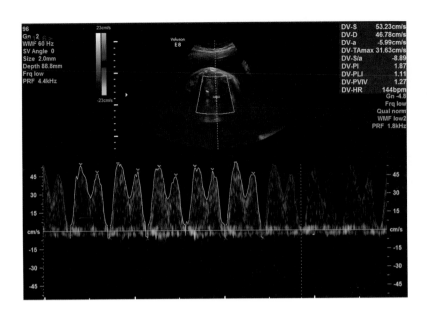

Figure 21.10 Absent a-wave in the ductus venosus waveform.

evaluation of the CTG through numerical indices, which is more reliable. Unlike conventional CTG, computerized CTG (cCTG) is more objective and consistent, and has been shown to reduce perinatal mortality, when compared with conventional CTG[17].

Special consideration has been given to the short-term variation (STV) in the analysis by cCTG, which is a reliable indicator of fetal wellbeing, and correlates with acidemia in the fetus (Figure 21.11). A decreasing STV correlated with earlier deliveries, lower birthweights, lower UA pH at birth, worse acid–base status at birth and worse postnatal outcome. Therefore, cCTG is commonly used in the monitoring of SGA fetuses and is one of the parameters used for timing delivery in a compromised fetus. An STV of ≤3 ms within 24 h of delivery is associated with higher metabolic acidemia (54.2% versus 10.5%) and early neonatal death (8.3% versus 0.5%), and is thus another parameter used to trigger delivery[18].

Management of fetal growth disorders

When risk factors for SGA are identified, aspirin should be started as soon as possible, as aspirin started prior to 16 weeks gestation halves the the risk of SGA[19]. If started later, it may not have an impact on fetal growth, but may be beneficial in the prevention of pre-eclampsia. There is as yet no treatment that has been proven to reduce SGA. Antithrombotic treatment with heparin appears promising but it has not been proven to improve perinatal mortality or reduce

preterm birth. In high-risk pregnancies identified for monitoring, serial growth scans and Doppler assessments should be arranged for throughout pregnancy and the frequency of monitoring tailored to the type of growth disorders.

After the diagnosis of SGA or LFD is made, investigations are carried out to try identifying a cause. When SGA is detected at an early gestation, karyotyping should be offered to exclude chromosomal abnormalities, particularly in the presence of other structural anomalies and normal UtA Dopplers. In high-risk populations, testing to exclude infection should be considered. If a chromosomal abnormality or infection is confirmed, those pregnancies are managed accordingly. A glucose tolerance test should be arranged for in LFD pregnancies, or if there is polyhydramnios.

Effective monitoring of fetal wellbeing remains a mainstay of current management. The aim is to identify signs of fetal compromise and then decide on the optimal timing for delivery. An ultrasound assessment is the most common tool used for monitoring as described above. The frequency of monitoring and number of parameters used will depend on whether the fetus is physiologically small, has late-onset FGR, early-onset FGR or is LFD (Figure 21.12).

Management of the constitutionally SGA fetus

A constitutionally SGA fetus may become FGR at any time point by showing reduced growth velocity,

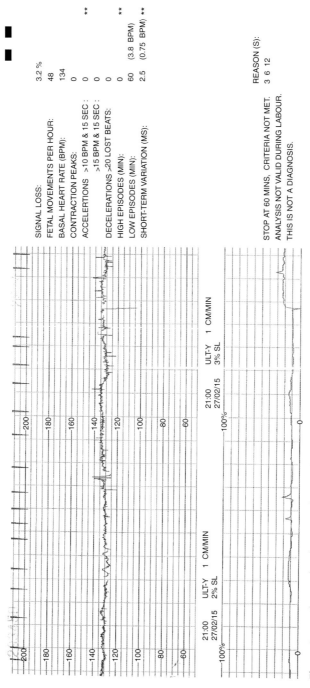

SIGNAL LOSS:	3.2 %
FETAL MOVEMENTS PER HOUR:	48
BASAL HEART RATE (BPM):	134
CONTRACTION PEAKS:	0
ACCELLERTIONS >10 BPM & 15 SEC :	0 **
>15 BPM & 15 SEC :	0
DECELERATIONS >20 LOST BEATS:	0
HIGH EPISODES (MIN):	0 **
LOW EPISODES (MIN):	60 (3.8 BPM)
SHORT-TERM VARIATION (MS):	2.5 (0.75 BPM) **

STOP AT 60 MINS, CRITERIA NOT MET.
ANALYSIS NOT VALID DURING LABOUR.
THIS IS NOT A DIAGNOSIS.

REASON (S):
3 6 12

Figure 21.11 Abnormal cardiotocography with short-term variation <3.

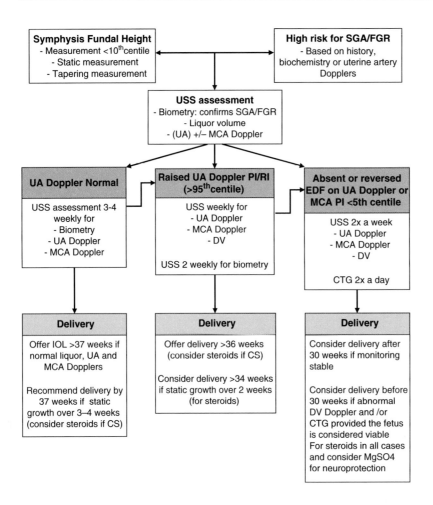

Figure 21.12 A suggested management pathway for small for gestational age (SGA) and fetal growth restriction (FGR).

CS, cesarean section;
CTG, cardiotocography;
DV, ductus venosus;
EDF, end-diastolic flow;
MCA, middle cerebral artery;
PI/RI, pulsatility/ resistance index;
UA, umbilical artery;
USS, ultrasound scan.

reduced liquor volume or abnormal Doppler waveforms. Thus, growth scans and UA Doppler should be carried out serially to ensure a normal growth velocity according to the centile that the fetus is on. There is rarely any significant morbidity in fetuses with EFW or AC <10th centile with normal Doppler indices and normal liquor volume. However, there is an inclination to offer induction near term for fear of an unlikely event of stillbirth. The Disproportionate Intrauterine Growth Intervention Trial At Term (DIGITAT) study randomized 650 women with suspected growth restriction after 36 weeks gestation to either induction of labor or expectant management with monitoring[20]. Although this trial included fetuses that were both FGR and constitutionally SGA, this is the only randomized trial investigating this subject. They reported that induction of labor did not increase the rates of instrumental delivery or cesarean section, and there was no difference in the rate of adverse neonatal

outcomes when compared with expectant management. Thus, it is reasonable to offer induction after 37 weeks to prevent possible neonatal morbidity and stillbirth. However, if women choose to, it is acceptable to await spontaneous labor if resources are available for intensive monitoring.

Management of late-onset FGR

Late-onset FGR is diagnosed when the fetus shows either tapering or static growth on the customized growth chart, or an abnormality in Doppler velocimetry, beyond 34 weeks' gestation. The UA Doppler is the standard test used to differentiate between SGA and FGR, but this is usually normal in late-onset FGR. In view of this, other vascular Dopplers have been explored. Late-onset FGR may show only mild growth restriction, have normal UA Dopplers, but have reduced MCA PI (<5th centile) secondary to vasodilation. This is associated with an increase in

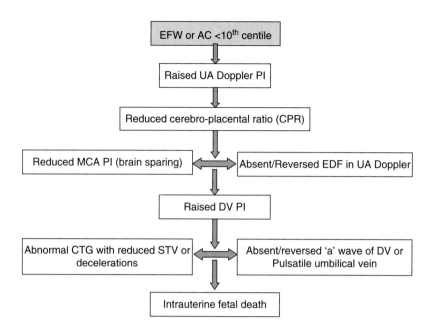

Figure 21.13 Sequential changes in tests of fetal wellbeing in fetal growth restriction.

CPR, cerebroplacental ratio;
CTG, cardiotocography;
DV, ductus venosus;
EDF, end-diastolic flow;
EFW, estimated fetal weight;
MCA, middle cerebral artery;
PI/RI, pulsatility/ resistance index;
STV, short-term variation;
UA, umbilical artery.

cesarean section for fetal reasons and neonatal acidosis. Thus, MCA PI may be used to time delivery in late-onset FGR[21]. The challenge is in the diagnosis of late-onset FGR as changes can be subtle. Thus, it is important to perform all Doppler studies during fetal surveillance scans.

Once late-onset FGR is diagnosed, the decision for delivery usually coincides with deterioration in any of the Doppler indices, CTG abnormalities discussed above, or if the pregnancy is beyond 36 weeks gestation. Although the DIGITAT study found no important differences in adverse outcomes between induction of labor and expectant monitoring after this gestation, the number of children with a birthweight below the 3rd percentile differed significantly between the induction of the labor group (12.5%) and the expectant monitoring group (31%), which suggests that a substantial number of children in the expectant monitoring group did not continue to grow along their own expected growth curves. Whilst this did not change the neonatal outcome, it could be a compelling reason for offering induction as severe FGR is associated with poorer long-term morbidity. Corticosteroids should be administered if delivery was before 36 weeks' gestation to help fetal lung maturity and reduce neonatal morbidity[22].

Management of early-onset or preterm FGR

The pathology for this group of FGR is placental insufficiency, and thus is diagnosed when the EFW or AC is <10th centile, or the growth is static with an abnormal UA Doppler. There is no treatment that alters the progression of FGR, and thus intensive ultrasound monitoring for growth velocity and Doppler studies are the mainstay of management. In all cases of early-onset FGR, close surveillance of maternal blood pressure is needed as there is a strong association of developing hypertensive disease.

Although there is no fixed temporal interval of fetal deterioration, there are sequential changes in fetal wellbeing tests of a compromised fetus (Figure 21.13)[23]. The amniotic fluid volume progressively decreases in early-onset FGR. This may be followed by progressive UA waveforms changes, as described above, and MCA vasodilation, resulting in a lower MCA PI. The presence of absent or reversed EDF occurs about the same time as MCA vasodilatation, which is about 1–2 weeks before acute deterioration. As FGR progresses, a pattern of retrograde a-wave in the DV, or pulsatile UV is observed, indicating advanced stages of fetal compromise. This change may coincide with the loss of STV in cCTG analysis (Figure 21.11 above). These changes are considered signs of fetal acidemia and have been used to time delivery in preterm FGR.

The challenge in fetal medicine is to decide on the optimal time for delivery of the severely FGR preterm fetus who is at risk of fetal hypoxia. A worsening condition in utero may lead to stillbirth, but if delivered there is a risk of complications from prematurity.

There is controversy about which test, or combination of tests that should be used to time delivery as there is no clear evidence available. The Growth Restriction Intervention Trial (GRIT) randomized 548 women where the clinician was uncertain about management for delivery in FGR pregnancies between 24 and 36 weeks gestation to immediate delivery or delayed delivery until the clinician is no longer uncertain about the decision for delivery[24]. There was a difference of 4 days in the time to delivery. The results showed that a delay in delivery resulted in more stillbirths, but this number was equivalent to the number of perinatal deaths in the immediate delivery group. There was no difference in the overall death rate, disability and cognitive development at 2 years of age between the two groups, and school-based evaluations of cognition, language, motor performance, and behavior between 6–13 years were also similar[25].

In FGR of gestations <30 weeks, the most significant determinant of intact survival remains gestational age. Counseling and management on an individual basis is important for these pregnancies. It may be best to delay delivery in situations of extreme prematurity despite the risk of IUD, particularly if the fetus is around the gestational age of viability. At slightly later gestations, it is common to deliver when there are signs of advanced fetal compromise, such as changes in DV, UV or STV on cCTG. The Trial of Randomised Umbilical and Fetal Flow in Europe (TRUFFLE) compared the decision for delivery between DV Doppler and CTG-STV monitoring and have completed recruitment[26]. The results may help to identify optimal parameters to inform decisions regarding the timing of delivery in these circumstances.

Similar to all preterm births, a course of antenatal corticosteroids should be completed prior to arranging for delivery as there are significant advantages to lung maturity. In these early gestations, magnesium sulfate has been shown to have a neuroprotective effect and reduces the incidence of cerebral palsy, and thus is recommended for deliveries prior to 30 weeks gestation[27]. Most of these fetuses are at high risk of intrapartum hypoxia and acidemia. Combined with the circumstances of prematurity, the mode of delivery for most of these fetuses would be cesarean section.

Management of LFDs

Most LFD fetuses have no identifiable risk factors. When it is diagnosed, it is imperative to exclude gestational diabetes, as most fetus that are LFD do not need additional antenatal surveillance or monitoring, except if it is secondary to poor glucose control in diabetic mothers. These macrosomic fetuses are at risk of IUD. The aim is therefore for optimal glycemic control in partnership with a diabetic team to prevent exponential growth velocity. It is known that macrosomic fetuses have augmented hemodynamic blood flow, but the role of Doppler studies in monitoring a LFD fetus is uncertain[28].

It was thought that intervening to deliver a LFD infant before it got too large would reduce perinatal and maternal morbidity and mortality. Unfortunately, a Cochrane systematic review has found that induction of labor for LFD fetuses in nondiabetic women do not alter the risks[29]. Similarly, in a retrospective population survey, induction for delivery prior to 40 weeks gestation in this group of women appears to increase the risks of cesarean section and neonatal and maternal morbidity[30]. Thus, expectant management until 40 weeks gestation in these pregnancies is not unreasonable and women need to be informed of the pitfalls of ultrasound in predicting macrosomia, and risks of interventions before term.

In the absence of clear management strategies that have been proven to reduce the risk of macrosomia, guidance about nutrition and physical activity, particularly in obese women, and good control of plasma glucose in women with diabetes is advisable.

Outcomes of fetal growth disorders

Immediate neonatal morbidity of FGR

The perinatal mortality rate in growth restricted fetuses is more than 10 times compared with those that are appropriately grown. These compromised fetuses are at risk of perinatal hypoxia and acidosis, regardless of the gestational age. Late-onset FGR may have slightly less complications as they are of a more advanced gestational age[31]. A common problem is hypoglycemia due to the depletion of glycogen store and possibly decreased production by the liver. They also have a problem with thermoregulation as they are not able to compensate for the excessive heat loss from the large body surface area and lack of subcutaneous tissue. Some babies may also have polycythemia induced by the chronic hypoxic state in utero, which induces erythropoietin production, leading to an increase in red cell mass.

Fetuses that have early-onset FGR are commonly delivered prematurely and have the highest morbidity and mortality[31]. These babies have an increased risk of sepsis, necrotizing enterocolitis, bronchopulmonary dysplasia, intraventricular or intraparenchymal hemorrhage, periventricular leukomalacia and retinopathy of prematurity). These complications have severe morbidity that may affect quality of life. Bronchopulmonary dysplasia may lead to chronic lung disease, and in severe forms may mean being oxygen dependent. Brain hemorrhages may have severe neurologic impairment, such as paraplegia or cerebral palsy. Many of these lead on to neurodevelopmental delay in later life. These complications arise mainly due to prematurity secondary to elective delivery for fear of further hypoxia or acidemia in utero. However, being growth restricted further increases the risks of these morbidities and possibly mortality as the rate of survival without severe morbidity in the TRUFFLE study of extremely preterm FGR babies was lower than the EPICure2 cohort of the same gestation[26]. Nonetheless, the overall outcomes were relatively good where two-thirds of these fetuses survived without severe neonatal morbidity. These favorable outcomes may be due to advances in neonatal medicine in managing complications of premature babies.

Long term morbidity of FGR

Apart from the neonatal complications at birth, FGR babies, particularly those born prematurely, have long-term health sequelae. Although most of those who survive are without severe disabilities at school age, many have serious difficulties in everyday life due to the burden of a spectrum of developmental abnormalities, behavioral and learning disorders. In addition, there are difficulties from neuromotor impairments, such as cerebral palsy, particularly in those that have early onset FGR and delivered preterm. The factors influencing neurodevelopmental outcomes are gestational age at delivery, fetal body and head size and abnormal Doppler flow in the UA and MCA[32].

Evidence shows that cardiovascular programming occurs prenatally as the fetus adapts to placental insufficiency[33]. This cardiovascular adaptation in utero persists in the form of subclinical cardiac and vascular dysfunction and remodeling in the newborn and children. Thus, FGR are associated with long-term problems, such as coronary heart disease, hypertension and type 2 diabetes. In another study, it was assumed that

constitutionally SGA babies were normal and did not have pathology[34]. However, cardiovascular remodeling appeared to occur in a large proportion of fetuses diagnosed as small near term, even if prenatal severity predictors of Doppler studies and neonatal outcome are normal. Although the cardiovascular function was worse in the FGR group compared with the SGA group, the concept that constitutionally SGA fetuses are normal needs to be further investigated from a cardiovascular morbidity point of view.

Complications of LFDs

LFD fetuses pose a risk to the mother at delivery, and are also at an increased risk of perinatal mortality and morbidity. The onset of spontaneous labor decreases with rising birthweights, which increases the need for intervention. For the mother of a macrosomic baby, there is an increased risk of cesarean section, vaginal trauma of third- and fourth-degree tears, postpartum hemorrhage, and the need for blood transfusions. Macrosomic babies themselves are at an increased risk of birth trauma, such as brachial plexus injury, shoulder dystocia and admissions to the neonatal unit[30]. Fetal macrosomia associated with diabetes indicates poor maternal glycemic control, and these fetuses are at an increased risk of stillbirth. However, even without diabetes, macrosomic fetuses have double the risk of stillbirths compared with fetuses of appropriate size.

Similarly to SGA fetuses, a fetus that is LFD is also at a risk of developing metabolic syndrome, which includes either glucose intolerance, hypertension, obesity or dyslipidemia in later life[35].

Summary

The aim of improving perinatal outcomes starts with the ability to identify a fetus that may develop a growth disorder. This will hopefully improve with the use of customized charts and screening strategies in place for high-risk pregnancies. More consideration is given to the SGA fetus and FGR, as fetuses that are small are more commonly encountered and carry higher morbidity and mortality risks than the larger fetus. It is important to differentiate between the SGA fetus that remains constitutionally small and the fetus that develops early-onset and late-onset FGR for different management strategies. Currently, there is still no treatment available to alter the course of FGR and close surveillance is the main management. Early-onset FGR has the greatest mortality and morbidity and future research should be directed at discovering treatments to improve placental blood flow and function in this group of fetuses. An example is the trial of sildenafil in these circumstances[36]. Another area of challenge in management of FGR is the lack of standard criteria upon which to decide the time of delivery, and the results of the TRUFFLE RCT is awaited. At present, each case needs to be carefully assessed and management individualized.

References

1. Kovo M, Schreiber L, Ben-Haroush A, et al. The placental factor in early- and late-onset normotensive fetal growth restriction. *Placenta* 2013; 34(4): 320–4.

2. Royal College of Obstetricians and Gynaecologists (RCOG). The investigation and management of the SGA fetus. RCOG Green-Top Guidelines No. 31. London: RCOG Press, February 2013.

3. Gardosi J, Chang A, Kalyan B, et al. Customised antenatal growth charts. *Lancet* 1992; 339(8788): 283–7.

4. Persson B, Stangenberg M, Lunell NO, et al. Prediction of size of infants at birth by measurement of symphysis fundus height. *Br J Obstet Gynaecol* 1986; 93(3): 206–11.

5. Gardosi J. Customised assessment of fetal growth potential: implications for perinatal care. *Arch Dis Child Fetal Neonatal Ed* 2012; 97(5): F314–7.

6. Papageorghiou AT, Ohuma EO, Altman DG, et al. International standards for fetal growth based on serial ultrasound measurements: the Fetal Growth Longitudinal Study of the INTERGROWTH-21st Project. *Lancet* 2014; 384(9946): 869–79.

7. Gagnon A, Wilson RD, Audibert F, et al. Society of Obstetricians and Gynaecologists of Canada Genetics Committee. Obstetrical complications associated with abnormal maternal serum markers analytes. *J Obstet Gynaecol Can* 2008; 30(10): 918–49.

8. Goetzinger KR, Cahill AG, Macones GA, et al. Echogenic bowel on second-trimester ultrasonography: evaluating the risk of adverse pregnancy outcome. *Obstet Gynecol* 2011; 117(6): 1341–8.

9. Chauhan SP, Cole J, Sanderson M, et al. Suspicion of intrauterine growth restriction: Use of abdominal circumference alone or estimated fetal weight below 10%. *J Matern Fet Neonatal Med* 2006; 19(9): 557–62.

10. Burd I, Srinivas S, Paré E, et al. Is sonographic assessment of fetal weight influenced by formula selection? *J Ultrasound Med* 2009; 28(8): 1019–24.

11. Nabhan AF, Abdelmoula YA. Amniotic fluid index versus single deepest vertical pocket as a screening test for preventing adverse pregnancy outcome. *Cochrane Database Syst Rev* 2008; (3): CD006593.

12. Cnossen JS, Morris RK, ter Riet G, et al. Use of uterine artery Doppler ultrasonography to predict pre-eclampsia and intrauterine growth restriction: a systematic review and bivariable meta-analysis. *CMAJ* 2008; 178(6): 701–11.

13. Bhide A, Acharya, G, Bilardo CM, et al. ISUOG Practice Guidelines: use of Doppler ultrasonography in obstetrics. *Ultrasound Obstet Gynecol* 2013; 41: 233–9.

14. Alfirevic Z, Stampalija T, Gyte GML. Fetal and umbilical Doppler ultrasound in high-risk pregnancies. *Cochrane Database Syst Rev* 2013; 11: CD007529.

15. Baschat AA, Gembruch U. The cerebroplacental Doppler ratio revisited. *Ultrasound Obstet Gynecol* 2003; 21(2): 124–7.

16. Baschat AA, Gembruch U, Weiner CP, et al. Qualitative venous Doppler waveform analysis improves prediction of critical perinatal outcomes in premature growth-restricted fetuses. *Ultrasound Obstet Gynecol* 2003; 22(3): 240–5.

17. Grivell RM, Alfirevic Z, Gyte GML, et al. Antenatal cardiotocography for fetal assessment. *Cochrane Database Syst Rev* 2010; (1): CD007863.

18. Serra V, Moulden M, Bellver J, et al. The value of the short-term fetal heart rate variation for timing the delivery of growth-retarded fetuses. *BJOG* 2008; 115(9): 1101–7.

19. Bujold E, Roberge S, Lacasse Y, et al. Prevention of preeclampsia and intrauterine growth restriction with aspirin started in early pregnancy: a meta-analysis. *Obstet Gynecol* 2010; 116(2): 402–14.

20. Boers KE, Vijgen SM, Bijlenga D, et al. DIGITAT Study Group. Induction versus expectant monitoring for intrauterine growth restriction at term: randomised equivalence trial (DIGITAT). *BMJ* 2010; 341: c7087.

21. Severi FM, Bocchi C, Visentin A, et al. Uterine and fetal cerebral Doppler predict the outcome of third-trimester small-for-gestational age fetuses with normal umbilical artery Doppler. *Ultrasound Obstet Gynecol* 2002; 19(3): 225–8.

22. Royal College of Obstetricians and Gynaecologists (RCOG). Antenatal corticosteroids to prevent respiratory distress syndrome. RCOG Green-Top Guidelines No. 7. London: RCOG, Press, October 2010.

23. Turan OM, Turan S, Gungor S, et al. Progression of Doppler abnormalities in intrauterine growth restriction. *Ultrasound Obstet Gynecol* 2008; 32(2): 160–7.

24. GRIT Study Group. A randomised trial of timed delivery for the compromised preterm fetus: short-term

outcomes and Bayesian interpretation. *BJOG* 2003; 110(1): 27–32.

25. Walker DM, Marlow N, Upstone L, et al. The Growth Restriction Intervention Trial: long-term outcomes in a randomized trial of timing of delivery in fetal growth restriction. *Am J Obstet Gynecol* 2011; 204(1): 34. e1–9.

26. Lees C, Marlow N, Arabin B, et al. TRUFFLE Group. Perinatal morbidity and mortality in early-onset fetal growth restriction: cohort outcomes of the trial of randomized umbilical and fetal flow in Europe (TRUFFLE). *Ultrasound Obstet Gynecol* 2013; 42(4): 400–8.

27. Crowther CA, Middleton PF, Bain E, et al; WISH Project Team. Working to improve survival and health for babies born very preterm: the WISH project protocol. *BMC Pregnancy Childbirth* 2013; 13: 239.

28. Ebbing C, Rasmussen S, Kiserud T. Fetal hemodynamic development in macrosomic growth. *Ultrasound Obstet Gynecol* 2011; 38(3): 303–8.

29. Irion O, Boulvain M. Induction of labor for suspected fetal macrosomia. *Cochrane Database Syst Rev* 2000; 2: CD000938.

30. Mulik V, Usha Kiran TS, Bethal J, et al. The outcome of macrosomic fetuses in a low risk primigravid population. *Int J Gynaecol Obstet* 2003; 80(1): 15–22.

31. Rosenberg A. The IUGR Newborn. *Seminars in Perinatology* 2008; 32(3): 219–24.

32. Baschat AA. Neurodevelopment following fetal growth restriction and its relationship with antepartum parameters of placental dysfunction. *Ultrasound Obstet Gynecol* 2011; 37(5): 501–14.

33. Barker DJ. Fetal and infant origins of disease. *Eur J Epidemiol* 1995: 25: 457–63.

34. Crispi F, Figueras F, Cruz-Lemini M, et al. Cardiovascular programming in children born small for gestational age and relationship with prenatal signs of severity. *Am J Obstet Gynecol* 2012; 207(2): 121.e1–9

35. Boney CM, Verma A, Tucker R, et al. Metabolic syndrome in childhood: association with birth weight, maternal obesity, and gestational diabetes mellitus. *Pediatrics* 2005; 115(3): e290–6.

36. Ganzervoort W, Alfirevic Z, von Dadelszen P, et al. STRIDER: Sildenafil Therapy In Dismal prognosis Early-onset intrauterine growth Restriction–a protocol for a systematic review with individual participant data and aggregate data meta-analysis and trial sequential analysis. *Syst Rev* 2014; 3: 23.

Chapter

22

Assessment of fetal wellbeing

Ai-Wei Tang and Umber Agarwal

Various modalities of surveillance equipment have been developed and used in the assessment and monitoring of fetal wellbeing in the antenatal and intrapartum period of high-risk pregnancies. These tests aim to identify fetuses at risk of hypoxia and acidemia for early intervention to prevent intrauterine death and minimize long-term complications. They are commonly used in cases of maternal medical problems, such as gestational hypertension, pre-eclampsia or diabetes, and in fetal conditions of suspected or known small for gestational age (SGA), antepartum hemorrhage, immune alloimmunization, decreased fetal movements, multiple pregnancies, fetal structural abnormalities, and postdates pregnancies. These tests include ultrasound evaluation of fetal biometry, Doppler assessment of fetal and uteroplacental circulation, liquor volume measurements, cardiotocography (CTG), fetal blood sampling (FBS) and fetal electrocardiogram (ECG). Most of these tests and interpretation of results are operator dependent, and thus it is of great importance that individuals are competent and guidelines are available to minimize measurement errors and improve reproducibility.

Ultrasound for fetal biometry

An estimated fetal weight can be obtained from ultrasound measurements of a few fetal parameters, such as head circumference, abdominal circumference and femur length, and forms the basic investigation for many high-risk pregnancies. It is used to monitor pregnancies that are SGA or are at risk of fetal growth restriction (FGR) secondary to maternal conditions, as discussed in Chapter 21. There is limited evidence for a routine growth scan after 24 weeks in an unselected or low-risk population as a Cochrane review has shown no improvements in overall perinatal mortality, and may be associated with a small increase in cesarean section rates[1].

Fetal biometry is also recommended as a screening tool to exclude SGA in women who have reduced fetal movements (RFM)[2]. A quality improvement programme in Norway for women with RFM included a clear guideline for managing RFM[3]. The management protocol included ultrasound for fetal biometry, anatomy and liquor volume within 2 h if they reported no fetal movements and within 12 h if there was RFM. The implementation was followed by a significant reduction in all stillbirths from 4.2–2.4% for women presenting with RFM. The study reported no increase in number of preterm births, infants requiring transfer to neonatal intensive care unit (NICU) or FGR. Although there was more than a doubling of ultrasound scans, there was a reduction in follow-up consultations and induction of labor.

Doppler ultrasound

Doppler evaluation of the fetoplacental circulation, using flow velocity waveforms to estimate flow resistance (pulsatility or resistance index (PI or RI), systolic/diastolic (S/D) velocity ratio) has been an important tool for the assessment of fetal wellbeing. The measurements should be obtained during fetal quiescence (absence of fetal breathing and body movements). Either power or color Doppler could be used to identify the vessels, with color Doppler having the advantage of visualizing direction of blood flow. The optimal techniques for assessing velocities and waveforms are[4] (Figure 22.1):

Fetal Medicine, ed. Bidyut Kumar and Zarko Alfirevic. Published by Cambridge University Press. © Cambridge University Press 2016.

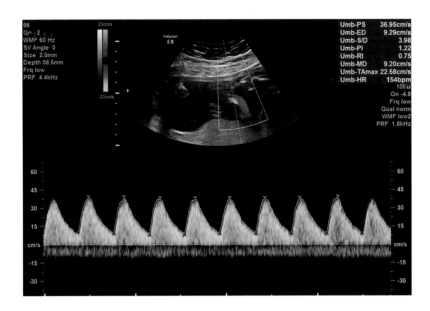

Figure 22.1 Example of a good Doppler.

- insonation in complete alignment with the blood flow, with the appropriate size gate similar to the width of the vessel (the gate indicator will lie perpendicular to the line of blood vessel)
- appropriate sweep speed (commonly 50–100 mm/s if the fetal heart rate (FHR) is 110–150 bpm) to have 3–10 consecutive waveforms recorded
- vessel wall filter or wall motion filter to be set as low as possible (<50–60Hz) (used to eliminate "noise/artefact" from movement of the vessel walls or other vessels)
- pulse repetition frequency (PRF) is the number of pulses transmitted by the transducer per minute time (1–10 kHz), and is adjusted to the velocity of the vessel studied (low PRF for low velocity flow – this will have a larger color jet, but at a risk of increased aliasing, particularly if there is higher flow velocity) and the waveform to fill about 75% of the Doppler screen.

Uterine artery Doppler

The uterine artery (UtA) Doppler assesses the placental flow on the maternal side of the circulation and is able to identify impaired placentation through abnormal flow velocity and increased resistance. The artery is identified at the cervicocorporeal junction with the help of color flow either transabdominally or transvaginally. It commonly crosses the external iliac artery anteriorly and superiorly, and is seen to ascend towards the uterine body. Both the left and right UtA PI should

be measured separately and the mean is reported. The presence of notching, unilateral or bilateral, should be noted[4] (see Chapter 21). There appears to be a progressive decrease in UtA mean PI from 11 weeks through to 34 weeks' gestation, and stabilizes until term[5].

UtA Doppler is used as a screening tool for FGR and pre-eclampsia in high-risk pregnancies (see Chapter 21). Abnormal UtA Doppler in the first or second trimesters is associated with perinatal complications. A recent systematic review reported that an abnormal 1st trimester UtA Doppler (PI or RI >90th centile or notching) is a highly specific test for predicting early-onset pre-eclampsia and early-onset FGR[6]. In the second trimester (20–24 weeks' gestation), UtA PI is not influenced by age, weight, height, method of conception, smoking, family history of pre-eclampsia, or pre-existing medical disorders such as chronic hypertension, diabetes mellitus, systemic lupus erythematosus or antiphospholipid syndrome. UtA Doppler is significantly higher in women of Afro-Caribbean racial origin and lower in South and East Asian women compared with Caucasians, higher in multiparous women with a previous history of pre-eclampsia and SGA, and decreases with gestational age. Thus, these characteristics need to be adjusted in a screening programme utilizing UtA Doppler. An abnormal UtA PI is also related to the severity of pre-eclampsia as there is a significant inverse association between uterine PI and the gestational age at delivery and fetal birthweight[7].

UA Doppler

The UA Doppler evaluates placental function and is the most commonly used parameter in the monitoring of fetal condition in high-risk pregnancies. Its use is associated with a reduction in perinatal death from 1.7% to 1.2%, with fewer inductions of labor and cesarean sections in high-risk pregnancies[8]. In a normal pregnancy, there should be a low-resistance system with forward flow throughout the cardiac cycle. There is a significant difference in the flow indices at the fetal end and placental end of the umbilical cord, with higher resistance in the fetal end. Thus, this test is best performed on a free loop of umbilical cord using color Doppler for consistency[4].

With increasing placental dysfunction, there is progressive change from a normal waveform, to increased vessel resistance flow, to absent end-diastolic flow (EDF), and/or reversed EDF (see Chapter 21). As discussed in Chapter 21, changes in the UA waveforms and resistance are used in the management of SGA/FGR. Similarly, an abnormal UA Doppler in other high-risk pregnancies, such as postdates, RFM or maternal diabetes, can be used to initiate further fetal surveillance testing, including other Doppler parameters and/or CTG. In cases of multiple pregnancies, there is a risk of assigning the wrong cord loop to the fetus, thus it is best to sample the UA just distal to the umbilical cord insertion at the fetal end[4]. It is important to remember that this segment of the cord has higher resistance compared to the placental end. Although there are published reference ranges for UA PI at different parts of the UA[9], it may be more useful to follow the umbilical cord and measure PI at different segments along the cord to obtain an average UA PI for interpretation of results when there is raised UA PI at the fetal end.

Middle cerebral artery

The fetal middle cerebral artery (MCA) is short and straight, and its Doppler flow indices are commonly used in the assessment of FGR (see Chapter 21 and in the diagnosis and management of fetal anemia (Chapter 15)). In addition to the techniques described above for obtaining reproducible Doppler signals, the gate for MCA Doppler assessment should be placed at the proximal third of the MCA, close to its origin from the internal carotid artery[4] (Figure 22.2). The angle between the ultrasound beam and direction of blood flow should be kept as close as possible to 0° and angle corrections should be avoided. This is especially important when using MCA in the diagnosis of fetal anemia as peak systolic velocity (PSV) changes according to the angle of insonation, and systolic velocity decreases with distance from the point of origin of MCA.

The exact mechanisms of reduced MCA resistance in FGR are not fully understood and are likely to be a combination of centralization of brain blood flow due to increased left ventricular cardiac output, and hypoxemia-induced vasodilatation in cerebral vasculature, resulting in the "brain sparing" effect. The proportional change may be first detected by the cerebroplacental ratio (see Chapter 21). An abnormal MCA Doppler increases the likelihood of neonatal compromise, and warrants further tests of fetal wellbeing, but does not necessarily mean an immediate need for delivery.

MCA Doppler is also used in the identification and management of fetal anemia secondary to conditions such as maternal–fetal alloimmunization, parvovirus infection, fetal–maternal hemorrhage, unexplained hydrops or twin anemia-polycythemia sequence. Fetuses with anemia have a high cardiac output and decreased blood viscosity, resulting in high blood-flow velocities in the MCA, giving an elevated MCA-PSV. The PSV can be measured with the autotrace function or using manual calipers of the maximum velocity (Figures 22.2 and 22.3). Fetal anemia that requires intervention is commonly diagnosed when the MCA-PSV is >1.5 multiples of the median for the gestation[10].

Ductus venosus

The ductus venosus (DV) is a high-velocity small vessel that connects the intra-abdominal umbilical vein to the inferior vena cava just below the diaphragm. This is the most common venous Doppler signal measured. Color Doppler shows aliasing due to the high velocity jet of blood through this narrow vessel, and can be used to identify its position either in the sagittal or transverse plane. Measurement is best done in the saggital plane, which allows alignment with the isthmus of DV without angle correction. DV is a four-phase waveform with a continuous forward flow towards the heart, varying according to different phases in the cardiac cycle. The waveforms consist of the "a" wave, synonymous with atrial contraction of the heart, followed by ventricular systole ("s" wave),

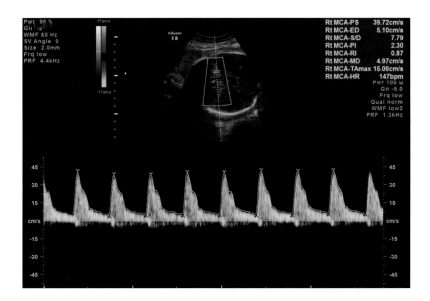

Figure 22.2 Middle cerebral artery peak systolic velocity using the autotrace function.

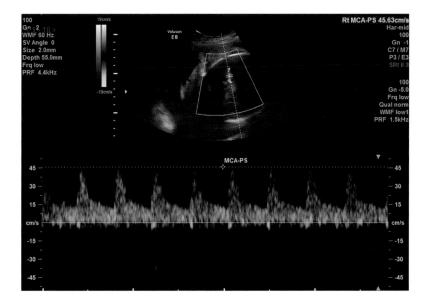

Figure 22.3 Middle cerebral artery peak systolic (MCA-PS) velocity using manual calipers.

then downward slope due to displacement of the mitral or tricuspid valve annulus ("y" descent), and then diastole ("d" wave) (Chapter 21). It is commonly used in the management of SGA/FGR (Chapter 21) to assess fetal cardiac function and in monitoring of twin-to-twin transfusion syndrome (TTTS) (Chapter 25). There may be myocardial impairment, and increased ventricular end-diastolic pressure resulting from an increase in right-ventricular afterload in FGR, which impacts forward flow of blood

through the heart. Thus, the a-wave becomes progressively decreased, absent or reversed secondary to the poor cardiac function. A reversed a-wave is a sign of fetal cardiac failure, and is almost always associated with UV pulsations.

In TTTS, the recipient twin suffers from a cardiac failure from vascular overload and DV Doppler is used to monitor diastolic impairment, demonstrated by increased DV PI and a high rate of abnormal end-diastolic flow[11].

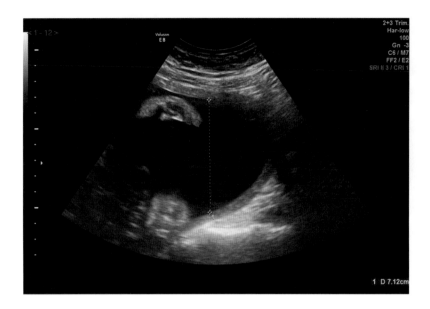

Figure 22.4 Measurement of the maximum pool depth.

Amniotic fluid volume assessment

The amniotic fluid is predominantly produced by the fetus from the second trimester, and thus is used as an indirect indicator of fetal wellbeing. Reduced urine production leading to olighydramnios can be a consequence of reduced renal perfusion due to the redistribution of the fetal cardiac output and shunting blood away from the kidneys to other organs.

Amniotic fluid volume is commonly estimated from a maximum pool depth (MPD), a single measurement of the deepest vertical pocket of liquor, or amniotic fluid index (AFI), the sum of vertical measurement of liquor in four quadrants of the uterus. The pocket of liquor measured needs to be free of umbilical cord loops and fetal parts (Figure 22.4). Diagnosis of oligohydramnios is more common when AFI is used and this leads to more labor inductions and more cesarean deliveries for fetal distress without evidence of improvements in adverse peripartum outcomes, such as admission to NICU, UA pH <7.1 and Apgar score <7 at 5 min[12]. For this reason, most current guidelines recommend that MPD is used for amniotic fluid volume assemment. Although the amount of liquor varies throughout pregnancy, the MPD should be >2 cm throughout pregnancy. Further evaluation of fetal wellbeing is warranted when the MPD is <2 cm as this could be due to prelabor preterm rupture of the membranes, or an early sign of FGR. Similarly, further investigations should be considered when MPD is increased, >10 cm.

Cardiotocography

Cardiotocography (CTG), a continuous simultaneous recording of FHR and uterine activity was introduced in the 1960s. This test aimed to identify fetuses with acute or chronic hypoxia through the interpretation of FHR patterns, which reflect fetal adaptation to hypoxia. Despite the lack of evidence in reducing perinatal mortality, and morbidity such as hypoxic-ischemic encephalopathy (HIE) and cerebral palsy, this method has been widely used in the antenatal and intrapartum period to assess fetal wellbeing[13]. It is commonly performed from 26 weeks' gestation, and sometimes even earlier if the fetus was deemed viable. The CTG assessment also forms a component of the formal biophysical profile (discussed below). The CTG is not recommended for low-risk populations, including as an admission test in early labor, as there is no apparent benefit of CTG over intermittent auscultation in reducing perinatal deaths and morbidity[14].

Interpretation of conventional CTG can be subjective, but development of computerized FHR analysis systems has allowed automated evaluation of the CTG through numerical indices, which is more reliable. Computerized CTG (cCTG) analyses are more objective and consistent. Compared to conventional CTG, cCTG has been shown to reduce perinatal mortality when used to monitor fetal wellbeing in high-risk pregnancies[13].

Table 22.1 Definitions in the Dawes–Redman criteria[16]

Criteria	Definition
High variation	A section of FHR trace in which the long-term variation exceeds a predefined threshold (threshold changes with gestational age)
Long-term variation	The average minute range during all or part of a FHR trace
Lost beats	The unit of measurement used to describe the size of a deceleration
Minute range	The difference in ms between the longest and shortest pulse intervals in 1 min of a FHR trace
Pulse interval	The time in ms (milliseconds) between two consecutive fetal heart beats
Reactive trace	A fetal heart rate trace that contains at least one episode of high variation
Short-term variation	The difference in ms between the mean pulse intervals in consecutive time periods of 1/16th of a minute, averaged over a FHR trace
Sinusoidal rhythm	A fetal heart pattern where the trace oscillates smoothly up and down

FHR, fetal heart rate.

Table 22.2 Dawes–Redman criteria for a CTG to be classified as reassuring[16]

An episode of high variation (above the 1st centile for gestational age
No decelerations (>20 lost beats)
Basal heart rate between 116–160 bpm
At least one fetal movement or three accelerations
No evidence of a sinusoidal FHR rhythm
STV >3 ms
Either an acceleration *or* variability in high episodes >10th centile and fetal movements >20
No errors or decelerations at the end of the record

Table 22.3 Codes of when criteria is not met for Dawes–Redman cCTG analysis[16]

Code	Reasons for not meeting the criteria
1	Basal heart rate outside normal range
2	Large decelerations
3	No episodes of high variation
4	No movements and fewer than three accelerations
5	Baseline fitting is uncertain
6	Short-term variation <3 ms
7	Possible error at the end of record
8	Decelerations at the end of record
9	High-frequency sinusoidal rhythm
10	Suspected sinusoidal rhythm
11	Long-term variations in high episodes below acceptable level
12	No accelerations

The world famous Dawes–Redman criteria was developed in Oxford University (Oxford, UK) as a computerized system that analyses antenatal CTG recording for fetuses between 26 and 42 weeks' gestation for 10–60 min, using a set of rules. The first analysis is made after 10 min and assesses a set of criteria including the basal heart rate, accelerations, decelerations, long-term variation, short-term variation (STV) and fetal movements (Table 22.1). The CTG will be classified as 'reassuring' when these criteria are met (Table 22.2). If not, the CTG is re-evaluated every 2 min until all the parameters are met, or until 60 min, whichever is sooner. When the CTG has not met the criteria, the reasons are listed to assess if further investigations are needed (Table 22.3).

Special consideration has been given to the STV in the analysis by cCTG. The machine divides each minute of CTG into 16 sections, equivalent to 3.75

s, which contains about 7–10 fetal heart beats, or 6–9 pulse interval (time between two consecutive heart beats). STV is calculated by the average change between these pulse intervals in 3.75 s. STV has been shown to be a reliable indicator of fetal wellbeing, and correlates with acidemia in the fetus. A decreasing STV correlated with earlier deliveries, lower birthweights, lower UA pH at birth, worse acid–base status at birth and worse postnatal outcome. An STV of ≤3 ms (Chapter 21) within 24 h of delivery is associated with higher metabolic acidemia and early neonatal death[15].

Table 22.4 BPP scoring system[17]

Biophysical variable	Normal (score – 2)	Abnormal (score – 0)
Gross body movements	≥2 discrete body or limb movements within 30 min	<2 episodes of body or limb movements within 30 min
Fetal breathing movements	≥1 episodes of breathing movement for 20 s within 30 min	Absent or fetal breathing movement for <20 s within 30 min
Fetal tone	≥1 episode of active extension with return to flexion of fetal limb(s) or trunk (opening or closing of hand included)	Slow extension with return to partial flexion or absent fetal movement
Amniotic fluid volume	≥1 vertical liquor pool depth of ≥2 cm	No measureable pool of liquor or vertical pool depth of <2 cm
Fetal heart rate monitoring with CTG	≥2 episodes of accelerations of >15 bpm for >15 s associated with fetal movements within 20 min	>1 episode of accelerations of <15 s within 20 min

Biophysical profile

The fetal biophysical profile (BPP) score refers to the sonographic assessment of four variables including fetal movements, fetal tone, fetal breathing and liquor volume, with or without assessment of the FHR on CTG (Table 22.4) – 2 points are awarded for each parameter that is present, yielding a maximum score of 10. However, if all of the ultrasonographic variable findings are normal, the FHR variable may be excluded. The presence of these features implies the lack of hypoxemia or acidemia at the time of testing[17]. A score of 8 or 10 is normal, a score of 6 is equivocal and a score of 4 or less is abnormal. However, if the MPD of liquor volume is <2 cm, further investigations of fetal wellbeing is warranted regardless of the composite score.

The use of BPP as a test of fetal wellbeing in high-risk pregnancies showed no significant difference in perinatal deaths and Apgar score of <7 at 5 min, and may lead to an increase in cesarean sections and labor inductions[18]. Studies have shown that Doppler ultrasound and cCTG are better predictors of acid–base status in the fetus, and thus have substituted BPP in the monitoring of high-risk pregnancies[19]. Therefore, BPP test is no longer routinely used in the assessment of fetal wellbeing.

Intrapartum assessments of fetal wellbeing

Labor is a stressful process that could lead to fetal hypoxia and result in permanent brain injury. Although numerous fetal monitoring tools have been developed, there is still no consensus on the ideal method for intrapartum monitoring or assessments to identify fetuses at risk of hypoxia and acidemia, or who require immediate delivery to avoid the risk of significant neonatal morbidity[20].

Intrapartum fetal heart monitoring

Intermitent ausculatation (IA) is defined as a systematic method of listening to the fetal heart, focusing on the rate, rhythm and variability for 1 min, with a hand-held ultrasound or acoustic device, commonly after a contraction. This is then repeated every 15 min during the first stage of labor, increasing to every 5 min in the second stage of labor[21]. This is the method of choice for intrapartum monitoring in the low-risk population due to the association of increased intervention with continuous electronic FHR monitoring[22].

Continuous electronic FHR monitoring through CTG is widely used as a screening test to detect the presence of fetal distress. There is an expectation that its use will lead to better neonatal outcomes when compared with IA. However, the evidence from randomized trials shows that its use is associated with a reduction in neonatal seizures, with no differences in the rates of neonatal death and/or cerebral palsy[22]. This is the case in both high- and low-risk pregnancies, and in preterm labors. Therefore, continuous intrapartum CTG is not recommended for routine use in all labors, and should be reserved for those with perceived risk factors, which increases the likelihood of fetal compromise in labor.

Although there are guidelines available in the interpretation of CTG patterns (Table 22.5), it is accepted

Table 22.5 Categorization of CTG interpretation[21]

Caterogy	Reassuring	Non-reassuring	Abnormal
Baseline rate	100–160 bpm	161–180 bpm	<100 or >180 bpm
Variability	>5 bpm	<5 bpm for 30–90 min	<5 bpm for >90 min
Decelerations	None	Variable decelerations: - dropping from baseline by <60 bpm and taking <60 s to recover, present for >90 min and occurring with >50% of contractions OR variable decelerations: - dropping from baseline by >60 bpm or taking over >60 s to recover, present for up to 30 min, and occurring with >50% of contractions OR late decelerations: - present for up to 30 min, occurring with >50% of contractions	Nonreassuring variable decelerations: - still observed 30 min after starting conservative measures occurring with >50% of contractions OR late decelerations: - present for >30 min do not improve with conservative measures occurring with >50% of contractions OR bradycardia or a single prolonged deceleration lasting 3 min or more

that there is significant intra- and interobserver variation in CTG interpretation due to the qualitative nature of information. However, the presence of reassuring components (e.g., accelerations and variability) indicate that there is no fetal hypoxia, acidemia or distress and confirms fetal wellbeing.

There are existing decision support software that extracts CTG parameters and present series of alarms or alerts for intervention depending on the severity of the abnormality. It is unclear if the addition of these computer based "intelligent" software to assist in the interpretation of intrapartum CTG have improved neonatal outcomes. This is being investigated in the INFANT (Intelligent Fetal Assessment) randomized controlled trial (RCT) trial (ISRCTN: 98680152). The primary outcome is mortality and significant neonatal morbidity (encephalopathy and any admissions to NICU within 48 h of birth for ≥48 h), with secondary outcomes including length of labor, length of hospital stays for mothers and their babies, and health service utilization. The trial has completed recruitment and results are currently awaited.

Stimulation tests

Various stimulation tests, such as fetal scalp stimulation and vibroacoustic stimulation, have been evaluated in labor in the presence of a nonreassuring FHR pattern on CTG. A response or acceleration of fetal heart after fetal scalp puncture, Allis clamp scalp stimulation, vibroacoustic stimulation, or digital

scalp stimulation may be useful for excluding fetal acidemia[23]. The effectiveness of vibroacoustic stimulation, however, has not been tested in a RCT[24]. When used, these assessments need to be repeatedly performed in the presence of continued nonreassuring FHR. A lack of response in any of these tests warrants further objective testing, such as fetal scalp sampling for pH.

Fetal pulse oxymetry

This method measures fetal oxygenation using a sensor attached to the top of the fetal head by suction, clip or a sensor pressed against the fetal cheek or fetal back. Results of fetal oximetry values ≥30% are considered reassuring, even when the CTG is nonreassuring, while values <30% may warrant an intervention. This method may be useful in reducing the cesarean section (CS) rate for nonreassuring fetal status, but not the CS rate overall[25].

Fetal blood sampling (FBS) for pH or lactate

FBS for pH is an objective measure of fetal acid balance and thought to be the "gold standard" in identifying intrapartum fetal hypoxia. The results of fetal pH and BE obtained will help assess the safety of continuing in labor, or whether immediate delivery is indicated (Table 22.6). Commonly, two samples are advised for confirmation of results. FBS is contraindicated in prematurity (<34 weeks gestation), fetal bleeding disorders (e.g., fetal and neonatal thrombocytopenia), or risk of maternal to fetal transmission

Table 22.6 Classification of FBS results[21]

Type	pH	Lactate (mmol/L)	Action required[a]
Normal	≥7.25	≤4.1	Repeat FBS no more than 60 min if abnormality persists, or sooner if additional non-reassuring or abnormal features are present
Borderline	7.21–7.24	4.2–4.8	Repeat FBS no more than 30 min if abnormality persists, or sooner if additional non-reassuring or abnormal features are seen
Abnormal	≤7.20	≥4.9	Plan for quickest mode of delivery within 30 min

[a] If the cardiotocogram remains unchanged and the FBS result is stable (lactate or pH is unchanged) after a second test, further samples may be deferred unless additional nonreassuring or abnormal features are seen. FBS, fetal blood sampling.

of infection (e.g., human immunodeficiency virus). Unfortunately, this is an invasive test, requires a relatively large amount of blood, and does not differentiate between respiratory or metabolic acidosis. Thus, fetal sampling for lactate, a metabolite of anaerobic metabolism was developed as this was a reflection of tissue hypoxia and required a smaller sample for analysis. However, results from FBS for pH or lactate could be affected by handling of the sample, aerobic contamination and through processing. A review of two RCTs showed no statistically significant differences between fetal pH and lactate analysis for low Apgar score at 5 min, admission to NICU, neonatal encephalopathy, or for metabolic acidemia[26]. There were also no significant differences in mode of delivery for nonreassuring fetal status, but there was a significantly higher success rate for lactate compared with pH estimation. Fetal acidosis reflects fetal hypoxia and anaerobic metabolism but its correlation with Apgar scores, development of HIE and cerebral palsy has not been very clear as it remains to be proved whether the adverse outcome is attributable to an acute hypoxic event occurring during labor or birth, or has been a chronic or intermittent hypoxia of longstanding duration of days or weeks. A cut-off point for defining pathologic fetal acidemia that correlates with an increased risk of neurologic deficit has been suggested to be a pH <7.0 and a base deficit of more than 12 mmol/l[27], and lactate >4.8 mmol/L as a cut-off for predicting either an Apgar score <4 at 5 min or moderate-to-severe HIE[28].

Fetal ECG

Fetal ECG, in addition to CTG, was another tool introduced with the aim to reduce neonatal hypoxia, HIE and unnecessary cesarean sections. Monitoring is used for term fetuses with ruptured membranes through a fetal scalp electrode alongside conventional CTG. The machine automatically analyses information of fetal ECG, such as length of the PR interval, amplitude of the T wave in relation to the QRS complex (T/QRS ratio) and shape of the ST waveforms. Any abnormalities in these parameters may indicate fetal myocardial dysfunction, which is thought to precede metabolic acidosis. Changes to any of the measurements are triggered as events by the machine, and require close observation or intervention. Systematic reviews have shown that fetal ECG significantly reduces the number of FBS taken during labor, fewer operative vaginal deliveries and less admissions to NICU[29,30]. However, the addition of fetal ECG monitoring made no difference to the number of cesarean deliveries, babies with metabolic acidosis, poor Apgar scores, neonatal encephalopathy or the requirement for neonatal intubation. Most of these trials were using ST segment analysis (STAN)[29]. Several ongoing RCTs aiming to assess the benefit of fetal ECG (STAN technology) in improving neonatal outcomes and their results should provide further insight into the role of fetal ECG.

Summary

It is important that pregnancies are stratified according to the risk status. Doppler ultrasound and CTG remain the mainstay of fetal monitoring. Unfortunately, no single intrapartum assessment tool has proven to be superior over the others. Current best practice rests on the use of a combination of tests to evaluate fetal wellbeing in both the antenatal or intrapartum periods.

References

1. Bricker L, Neilson JP, Dowswell T. Routine ultrasound in late pregnancy (after 24 weeks' gestation). *Cochrane Database Syst Rev* 2008; CD001451.

2. Royal College of Obstetricians and Gynaecologists (RCOG). Reduced fetal movements. RCOG Green-Top Guidelines No.57. London: RCOG Press, February 2011.

3. Tveit JV, Saastad E, Stray-Pedersen B, et al. Reduction of late stillbirth with the introduction of fetal movement information and guidelines – a clinical quality improvement. *BMC Pregnancy Childbirth* 2009; 9: 32.

4. Bhide A, Acharya, G, Bilardo CM, et al. ISUOG Practice Guidelines: use of Doppler ultrasonography in obstetrics. *Ultrasound Obstet Gynecol* 2013; 41: 233–9.

5. Gómez O, Figueras F, Fernández S, et al. Reference ranges for uterine artery mean pulsatility index at 11–41 weeks of gestation. *Ultrasound Obstet Gynecol* 2008; 32(2): 128–32.

6. Velauthar L, Plana MN, Kalidindi M, et al. First-trimester uterine artery Doppler and adverse pregnancy outcome: a meta-analysis involving 55,974 women. *Ultrasound Obstet Gynecol* 2014; 43(5): 500–7.

7. Gallo DM, Poon LC, Akolekar R, et al. Prediction of preeclampsia by uterine artery Doppler at 20–24 weeks' gestation. *Fetal Diagn Ther* 2013; 34(4): 241–7.

8. Alfirevic Z, Stampalija T, Gyte GML. Fetal and umbilical Doppler ultrasound in high-risk pregnancies. *Cochrane Database Syst Rev* 2013; (11): CD007529.

9. Acharya G, Wilsgaard T, Berntsen GK, et al. Reference ranges for serial measurements of blood velocity and pulsatility index at the intra-abdominal portion, and fetal and placental ends of the umbilical artery. *Ultrasound Obstet Gynecol* 2005; 26(2): 162–9.

10. Mari G, Deter RL, Carpenter RL, et al. Noninvasive diagnosis by Doppler ultrasonography of fetal anemia due to maternal red-cell alloimmunization. Collaborative Group for Doppler Assessment of the Blood Velocity in Anemic Fetuses. *N Engl J Med* 2000; 342(1): 9–14.

11. Stirnemann JJ, Mougeot M, Proulx F, et al. Profiling fetal cardiac function in twin-twin transfusion syndrome. *Ultrasound Obstet Gynecol* 2010; 35(1): 19–27.

12. Nabhan AF, Abdelmoula YA. Amniotic fluid index versus single deepest vertical pocket as a screening test for preventing adverse pregnancy outcome. *Cochrane Database Syst Rev* 2008; 3: CD006593.

13. Grivell RM, Alfirevic Z, Gyte GML, et al. Antenatal cardiotocography for fetal assessment. *Cochrane Database Syst Rev* 2012; 2: CD007863.

14. Devane D, Lalor JG, Daly S, et al. Cardiotocography versus intermittent auscultation of fetal heart on admission to labour ward for assessment of fetal wellbeing. *Cochrane Database Syst Rev* 2012; 2: CD005122.

15. Serra V, Moulden M, Bellver J, et al. The value of the short-term fetal heart rate variation for timing the delivery of growth-retarded fetuses. *BJOG* 2008; 115(9): 1101–7.

16. Huntleigh Healthcare Ltd. Sonicaid Team Operator's Manual. Cardiff: Huntleigh Healthcare Diagnostic Products Division, 2005.

17. Manning FA. Fetal biophysical profile. *Obstet Gynecol Clin North Am* 1999; 26(4): 557–77.

18. Lalor JG, Fawole B, Alfirevic Z, et al. Biophysical profile for fetal assessment in high risk pregnancies. *Cochrane Database Syst Rev* 2008; 1: CD000038.

19. Turan S, Turan OM, Berg C, et al. Computerized fetal heart rate analysis, Doppler ultrasound and biophysical profile score in the prediction of acid-base status of growth-restricted fetuses. *Ultrasound Obstet Gynecol* 2007; 30(5): 750–6.

20. Hill JB, Chauhan SP, Magann EF, et al. Intrapartum fetal surveillance: review of three national guidelines. *Am J Perinatol* 2012; 29(7): 539–50.

21. National Institute for Health and Care Excellence (NICE). Intrapartum care: care of healthy women and their babies during childbirth. CG190. London: NICE, December 2014.

22. Alfirevic Z, Devane D, Gyte GML. Continuous cardiotocography (CTG) as a form of electronic fetal monitoring (EFM) for fetal assessment during labour. *Cochrane Database Syst Rev* 2013; 5: CD006066.

23. Skupski DW, Rosenberg CR, Eglinton GS. Intrapartum fetal stimulation tests: a meta-analysis. *Obstet Gynecol* 2002; 99(1): 129–34.

24. East CE, Smyth RMD, Leader LR, et al. Vibroacoustic stimulation for fetal assessment in labour in the presence of a nonreassuring fetal heart rate trace. *Cochrane Database Syst Rev* 2013; 1: CD004664.

25. East CE, Chan FY, Colditz PB, et al. Fetal pulse oximetry for fetal assessment in labour. *Cochrane Database Syst Rev* 2007; 2: CD004075.

26. East CE, Leader LR, Sheehan P, et al. Intrapartum fetal scalp lactate sampling for fetal assessment in the presence of a non-reassuring fetal heart rate trace. *Cochrane Database Syst Rev* 2010; 3: CD006174.

27. MacLennan A. A template for defining a causal relation between acute intrapartum events and cerebral

palsy: international consensus statement. *BMJ* 1999; 319(7216): 1054–9.

28. Kruger K, Hallberg B, Blennow M, et al. Predictive value of fetal scalp blood lactate concentration and pH as markers of neurologic disability. *Am J Obstet Gynecol* 1999; 181(5): 1072–8.

29. Neilson JP. Fetal electrocardiogram (ECG) for fetal monitoring during labour. *Cochrane Database Syst Rev* 2013; 5: CD000116.

30. Becker JH, Bax L, Amer-Wåhlin I, et al. ST analysis of the fetal electrocardiogram in intrapartum fetal monitoring: a meta-analysis. *Obstet Gynecol* 2012; 119(1): 145–54.

Multiple pregnancy: pathology and epidemiology

Leanne Bricker

Multiple pregnancy rates are rising and a significant amount of fetal medicine workload is dedicated to the care of multiple pregnancy. It is important to understand the different types of multiple pregnancy, factors which influence multiple pregnancy rates, fetal, maternal and perinatal risks and impact on women, their familes and society at large.

Zygosity

There are two types of twin pregnancy – dizygotic and monozygotic.

(1) Dizygotic twins occur when two ovum are fertilized and have separate amnions, chorions and placentas (dichorionic diamniotic). The placentas may fuse if the implantation sites are close together. The majority of twin pregnancies are dizygotic (about 70%).

(2) Monozygotic twins develop when a single fertilized ovum or zygote divides after conception (Figure 23.1). Early division of the zygote (within 2 days of fertilization) results in separate chorions and amnions (dichorionic diamniotic twins). This occurs in approximately 30% of monozygotic twins. Later division (3–8 days after fertilization) results in a shared chorion and placentation and occurs in approximately 70% of monozygotic twins (monochorionic diamniotic twins). Division of the zygote between 9–12 days after fertilization results in a shared chorion, amnion and placentation and is rare, occurring in only 1% of monozygotic twins (monochorionic monoamniotic twins). If twinning occurs more than 12 days after fertilization, then the monozygotic fertilized ovum only partially divides resulting in conjoined twins. This is

extremely rare occurring in 1 in 50,000 to 100,000 twin pregnancies[1]. The factors associated with timing of division are not known.

Triplet pregnancies may result from various fertilization and division scenarios involving ovum and sperm. Triplets can be trizygotic, dizygotic and monozygotic. Zygosity in higher order multiples (quadruplets or more) also varies.

In any scenario where there is shared placentation, and hence vascular anastamoses in the placenta, there is an increased risk of complications due to this configuration.

The evaluation of the membranes (amnion and chorion) and placenta(s) after the birth is important in all multiple pregnancies, but it does not always help determine zygosity.

Epidemiology

Twins and triplets occur naturally in about 1 in 80 and 1 in 8,000 pregnancies, respectively. There are familial and genetic factors that contribute to the risk of having naturally occurring twins, which are most commonly nonidentical twins (fraternal; dizygotic) and occur due to multiple ovulation; therefore, the chance of having twins runs down the maternal line. There are some families (few) who have a pedigree of recurrent monozygotic twinning but this is rare.

Currently, multiple pregnancies account for about 3% of births and about 15% of infant mortality. In the developed world, multiple birth rates started declining in the 1959s reaching a nadir in the 1970s but rising since then. From the late 1990s while triplet rates began to decline, twin rates continued to rise.[2]

The incidence of multiple pregnancy, and in particular twin pregnancy, varies between populations

---

Fetal Medicine, ed. Bidyut Kumar and Zarko Alfirevic. Published by CAMBRIDGE UNIVERSITY PRESS. © Cambridge University Press 2016.

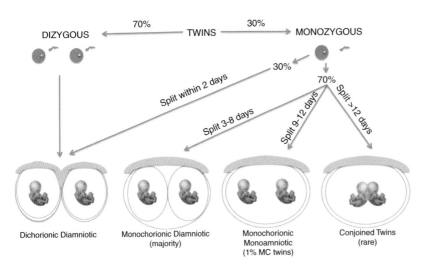

Figure 23.1 Zygosity, chorionicity and amnionicity.

and over time. The population differences are mainly due to variation in dizygous twinning as monozygous twinning rates remain relatively constant. Variation over time relates to changes in factors that are known to influence twinning rates.

Factors influencing twinning rates

Population variation

As there are familial/genetic factors involved in dizygotic twinning, there are variations by race, and hence parts of the world with Asians having the lowest rate (Japan has the lowest rate) and Europeans and most other populations intermediate rates, but some Africans very high rates (Nigeria has the highest rate) [3].

Maternal age

Women of an older age (35–39 years) are at higher risk of multiple pregnancy and this is thought to be due to a rise in the level of gonadotrophins with age, with maximum stimulation of follicles occurring at age 35–39 years. Delayed childbearing and the increased use of assisted reproductive therapy (ART) with advancing age also contributes to multiple pregnancy rates[3].

Parity

The chance of twinning has been noted to be associated with increasing parity. One theory is that women who are more fertile, and hence have many pregnancies, are more likely to conceive twins or more. Others think this is due to the maternal age effect[3].

Socioeconomic, constitutional and maternal lifestyle factors

In the literature, some studies suggest lower social class, greater maternal height, obesity, heavy smoking and possibly different dietary habits contribute to twinning rates, but there is conflicting evidence and these associations are not clear[3].

Family history

There is consistent evidence in the literature that if a first-degree relative has had twins, there is an increased chance of twinning, particularly dizygous twins. Twinning seems to run down the maternal line[3].

Oral contraceptive use

There is conflicting evidence whereby some studies suggest lower twinning rates with recent oral contraceptive use, some higher rates and some no association.

Assisted reproductive technology

Up to two-thirds of the increase in multiple gestations have been attributed to the use of in-vitro fertilization (IVF) and ovulation induction making ART the largest contributor to the rising multiple pregnancy rate. In Europe, a quarter of deliveries following IVF are multiple pregnancies[4]. The rates are even higher in the USA and Canada.

It is possible to reduce multiple pregnancy rates from ART by cautious use of ovulation induction agents and reducing embryo transfer number, but there are complex factors worldwide that affect the widespread adoption of single embryo transfer (SET) policies[5]. Furthermore, monozygotic twinning (70% of which will be monochorionic with shared placentation and highest risk) still occurs with ART and SET, particularly since the introduction of day 5 blastocyst transfer, which optimizes successful pregnancy rates. There are theories about why blastocyst transfer is associated with higher rates, but there is no definitive explanation[6].

Maternal risks

Multiple pregnancy is associated with increased incidence of all maternal complications (apart from post-term pregnancy and macrosomia), including hypertensive disorders (gestational hypertension and pre-eclampsia), gestational diabetes, obstetric cholestasis, antepartum hemorrhage, postpartum hemorrhage, and incidence and complications of operative delivery, Maternal mortality is more than double that of singleton pregnancy[7]. Women who have multiple pregnancy are at increased risk of postpartum depression and this has an impact on other children and the family.

Fetal risks

Fetal loss/miscarriage

There is a higher risk of fetal loss and miscarriage (pregnancy loss before 24 weeks gestation) in multiple pregnancy, with risks increasing with number of fetuses. The higher fetal loss rates are mainly explained by the increased risk of poor implantation, fetal abnormality (aneuploidy and structural), extreme preterm labor and in monochorionic twins, complications of shared placenta.

Fetal abnormality

Fetuses in multiple pregnancy are at increased risk of structural abnormalities and this is thought to be mainly due to abnormal cleavage in monozygotic twinning. In the majority of cases, only one fetus is affected. If more than one is affected (rare), the severity can be variable with one severely affected and another not as severely affected.

Fetuses in multiple pregnancy are not individually at increased risk of chromosomal abnormality, but the risk of chromosomal abnormality is higher because of the additive effect, i.e., because the more fetuses the more chance there is an abnormality, e.g., in twins it is doubled and in triplets it is tripled.

There are also abnormalities that are unique to multiple pregnancy, namely conjoined twins, acardiac twin in twin reversed arterial perfusion sequence.

Preterm birth

The most common complication for the fetus of multiple pregnancy is preterm delivery, which is associated with increased perinatal morbidity and mortality[8]. Up to 60% of twins deliver before 37 weeks' gestation (10% before 32 weeks) and the rates are higher for triplets and higher orders, i.e., with increasing number of fetuses gestational age at delivery decreases. The vast majority of higher order multiples do not reach 34 weeks, let alone term. The causes of preterm birth fall into three categories: iatrogenic (clinically indicated), spontaneous preterm labor or premature rupture of the amniotic membranes. In twins, about 50% are iatrogenic, one-third after spontaneous preterm labor and 10% after premature rupture of the amniotic membranes[9].

Although only about 2–3% of births are multiples (mainly twins), up to 30% of admissions to neonatal units are multiples. It is important not to be complacent about this as although modern neonatal care has resulted in increased survival rates for extreme preterm babies, there has not been a dramatic effect on long-term outcomes, and it is now known that even late preterm and early term births are associated with more long-term morbidity than previously thought[10]. Some studies have suggested that preterm multiples have poorer outcome compared with weight and gestation-matched singletons.

Abnormal growth

Whilst fetal growth in multiple pregnancy is thought to mirror that of singleton growth in the first and second trimester, some studies describe slower growth in the third trimester[11].

Multiple pregnancies also have higher rates of intrauterine growth restriction. This is probably due to both abnormal placentation and increased metabolic demands. Growth restriction is a major risk factor for adverse perinatal outcome.

Even if not growth restricted due to placental dysfunction, twins and other multiples are more likely to be small for gestational age (SGA). SGA neonates are also at risk of morbidity requiring neonatal intervention, e.g., hypoglycemia, jaundice, hypothermia, polycythemia and impaired immune function.

Shared placentation complications

Monochorionic multiple pregnancies (usually twins) are at risk of serious complications unique to shared placental vascular anastomoses connecting the fetal circulations. The shared vascular connections allow intertwin blood transfusion, which if balanced, is a normal physiologic phenomenon. However, if there is imbalance, i.e., net flow in one direction, twin-to-twin transfusion syndrome or twin anemia-polycythemia sequence occurs. If the placenta is shared unequally, selective fetal growth restriction can occur (where one fetus is growth-restricted and the other normally grown), which is pathologically different to growth restriction in singleton pregnancy or discordant growth in dichorionic twin pregnancy because the shared circulation results in a clinically unique pathophysiologic process. It is thought that imbalanced blood flow through particular types of vascular anastomoses early in pregnancy resulting in reversed arterial flow is what causes twin reversed arterial perfusion sequence.

Perinatal outcome

Epidemiologic studies show that twins and triplets have increased rates of stillbirth as pregnancy progresses, and in twins this rate becomes significantly different to singletons from 37 weeks' gestation[12], whereas in triplets this significant difference occurs earlier (33–35 weeks). Monochorionic twins have much higher rates of fetal death in utero compared with dichorionic twins and this is thought to be mainly due to complications related to shared placental circulation, but not exclusively[13].

Neonatal mortality rates are similarly higher in multiples but this is mainly due to the fact that preterm birth rates are higher. As with increasing number of fetuses average gestational age at delivery decreases so neonatal mortality rates increase.

Adverse neurodevelopmental outcome is also increased in multiples, and this again is a function of higher preterm birth and abnormal growth rates. Cerebral palsy rates in are up to 6 times higher in twins and 24 times higher in triplets compared with singletons[14].

Another factor to consider is that multiples are at increased risk of adverse outcome secondary to intrapartum complications. Furthermore, it is well known that second twins are born in poorer condition compared with first twins no matter how they are delivered[15].

Impact of multiple pregnancy

Multiple pregnancies are often seen as special and at times even coveted. Often women and their families are not aware of the potential adverse events and the impact thereof.

In the context of ART, there are particular challenges in that the majority of triplet and higher order pregnancies result from ART and management in these cases can be very complex: parental expectations are high and they do not necessarily perceive multiple pregnancy, particularly twins, to be a negative situation; levels of anxiety are high even if pregnancy progressing normally; and there can be ethical, cultural and psychologic dilemmas relating to prenatal diagnosis and fetal complications and management thereof, including complex decisions to be made in the event of discordant abnormality/pathology and higher order multiples (quadruplets or more).

A UK economic analysis showed that multiple births disproportionately contribute to healthcare costs particularly in the first year of life[16]. In the USA in the year 2000, it was estimated that multiple births from ART resulted in costs of 640 million dollars[17].

Often ART specialists are focused on achieving pregnancy, obstetricians on live birth and neonatologists on live discharge. The rising multiple birth rates, and in particular of triplets and higher order multiples (quadruplets or more), contributes to the burden of childhood disease and educational special needs, which is a worrying phenomenon and it is important to shift the focus to optimizing long-term outcomes.

Summary

The rate of multiple births is increasing and this is due to increasing use of ART and advancing maternal age. There are geographic and population variations in rates of multiple pregnancy due to a number of different factors. Multiple pregnancies can be dizygotic or monozygotic, and monozygotic twins or higher order combinations have the highest risk of complications and adverse outcomes due to complications of shared placentation. The most common complication of multiple pregnancy is preterm birth and this risk increases with increasing number of fetuses. Morbidity and mortality rates are higher in multiple pregnancy compared with singleton pregnancy due to increased rates of prematurity, abnormal growth, low birthweight, congenital abnormality and obstetric complications. Adverse neurodevelopmental outcomes, including cerebral palsy, is increased in multiple births compared with singletons. Multiple births have a significant psychosocial and financial impact on families and society in general.

References

1. Mutchinick OM, Luna-Muñoz L, Amar E, et al. Conjoined twins: a worldwide collaborative epidemiological study of the International Clearinghouse for Birth Defects Surveillance and Research. *Am J Med Genet C Semin Med Genet* 2011;157C(4): 274–87.

2. Collins J. Global epidemiology of multiple birth. *Reprod Biomed Online* 2007; 15 Suppl 3: 45–52.

3. Bortolus R, Parazzini F, Chatenoud L, et al. The epidemiology of multiple births. *Human Reproduction Update* 1999; 5(2): 179–87.

4. European Society of Human Reproduction and Embryology (ESHRE). Assisted reproductive technology in Europe 2002. Results generated from European registers by ESHRE. *Human Reprod* 2006; 21: 1680–97.

5. Bhattacharya S, Kamath MS. Reducing multiple births in assisted reproduction technology. *Best Pract Res Clin Obstet Gynaecol* 2014; 28(2): 191–9.

6. Vitthala S, Gelbaya TA, Brison DR, et al. The risk of monozygotic twins after assisted reproductive technology: a systematic review and meta-analysis. *Human Reprod Update* 2009; 15(1): 45–55.

7. Lewis G, ed. Why Mothers Die 2000–2002. Report on Confidential Enquiries into Maternal Deaths in the United Kingdom, 8th edn. London: RCOG Press, 2004.

8. Tucker J, McGuire W. Epidemiology of preterm birth. *BMJ* 2004; 329: (7467): 675–8.

9. Ananth CV, Joseph KS, Demissie K, et al. Trends in twin preterm birth subtypes in the United States, 1989 to 2000: impact of perinatal mortality. *Am J Obstet Gynecol* 2005; 193: 1076–82.

10. Boyle EM, Poulsen G, Field DJ, et al. Effects of gestational age at birth on health outcomes at 3 and 5 years of age: population based cohort study. *BMJ* 2012; 344: e896.

11. Alexander GR, Kogan M, Martin J, et al. What are the fetal growth patterns of singletons, twins, and triplets in the United States? *Clin Obstet Gynecol* 1998; 41: 114.

12. Minakami H, Sato I. Reestimating date of delivery in multifetal pregnancies. *J Am Med Assoc* 1996; 275(18): 1432–4.

13. Hack KE, Derks JB, Elias SG, et al. Increased perinatal mortality and morbidity in monochorionic versus dichorionic twin pregnancies: clinical implications of a large Dutch cohort study. *BJOG* 2008; 115(1): 58–67.

14. Pharoah PO, Cooke T. Cerebral palsy and multiple births. *Arch Dis Child Fetal Neonatal Ed* 1996; 75: F174–7.

15. Rossi AC1, Mullin PM, Chmait RH. Neonatal outcomes of twins according to birth order, presentation and mode of delivery: a systematic review and meta-analysis. *BJOG* 2011; 118(5): 523–32.

16. Henderson J, Hockley C, Petrou S, et al. Economic implications of multiple births: inpatient hospital costs in the first 5 years of life. *Arch Dis Child Fetal Neonatal Ed* 2004; 89: F542–5.

17. Collins J, Graves G. The economic consequences of multiple gestation pregnancy in assisted conception cycles. *Hum Fertil* 2000; 3: 275–83.

Chapter

24

Multiple pregnancy: diagnosis and screening

Leanne Bricker

It is generally accepted that in pregnancy, antenatal care is a prerequisite for optimizing outcomes. This premise is no different for multiple pregnancies, but given the higher risk of complications and the fact that the pathophysiology of some complications and conditions are unique to multiple pregnancy, there are additional considerations to enable accurate diagnosis and effective screening. A prerequisite is early diagnosis and appropriate assignation of level of risk.

Diagnosis of multiple pregnancy

Ideally multiple pregnancy should be diagnosed early. Obstetric sonography in early pregnancy is widespread and advocated to improve gestational dating, thus reducing induction of labor for postmature pregnancy and it also improves early detection of multiple pregnancy[1]. Early detection of multiple pregnancy and accurate dating in multiple pregnancy is desirable for several reasons: i) it allows accurate amnionicity and chorionicity determination; ii) which in turn allows appropriate planning of care, including discussion about screening for aneuploidy and other fetal complications such as fetal abnormality, twin-to-twin transfusion syndrome (TTTS) and fetal growth restriction (FGR); iii) allows labeling of each fetus according to lateral or vertical orientation to enable consistent assessment when serial ultrasound monitoring is undertaken and when undertaking/interpreting screening and diagnostic tests; and iv) it allows time for discussion about the risks of higher order multiple pregnancy and consideration of multifetal reduction (in settings where this is acceptable).

Gestational dating

There is uncertainty about whether singleton crown–rump length (CRL) charts can be used reliably for gestational dating in twin, triplet and higher order multiple pregnancies, and if so, whether to date according to CRL for larger, smaller or average of the CRL of the fetuses. There are no validated first-trimester CRL charts for multiple pregnancy. Studies have evaluated accuracy of dating using singleton charts of ultrasound parameters in twins conceived with assisted reproduction, as actual gestation is known in these pregnancies. The findings are conflicting but a recent study found that i) singleton charts can be used to accurately date twin pregnancy and ii) there was no significant difference in smaller CRL or mean CRL in twins compared with singletons[2]. Furthermore, a difference in twin CRLs is a common finding in twin gestations regardless of chorionicity and seems to reflect a physiologic variation rather than pathology. However, as reduced CRL may reflect a fetal growth problem secondary to fetal abnormality, UK National Institute for Health and Care Excellence (NICE) guidelines[3] recommend dating by the largest CRL to avoid estimating it from a fetus with early growth pathology, albeit that it is recognized that this may exaggerate this risk causing anxiety. By similar logic, head circumference measurement of the larger fetus may be used to date multiple pregnancies in the second trimester.

Pregnancies conceived with assisted reproduction should be dated from oocyte retrieval date but add 14 days. When replacing frozen embryos, the clock stops at time of freezing and add remaining days. For example, if embryos frozen on day 3 add 11 days, if embryos frozen on day 5 add 9 days.

Fetal Medicine, ed. Bidyut Kumar and Zarko Alfirevic. Published by Cambridge University Press. © Cambridge University Press 2016.

Amnionicity and chorionicity determination

Appropriate amnionicity and chorionicity determination is key to providing optimal antenatal care. This should be carried out in the first trimester and if it cannot be determined, the woman should be referred for specialist review to clarify the matter, and if still indeterminate, the pregnancy should be treated as monochorionic until proven otherwise.

Several methods of chorionicity determination have been described, namely number of placentas, fetal sex determination (whereby discordant gender is diagnostic of dichorionicity), the presence and thickness of the intertwin membrane, and the presence of "lambda" or "twin peak" sign in case of dichorionic and "T" sign in case of monochorionic twins. Ultrasound determination of amnionicity and chorionicity is best achieved in the first trimester by examining the intertwin membrane at its placental attachment and identifying the lambda or T sign. The lambda sign is seen in dichorionic twin pregnancy and appearances are of a triangular tissue projection extending from the base of the intertwin membrane giving the characteristic appearance of the Greek letter lambda (λ). It is produced by extension of chorionic villi into the interchorionic space where the two separate placentas and chorionic attachments meet. In monochorionic diamniotic pregnancies, the T sign occurs when there is no triangular chorionic projection and the two amnions meet perpendicularly to the shared placenta (Figure 24.1). In monochorionic monoamniotic preganancies, there will be no intertwin membrane, but caution is advised as if the membrane is lying in the horizontal plane it may not be seen unless the sonographer scans laterally and angles in at the sides of the uterus. Typically in monoamniotic twins, the placental cord insertions are close together and this may be helpful in diagnosing this rare type of monochorionic twin pregnancy.

The most recent and largest study to date on the accuracy of amnionicity and chorionicity determination using lambda and T signs and number of placental masses of 613 pregnancies, reported a sensitivity of 100% and specificity of 99.8% when ultrasound was undertaken between 11 and 14 weeks gestation[4]. In the second trimester, the lambda sign gradually disappears limiting its use, and therefore if amnionicity and chorionicity have not been determined in the first trimester, fetal sex determination may help but is limited as a good number of dichorionic twins may be same sex. Although measuring intertwin membrane thickness has been described (membrane thickness of >1.5 mm used to diagnose dichorionicity), it is not as reliable as using lambda and T sign, technically more challenging and affected by inter and intraobserver variability in the second and third trimesters[5].

Monoamniotic twins can be diagnosed erroneously in the second trimester when there is severe

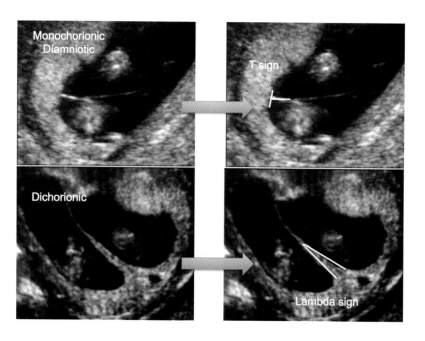

Figure 24.1 Ultrasound features of dichorionic versus monochorionic twins.

TTTS. Therefore, if not diagnosed in the first trimester and monoamnioticy suspected, the sonographer needs to look carefully to exclude a collapsed amniotic membrane around a donor fetus with an absent bladder, and it is also worthwhile assessing whether the cord insertions are close together or not.

Importance of labeling fetuses

It is known that labeling twins by assigning numbers (twin 1 and twin 2) and allocating the label "twin 1" to the fetus closest to the cervix in early pregnancy, does not accurately determine which will be the leading twin as pregnancy progresses or indeed birth order. This is particularly true for laterally orientated twins, i.e., left and right twins where 8.5% change presenting order between the first and last scans, and 20.3% delivered by cesarean versus 5.9% delivered vaginally change birth order (i.e., the twin labelled "twin 2" delivers first)[6]. Correct labeling according to orientation in relation to the mother as lateral maternal left and maternal right or vertical upper and lower, is better than assigning a fetus number as it enables consistency with longitudinal biometric assessment, accuracy when interpreting screening results and undertaking invasive diagnostic tests where necessary, and avoids misconception about birth order ensuring the parents and pediatric team are aware of the possibility of peripartum switch (i.e., possible change in birth order). This is particularly important if one fetus has an abnormality that is not outwardly obvious, e.g., cardiac abnormality.

Screening for aneuploidy

Down's syndrome and other aneuploidy screening in multiple pregnancy is complicated because i) there is a higher risk of aneuploidy, ii) the sensitivity (i.e., detection rate (DR)) of screening tests is probably lower compared with singleton screening, iii) the false-positive rate (FPR) is higher, iv) the likelihood of being offered invasive diagnostic testing is higher as is the risk of complications of invasive diagnostic testing, and v) in the event of an affected fetus, the options are complex including selective reduction and risks to the surviving normal fetus or fetuses. The published literature on first-trimester screening in multiple pregnancy is of poor quality and there is limited published literature on second-trimester screening in multiple pregnancy.

The UK NICE guideline reviewed nine studies that evaluated first-trimester screening[3], three evaluated combined screening – nuchal translucency (NT), maternal age, other maternal factors, and serum screening using beta-human chorionic gonadotrophin and pregnancy-associated plasma protein-A, three evaluated NT and maternal age and six evaluated NT alone. Two of these studies included triplets but did not report separate data for twins versus triplets. One only evaluated monochorionic twins. For twins, all methods have high sensitivities but combined screening overall performs best and should be offered.

For dichorionic twin pregnancies, each fetus has an individual risk of Down's syndrome or other aneuploidy and therefore the risk should be calculated for each fetus separately, i.e., fetus specific risk. It should be noted that about 10% of dichorionic twins are monozygotic but clinically it is not possible to determine if this is the case.

For monohorionic twins each fetus has the same risk of being affected with Down's syndrome or other aneuploidy (unless there is heterokaryotypia, which is extremely rare) and the overall risk is the same as in a singleton pregnancy. Therefore, the NT measurement should be averaged and used to calculate a pregnancy specific risk.

For triplets or higher order multiple pregnancies, there are no normograms for serum screening, and therefore NT and maternal age is the only available screening (Table 24.1).

It is also important to note that if there has been a 'vanishing twin', i.e., the pregnancy started as multiple but then naturally reduced to singleton in the first trimester, serum markers may be higher than in singleton pregnancy and the results of screening using serum markers not as accurate. Women need to be fully informed about the higher risks with screening and need to be aware that decision making and options are complex if the screening test is positive. This requires experienced professionals providing information and counseling before the screening test, and indeed afterwards if the result is positive. Furthermore, if the test is positive and the woman opts for invasive diagnostic testing, this should be performed by a specialist who has the expertise to subsequently perform selective termination of pregnancy if required[7].

If first-trimester screening is not possible (e.g., the woman presents too late), there is limited published evidence to enable recommendations but the NICE guideline[3] recommends offering second-trimester serum screening for twins. With the triple test, the DR is 63% but FPR high at 10.8% (which may be improved by using the quadruple test)[8]. For triplet or higher

Table 24.1 Down's syndrome screening test options in multiple pregnancy

Type of multiple pregnancy	First Trimester	Second Trimester
Dichorionic twins	Combined NT test Calculate fetus specific risk	Serum screening Calculate pregnancy specific risk
Monochorionic twins	Combine NT test Calculate pregnancy specific risk by using average NT	Serum screening Calculate pregnancy specific risk
Triplets or higher order	NT and maternal age alone	No available test
Vanishing twin	Combined NT test but note not as accurate	Serum screening but note not as accurate

NT, nuchal translucency.

order pregnancy, there are no second-trimester screening options.

Recently, noninvasive prenatal testing has become commercially available for screening for trisomies 21, 18 and 13; monosomy X and sex determination with high levels of accuracy and low false-positive and false-negative rates. Many women are opting for this test and it is predicted that other forms of screening will become obsolete in the not too distant future in singleton pregnancy. In mulitiple pregnancy, however, there is little robust published evidence about accuracy and false-positive or negative rates and although available commercially for multiple pregnancies, further research is needed to quantify these issues. Of course even if this form of screening becomes the norm in the future, in multiple pregnancy where chromosomal abnormality is likely to be discordant (particularly if there is dizygosity or polyzygosity), detailed ultrasound and, in cases where it is not obvious (i.e., no visible structural features aiding identification of the affected fetus), invasive testing will be required to identify and confirm diagnosis of an affected fetus.

Screening for fetal anomalies

Structural abnormalities, particularly cardiac abnormalities, are more common in twin and higher order pregnancies. This is mainly because of the higher incidence of abnormalities in monozygotic twins (owing to the unusual nature of the cleavage of the conceptus) compared with dizygotic twins[9,10].

The management of these pregnancies where one fetus has an abnormality is complex. Timely diagnosis enables more choices, time to prepare, optimizing fetal surveillance depending on the anomaly, involvement of other specialists (e.g., genetics team, pediatric surgeons) and appropriate birth planning (place, timing

and mode), including access to intrauterine therapy where it is possible.

There is limited published evidence about screening for structural abnormalities in twin or higher order pregnancies. Logic suggests that the scan will take longer and that visualization at scan may be limited depending on fetal lies, but there is little reason to expect midtrimester ultrasound to be significantly less or more effective in multiple pregnancy. The limited evidence suggests DRs for twin pregnancy is similar to published data for singletons[9,11]. Therefore, routine anomaly screening by ultrasound between 18 weeks and 20+6 weeks gestation as in singleton pregnancy is recommended.

Abnormalities specific to monozygotic twins are midline, such as holoprosencephaly and neural tube defects, and cardiac abnormalities. Therefore, the value of fetal echocardiography in addition to routine anatomy scan is questioned. As not all monozygotic twins are monochorionic, this policy would need to be applied to all twins irrespective of chorionicity unless one were to undertake fetal sexing and exclude discordant sex twins, which can complicate matters (as couples may not want to know sex of the babies). A Scandanavian study of twin pregnancies[11] where women had a package of scans (NT scan, anomaly scan at 19 weeks, fetal echocardiography at 21 weeks and a cervical length at 23 weeks), found that 0.5% of the fetuses had cardiac anomalies, 80% of which were detected at the 19-week anomaly scan (i.e., before fetal echocardiography), and therefore concluded that formal fetal echocardiography is not justified.

Screening for FGR

Fetuses of multiple pregnancies are at increased risk of being small for gestational age (SGA) and, if there is placental dysfunction, intrauterine growth restricted

(IUGR). Both SGA and IUGR fetuses and babies have poorer perinatal outcomes and therefore identifying growth problems is important.

Symphysis-fundal height measurement is not effective in identifying growth problems in twin pregnancy, and serial ultrasound scans are required to identify both small babies but also a significant size difference between fetuses.

The problem with interpreting the published literature to inform the best parameters to use is that criteria for abnormality and definitions of SGA or IUGR or growth discordance are variable and one is often not comparing like with like. The NICE guideline presents a review of 26 studies of ultrasound parameters in twin pregnancies, including various fetal biometric measurements, estimated fetal weight (EFW) based on formulae of ultrasound parameters, Doppler ultrasound of the umbilical cord and composite screening strategies[3]. Acknowledging that most of the evidence is low or very low quality, the conclusions were: i) any single fetal biometric parameter is a poor a predictor of IUGR or birthweight discordance; ii) an EFW ≤10th centile is a moderately useful predictor of IUGR, defined as birthweight ≤10th centile; iii) the best cut-off for intertwin birthweight discordance is an EFW difference of 25% or more; iv) the best EFW is derived when applying a formula that includes at least two biometric parameters; v) the best predictor of IUGR or discordance between twins is an ultrasound carried out within 28 days of birth; vi) there is no strong evidence supporting the routine use of umbilical artery (UA) Doppler for the prediction of IUGR or birthweight discordance; and vii) there is no strong evidence that any composite screening strategy detects IUGR in twin pregnancy. No studies addressed the value of amniotic fluid volume assessment or middle cerebral artery (MCA) Doppler examination. No studies addressed timing and frequency of scanning. There was no evidence to guide management of triplet pregnancies, but it seems logical to apply the conclusions to triplets and higher order pregnancies. On the basis of the detailed review, the recommendation is that EFW discordance should be calculated using two biometric parameters from 20 weeks' gestation, scans should be undertaken at intervals of <28 days, a ≥25% EFW discordance should be considered significant, and UA Doppler should not be used to monitor for IUGR or birthweight differences in twin and triplet pregnancies[3].

More recently, a large UK cohort study of 2161 twin pregnancies (302 monochorionic and 1859 dichorionic

twin pregnancies) has shown that EFW discordance is accurate in predicting birthweight discordance, both EFW and birthweight discordance are good predictors of adverse outcome and that the optimal cut-off for the prediction of perinatal mortality irrespective of chorionicity or individual fetal size is an EFW discordance of ≥25%[12].

Note: the formula for calculating EFW discordance percentage is:

$$\text{EFW larger fetus} - \text{EFW smaller fetus/EFW larger fetus} \times 100$$

e.g., 600 g – 400 g/600 g × 100 = 33%.

Screening for complications of shared placentation

Twin-to-twin transfusion syndrome

About 10–15% of monochorionic pregnancies with shared placentation develop TTTS where the outcome is significantly improved if treated with laser ablation. Given that there is available treatment, it is important to screen for TTTS to allow timely access to this treatment.

It is worth noting that the chronic form of TTTS (most common form) usually presents between 16 and 24 weeks' gestation and treatment is recommended from 16 weeks' gestation, therefore earlier screening would need to be very effective to advocate its use.

The NICE guideline[3] reviewed several studies evaluating first-trimester parameters for TTTS screening, namely NT and/or CRL and/or ductus venosus Doppler blood flow. They all showed low sensitivity and variable specificity. As these parameters are not predictive and there is potential to cause unnecessary anxiety, first-trimester screening for TTTS is not advised.

Whilst it is known that serial ultrasound scans are necessary to identify TTTS by looking for the obvious features, there is little published evidence about how often to undertake the scans or what preclinical features are worrying. Intertwin membrane folding and amniotic fluid discordance have been shown to have better sensitivity than the aforementioned first-trimester parameters but poorer specificity, and therefore should warrant a step-up in the frequency of scans but also continued vigilance in those pregnancies without these features. The NICE guideline recommends a scan every 2 weeks from 16–24 weeks to screen for TTTS but a

Table 24.2 Quintero staging of TTTS [14]

Stage	Description
I	Discrepancy in amniotic fluid volume with oligohydramnios of a MPD ≤2 cm in one sac and polyhydramnios in other sac (MPD ≥8 cm). The bladder of the donor twin is visible and Doppler studies are normal.
II	The bladder of the donor twin is not visible (during length of examination, usually around 1 h) but Doppler studies are not critically abnormal.
III	Doppler studies are critically abnormal in either twin and are characterized as abnormal or reversed end-diastolic velocities in the umbilical artery, reverse flow in the ductus venosus or pulsatile umbilical venous flow in either twin.
IV	Ascites, pericardial or pleural effusion, scalp edema or overt hydrops present in recipient twin.
V	One or both babies are dead.

MPD, maximum pool depth.

step-up to weekly scans if there is intertwin membrane folding or liquor discordance[3].

The diagnosis of TTTS is based on several ultrasound criteria: the presence of a shared placentation, i.e., monochorionicity (ideally diagnosed in first trimester by identification of single placental mass and T sign); oligohydramnios with maximum vertical pocket (MVP) <2 cm in one sac and polyhydramnios in the other sac (MVP ≥8 cm) (note: in Europe the diagnosis is ≥8 cm at ≤20 weeks and ≥10 cm over 20 weeks)[13]; discordant bladder appearances, where in severe TTTS the donor fetus's bladder is not visible; and hemodynamic and cardiac compromise in severe TTTS. Quintero et al. published a classification system for staging TTTS, which has been widely used [14] (Table 24.2). It is important to note, however, that while this staging system is useful in describing appearances and classifying the stage at diagnosis, it does not help with predicting the natural history or progression of the disease.

Several studies of TTTS have shown that disease severity at presentation is one of the determinants of fetal outcome, and therefore early diagnosis and timely referral to a specialist who can offer intervention is essential.

Very rarely, TTTS can present late, i.e., in the third trimester. In these cases, it is usually very acute and rapidly progressive and may require delivery soon after diagnsosis.

Selective growth restriction (SGR)

Unequal placental sharing and peripheral, velamentous cord insertions are common in monochorionic multiple pregnancies and on occasion result in discordant fetal growth where one fetus is usually normal size and the other SGA (defined as EFW <10th centile). However, even if both fetuses' EFW are >10th

Table 24.3 Ultrasound features of TTTS versus SGR

TTTS	SGR
Size discordance	Size discordance
Oligohydramnios polyhydramnios sequence In severe cases "stuck" twin	Liquor discordance But normal liquor volume in larger twin's sac
May be abnormal UA Doppler in smaller fetus	May be abnormal UA Doppler is smaller fetus
May be abnormal DV Doppler in larger fetus	May be abnormal DV Doppler in smaller fetus
Bladder may not be visible in donor fetus Bladder may be large in recipient fetus	Bladder visible in both fetuses

DV, ductus venosus; SGR, selective growth restriction; TTTS, twin-to-twin transfusion syndrome; UA, umbilical artery.

centile, there may be significant size discordance. This is termed selective growth restriction (SGR).

SGR (by this definition) is encountered in approximately 10% of all monochorionic multiple pregnancies. The pathophysiology and natural history of this condition are different to growth discordance in dichorionic multiple pregnancy. The prospective diagnosis initially may be difficult as there may be diagnostic "overlap" between mild TTTS and SGR. For example, liquor volumes in TTTS syndrome may differ between the fetuses because of polyhydramnios in one of the amniotic sacs and oligohydramnios in the other amniotic sac (see above), but in SGR this may differ between the fetuses because of oligohydramnios in one of the amniotic sacs and normal liquor in the other amniotic sac. With serial scans the diagnosis often becomes clearer but if diagnosis remains unclear, tertiary level opinion should be sought. See Table 24.3 for the difference in ultrasound features of TTTS versus SGR.

In a recently published prospective multicenter cohort study, which included 1,028 unselected twin pairs recruited over a 2-year period, participants underwent 2-weekly ultrasonographic surveillance from 24 weeks of gestation with surveillance of monochorionic twins 2-weekly from 16 weeks[15]. Perinatal outcome data were recorded for 977 patients (100%) who continued the study with both fetuses alive beyond 24 weeks, including 14 cases of TTTS. Adjusting for gestation at delivery, twin order, gender and growth restriction, perinatal mortality, individual morbidity, and composite perinatal morbidity were all seen to increase with birthweight discordance exceeding 18% for monochorionic twins without TTTS (hazard ratio 2.6, 95% CI 1.6–4.3, P <0.001). A minimum twofold increase in risk of perinatal morbidity persisted even when both twin birthweights were appropriate for gestational age. However, others have noted that prenatal risk does not increase until the difference in EFW is >25%[3,12]. A compromise cut-off of diagnosis of SGR is taken of >20%.

Twin anemia-polycythemia sequence

Twin anemia polycythemia sequence (TAPS) is a form of chronic fetofetal transfusion, characterized by large intertwin hemoglobin differences, without signs of twin oligo-polyhydramnios sequence (TOPS). TAPS may occur spontaneously or after laser surgery for TTTS (postlaser form). The spontaneous form complicates approximately 3–5% of monochorionic twin pregnancies, whereas the post-laser form occurs in up to 13% of TTTS cases[16]. The pathogenesis of TAPS is based on the presence of few, minuscule arteriovenous placental anastomoses (diameter <1 mm) allowing a slow transfusion of blood from the donor to the recipient and leading gradually to highly discordant hemoglobin levels.

The diagnosis can be reached either antenatally or postnatally. Antenatal diagnosis of TAPS is based on Doppler ultrasound abnormalities showing an increased middle cerebral artery peak systolic velocity (MCA-PSV) in the donor twin, suggestive of fetal anemia (>1.5 multiples of the median (MoM)), and a decreased MCA-PSV in the recipient twin, suggestive of polycythemia (<1.0 MoM), in the absence of signs of TOPS. Postnatal diagnosis of TAPS is based on the presence of (chronic) anemia in the donor (including reticulocytosis) and polycythemia in the recipient. Postnatal hematologic criteria include an intertwin hemoglobin difference >8 g/dL and a reticulocyte count ratio >1.7. Antenatal TAPS may therefore complicate even apparently uncomplicated MC twin pregnancies. Some experts recommend screening for this condition by the use of serial MCA-PSV from 20 weeks of gestation (at 2-weekly intervals as part of the ultrasound scan to detect SGR). As there are no agreed and recognized evidence-based treatment options for TAPS, the value of routinely screening remains debateable (this is discussed in more detail in Chapter 25). It is important to note that TAPS is pathologically different to TTTS and is not a recognized precursor of TTTS.

Twin-reversed arterial perfusion sequence

Twin-reversed arterial perfusion (TRAP) sequence occurs when one twin, lacking a functioning cardiac system ("acardiac" twin), receives deoxygenated blood from the normally developing "pump" twin via an arterial anastamosis in a monochorionic pregnancy. The acardiac twin gets circulation to the lower part of its body and little or no perfusion of the upper torso and head, and therefore develops anomalously – most commonly it has an absent thorax and head (acardiac acephalus) but can also develop only a head (acardius acormus), be a mass with no recognizable human parts (acardius amorphous) or be a head with one or more partially developed limbs (acardius myelacephalus). The pump twin is usually structurally normal but at significant risk for cardiac failure and, if left untreated, will die in 50–75% of cases. It is rare, occurring in 1 in 35,000 births.

Diagnosis of TRAP sequence can be difficult and it is often missed because on ultrasound, if only one fetal heartbeat is seen, an assumption of simple single fetal death is made. Therefore, if fetal cardiac activity is not seen in a fetus of a twin pregnancy, it is important to examine the nonviable fetus using color Doppler to i) determine whether there are features of an acardiac fetus, i.e., underdeveloped head and upper body, edema and ii) demonstrate reversed blood flow in the aorta and/or umbilical cord[17].

Conjoined twins

If conjoined twinning is suspected in early pregnancy, transvaginal sonography may help determine the type of fusion and whether there is cardiovascular involvement. Ultrasound features include fixed position of fetal heads, inability to detect separate bodies or skin contours and lack of dividing membrane.

Conjoined twins are classified according to site of the most prominent area of fusion, which is ventral in the majority of cases. The type of fusion is named with the suffix "pagus," which means fixed. Ventral unions/fusions include paraphagus 28% (pelvic and variable trunk), thoracopagus 19%, omphalopagus 18%, cephalopagus 11% and ischiopagus 11%. Dorsal unions or fusions include pyopagus 6% (sacrum), craniopagus 5% and rachiopagus 2% (vertebral column)[18].

It is important to determine type and severity to inform discussions about prognosis and management.

Predicting preterm labor and delivery

Several factors/tests have been studied with regard to diagnostic accuracy as a predictor of spontaneous preterm birth in twin and triplet pregnancies, namely ultrasonographic cervical length (CL) measurements, fetal fibronectin test (FFT), home uterine activity monitoring, past obstetric history of preterm birth and composites of these approaches.

A systematic review of 21 studies[19] comprising 3,523 twin pregnancies concluded that transvaginal CL at 20–24 weeks' gestation is a good predictor of spontaneous preterm birth in asymptomatic women with twin pregnancies. The NICE guideline, having reviewed all the evidence including the aforementioned systematic review, concluded that a CL of <25mm at 18–24 weeks' gestation is a good predictor of spontaneous preterm delivery in twin pregnancy and a CL measurement of <25mm at 14–20 weeks' gestation is a good predictor of spontaneous preterm birth in triplet pregnancy[3].

Studies of FFT in twin pregnancies showed there was no association between a positive test and risk of spontaneous preterm delivery. However, when combined with CL assessment, FFT can predict preterm delivery.

A systematic review of six randomized trials of home uterine activity monitoring showed this intervention to be ineffective in predicting spontaneous preterm delivery[20].

An effective predictor is a history of previous preterm delivery, although this is not helpful in primigravidae.

Whilst some approaches for prediction of preterm delivery are effective, strategies for prevention remain limited, and therefore there is much debate about whether screening to predict preterm labor and delivery in multiple pregnancy where there or no other risk factors should be routine.

Summary

Twin, triplet and higher order pregnancies are high risk for both mother and babies, and these pregnancies require accurate and appropriate diagnosis and screening to optimize outcomes. Early pregnancy care should include a scan to date the pregnancy and determine chorionicity and amnionicity. An individualized care pathway should be developed based on chorionicity, amnionicity and other risk factors specific to the woman. Screening for fetal abnormalities and complications should be offered along with specific information about the complex clinical issues and decisions that may result from such screening. Screening strategies for fetal complications should be such that accurate and as early as possible diagnosis occurs to enable timely referral to fetal medicine specialists with knowledge and expertise to provide optimal clinical management.

References

1. Whitworth M, Bricker L, Neilson JP, et al. Ultrasound for fetal assessment in early pregnancy. *Cochrane Database Syst Rev* 2010; 4: CD007058.

2. Dias T, Mahsud-Dornan S, Thilaganathan B, et al. First-trimester ultrasound dating of twin pregnancy: are singleton charts reliable? *BJOG* 2010; 117(8): 979–84.

3. National Collaborating Centre for Women's and Children's Health. Multiple pregnancy: the management of twin and triplet pregnancies in the antenatal period. London: RCOG Press, 2011.

4. Dias T, Arcangeli T, Bhide A, et al. First-trimester ultrasound determination of chorionicity in twin pregnancy. *Ultrasound Obstet Gynecol* 2011; 38(5): 530–2.

5. Stagiannis KD, Sepulveda W, Southwell D, et al. Ultrasonographic measurement of the dividing membrane in twin pregnancy during the second and third trimesters: a reproducibility study. *Am J Obstet Gynecol* 1995; 173: 1546–50.

6. Dias T, Ladd S, Mahsud-Dornan S, et al. Systematic labeling of twin pregnancies on ultrasound. *Ultrasound Obstet Gynecol* 2011; 38: 130–3.

7. Royal College of Obstetricians and Gynaecologists (RCOG). Amniocentesis and chorionic villus sampling. RCOG Green-Top Guideline No. 8. London: RCOG Press, 2010.

8. Garchet-Beaudron A, Dreux S, Leporrier N, et al; ABA Study Group; Clinical Study Group. Second-trimester Down syndrome maternal serum marker screening: a

prospective study of 11 040 twin pregnancies. *Prenat Diagn* 2008; 28(12): 1105–9.

9. Edwards MS, Ellings JM, Newman RB, et al. Predictive value of antepartum ultrasound examination for anomalies in twin gestations. *Ultrasound Obstet Gynecol* 1995; 6: 43–9.

10. Schinzel AA, Smith DW, Miller JR. Monozygotic twinning and structural defects. *J Pediatr* 1979; 95: 921–30.

11. Sperling L, Kiil C, Larsen LU et al. Detection of chromosomal abnormalities, congenital abnormalities and transfusion syndrome in twins. *Ultrasound Obstet Gynecol* 2007; 29(5): 517–26.

12. D'Antonio F, Khalil A, Dias T, et al. on behalf of the Southwest Thames Obstetric Research Collaborative (STORK). Weight discordance and perinatal mortality in twins: analysis of the Southwest Thames Obstetric Research Collaborative (STORK) multiple pregnancy cohort. *Ultrasound Obstet Gynecol* 2013; 41: 643–8.

13. Senat MV, Deprest J, Boulvain M, et al. Endoscopic laser surgery versus serial amnioreduction for severe twin-to-twin transfusion syndrome. *N Engl J Med* 2006; 8: 136–44.

14. Quintero RA, Morales WJ, Allen MH, et al. Staging of twin-twin transfusion syndrome. *J Perinatol* 1999; 19: 550–5.

15. Breathnach FM, McAuliffe FM, Geary M, et al; Perinatal Ireland Research Consortium. Definition of intertwin birth weight discordance. *Obstet Gynecol* 2011; 118(1): 94–103.

16. Slaghekke F, Kist WJ, Oepkes D, et al. Twin anemia-polycythemia sequence: diagnostic criteria, classification, perinatal management and outcome. *Fetal Diagn Ther* 2010; 27(4): 181–90.

17. Sueters M, Oepkes D. Diagnosis of twin-to-twin transfusion syndrome, selective growth restriction, twin anaemia-polycythaemia sequence, and twin reversed arterial perfusion sequence. *Best Pract Res Clin Obstet Gynaecol* 2014; 28(2): 215–26.

18. Spencer R. Anatomic description of conjoined twins: a plea for standardized terminology. *J Pediatr Surg* 1996; 31: 941–4.

19. Conde-Agudelo A, Romero R, Hassan SS et al. Transvaginal sonographic cervical length for the prediction of spontaneous preterm birth in twin pregnancies: a systematic review and meta-analysis. *Am J Obstet Gynecol* 2010; 203(2): 128.e1–128.c12.

20. Colton T, Kayne HL, Zhang Y et al. A metaanalysis of home uterine activity monitoring. *Am J Obstet Gynecol* 1995; 173(5): 1499–505.

Multiple pregnancy: management and outcomes

Leanne Bricker

In twin, triplet and higher order multiple pregnancy, the mother and babies are at increased risk of many complications. This chapter will address clinical strategies to minimize the risk and manage the complications.

Multifetal pregnancy reduction

To optimize perinatal outcome, multifetal pregnancy reduction (MFPR) in the late first trimester has been used in the last 20–25 years to reduce higher order multiple pregnancies (quadruplets or more) to twins. The value of MFPR in higher order multiple pregnancies is undisputed, but for triplets this option has been more controversial although outcomes are improved. Reduction from twins to singleton is even more controversial.

For MFPR in triplet pregnancy, there are no randomized controlled trials. A meta-analysis of 14 studies published between 1984 and 2005 of 20 or more cases who underwent MPFR from triplets to twins (2641 cases) compared the outcome with 17 comparable studies of unreduced triplets of 20 more cases published in the same period (1041 cases)[1]. The cut-off of 20 cases or more was to limit inexperience bias in both the technique of MFPR and in caring for triplet pregnancies. There was no significant difference in the pregnancy loss rate before 24 weeks or take-home-baby rate, but preterm delivery before 28 and 32 weeks and perinatal mortality was significantly reduced when triplets were reduced to twins. The limitations of this meta-analysis were that it compared data from different retrospective studies, and the unreduced triplet studies did not differentiate between trichorionic triplets and those where there may have been shared placentation, and hence at greater risk of poor outcome.

Of course if there is shared placentation (monochorionicity) in triplet or higher order multiple pregnancies, it is not advisable to reduce one of a monochorionic pair, e.g., a dichorionic triplet pregnancy could not be reduced to dichorionic twins, as there is a significant risk of damage to the other fetus of the monochorionic pair if it survives the reduction. In these cases, the options would be to reduce the singleton keeping the monochorionic twin pair or reduce the monochorionic twin pair resulting in a singleton pregnancy. If the former is opted for, there remains the risk of monochorionic placentation problems later in pregnancy.

With MFPR, not only are there ethical considerations, but also significant psychologic impact on the parents, including emotional distress, fear, feelings of regret and guilt. This is often compounded by the fact that the pregnancy is the result of assisted conception and the pregnancy long awaited and much wanted. Religious and other cultural beliefs may also influence their decision making. Given that it is best to perform these procedures at 11–14 weeks' gestation and the aforementioned issues are complex, it is very important that detailed counseling is undertaken and appropriate time given for couples to consider all the issues, including the perinatal outcome and the potential psychologic impact. It is therefore crucial that discussion occurs early and referral to a clinician with the expertise timely.

The consensus views from the UK Royal College of Obstetricians and Gynaecologists 50th Study Group on mutliple pregnancy stated that "parents of high-order multiple pregnancies (≥3) should be counseled and offered multifetal pregnancy reduction (MFPR) to twins in specialist centres"[2].

The procedure is performed between 11–14 weeks gestation as spontaneous reduction may occur before this ("vanishing" fetus) and a detailed scan,

Fetal Medicine, ed. Bidyut Kumar and Zarko Alfirevic. Published by Cambridge University Press. © Cambridge University Press 2016.

including nuchal translucency (NT) measurement to exclude anomalies or features of aneuploidy, may guide selection of fetuses for reduction, aiming to keep the healthiest fetuses. The procedure is performed by transabdominal ultrasound guided intracardiac injection of potassium choride, normal saline or aspirated amniotic fluid into the targeted fetus using a 20-gauge needle. To minimize the risk of infection and miscarriage if there is normal scan and NT, the fetus furthest from the cervix and most easy to access transabdominally is targeted. If one fetus is smaller or appears abnormal it is targeted. Antibiotics may be given to reduce the risk of infection and miscarriage. Chorionic villus sampling may be considered prior to reduction to optimize targeting abnormal fetuses/keeping normal fetuses, but nowadays this is not commonly performed as scan and NT assessment are relatively accurate, invasive testing complex (particularly as there is a risk of contamination and inaccurate results) and invasive testing would add to the risk of whole pregnancy loss. After reduction before 14 weeks, the risk of miscarriage is about 3–5% and this has been shown to be operator dependent, hence this should be undertaken in specialist fetal medicine units by experienced practitioners. If reduction is undertaken after 14 weeks, the risk of miscarriage is substantially higher – about 10–15%.

General management of multiple pregnancy

How, where and when to deliver care

Given the extra elements required to deliver optimal antenatal care in multiple pregnancy, it seems logical that this should be provided in a dedicated service, whether it be in a clinic staffed by a dedicated multidisciplinary team or delivered by a core team in a specialized model.

There are no randomized controlled trials (RCTs) addressing the effectiveness of specialist care in preventing adverse fetal outcomes. There is conflicting evidence from other studies conducted in the USA about the value of specialist multiple pregnancy care or clinics. A review of studies showed that specialist care has an impact on some of the important outcomes including fewer women with pre-eclampsia, less preterm birth, fewer low birthweight babies, fewer perinatal deaths, less major neonatal morbidity and lower infant mortality[3]. The conclusions from this limited evidence are that i) there is a potential for bias, for example, women at lower risk may have had better access to this care (for

financial, educational or other reasons), ii) it is not clear whether it is the actual elements of care (and if so which elements) or the continuity and specialist knowledge of the caregivers that makes the difference and iii) as the evidence comes from one healthcare setting (i.e., USA) where in particular there is little midwifery input, it may not be reproducible in other settings. What appears to be clear is that continuity and consistency of care by the same experienced and knowledgeable professionals contributes to better outcomes. Further research using methodologies that minimize bias in different health settings is needed to corroborate these findings.

Given that better outcomes may result from continuity and consistency of care provided by the same experienced and knowledgeable professionals, the UK National Institute for Health and Care Excellence (NICE) guideline recommends that "clinical care for women with twin and triplet pregnancies should be provided by a nominated multidisciplinary team consisting of a core team of named specialist obstetricians, specialist midwives and ultrasonographers, all of whom have experience and knowledge of managing twin and triplet pregnancies"[4].

The guideline goes on to specify a schedule of appointments including timing of ultrasound scans depending on whether twin or triplets and based on chorionicity and amnionicity (Table 25.1). It also specifies when to offer delivery, i.e., recommended timing of delivery. It is recognized that this is a minimum requirement/recommendation, and if there are comorbidities or complications there may be a need to deviate from the schedule.

For higher order multiple pregnancy, it is advised that antenatal care should be delivered by fetal medicine specialists and should involve regular serial ultrasound but there is no published literature to guide this care and it would need to be individualized.

Information and emotional support

The risks of multiple pregnancy and the additional elements of antenatal care required to mitigate and identify them can lead to a certain level of anxiety for the woman and her partner/family. In today's world, women also have access to a wide range of information from various sources (internet, media, etc.) some of which may be poor or misleading. It is important to ensure women are given good information, are guided to reputable sources of further information, and have the opportunity to clarify matters that are unclear to

Table 25.1 Recommended schedule of antenatal appointments for uncomplicated twin and triplet pregnancy according to chorionicity and amnionicity [4].

Dichorionic diamniotic twins	Offer women with uncomplicated dichorionic twin pregnancies at least eight antenatal appointments with a healthcare professional from the core team.
	At least two of these appointments should be with the specialist obstetrician.
	Combine appointments with scans when crown–rump length measures from 45 mm to 84 mm (at approximately 11 weeks, 0 days to 13 weeks, 6 days) and then at estimated gestations of 20, 24, 28, 32 and 36 weeks.
	Offer additional appointments without scans at 16 and 34 weeks.
	Offer delivery from 37 weeks' gestation.
Monochorionic diamniotic twins	Offer women with uncomplicated monochorionic diamniotic twin pregnancies at least nine antenatal appointments with a healthcare professional from the core team.
	At least two of these appointments should be with the specialist obstetrician.
	Combine appointments with scans when crown–rump length measures from 45 mm to 84 mm (at approximately 11 weeks, 0 days to 13 weeks, 6 days) and then at estimated gestations of 16, 18, 20, 22, 24, 28, 32 and 34 weeks.
	Offer delivery from 36 weeks' gestation.
Triamniotic triamniotic triplets	Offer women with uncomplicated trichorionic triamniotic triplet pregnancies at least seven antenatal appointments with a healthcare professional from the core team.
	At least two of these appointments should be with the specialist obstetrician.
	Combine appointments with scans when crown–rump length measures from 45 mm to 84 mm (at approximately 11 weeks, 0 days to 13 weeks, 6 days) and then at estimated gestations of 20, 24, 28, 32 and 34 weeks (see 55).
	Offer an additional appointment without a scan at 16 weeks.
	Offer delivery from 35 weeks' gestation.
Monochorionic triamniotic and dichorionic triamniotic triplets	Offer women with uncomplicated monochorionic triamniotic and dichorionic triamniotic triplet pregnancies at least 11 antenatal appointments with a healthcare professional from the core team.
	At least two of these appointments should be with the specialist obstetrician.
	Combine appointments with scans when crown–rump length measures from 45 mm to 84 mm (at approximately 11 weeks, 0 days to 13 weeks, 6 days) and then at estimated gestations of 16, 18, 20, 22, 24, 26, 28, 30, 32 and 34 weeks.
	Offer delivery from 35 weeks' gestation.
Any twin or triplet pregnancy where there is a shared amnion	Women with twin and triplet pregnancies involving a shared amnion should be offered individualised care from a consultant in a tertiary level fetal medicine centre.

them. They should be encouraged to explore socio-economic issues related to caring for and supporting more than one child. This process of information giving is ongoing and can be delivered in a number of formats.

Nutritional supplements, diet and lifestyle advice

In multiple pregnancy, as the metabolic rate of the mother is greater than in singleton pregnancy, it has been suggested that a high-calorie diet may help maintain her nutritional state. The counterargument is that boosting weight gain might not be advantageous. There are no RCTs to advise whether specific dietary advice for women with multiple pregnancy does more good than harm.

The NICE guideline group reviewed the limited literature on nutritional supplements and dietary advice

in multiple pregnancy and concluded that the few published studies were of very low quality and there was no evidence to give different advice to that given in singleton pregnancy[4]. However, they emphasized it is important to be aware of the higher incidence of anemia and recommended checking the full blood count at 20–24 weeks to identify women who may need iron and folic acid supplementation.

There is no evidence in the literature to inform specific advice about other lifestyle issues, e.g., work patterns, sexual activity and exercise in multiple pregnancy.

Use of corticosteroids

It is well known that antenatal corticosteroids reduce neonatal complications in preterm babies. Even though it is thought that corticosteroids are less effective in multiple pregnancy the question arises, given the substantial risk of preterm delivery in multiple pregnancy, as to whether giving an untargeted course of steroids routinely at a given gestation or whether giving multiple courses at regular intervals may be beneficial. The problem with giving a single course routinely would be that the time of administration may be remote from delivery and the effect dampened. Multiple courses are associated with potential harm, i.e., lower birthweight and reduced head circumference. On this basis, it is better to avoid untargeted routine single or multiple courses of steroids and to advocate targeted steroids when indicated, i.e., when preterm labor or birth is imminent, and therefore to shift the focus towards informing all women with twin and triplet pregnancies of the increased risk of preterm birth and the benefits of targeted steroids, and provide information about symptoms and signs to be aware of so that they can present in a timely manner.

Timing of delivery

Up to 60% of twins and more triplets and higher order pregnancies deliver preterm (i.e., before 37 weeks' gestation). For those that are undelivered, appropriate timing of delivery is aimed at optimizing gestation but avoiding stillbirth. For triplets and higher orders, it is rare to get beyond 35 weeks' gestation. Epidemiologic studies show that perinatal mortality of twins increases significantly after 37 weeks' gestation. Therefore, for uncomplicated twin pregnancies delivery should be considered from 37 weeks' gestation. Slightly earlier delivery is advocated for monochorionic diamniotic (MCDA) twins because even in uncomplicated MCDA twins, the risk of stillbirth is higher than dichorionic twins at all gestations, and on balance of risks, given advances in neonatal care, earlier delivery seems logical. A systematic review concluded that elective delivery from 36 completed weeks may be the best current strategy to decrease fetal mortality in MCDA twins[5]. The important point to make is that uncomplicated MCDA twins do not need to be delivered before 36 weeks' gestation, and if uncomplicated and the woman wishes delivery could be considered after 37 completed weeks (bearing in mind the risk of stillbirth and consequences remains present).

The UK NICE guideline recommends delivery of dichorionic twins from 37 completed weeks' gestation, monochorionic twins from 36 completed weeks' gestation and triplets from 35 weeks' gestation[4].

Timing of delivery for monoamniotic twins will be discussed later in this chapter.

Mode of delivery

With regard to absolute indications for cesarean section (CS), it is generally recommended that monoamniotic twins, conjoined twins and triplets or more are delivered by elective CS[6]. Also, most clinicians would advise that if the first twin is nonvertex, delivery is by CS; this is partly due to the findings of the term breech trial[7] (although that trial applied to singleton pregnancy) and concerns about the rare complication of locked twins, which carries a high mortality rate. There is now good evidence from a large international multicenter randomized trial (Twin Birth Study)[8] – 2804 uncomplicated twin pregnancies where the leading twin was vertex recruited after 32 weeks' gestation and randomized to planned vaginal birth versus planned CS – that planned elective CS is not advantageous for the fetuses, and this finding applies to both dichorionic and monochorionic diamniotic twins. The authors did emphasise requirements to optimize outcomes were that the deliveries were carried out by skilled clinicians, particularly in vaginal breech delivery (if the second twin nonvertex), and there was access to facilities for emergency CS without delay. The evidence to guide mode of delivery for preterm twins <32 weeks is not robust and conflicting. There is some evidence to support CS when the fetal weight range is 500–1500 g; however, vaginal delivery is an acceptable practice if the first twin is vertex until more robust data come available[7].

Prevention of preterm labor and delivery

Interventions that have been studied to prevent spontaneous preterm labor, and hence delivery, in twin and triplet pregnancies include bed rest, progesterone (intramuscular or vaginal), cervical cerclage and tocolytics (oral betamimetics). Sexual abstinence has never been studied in multiple pregnancy.

A systematic review of seven RCTs (five of twins, two of triplets) of bed rest found no evidence to support this intervention to reduce preterm delivery[9].

Several RCTs have evaluated the clinical effectiveness of progesterone (intramuscular or vaginal) versus placebo in the prevention of preterm birth in women with twin and triplet pregnancies. None have shown this intervention to be effective[4]. A systematic review and meta-analysis of individual patient data from five RCTs considering the impact of vaginal progesterone in women with asymptomatic short cervix (defined as 25 mm or less on midtrimester ultrasound) included only 52 twin pregnancies[10]. Whilst there was a significant reduction in preterm birth in singleton pregnancy, there was no such effect in twin pregnancies. However, there was a reduction in composite neonatal morbidity and mortality, and it is believed that these findings need to be confirmed in a prospective randomized trial of progesterone for women with twin pregnancy and short cervix[11].

One RCT and one observational study (prospective) of twin pregnancies and four observational studies (retrospective) of triplet pregnancies evaluated the effectiveness of cervical cerclage in the prevention of preterm birth. None showed this intervention to be effective[4]. More recently, the cervical pessary (Arabin pessary) has been studied in women with short cervix and while the preliminary results are promising, results of appropriately powered trials are awaited[11].

A systematic review of five RCTs evaluating the effectiveness of betamimetics found no evidence to support this intervention to reduce preterm delivery[12].

Therefore, in the absence of an effective intervention routine screening to predict, preterm delivery is not recommended in twin and triplet pregnancy. There is no evidence to guide management in higher order pregnancies or for those who have twin and triplet pregnancies and have other risk factors apart from the multiple pregnancy, and therefore this management should be individualized.

Management of complicated multiple pregnancy
Discordant fetal anomaly
Fetal anomalies are more common in twins and higher order pregnancies compared with singletons. In monochorionic twins, the rate of structural anomaly is even higher although discordant aneuploidy is very rare. If the abnormality is associated with chromosomal abnormality, invasive prenatal diagnosis may be offered. Invasive prenatal diagnosis in multiple pregnancy should ideally be undertaken by a specialist who has the expertise to undertake selective reduction should the need arise as it is very important, particularly where there are no obvious features to identify

the abnormal fetus, that the pregnancy is carefully mapped. If the condition is severe or lethal, selective termination of pregnancy is an option, but the technique used will depend on whether there is shared placentation.

In dichorionic twins where selective termination is planned, fetocide using medical therapeutics can be undertaken. It is recommended that this is either undertaken before 14 weeks' gestation or after 32 weeks' gestation. This is because, if undertaken before 14 weeks' gestation, the outcomes are better, in particular gestation at delivery of the surviving normal fetus[13]. Therefore, if the window of opportunity to intervene before 14 weeks is lost, the delay until 32 weeks is advocated to afford the normal fetus the best chance of a normal outcome. This can be a very difficult concept for couples and requires expert counseling and good emotional support. If the woman insists on selective reduction before 32 weeks, she needs to be aware of the risks to the normal fetus of preterm delivery secondary to procedure-related ruptured membranes, infection and preterm labor.

In monochorionic twins, as the fetal circulations are connected, selective termination cannot be undertaken with medical therapeutics because of the risk of death and neurologic damage to the co-twin. Invasive techniques, such as cord occlusion or interstitial ablation, are required and these techniques are challenging, high-risk procedures and require specific expertise.

Discordant fetal growth
In dichorionic twins where there is growth restriction in one fetus, the management in terms of surveillance does not differ from that in singleton fetal growth restriction. However, when timing delivery, the risks for the normal fetus need to be carefully considered. If there is severe growth restriction at extremes of gestation (24–28 weeks), the woman and her partner may need to consider allowing the growth-restricted fetus to die in utero to gain optimal gestation and outcome for the normal fetus. Monochorionic twin growth discordance will be addressed later in this chapter.

Single fetal death
Single fetal death in the first trimester is relatively common and is termed "vanishing twin syndrome." It is a low-risk situation for the surviving fetus and the woman, and her family can be reassured that there are unlikely to be long-term consequences. The

ongoing pregnancy can be treated as a routine single-ton pregnancy.

After the first trimester, single fetal death is a high-risk situation for the surviving fetus in mono-chorionic and dichorionic twin pregnancy. The risks are, however, much higher for monochorionic twins. A systematic review of 22 studies showed that the rates of co-twin death, preterm delivery, abnormal post-natal cranial imaging and rate of neurodevelopmental impairment after single fetal death were 15%, 68%, 34% and 26% in monochorionic versus 3%, 54%, 16% and 2% in dichorionic twins[14]. Monochorionic twins will be discussed below. What is unclear is whether preterm delivery was spontaneous or iatrogenic, and if iatrogenic what the indication for delivery was. Therefore, some of the morbidity in dichorionic twins may be secondary to clinicians deciding to deliver the surviving fetus preterm for fear of it succumbing to the unknown pathology that caused one twin's death, and the morbidity secondary to preterm delivery.

In current practice in dichorionic twins, if there is co-twin demise, delivery is not recommended unless there are signs of surviving twin compromise (e.g., abnormal cardiotocography (CTG)). There is no evi-dence to guide ongoing monitoring in this situation but it seems sensible to undertake a CTG at the time of single death diagnosis (only at a gestation where CTG is advocated, i.e., not before 24–26 weeks), and there-after, if clinically indicated, e.g., reduced fetal move-ments. Continuing the pregnancy to afford a better gestation can be difficult for the anxious woman, her partner and family, and in addition to requiring emo-tional support, regular clinical review including ultra-sound at least every 2 weeks is advocated.

Complications of shared placentation

Single fetal death

If one of a monochorionic twin pair dies, damage to the surviving twin is thought to occur due to acute hemo-dynamic changes around the time of death, with the survivor losing part of its circulating volume into the circulation of the dying/dead twin. This causes hypo-tension and low perfusion leading to ischemic organ damage, which if persistent, can lead to the death of the surviving fetus, but if transient, survival but organ damage, particularly but not exclusively brain damage.

If single fetal death occurs, by the time it has been diagnosed, the damage has been done and rapid deliv-ery is usually unwise unless the pregnancy is advanced, i.e., term (37+ weeks' gestation) or there is evidence of acute compromise (abnormal CTG) in the surviving fetus. Clinical management is complex as apart from the risks to the surviving fetus, the emotional effects and psychologic consequences for the woman, her partner and family are significant.

Some advocate assessing for fetal anemia in the surviving fetus using middle cerebral artery Doppler peak systolic velocity measurements, and intrauterine transfusion in such cases has been described but the clinical value of this intervention is not established.

Serial brain ultrasound imaging is advised and planning fetal magnetic resonance imaging (MRI) no earlier than 4 weeks after the event to assess for ser-ious cerebral morbidity is recommended[15]. Fetal MRI provides more detailed information about hem-orrhagic or ischemic brain lesions that may not be seen on ultrasound. In circumstances where there is brain damage depending on the prognosis, termination of pregnancy may become an option.

As clinical management is difficult and need for detailed counseling is required, it is recommended that such cases are seen by fetal medicine experts who have the knowledge and expertise to provide this complex care.

There is no evidence to guide when to deliver the surviving fetus, but it seems logical to advise planned delivery at 37–38 weeks unless there is an indication to deliver sooner.

Twin-to-twin transfusion syndrome

Where there is mild-to-moderate TTTS (oligohy-dramnios polyhydramnios sequence, but visible donor bladder and normal umbilical artery Dopplers in both fetuses – Quintero stage I, see Table 24.2 in Chapter 24) it may progress but many remain stable, and unless there is progression invasive treatment, is not advised. Therefore, weekly ultrasound monitoring in these cases is required and women should be warned to report symptoms of progression, including increasing abdominal discomfort, shortness of breath and palpa-tations. Clinicians should also be educated to consider TTTS in women with monochorionic twin pregnancy reporting these symptoms.

Severe TTTS (oligohydramnios polyhydramnios sequence, absent donor bladder and/or abnormal umbilical artery (UA) Doppler in donor or ductus venosus (DV) Doppler in recipient and or hydrops of recipient – Quintero stage II–IV; see Table 24.2 in Chapter 24) is associated with poor outcomes, including pregnancy loss in up to 85–90% of cases and significant risk of neurologic damage, cardiovascular and renal consequences in survivors. In the past, available treatment options were amnioreduction, septostomy and fetoscopic laser coagulation of placental vascular anastomoses. It is now known that fetoscopic laser is the treatment of choice and is associated with better outcomes compared with amnioreduction for severe TTTS between 16 and 26 weeks' gestation[16] – more survivors, later gestation at delivery and less neurologic morbidity. Nowadays some experts advocate laser in selected cases presenting as early as 15 weeks (but there are higher procedure-related pregnancy loss rates as amnion and chorion may not be fused) and as late as 28–29 weeks' gestation. The procedure is accompanied by amnioreduction at the end to relieve uterine over-distension.

Fetoscopic laser ablation is a technically challenging procedure, particularly if the women is overweight or obese, the placenta is anterior, the amniotic fluid turbid (requiring amnioinfusion during the procedure) and the pregnancy triplet or higher order. It is undertaken in specialist centers with specific expertise, and therefore early diagnosis and timely referral is important. There are various techniques and much recent research has concentrated on reducing recurrence of TTTS and occurrence of postlaser twin anemia polycythemia sequence (TAPS), including reducing procedure-related complications. The procedure-related risk of ruptured membranes and/or miscarriage is about 7%, and delivery occurs at a median gestational age of about 34 weeks. The use of elective cervical cerclage at the time of laser has been shown to be ineffective, but some specialists do insert a cerclage if the cervical length is less than 20 mm at the time of diagnosis of TTTS, but this needs further evaluation.

A trial of fetoscopic laser for stage 1 TTTS is underway.

If TTTS recurs, it may be managed by repeat laser or amnioreduction depending on severity and gestation. In recurrence at advanced gestation, i.e., >28 weeks' delivery may be considered.

Selective growth restriction

When selective growth restriction (SGR) is diagnosed, there is limited evidence to provide guidance for the clinical care of these complex cases, but experts agree that these pregnancies should be managed by fetal medicine specialists using advanced ultrasound techniques to monitor fetal growth and wellbeing (using Doppler of placental and fetal circulation and computerized CTG). The management goal is to prolong pregnancy in favor of the normally grown fetus, but avoid single fetal death of the growth restricted fetus and potential consequences thereof for the normally grown fetus.

If there is deterioration in fetal wellbeing of the growth-restricted fetus, preterm delivery may be offered. In severe cases, if it is diagnosed prior to viability (<24 weeks) and there is evidence of significant compromise in the growth-restricted fetus, and thus a high risk of fetal death, selective termination may be considered. Selective termination may also be considered in cases where there is significant risk of fetal demise <26 weeks and a desire to optimize outcome for the normally grown fetus. Selective termination would need to be undertaken using cord occlusive techniques given the shared circulation and requires specific expertise.

SGR is divided into three subtypes depending on whether there is UA waveform abnormality, and if so what the abnormality is. Perinatal outcome differs in these three subtypes[17]. In type 1 SGR, the lowest risk type, there is positive end-diastolic flow in the UA waveform of the growth-restricted fetus, and if this persists, the outcome can be good with over 90% survival. In type II SGR, there is persistent absent or reversed end-diastolic flow in the UA waveform of the growth-restricted fetus, and there is a risk of fetal death of either twin in up to 29% and neurologic sequelae in 15% of cases born before 30 weeks. In type III SGR, there is intermittent present, absent and reversed end-diastolic flow in the UA waveform of the growth-restricted fetus and a 10–20% risk of sudden death of the growth-restricted fetus (even if stable ultrasound and/or normal computerized CTG hours or days before), and a high rate of neurologic morbidity (up to 20%) in the larger twin (even if the smaller twin is liveborn).

In these cases, the presence of placental vascular anastomoses are both protective and dangerous. Protective because, paradoxically, transfusion from the larger to smaller twin may compensate for the placental insufficiency and prolong survival, resulting in a longer latency from diagnosis to deterioration and delivery (10 weeks versus 3–4 weeks in singleton growth restriction). Dangerous because there can be acute transfusional events, which are neither predictable nor preventable, resulting in fetal death and fetal compromise with long-term consequences if survival.

With regular and intensive surveillance, the aim is to get the pregnancy to 34 weeks' gestation. Triggers to deliver earlier would be lack of/significantly suboptimal fetal growth and/or abnormal DV Doppler waveforms (absent or reversed end-diastolic flow) and/or abnormal computerized CTG (overt decelerations or short term variation <4.0).

Twin anemia polycythemia sequence

While TAPS is a recognized morbid condition, currently our knowledge of the natural history, fetal and neonatal implications, and optimal surveillance and treatment is lacking. There are case series and case studies in the literature describing a range of treatment options and outcomes. The treatment options described are expectant management, delivery, intra-uterine blood transfusion of the anemic fetus with or without partial exchange transfusion of the polycythemic fetus, selective fetocide or fetoscopic laser. None of these interventions have been subject to robust prospective evaluation in the research setting. Perinatal outcome may range from double intra-uterine fetal death to the birth of two healthy babies with hemoglobin discordance. Mortality and short, medium and long-term morbidity data again is based on case reports and small case series. Cases of cerebral injury have been described. As there is limited guidance, there remains debate about whether to screen for this condition and if so, what to do if screening is positive. However, experts agree that when the condition is diagnosed, tertiary level fetal medicine opinion should be sought and clear decisions about management will depend on gestation at diagnosis and local expertise.

Twin-reversed arterial perfusion sequence

If a diagnosis of twin-reversed arterial perfusion (TRAP) sequence is made, it is important to evaluate the anatomy and cardiac function of the surviving fetus, and management options include expectant management with regular surveillance or invasive techniques to interrupt the vascular anastamoses between the twins. Invasive techniques that have been described include cord occlusion using bipolar diathermy, intrafetal laser ablation or radiointerstitial thermal ablation. Poor prognostic indicators are: i) if the relative size of the acardiac twin is >50% of the pump twin and ii) if the pump twin is showing signs of cardiovascular compromise. The advocates of selecting cases for invasive treatment argue that in some cases the flow to the acardiac twin ceases naturally and

procedure-related complications can be avoided, and there are reported cases of good outcomes with expectant management. Those who advocate treating all cases argue that overall outcomes are better (80% survival of the pump twin) and monitoring for deterioration (persistent growth of the acardiac fetus or cardiovascular compromise in the pump twin) may identify some at risk, but there are still unpredictable deaths that occur due to acute pathologic processes. Studies have shown that optimal outcomes are achieved if the procedure is performed before 16 weeks[18], which is another reason why some advocate treating all as with expectant management and selective treatment this gestational threshold is breached.

Conjoined twins

The prognosis for conjoined twins depends on the type of fusion but is often very guarded, and nowadays a number of women opt for termination of pregnancy. If the pregnancy is to continue, the management is complex, often requires other imaging and requires involvement of a very specialist multidisciplinary team, including fetal medicine experts and various medical and surgical pediatric specialities. Delivery by cesarean is advocated (but vaginal delivery has been described) and may need to be undertaken preterm if there is evidence of fetal compromise and live birth desirable. In some cases, emergency separation after birth is required (if one dies or has a life-threatening condition) but in most cases separation is planned electively after extensive evaluation and planning involving the relevant clinicians.

Monoamniotic twins

Monochorionic monoamniotic twin pregnancies are at very high risk of fetal loss and this is classically thought to be due to complications of cord entanglement, but there are also important contributions from TTTS, twin-reversed arterial perfusion sequence and congenital anomalies. It is important to note that cord entanglement is universally present and it is critical (i.e., occlusive) cord entanglement, which is the major concern (Figure 25.1). The published literature undoubtedly confirms the high loss rates but unfortunately, given the rarity of this type of twin pregnancy (only 1% of monochorionic twins), is underpowered to address management strategies that may reduce this risk. Clinical management is aimed at preventing fetal loss but optimizing gestation at delivery. Intensive fetal surveillance is advocated and some even recommend

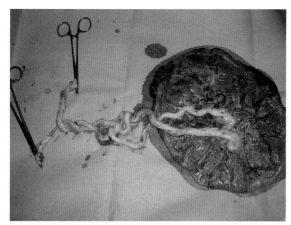

Figure 25.1 Monoamniotic placenta and cords demonstrating loose cord entanglement found at elective cesarean section.

inpatient care in the third trimester. There are, however, several case series that show acceptable outcomes with outpatient care. Intensive fetal surveillance described is regular ultrasound and CTG but the optimal regimen, i.e., how often to undertake these modalities, is not known and there is no robust evidence that intense surveillance makes a difference. It seems logical to conclude that cord entanglement may become critical at any time, and therefore unless there is continuous surveillance, a sudden fetal loss may occur even if ultrasound or CTG were normal a few hours or days beforehand. In the past some have advocated the use of Sundilac (a nonsteroidal anti-inflammatory drug) to reduce fetal renal blood flow, and hence liquor volume, i.e., medical amnioreduction, and avoid cord entanglement or critical cord entanglement, but this strategy has largely been abandoned due to lack of convincing evidence of efficacy and concerns about the potential adverse fetal effects of the drug. A more recent literature review of 10 studies comprising 378 monoamniotic pregnancies suggests that the majority of losses occur before 24 weeks and those that occur later are secondary to fetal congenital abnormaility[19]. Interestingly, the most common cardiac anomaly in monoamniotic twins is transpositon of the great arteries. A recent relatively large retrospective cohort study (Canada, Switzerland and Belgium) of 193 monoamniotic twin pregnancies, managed either as inpatients or with intensive outpatient surveillance from 26–28 weeks, showed that overall fetal death occurred in 18% of cases but if both twins survived to 23 weeks and beyond, the chance of survival was around 96%[20]. Type of surveillance (i.e., inpatient or outpatient) did

not significantly affect the outcome. They also showed that the prospective risk of fetal death was higher than nonrespiratory neonatal complication rates after 32+4 weeks, and therefore, this group's recommendation was to deliver monochorionic twins at 33–34 weeks' gestation. Elective cesarean delivery is recommended to avoid cord accidents and the rare complication of locked twins.

Summary

Twin, triplet and higher order multiple pregnancies are high risk and these sometimes complex pregnancies require additional elements of care to identify and manage complications effectively and optimize outcomes. This care needs to be delivered by health professionals with specific knowledge and expertise ensuring consistency and continuity, and this may be best delivered in the context of a specialist clinic or service. Knowledge of chorionicity and amnionicity is essential to guide care plans and management of complications. The evidence to guide management of higher order pregnancies is lacking but multifetal pregnancy reduction should be discussed. If invasive diagnosis is required, this should be performed by a clinician who can map the pregnancy and is able to offer selective termination if the need arises. Preterm delivery prevention options are limited, and the focus should be on ensuring women know signs and symptoms to enable timely presentation to get corticosteroids on board. Complications that arise require a high level of expertise and should be discussed with and, if appropriate, referred to specialists in fetal medicine. These complex cases include discordant fetal anomaly, discordant growth, single fetal death, complications of shared placentation (TTTS, SGR, TAPS, TRAP sequence and conjoined twins), triplets and higher order pregnancies with shared placentation. Attention should be given to relevant and accurate information provision and emotional support required to mitigate the stress and anxiety associated with complications. There are a number of areas of care that require further research to establish a more robust evidence base, but where the evidence is lacking, a more pragmatic and sensible approach is advocated.

References

1. Wimalasundera RC. Selective reduction and termination of multiple pregnancies. In: Kilby M, Baker PN, Critchley H, Field DJ, eds. *Multiple Pregnancy* London: RCOG Press, 2006; 95–108.

2. Royal College of Obstetricians and Gynaecologists (RCOG). Consensus views arising from 50th Study Group: Multiple Pregnancy. In: Kilby M, Baker PN, Critchley H, Field DJ, eds. London: RCOG Press, 2006; 283–5.

3. Bricker L, Optimal antenatal care for twin and triplet pregnancy: The evidence base, *Best Pract Res Clin Obstet Gynaecol* 2014; 28(2): 305–17.

4. National Collaborating Centre for Women's and Children's Health. Multiple pregnancy: the management of twin and triplet pregnancies in the antenatal period. London: RCOG Press, 2011.

5. Danon D, Sekar R, Hack KE, et al. Increased stillbirth in uncomplicated monochorionic twin pregnancies: a systematic review and meta-analysis. *Obstet Gynecol* 2013; 121: 1318–26.

6. Barrett JFR. Twin delivery: method, timing and conduct. *Best Pract Res Clin Obstet Gynaecol* 2014; 28(2): 327–38.

7. Hannah ME, Hannah WJ, Hewson SA et al. Planned caesarean section versus planned vaginal birth for breech presentation at term: a randomised multicentre trial. Term Breech Trial Collaborative Group. *Lancet* 2000; 356(9239): 1375–83.

8. Barrett, JF, Hannah ME, Hutton EK, et al. for the Twin Birth Study Collaborative Group. A randomized trial of planned cesarean or vaginal birth for twin pregnancies. *NEJM* 2013; 369: 1295–305.

9. Crowther CA, Han S. Hospitalisation and bed rest for multiple pregnancy. *Cochrane Database Syst Rev* 2010; (7): CD000110.

10. Romero R, Nicolaides K, Conde-Agudelo A, et al. Vaginal progesterone in women with an asymptomatic sonographic short cervix in the midtrimester decreases preterm delivery and neonatal morbidity: systematic review and meta-analysis of individual patient data. *Am J Obstet Gynecol* 2012; 206: 124.e1–19.

11. Rode L, Tabor A. Prevention of preterm delivery in twin pregnancy. *Best Pract Res Clin Obstet Gynaecol* 2014; 28(2): 273–83.

12. Yamasmit W, Chaithongwongwatthana S, Tolosa JE, et al. Prophylactic oral betamimetics for reducing preterm birth in women with a twin pregnancy. *Cochrane Database Syst Rev* 2012; 9: CD004733.

13. Yaron Y, Johnson KD, Bryant-Greenwood PK, et al. Selective termination and elective reduction in twin pregnancies: 10 years experience at a single centre. *Human Reproduction* 1998; 13(8): 2301–4.

14. Hillman SC, Morris RK, Kilby MD. Co-twin prognosis after single fetal death: a systematic review and meta-analysis. *Obstet Gynecol* 2011; 118(4): 928–40.

15. Shek NW, Hillman SC, Kilby MD. Single-twin demise: Pregnancy outcome. *Best Pract Res Clin Obstet Gynaecol* 2013; S1521–6934(13): 00154–5.

16 Roberts D, Neilson JP, Kilby MD, et al. Interventions for the treatment of twin-twin transfusion syndrome. *Cochrane Database Syst Rev* 2014; 1: CD002073.

17. Gratacós E, Lewi L, Muñoz B, et al. A classification system for selective intrauterine growth restriction in monochorionic pregnancies according to umbilical artery Doppler flow in the smaller twin. *Ultrasound Obstet Gynecol* 2007; 30(1): 28–34.

18. Pagani G, D'Antonio F, Khalil A, et al. Intrafetal laser treatment for twin reversed arterial perfusion sequence: cohort study and meta-analysis. *Ultrasound Obstet Gynecol* 2013; 42(1): 6–14.

19. Dias T, Thilaganathan B, Bhide A. Monoamniotic twin pregnancy. *The Obstetrician & Gynaecologist* 2012; 14: 71–8.

20. Van Mieghem T, De Heus R, Lewi L, et al. Prenatal management of monoamniotic twin pregnancies. *Obstet Gynecol* 2014; 124(3): 498–506.

Chapter

26

Placenta, amniotic membrane and amniotic fluid

Bidyut Kumar and Ezechi Cally Nwosu

Placental development

Human placenta development is a highly organized process due to the significant role it plays in pregnancy in establishing appropriate interface for fetal nutrition, gas exchange, disposal of waste products and fetomaternal circulation. It ensures maternal recognition of pregnancy by altering local environment immunity to prevent fetal allograft rejection and plays an important part in producing pregnancy hormones.

About 3 days after fertilization, a 16-cell morula is formed. It contains an *inner cell mass* and a surrounding layer of cells called the *outer cell mass*. Gradually intercellular spaces appear within the inner cell mass, which become confluent with adjoining spaces to produce a single cavity. The cell is now called a *blastocyst*. Cells of the inner cell mass, now called *embryoblast* become clustered at one pole of the blastocyst, and those of the outer cell mass form the epithelial wall of the blastocyst, which would form the future trophoblast. Trophoblastic cells over the embryoblast pole begin to penetrate between the epithelial cells of the decidual epithelium about the 6th day after fertilization. The blastocyst is partially imbedded in the endometrial or decidual stroma on the 8th day and the area over the embryoblast differentiates into (i) an inner mononucleated cell layer called the *cytotrophoblast* and (ii) an outer multinucleated layer called the *syncytiotrophoblast*. Cytotrophoblast cells undergo mitosis and migrate into the syncytiotrophoblast where they fuse and lose their individual cell membranes.

The embryoblast differentiates into two layers, called the *hypoblast* and *epiblast*. These two layers form a flat disc, which later gives rise to the embryo. A small cavity appears within the epiblast, which enlarges to become the amniotic cavity. Epiblast cells adjacent to the cytotrophoblast are called *amnioblasts*, which together with the rest of the epiblast line the amniotic cavity.

By the 12th day, the blastocyst is completely embedded in the endometrial stroma. The trophoblast is now characterized by lacunar spaces in the syncytiotrophoblast that form an intercommunicating network, which is particularly evident at the embryonic pole. The cells of syncytiotrophoblast penetrate deeper into the stroma and erode the endothelial lining of the maternal capillaries giving rise to dilated sinusoids. The lacunar spaces in the syncytiotrophoblast now become continuous with the sinusoids and maternal blood enters the lacunar system. As the trophoblast continues to erode more and more sinusoids, maternal blood begins to flow through the trophoblastic system, establishing the uteroplacental circulation.

The cytotrophoblast, syncytiotrophoblast, extraembryonic mesoderm, the lacunar spaces and sinusoids give rise to the placenta.

Trafficking

Healthy fetal growth depends on the availability of adequate transfer channels between the placenta and fetus and adequate nutrients, which in turn depends on the capacity to transport nutrients. The activity of a range of nutrient transporters is known to affect fetal growth. Several factors influence transport across the placenta such as uteroplacental blood flow, area available for exchange, physical metabolism, activity and expression of specific transporter proteins in the placental barrier.

Transfer of highly permeable molecules, such as oxygen and carbon dioxide, are particularly influenced by blood flow. For less permeable substrates, the

Fetal Medicine, ed. Bidyut Kumar and Zarko Alfirevic. Published by Cambridge University Press. © Cambridge University Press 2016.

placenta possesses both passive and active transport concentration gradients. Glucose crosses the placenta by facilitated diffusion. Net glucose transfer is therefore highly dependent on maternal–fetal concentration gradients. Other nutrients, such as calcium, are transported by primary active transport; a process directly linked to hydrolysis of adenosine triphosphate. A wide range of nutrients, such as amino acids, phosphorous and lactate, are transported across the placenta, mediated by secondary active transport utilizing energy provided by ion gradients, such as sodium, chloride and protons. Changes in energy availability or ion gradients can profoundly influence net transfer of substrates transported by active mechanism.

Placental transfer of maternal immunoglobulin G (IgG) antibodies to the fetus is an important mechanism providing protection to the fetus whilst fetal humoral response is inefficient. IgG is the only class of maternal antibody that significantly crosses the human placenta. Fetal receptor antigen, expressed by syncytiotrophoblast cells, mediates this crossing. IgG transfer from mother to fetus depends on gestational age with transfer beginning as early as 13 weeks in a linear fashion, progressing to the largest amount in the third trimester.

Iron transport from mother to fetus is crucial for fetal development, but the exact mechanism is uncertain and transfer has to be regulated because of its toxicity. It is suggested that transport across the placenta occurs directly via transferring, present on the surface of trophoblasts directly in contact with maternal blood or possibly by trophoblastic erythrophagocytosis in the hemophagous area of the placenta and also in endometrial glands. In the developing fetus, iron is accumulated against a concentration gradient and in the case of maternal iron deficiency, the placenta protects the iron transport to fetus through increased expression of placental transferrin receptor together with a rise in divalent metal transporter.

Placental developmental abnormality

Circumvallate placenta

Circumvallate placenta is a rare placental condition in which the fetal membranes (chorion and amnion) "double back" on the fetal side around the edge of the placenta. Prevalence is estimated to be around 1–7%[1] On antenatal ultrasound the placenta may show a thick peripheral rim of chorionic tissue appearing as an echo dense ridge, although it may be only be apparent following delivery.

It is associated with higher incidence of perinatal complications, such as premature delivery (64.1%), placental abruption (10.9%), small for gestational age (36.9%), neonatal death (8.9%), neonatal intensive care admission (55.4%), chronic lung disease (33.9%), oligohydramnios, abnormal cardiotocogram (CTG), intrauterine fetal death and miscarriage[2–4]. The odds ratio for placental abruption in patients with circumvallate placenta is reported as 13.1 (95% confidence interval, 5.65–30.2)[3].

When vaginal bleeding during the second trimester and premature chemical rupture of membranes were both used as predictive factors for circumvallate placenta, the sensitivity was 28.8% and specificity was 99.9%.

Battledore placenta

Battledore placenta is a situation where the umbilical cord is attached at the border of the placenta – so called because of the putative resemblance to the racquet in battledore, a precursor to badminton. The shortest distance between the cord insertion and placental edge is within 2 cm. Although risks associated with battledore placentation are rare, complications such as fetal distress, intrauterine growth restriction, preterm labor and cord prolapse have been described[5–7].

Velamentous insertion of cord and vasa praevia

Velamentous insertion of umbilical cord is an abnormality where the umbilical cord inserts into the fetal membranes resulting in the fetal blood vessels from the umbilical cord coursing through the membranes between the amnion and chorion to the placenta.

When such blood vessels cross over the internal cervical os and below the fetal presenting part, unprotected by placental tissue or the umbilical cord, the condition is called *vasa praevia*. In this condition, the vessels close to the cervical os are likely to rupture at spontaneous rupture of membranes or during artificial rupture of membranes resulting in fetal bleeding. Incidence is reported to be between 1 in 2,000 to 6,000 pregnancies. Associated risk factors are placenta praevia, bilobed placenta or a placenta with succinturiate lobe and multiple pregnancies. Usually there is no major maternal risk.

Diagnoses maybe difficult antenatally, but may be possible in labor if the cervix is dilated and blood vessels are felt on vaginal examination. During the antenatal period, it is possible to diagnose vasa praevia with transvaginal ultrasound scan aided by color Doppler. If the diagnosis is at term, then delivery by elective cesarean section is indicated. If diagnosis is suspected in the second trimester, imaging should be repeated in the third trimester to confirm or refute the diagnosis. If diagnosis is confirmed in the third trimester, the usual and safe practice is to advise prophylactic administration of corticosteroids for fetal lung maturation and admission at 28–32 weeks of gestation to a unit with appropriate facilities for neonatal resuscitation, in the event of necessity of emergent preterm delivery.

Where undiagnosed during antenatal period, vasa praevia often presents with fresh vaginal bleeding at rupture of membrane and fetal heart rate abnormalities on CTG. It is rare but the risk of fetal mortality is about 60%. Given that fetal blood volume is around 80–100 mL/kg, the loss of relatively small amounts of blood can have major implications for the fetus, and hence, rapid delivery by category 1 cesarean section and intensive resuscitation of newborn is essential[8].

Placenta praevia

Placenta praevia is a condition in pregnancy, from fetal viability until delivery, where the placenta is inserted wholly or partly in the lower segment of the uterus and may cover all or part of the internal cervical os. The incidence at delivery varies widely. It is estimated that it affects 0.4–0.5% of all labors. There are several risk factors that influence placenta praevia, which include increased maternal age, smoking, abnormal uterus and increased parity.

Diagnosis is by ultrasound and it is clinically classified into major and minor praevia. Major placenta praevia is inserted in the lower segment of the uterus and covers the internal cervical os while minor, or partial, exists if the leading placental edge is implanted in the lower segment of the uterus. Clinical suspicion of praevia should be raised in all bleeding after 20 weeks' gestation. A high presenting part, abnormal lie and painless or unprovoked bleeding, irrespective of previous imaging reports are more suggestive of a low-lying placenta, although may not be present. Definitive diagnosis usually relies on ultrasound imaging abdominal and transvaginal[8].

Transvaginal scans are safe, improve acurracy and are well-tolerated by women if abdominal sonography is inconclusive or antepartum hemorrhage continues despite satisfactory abdominal ultrasound examination. Women with placenta praevia in the third trimester of pregnancy should be counseled in the risks of preterm delivery and obstetric hemorrhage. Care should be tailored to individual needs. Care can be managed at home at a woman's request, however, she and her partner should be encouraged to ensure they have safety precautions in place, including having someone available to help should the need arise and, particularly, having ready access to the hospital. Prior to delivery, all women with praevia and their partners should be counseled and decision reached regarding delivery, blood transfusion and hysterectomy.

The UK Royal College of Obstetricians and Gynaecologists (RCOG) does not recommend delivery by elective cesarean delivery in an asymtomatic woman before 36–37 weeks' gestation. The mode of delivery should be based on clinical judgement supplemented by sonographic information. Placental edge <2 cm from internal os at 36 weeks in the third trimester is likely to need cesarean section, particularly if the placenta is thick, but the evidence for this is poor and further research is needed. Timing of delivery depends upon maternal and fetal risk and gestational age. Involvement and discussion with a senior anesthetist should take place as soon as possible, regarding timing of delivery and appropriate anesthesia. Placenta praevia with or without risk of previous cesarean section carries the risk of massive hemorrhage, and therefore hysterectomy and delivery should be carried out in a unit with adequate access to a blood bank and facilities for high-dependency care. Blood crossmatching and blood products should be readily available in anticipation of massive hemorrhage.

Placenta vascular abnormality

Choriangioma

Placental chorangiomas are rare nontrophoblastic benign harmatoma-like growths in the placenta consisting of blood vessels, reported to be present in about 1% of placentas examined by microscopy. They are often found on the surface of the placenta or in the placental parenchyma. Most chorangiomas are small and are of no clinical significance. However, clinically significant chorangioma or multiple chorangiomas may be associated with fetal anemia, polyhydramnios, hydrops fetalis, antepartum hemorrhage, pregnancy-induced hypertension and unexplained fetal death attributed to shunting of blood through the hemangiomas, preterm birth, fetal growth retardation, postpartum hemorrhage, thrombocytopenia and disseminated intravascular coagulation. Chorionagiomas are usually located on the fetal surface of the placenta, although they may occur inside the placental tissue or bulge from the maternal surface. Masses are rarely located in the membrane. Sonographically, chorioangiomas are a well-circumscribed placental mass of relatively homogeneous structure with echogenicity different from placental tissue. Color flow and power Doppler help diagnosis by allowing the vascularity of the tumor to be assessed and may allow the detection of angiomatous cellular and degenerative changes. Antenatal magnetic resonance imaging (MRI) of placenta for imaging of chorioangiomas has been reported but it remains uncertain whether it adds to the diagnostic information obtained by ultrasound.

Histologic examination of chorangioma indicates they are heterogeneous structures with a capsule and vessels. Microscopically, they are composed of numerous proliferative blood vessels in various stages of differentiation, capillary-type blood vessels, carvenous, endotheliosis, fibrosis, cellularity, solid areas and focal necrosis. However, atypical lesions with increased predominance of tissue types of blood vessels, carvenous areas and mitosis are associated with complications.

Whether the size of chorioangiomas is of any clinical significance remains undecided. Some authors have considered 4 cm as the cut-off measurement above which chorioangiomas have been said to be clinically significant. Others have suggested a cut-off of 5 cm or more. In a systematic review of 112 cases, in 99 cases a size of the chorioangioma was reported. In 78 of these cases the chorioangioma was reported to be >5 cm (78%). In this cohort, the fetal and perinatal mortality was 28.2%. When the placental tumor was reported to be between 4 and 5 cm (12/99; 12.2%) all had perinatal complications and in three this was associated with a stillborn baby (25%)[9].

Several different treatment modalities have been tried but none has proven superior to any other. The use of the cyclooxygenase-2 inhibitor sulindac can reduce polyhydramnios, thereby leading to prolongation of gestation and improved survival of babies. Amnioreduction, laser ablation of placental vessels, embolization of placental vessel, ligation of feeding vessel to chorioangioma, in-utero alcohol injection and intrauterine fetal transfusion have been reported. Conservative management remains a viable option because there is no good evidence to demonstrate that any kind of treatment is better than conservative methods[10].

Gestational trophoblastic diseases

Gestational trophoblastic disease (GTD) forms a group of disorders that range from molar pregnancies to malignant conditions such as choriocarcinoma. It encompasses a continuum of a neoplastic process that arises from the fetal chorion of the placenta (trophoblast). This group of disorders consists of diseases with a varying propensity for local invasion and metastasis. The World Health Organization (WHO) has classified GTD as two premalignant diseases consisting of complete or classical hydatidiform mole (CHM) and partial hydatidiform mole (PHM) and three malignant disorders consisting of invasive mole, choriocarcinoma and placental site trophoblastic tumor (PSTT). The last three conditions are often collectively referred to as gestational trophoblastic neoplasia (GTN).

Estimates for the incidence of various forms of GTD vary in different regions of the world. In Western countries, the incidence is about 1:1,000–1,500 pregnancies with incidental findings of approximately 1 in 600 in therapeutic abortions. In South East Asia and some developing countries, the rate is reported as much as 15 times higher than in the USA and UK. Japan has a reported rate of 2 per 1,000 pregnancies. In the Far East, some sources estimate the rate as high as 1:120 pregnancies. In the UK, the calculated incidence is 1:714 of live births. Twenty per cent of patients with hydatidiform mole will develop trophoblastic malignancy, 15% uterine invasion and in 4% metastasis. No cases of choriocarcinoma have been reported after partial molar pregnancy, although 4% of patients develop persistent nonmetastatic trophoblastic disease requiring chemotherapy[11–13].

In normal pregnancy, half the chromosomes come from the mother and half from the father. In *complete* molar pregnancy, all the genetic material is commonly from the father with an empty oocyte lacking fertilized maternal genes. In 75–80% of cases, a single sperm undergoes duplication within the empty ovum. Less often, an empty ovum is fertilized by two sperms and there is no fetal tissue. In patients with complete molar pregnancy, the main complaints are hyperemesis and vomiting, probably related to extremely high levels of human chorionic gonadotropin (hCG), and vaginal bleeding. The uterus is often distended and incompatible with gestation due to large amounts of blood with patients occasionally passing a jelly like substance similar to a "bunch of grapes." Pregnancy-induced hypertension occurs in 27% of patients along with proteinuria and edema. Theca lutein ovarian cysts >6 cm in size may accompany ovarian enlargements.

In *partial* molar pregnancies, the trophoblast cells have three sets of chromosomes (triploid). Two sperms are believed to fertilize the ovum at the same time leading to one set of maternal and two of paternal chromosome. Around 10% of partial moles are tetraploid or mosaic in nature. Usually, there is no evidence of fetal tissue or blood in a partial molar pregnancy. An embryo may be present at the start but becomes nonexistent as pregnancy progresses. Various abnormal fertilizations occur giving rise to fetuses with abnormal chromosomes, such as triploidy, tetraploidy etc. Patients with partial mole do not have the same clinical features as complete mole. Symptoms and signs are often consistent with incomplete or missed abortion, vaginal bleeding and absence of fetal heart. Uterine enlargement has been reported in 3% of cases with theca lutein cysts, hyperemesis and hyperthyroidism in 7% of cases.

Invasive mole can develop from complete mole invading the myometrium. Choriocarcinoma commonly follows molar and partial molar pregnancy but can arise from placenta of ectopic pregnancy, and hence ectopic pregnancy should be considered when bleeding persists after the usual and appropriate management. Invasive malignancies can develop after normal or abnormal pregnancies, often presenting with persistent vaginal bleeding before metastasis. Risk factors of malignancy include previous molar pregnancy, women under 16 years and over 45 years who conceive.

GTD should be suspected in a woman with vaginal bleeding, hCG levels higher than normal, ultrasound picture of snowstorm appearance of the placenta usually with or without a fetus.

Management of patients with any of the conditions involves stabilizing the patient for surgery, blood transfusion, if required, correction of coagulopathy and treatment of hypertension. Blood investigations include liver function tests, urea and creatinine and thyroid function tests. Ultrasound scan is the gold standard for identifying complete and partial moles, whilst chest X-ray is important for baseline assessment to determine metastasis to the lungs, usually the primary site of metastasis for malignant trophoblastic tumors.

Surgical care involves evacuation of the uterus by suction curettage. Histologic examination is necessary to confirm diagnosis from obtained tissues. In the case of PHM, suction curettage may become difficult or impossible because of the size of fetal parts and medical evacuation may have to be considered. Medical evacuation of CHM should be avoided if possible because of concerns about the use of potent oxytocic agents and the risk of dissemination of trophoblastic tissue emboli through the venous system. Intravenous oxytocin infusion is not recommended before dilatation of the cervix and initiation of evacuation of molar tissue, but should be started after dilatation of the cervix and continued postoperatively to reduce risk of hemorrhage. Other uterotonic agents may be used to ensure reduced postoperative bleeding.

There are conflicting views about administration of anti-D Ig after the evacuation of molar tissue. The American College of Obstetricians and Gynecologists recommends its administration, even though fetal blood cells should not be present in CHM[14]. The RCOG guideline of 2010 states that anti-D prophylaxis is not required in CHM but should be administered after evacuation of PHM[15]. In the case of PHM, anti-D prophylaxis should be given after evacuation because of the presence of fetal red blood cells in the conceptus.

Pulmonary complications may occur around the time of evacuation of molar pregnancy among patients with markedly enlarged uterus. Trophoblastic embolization is quoted as one of the common causes for respiratory distress. The other possible causes are high-output congestive heart failure due to anemia, hyperthyroidism, pre-eclampsia or iatrogenic fluid overload. Hyperthyroidism and pregnancy-induced hypertension usually abate promptly after evacuation of the mole and may not require specific therapy. Theca lutein cysts may take several months to resolve after evacuation of molar tissue but very rarely need to be removed. Surgical intervention should be reserved for rupture or torsion of ovary, which is rare.

In carefully selected women who do not wish to preserve childbearing capacity, hysterectomy may be an alternative form of treatment. It reduces the risk of GTN when compared with suction curettage. However, the risk of postmolar GTN after hysterectomy remains approximately 3–5% and these patients should be monitored postoperatively with serial hCG estimation.

Follow-up after GTD

After evacuation of molar pregnancy, it is important to monitor all women carefully in order to diagnose and treat malignant sequelae promptly. All women diagnosed with GTD should be provided with written information about the condition, and the need for referral for follow-up to a trophoblastic screening center should be explained. Registration of women with GTD represents a minimum standard care. After registration, follow-up consists of serial estimation of hCG levels, either in blood or urine specimens. Quantitative serum hCG determination should be performed using commercially available assays capable of detecting beta-hCG to baseline values of less than 5 mIU/mL. If the hCG falls to normal within 8 weeks of evacuation, the monitoring can be stopped at 6 months postevacuation. If the hCG falls more slowly, monitoring can stop at 6 months after the first normal value after normalization. After normalization of the serum hCG, the monitoring is by urine hCG. This means that pregnancy should be avoided for a minimum of 6 months after hCG levels return to normal.

All patients are advised to avoid the use of estrogen-containing oral contraceptive pills (OCP) whilst hCG levels are elevated as there is a theoretical risk of inducing metastatic or drug resistant disease. Intrauterine devices should not be inserted until the hCG normalizes because of the risk of uterine perforation, bleeding and infection if residual tumor is present. Use of barrier methods of contraception is advisable until hCG levels revert to normal. There is no evidence as to whether single agent progestogens have any effect on GTN. Combined OCP may be used after the hCG levels have returned to normal. If OCP had been started before the diagnosis of GTD was made, the woman can be advised to remain on OCP, but she should be advised that there is a potential but low increased risk of developing GTN.

Patients with prior partial or complete moles have a 10-fold increased risk (1–2% incidence) of a second hydatidiform mole in a subsequent pregnancy. Therefore, all future pregnancies should be evaluated by early obstetric ultrasonography. All women should notify the screening center at the end of any future pregnancy, whatever the outcome of the pregnancy, hCG levels are measured 6–8 weeks after the end of the pregnancy to exclude disease recurrence.

Management of GTN

There is no role for chemotherapy if serum hCG levels keep decreasing after evacuation of molar pregnancy.

The diagnosis of malignant sequelae as indicated by the need for chemotherapy include the plateau or increase of hCG levels after evacuation of hydatidiform mole, the histologic diagnosis of choriocarcinoma or invasive mole on the basis of findings from uterine curettage or identification of clinical or radiographic evidence of metastases. Repeat curettage is not recommended because it does not often induce remission or influence treatment and may result in uterine perforation and hemorrhage.

In order to diagnose postmolar trophoblastic disease, the International Federation of Gynecologists and Obstetricians (FIGO) have recommended standardized hCG criteria. Based on consensus committee recommendations from the Society of Gynecologic Oncology, the International Society for the Study of Trophoblastic Disease, and the International Gynecologic Cancer Society, the following criteria were proposed by FIGO[16].

- An hCG level plateau of four values ±10% recorded over a 3-week duration (days 1, 7, 14 and 21).
- An hCG level increase of >10% of three values recorded over a 2-week duration (days 1, 7 and 14).
- Persistence of detectable hCG for more than 6 months after molar evacuation.
- If hCG values do not fall as expected, then a new intrauterine pregnancy should be excluded on the basis of hCG levels and ultrasonography, particularly when there has been a long delay in follow-up of serial hCG levels and noncompliance with contraception.

FIGO anatomic staging for GTN

Gestational trophoblastic neoplasia (GTN) stage	Description
Stage 1	Disease confined to uterus. Persistently elevated hCG.
Stage 2	GTN extends outside of the uterus, but is limited to the genital structures (adnexa, vagina, broad ligament).
Stage 3	GTN extends to the lungs with or without known genital tract involvement.
Stage 4	Far advanced disease with involvement of the brain, liver, kidneys or gastrointestinal tract.

To allow objective comparison of reported information as well as of treatment results, FIGO reports data on GTN using an anatomic staging system as shown below[17].

Stage 4 tumors generally have the histologic pattern of CCA and commonly follow a nonmolar pregnancy, with protracted delays in diagnosis and large tumor burdens.

In order to predict the likelihood of drug resistance and to assist in selecting appropriate chemotherapy, a modified WHO prognostic scoring system was recommended by FIGO in year 2000. In general, patients with stage 1 disease have a low-risk score and patients with stage 4 disease have a high-risk score. Therefore, the distinction between low and high risk applies to stages 2 and 3.

Women are assessed before chemotherapy using this scoring system. Women with scores ≤6 are at low risk and are treated with single agent intramuscular methotrexate alternating daily with folinic acid for 1 week followed by 6 rest days. Women with scores ≥7 are at high risk and are treated with intravenous multiagent chemotherapy, which includes combinations of methotrexate, dactinomycin, etoposide, cyclophosphamide and vincristine. Treatment is continued in all cases until the hCG level has returned to normal and then for a further 6 consecutive weeks. The need for chemotherapy following a CHM is 15% and 0.5% after a PHM. The development of postpartum GTN requiring chemotherapy occurs at a rate of 1 in 50,000 births. The cure rate for women with a score of less than or equal to 6 is almost 100% and for those with a score of ≥7 or more is 95%(15).

PSTT are rare and are generally not sensitive to chemotherapy as with other forms of malignant gestational trophoblastic disease. It is therefore important to distinguish these tumors histologically. They are characterized by the absence of villi with proliferation of intermediate trophoblast cells. The number of syncytiotrophoblast cells observed is decreased in PSTT, with relatively lower levels of hCG secreted by these tumors. Surgery is an important modality in the treatment of PSTT and fortunately most patients have disease confined to the uterus and are cured by hysterectomy.

Women who undergo chemotherapy should be advised not to conceive for 1 year after completion of treatment. In women who conceive within 12 months of completing chemotherapy there may be an increased risk of miscarriage, higher rate of termination of pregnancy and an increased rate of stillbirth compared with normal population[17].

Following completion of chemotherapy for GTN once hCG remission has been achieved, patients should undergo serial determinations of hCG levels at 2-week intervals for the first 3 months of remission and then at 1-month intervals until monitoring has shown 1 year of normal hCG levels. The risk of recurrence after 1 year of remission is less than 1% but late recurrences have rarely been observed. Patients should be advised to use a reliable form of hormonal contraception during the first year of remission[16].

Management of hydatidiform mole and a coexistent fetus

Both complete and partial moles with coexistent fetuses have been reported. This occurs in 1 in 22,000 to 1 in 100,000 pregnancies. Most of these pregnancies are diagnosed antepartum by ultrasound findings of a complex,

Modified WHO prognostic scoring system as adapted by FIGO (2000)[18]

Scores	0	1	2	4
Age	<40 years	>40 years	—	—
Antecedent pregnancy	Mole	Abortion	Term	—
Interval months from index pregnancy	<4	4 to <7	7 to <13	≥13
Pretreatment serum hCG (IU/L)	<1,000	>10,000	<100,000	>100,000
Largest tumor size, including uterus (cm)	<3	3 to <5	≥5	—
Site of metastases	Lung	Spleen/kidney	gastrointestinal	Liver/brain
Number of metastases	—	1–4	5–8	>8
Previous failed chemotherapy	—	—	Single drug	Two or more drugs

cystic placental component distinct from the fetoplacental unit, but in some cases, the diagnosis is not suspected until examination of the placenta following delivery. Complications of hydatidiform mole with a coexistent fetus appear to be increased and include hyperthyroidism, hemorrhage, preterm labor and pregnancy-induced hypertension. In some studies, compared with singleton hydatidiform moles, twin pregnancies with a fetus and a mole were found to carry an increased risk for postmolar gestational trophoblastic disease with a higher proportion of patients having metastatic disease and requiring multiagent chemotherapy[16].

There are no clear guidelines for management of such patients, and so advice should be sought from the regional fetal medicine unit and the relevant trophoblastic screening center. The ultrasound examination should be repeated to exclude retroplacental hematoma, other placental abnormalities or degenerating myoma, and to fully evaluate the fetoplacental unit for evidence of a partial mole or gross fetal malformations. If the diagnosis is still suspected and continuation of pregnancy is desired, fetal karyotyping should be considered. A chest X-ray may be also considered to screen for metastases and serial serum hCG values monitored. After delivery, the placenta should be histologically evaluated and the patient followed closely with serial hCG values, similar to management of a woman with a singleton hydatidiform mole.

Placental abruption

Placental abruption is a complication of pregnancy resulting from placental separation from the uterus before birth of the baby. It is amongst the most common causes of antepartum hemorrhage (APH) in the third trimester and is a significant contributor of maternal and fetal mortality worldwide. In the 2009–2012 report on confidential enquiry in to maternal death, hemorrhage was the third most common direct cause of maternal death in the UK[19]. Of the 17 maternal deaths due to hemorrhage, three were due to APH. Maternal and fetal outcome depends on early diagnosis, skilled intervention, severity of abruption, gestational age and speed of intervention. The estimate of incidence of placental abruption is about 6.5 per 1,000 births.

Etiology

Etiology is unknown but known risk factors include trauma (road traffic accident, domestic violence and external cephalic version, pre-eclampsia, multiparity,

previous abruption, previous cesarean section, smoking, cocaine use, multiple pregnancy, thrombophilia, intrauterine infections, polyhydramnios and assisted reproductive technique. Of the risk factors, the most predictive is abruption in a previous pregnancy. A study from Norway reported a 4.4% incidence of recurrent abruption[20]. It recurs in 19–25% of women who have had two previous pregnancies complicated by abruption[21]. Bleeding and sonographic detection of intrauetrine hemotaoma in the first trimester increases the risk of subsequent placental abruption.

Placental abruption is concealed in 20% of cases where there is no external bleeding. In concealed abruption, blood pools behind the placenta becoming evident at the time of or after delivery.

Abruptions can be mild without symptoms, with blood clots seen after delivery at routine placental examination. The mother may present with vaginal bleeding with mild uterine contractions and tenderness, with or without tetany and no evidence of abnormality on CTG and normal neonatal outcome, only for abruption to be confirmed on placental examination. In women with significant abruption, vaginal bleeding may or may not be enough to cause hemodynamic shock and abnormality on CTG. Abruption in such cases is often evident after delivery of the infant followed by significant placental bleeding. In severe classical placental abruption, the mother presents with shock, vaginal bleeding, rigid tense abdomen (board-like rigidity) and fetal death. These cases may be associated, immediately or shortly after presentation, with disseminated intravascular coagulation. In some cases of significant abruption, blood arising from separation of placenta, trying to force its way through the uterine wall into the serosa, turns the uterus bluish in a condition known as "couvelaire uterus."

Diagnosis and treatment

Placental abruption suspicion should be made when a pregnant woman presents with a sudden localized abdominal pain with or without vaginal bleeding. The fundus may be large for date suggesting bleeding. Abdomen examination may reveal gradually progressing tenderness and rigidity of the uterus. Initially, CTG could be normal but gradually becomes abnormal due to fetal distress. Placental abruption is a clinical diagnosis and there are no sensitive or reliable diagnostic tests available. Ultrasound has limited sensitivity in the identification of retroplacental hemorrhage. The Kleihauer test is not a sensitive test for diagnosis of abruption.

Treatment depends on the amount of blood lost and fetal status. If the fetus is preterm and neither mother or fetus are in distress, immediate delivery should be kept on hold for steroid administration to optimize fetal lung maturity while maternal and fetal monitoring is in progress, with immediate surgical delivery avaialble if fetal or maternal distress occurs. In the course of monitoring, blood volume replacement to maintain blood pressure and plasma replacement should be initiated. Vaginal birth is preferred over cesarean, if possible, unless evidence of progressive distress becomes evident. Cesarean section is contraindicated in the presence of disseminating coagulopathy, which must be corrected before surgical inervention.

In severe cases, postdelivery monitoring should be performed in a high-dependency unit.

Anti-D administration should be undertaken in Rhesus-negative women with a Rhesus-positive fetus.

Morbidly adherent placenta

Morbidily adherent placentation occurs when the placenta invades the uterus making it difficult to remove following delivery of the infant.

Three grades of abnormal placental adhesion are described based on degree of invasion of the uterus – accreta, increta and percreta.

In *accreta*, placental invasion of the myometrium is diffuse rather than being restricted within the decidua basalis, and is inseparable from the uterine wall.

With *increta*, placental invasion extends to the myometrium and serosa.

In *percreta*, placental invasion extends beyond the uterine wall to the pertoneum. It is associated with significant maternal and fetal mortality and morbidity. Hemorrhage and its consequences mainly affect the mother, and for the fetus the main risk arises from consequences of prematurity.

Risk factors include previous uterine scar, damage to myometrium due to previous placenta praevia, maternal age and multiparity. Other risk factors are uterine ablations, previous uterine curettage, Asherman's syndrome, myomectomy and surgical termination of pregnancy, and congenital uterine abnormalities. Women at risk should have ultrasound at 20 weeks' gestation, if necessary complemented with MRI in equivocal cases, although accuracy of MRI over ultrasound scan is controversal[22–24].

Diagnosis

The prevalence of placental accreta is on the increase because of rising cesarean section rates. A high index of suspicion should be exercised about morbidly adherent placenta at the routine 20 weeks' anomaly scan in women at risk if the placenta is located in the lower uterine segment or overlaps the internal cervical os at this gestation. A transvaginal scan can help localize the placenta more accurately. Risk factors of morbid adhesion of placenta include previous placental adhesion, previous cesarean section(s) and traumatic injuries or surgery to the uterus such as myomectomy. Firm diagnosis is crucial to enable determination of appropriate management due to the potential risk of life-threatening hemorrhage. Clarification of diagnosis is therefore necessary by 32 weeks. Definitive diagnosis is made at the time of surgery.

Antenatal imaging techniques, which can help raise strong suspicion of morbidly adherent placenta are grey-scale ultrasound, color Doppler and MRI.

Criteria for diagnosis of morbid adhesion of placenta is shown in table 1 [25, 26, 27, 28, 29].

Because of variations in nomenclature and inter-observer perception of ultrasound findings, a standard reporting system is useful. This will help comparative analysis and clinical audit of diagnostic methods and outcome. For an example of a standard proforma for reporting ultrasound findings in suspected abnormally invasive placenta, the reader is referred to the work by Alfirevic et al [30, 31].

MRI is more costly than abdominal ultrasound, requiring experience and expertise in evaluation of placental invasion. Several studies have suggested comparable diagnostic accuracy with ultrasound. The role of MRI in diagnosing placenta accrete is still debated; however, many studies recommend MRI for women in whom ultrasound findings are inconclusive. MRI is particularly helpful when there is a risk of morbid adhesion of a posterior positioned placenta. Several MRI findings have been described with the main features of MRI consisting of uterine bulging or widening of the lower uterine segment producing an hourglass-shaped uterus, heterogeneous signal intensity within the placenta or increased placental vascularity, tenting of the urinary bladder, direct invasion of adjacent pelvic structures by placental tissue, interruption of the normal layered appearance of the myometrium and dark intraplacental bands on T2-weighted imaging. On most occasions, when MRI is used, it is usually used in conjunction with ultrasound for such diagnosis[32].

Table 26. 1 Features of normal and morbidly adherent placenta

Type of placenta	Grey scale ultrasound features	Two dimensional colour Doppler ultrasound features
Normal	Homogeneous appearance. (See figure 26.1.)	Linear flow near basal plate and the fetal surface.
	Retro-placental sonolucent area. (See figure 26.1.)	No or minimal vascular projections in to the interface of uterine serosa and urinary bladder.
	Well defined echogenic interface of uterine serosa and bladder. (See figure 26.1.)	
	Vascular flow parallel to basal plate.	
	Absence of irregular projection or bulge in to bladder.	
Morbidly adherent placenta	Loss of or irregular retro-placental hypoechoic area. (See figure 26.2.)	Diffuse or focal lacunar flow. (See figure 26.3.)
	Placenta filled with prominent lacunae. (See figure 26.3.)	Vascular lakes with turbulent flow (peak systolic velocity over 15 cm/sec). (See figures 26.4 and 26.7.)
	Thinning or disruption of the echogenic interface between uterine serosa and bladder. (See figure 26.2.)	Hyper-vascular serosa-bladder interface. (See figure 26.4.)
	Presence of focal exophytic mass invading urinary bladder. (See figures 26.4, 26.6 and 26.7.)	Markedly dilated and aberrant blood vessels in the peripheral sub-placental zone. (See figure 26.5 and 26.6.)
	Area of placental implantation in lower segment bulging in to urinary bladder. (See figure 26.8.)	

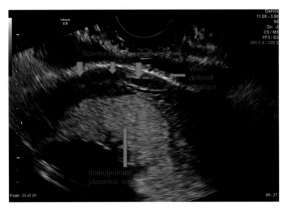

Figure 26.1

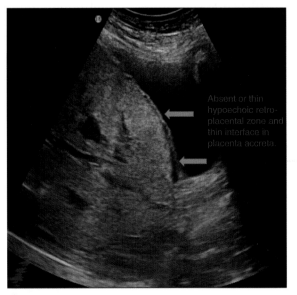

Figure 26.2

Management

Management involves the prevention and treatment of anemia during the antenatal period in all women with placenta praevia. All at-risk women should be counseled in the risk of preterm labor and obstetric hemorrhage that could lead to cesarean hysterectomy to save

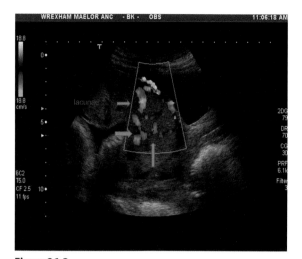

Figure 26.3

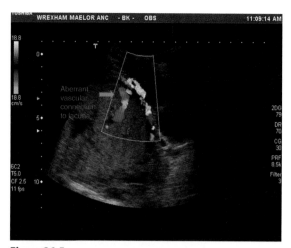

Figure 26.5

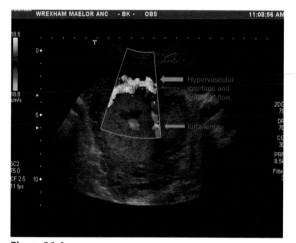

Figure 26.4

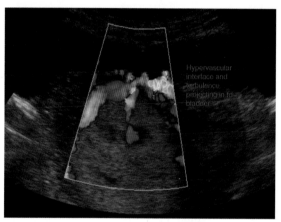

Figure 26.6

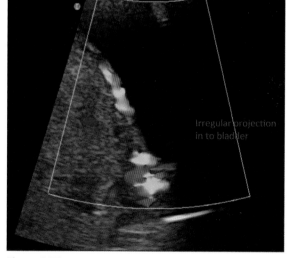

Figure 26.7

their lives, although management would be tailored to individual cases. In the case of confirmed asymptomatic major or pathological accreta, such patients should be transferred for delivery in a unit well equipped for management of such cases and in provision of intensive neonatal care. It is preferable such patients are admitted from diagnosis, although in the appropriately selected case, home management is acceptable on the provision that home is in close proximity to the hospital, there is constant presence of a companion and fully informed consent by the woman is available.

Prolonged inpatient care can be associated with increased risk of thromboembolism: therefore, mobility should be encouraged together with the use of

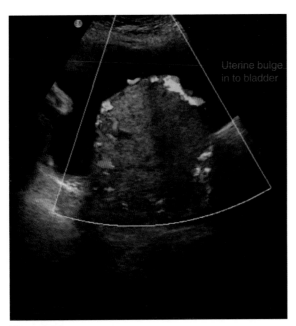

Uterine bulge in to bladder

Figure 26.8

thromboembolic stockings and hydration. Use of anticoagulation can be hazardous and should be limited to women with a very high risk of thromboembolism. Transfer of the patient to a tertiary perinatal unit should be considered and discussed with the patient and her partner as soon as possible and the risks with possible outcomes discussed.

Delivery should involve an experienced multidisciplinary team (MDT) involving an obstetrician, anaesthetist, surgeons, intensive care unit, interventional radiologist, urologist, neonatologist patient and neonatologist. Due to risk of massive hemorrhage, blood and blood products should be made available following liaison with a hematologist and blood bank in advance of surgery. Cell saver should be used especially in patients who refuse blood transfusion. Crossmatched blood should be ready at all times in anticipation of massive hemorrhage. Due to associated risk of preterm labor patients should be given prophylactic steroids to optimize fetal lung maturity and to improve neonatal outcome.

Delivery

Timing of delivery should be decided with appropriate members of the MDT and recorded in the case notes. Before cesarean section, the patient should be catheterized and the indwelling catheter left in place. A senior obstetrician should carry out the cesarean section. The choice of skin incision depends on the location of the placenta and to ensure adequate exposure. If possible, incision on the uterus should be at a site distant from the placenta in order to deliver the baby without disturbing the placenta, so that conservative management of the placenta or elective hysterectomy could be considered if the placenta does not separate easily, and hence placenta accreta is confirmed. Going through the placenta to deliver the baby is associated with more bleeding and a high chance of hysterectomy, and should therefore be avoided. If the placenta fails to separate with usual measures, leaving it in place and closing the uterus and, where appropriate, proceeding to a hysterectomy, are associated with less blood loss than trying to separate it. If the placenta separates, it needs to be delivered and hemorrhage that occurs needs to be dealt with in the usual way.

If the placenta partially separates, the separated portions(s) need to be delivered and hemorrhage that occurs needs to be dealt with in the usual way. Adherent portions can be left in place, but blood loss in such situations can be significant and massive hemorrhage management needs to follow in a timely fashion. Conservative management of placenta accreta when the woman is already bleeding is unlikely to be successful and risks wasting valuable time. Appropriately experienced surgeons should perform surgical manoeuvres required in the face of massive hemorrhage associated with placenta praevia. Calling extra help early should be encouraged and not seen as "losing face." Following delivery, supportive care should be carried out in appropriate units and intensive care unit, and routine antibiotics given in-keeping with unit protocol.

Following delivery and recovery, surgical procedures undertaken should be fully explained to the woman and her partner. Where the placenta is left in situ, the woman should be warned of the risks of bleeding, and infection and antibiotics continued during her recovery period and the immediate postpartum period. Neither methotrexate nor arterial embolization reduces these risks and neither is recommended routinely. Follow-up of the woman using ultrasound should supplement beta-human serum hCG measurements. An incident report form should be completed regarding severe hemorrhage and cesarean hysterectomy as appropriate.

Amniotic fluid

Amniotic fluid serves several functions, such as cushioning the baby from injury throughout gestation to optimize growth, and prevents the fetal umbilical cord from being compressed against the uterine wall, hence ensuring adequate fetal nutrition and oxygenation at all times. In surrounding the fetus, it ensures optimal temperature maintainenance around the fetus at all times and an equal distribution of nutrients around the baby, and it provides bacteriostatic qualities that enable growth in infection-free environment.

Amniotic fluid production

Two fluid sacs (extracoelomic and coelomic) containing fluid relative to the size of the fetus surround the embryo from 7–12 weeks' gestation during which they fuse to become the amniotic cavity. Despite extensive assessment of contents, the mechanism of production of fluid remains unclear.

Amniotic fluid volume production is a dynamic physiologic process involving the fetus, placental surface, amnion and mother. Mechanism of production in the early first trimester is uncertain, although it is believed to result from the active transport of solutes across the amnion into amniotic space, with water following down a chemical gradient. In the second and third trimesters, fetal kidneys become a major source of fluid entering the amniotic sac. Fetal urine first enters the amniotic sac at 8–11 weeks. Smaller contributions occur across vessels on the fetal surface, umbilical cord and fetal skin. Transcutaneous fetal flow ceases after keratinization at 22–24 weeks. At term, the main sources of amniotic fluid production are fetal urine and fluid exudates from the lungs, whilst clearance is mainly by fetal swallowing and intermembraneous exchange. It is estimated fetal urine flow rate averages 500–600 mL/day.

Assessment of amniotic fluid

Amniotic fluid volume changes with gestational age. Aberrations in control may cause increased (polyhydramnios) or reduced (oligohydramnios) volumes often associated with poor perinatal outcomes. Amniotic fluid volume can be estimated subjectively or objectively by experienced clinicians with comparable accuracy. Subjective assessment lacks consistency although this depends on the examiner. Quantification of amniotic fluid is said to be preferred because of ease of mesurement, consistency, reproducibility and its inclusion criteria in biophysical profile (BPP) in assessment of fetal wellbeing, but this has become debatable. Several authors have tried to create gestation-specific amniotic fluid volume charts. The commonly employed

methods of measuring amniotic fluid volume are by assessing amniotic fluid index (AFI) or by measuring the maximum pool depth (MPD). AFI is measured in centimeters by adding the maximum vertical pool depth in each quadrant of the uterus. MPD is the single deepest vertical pool of fluid identified by ultrasound in centimeters. At the present time, there is no accurate method of measuring the amniotic volume. Studies comparing the two methods conclude that MPD is preferred because reliance on AFI alone increases detection rates of oligohydramnios, resulting in increased intervention (induction of labor) without improving neonatal outcome. Measurement of AFI and MPD are used in BPP, which aims to identify babies inadequately oxygenated. Oligohydramnios is defined as a value of AFI <5 cm or MPD <2 cm[33–36].

Polyhydramnios

Polyhydramnios is a pathologic increase in amniotic fluid volume, occurring in 1–2% of pregnancies, and is associated with increased maternal and fetal mortality and morbidity. Quantitatively, it is diagnosed when AFI is >24 cm or MPD is >8 cm.

Etiology

The majority of cases are idiopathic and common associations are maternal diabetes, multiple pregnancy, twin–twin transfusion syndrome (TTTS), fetal anatomic or neurologic abnormalities preventing fetal swallowing, fetal congenital cystic adenoid malformation of the lungs, fetal aneuploidy (trisomy 18 and 21), rhesus isoimmunization and Bartter's syndrome (a rare inherited fetal disorder, where the kidneys are unable to regulate electrolyte excretion resulting in diuresis). Infections, such as parvovirus, rubella and cytomegalovirus, may be associated with increased amniotic fluid volume. Fetal compromise, which might result from polyhydramnios, includes cord prolapse and prematurity with associated complications. Maternal problems include placental abruption leading to hemorrhage due to rapid decompression and uterine atony.

Diagnosis

Polyhydramnios can be mild, moderate or severe depending on the speed of accumulation of amniotic fluid. Polyhydramnios is suspected on examination when the uterus feels large for date and fetal parts are difficult to palpate. Occasionally, the pregnant woman has respiratory symptoms due to upward splinting of the diaphragm. Acute polyhydramnios is more common with monochorionic twins and progressive with TTTS. Diagnosis of polyhydramnios with AFI is amniotic fluid volume >25 cm whilst MPD is >8 cm.

Investigations

Investigations should include a comprehensive ultrasound examination of the fetus and placenta to identify any detectable cause. Maternal blood should be tested to exclude diabetes. Urea and electrolytes and urine osmolality should be performed to exclude diabetes insipidus in suspected cases (rare). When hydrops fetalis is visible on ultrasound (with excessive fluid in one or more fetal compartments, such as the pleura or abdominal space), hemolytic disease should be suspected and the Kleiheur test should be performed, as well as screening for maternal antibodies against red blood cells. Investigation for a maternal infection screen is controversial because some authors recommend testing for TORCH [toxoplasma, others (syphilis, varicella–zoster, parvovirus B19), rubella, cytomegalovirus and herpes virus], whilst others advise that a TORCH test is not beneficial in women where polyhydramnios is an isolated finding, particularly when diagnosed in the third trimester[37,38].

Management

Management depends on the cause and gestational age, and hence the importance of assessment and investigation. Depending on gestational age, prophylactic steroid injection should be considered to optimize fetal lung maturation in case preterm birth takes place. If fetal abnormality is suspected or detected, then consideration should be made for transfer of the patient to a tertiary unit.

Counseling with a neonatologist should involve explaining the risks of polyhydramnios to the woman and baby. Mild polyhydramnios can be monitored and managed conservatively on an outpatient basis if the woman is asymptomatic, understands the risk of the condition and accepts special regular monitoring for her pregnancy. Preterm labor is commonly due to overdistension of the uterus and measures should be initiated to minimize risk, including avoidance of stressful activity. Depending on etiology, serial ultrasound scan with BPP may be necessary at regular intervals. If fetal hydrops is present due to either infection or rhesus immunization, consideration should be given to

transfer of care to a tertiary centre for further inestigation and possible in-utero transfusion if indicated. This reduces the likelihood of fetal congestive heart failure, thereby allowing prolongation of the pregnancy and improving fetal survival. If diabetes is diagnosed, optimizing glycemic control should be the key to reducing amniotic fluid production, which is usually done with dietary manipulation and insulin if required.

Amniotic fluid reduction

Indomethacin is the drug of choice for women who are symptomatic. It is believed to be very effective, particularly in cases where the condition is associated with increased fetal urine production, with the mechanism of action being reduction of urine production by fetal kidney, possibly by the effect of vasopressin. However, it does not appear to be effective in cases where the underlying cause is neuromuscular disease affecting fetal swallowing or hydrocephalus. It is contraindicated in TTTS or after 35 weeks' gestation as the adverse effects outweigh the benefits.

Amniocentesis is not recommended where indomethacin is contraindicated in severe polyhydramnios as above, where immediate symptomatic relief is not required, or in patients with evidence of chorioamnionitis. Beyond 35 weeks, it may be safer to deliver rather than aim to gain a few more days in utero for the fetus. An experienced clinician should perform induction of the labor by forewater amniotomy, with consent obtained from the patient to proceed to emergency cesarean section if required. Polyhydramnios associated with TTTS may benefit from laser ablation of the connecting placental vessels (see Chapter 25). The NSAID sulindac has been used by researchers with good effect in amniotic fluid reduction, with less constrictive effect on the fetal ductus; however, its use has not been recommended outside a controlled research environment. Following delivery of the infant complicated by polyhydramnios, a thorough examination of the newborn is necessary, including consideration of karyotype to identify the cause for the polyhydramnios.

Anhydramnios

Anhydramnios is a complete absence of amniotic fluid around the fetus and can occur at any stage of the pregnancy. Visualization of fetal structures can sometimes be very difficult due to the absence of amniotic fluid. Presence of anhydramnios in the first trimester is often associated with congenital malformation, such as renal agenesis. Careful ultrasound assessment with the use of Doppler studies is crucial in identfying the cause in order to determine management and decide counseling.

Oligohydramnios progressing to anhydramnios may arise from chronic spontaneous rupture of membranes (SROM) due to several factors, such as congenital malformations, infection and fetal growth restriction (FGR). Oligohydramnios and anhydramnios are commonly associated with poor pregnancy outcome. Before 20 weeks' gestation, fetal demise is often due to pulmonary hypoplasia, spontaneous miscarriage or intrauterine infection. At term, oligohydramnios is commonly associated with chronic SROM and/or FGR. Outcome in pregnancies beyond 34 weeks is usually good with optimum management. Doppler ultrasonography of fetal vessels is an important adjunct in investigating fetuses affected by FGR.

Amniotic band syndrome

Amniotic band syndrome (ABS) is a rare group of disorders in pregnancy with an incidence of 1:1,200–15,000 live births. Although etiology is uncertain, it is believed to occur when the inner membrane (amnion) ruptures or tears without injury to the outer membrane (chorion), exposing several fibrous strands or "bands" floating in amniotic fluid. The fibrous bands can entrap parts of the active fetus and cause progressive constriction of fetal body parts preventing blood flow, edema, and on some occasions result in amputation of the affected part. The degree of injury caused to the fetus by entrapment is variable, varying from minor to lethal. The progress of pregnancy is not affected. The most severe life-complicating situation is when the fibrous bands wrap around vital areas, such as the head or the umbilical cord, causing growth retardation and fetal death in utero. ABS can involve entrapment of upper extremities, distal limbs and longer digits. Fetal hands are affected in almost 90% of cases. There is no racial or sexual predilection or risk of recurrence in patients with previously affected pregnancies, and it does not run in families. ABS poses no risk to mother in pregnancy.

Diagnosis with ultrasound or MRI is difficult unless there is obvious edema distal to progressive constriction. Routine ultrasound evaluation of the fetus in the second trimester can detect amputation of fetal extremities, including hands and feet. Detailed assessment of these areas is crucial. Most defects are detected at birth, including identification of fibrous bands, short or absent fingers or toes, cleft lip, cleft palate and club-foot. Misdiagnosis is also common, and when there are suggestive signs of amniotic band syndrome, further detailed assessment with three-dimensional ultrasound and MRI should be considered to confirm diagnosis and severity.

Surgical management (particularly reconstructive) is the best option for cases detected at birth, such as correcting deep constriction grooves, fused fingers or toes, cleft lip or palate and other physical deformities.

References

1. Harris RD, Barth RA. Sonography of the gravid uterus and placenta: current concepts. *AJR Am J Roentgenol* 1993; 160(3): 455–65.

2. Taniquchi H, Aoki S, Sakamaki K, et al. Circumvallate placenta: associated clinical manifestations and complications – a retrospective study. *Obstet Gynecol Int* 2014; 986230.

3. Harris RD, Wells, W A, Black WC, et al. Accuracy of prenatal sonography for detecting circumvallate placenta. *AJR Am J Roentgenol* 1997; 168(6): 1603–8.

4. Suzuki S. Clinical significance of pregnancies with circumvallate placenta. *J Obstet Gyneacol Res* 2008; 34(1): 51–4.

5. Tufail S, Nawaz S, Sadaf M, et al. Association between battledore placenta and perinatal complications. *J Rawalpindi Med College* 2012; 16(2): 159–61.

6. Di Salvo DN, Benson CB, Laing FC, et al. Sonographic evaluation of the placental cord insertion insertion site. *AJR Am J Roentgenol* 1998; 170: 1295–8.

7. Alfirevic Z, Stampalija T, Gyte GML. Fetal and umbilical ultrasound in high-risk pregnancies. *Cochrane Pregnancy and Childbirth Group. Cochrane Database Syst Rev* 2013; 11: CD007529.

8. Royal College of Obstetricians and Gynaecologists (RCOG). Placenta praevia, placenta accreta and vasa praevia: diagnosis and management. RCOG Green-Top guideline No. 27. London: RCOG Press, 2005.

9. d'Ercole C, Cravello L, Boubli L, et al. Large choriangioma associated with hydrops fetalis: pren diagnosis and management. *Fetal Diagn Ther* 1996; 11: 357–60.

10. Al Wattar BH, Hillman SC, Marton T, et al. Placetal chorioangioma: a rare case and systematic review of literature. *J Matern Fetal Neonatal Med* 2014; 27(10): 1055–63.

11. Secki MJ, Sebire NJ, Berkowtitz RS. Gestational trophoblastic disease. *Lancet* 2010; 376(9742): 717–29.

12. Moodley M, Tunkyi k, Moodley J. Gestational trophoblastic syndrome: an audit of 112 patients. A South African experience. *Int J Gyn Cancer* 2003; 13(2): 234–9.

13. Sivanesaratnam V. Management of gestational trophoblastic disease in developing countries. *Best Pract Res Clin Obst Gynaecol* 2003; 17(6): 925–42.

14. American College of Obstetricians and Gynecologists (ACOG). Prevention of RhD alloimmunization. Gynecology & Obstetrics ACOG Practice Bulletin No. 4, May 1999. *Int J Gynecol Obstet* 1999;66:63–70.

15. Royal College of Obstetricians and Gynaecologists (RCOG). The management of gestational trophoblastic disease. Green-Top Guideline No 38. London: RCOG Press, February 2010.

16. American College of Obstetricians and Gynecologists (ACOG). Diagnosis and treatment of gestational trophoblastic disease. ACOG Practice Bulletin – Clinical Management Guidelines for Obstetrician–Gynecologists, No. 53. *Obstet Gynecol* 2004; 103(6): 1365–77.

17. Berkowitz RS, Goldstein DP. Current management of gestational trophoblastic diseases. *Gynecol Oncol* 2009; 112: 654–62.

18. Royal College of Obstetricians and Gynaecologists (RCOG). The management of gestational trophoblastic disease. RCOG Green-Top Guideline No. 38, London: RCOG Press, February 2010.

19. Knight M, Kenyon S, Brocklehurst P, et al. (eds) on behalf of MBRRACE-UK. Saving Lives, Improving Mothers' Care – Lessons learned to inform future maternity care from the UK and Ireland confidential enquiries into maternal deaths and morbidity 2009–12. Oxford: National Perinatal Epidemiology Unit, University of Oxford, 2014.

20. Rasmussen S, Irgens LM. Occurrence of placental abruption in relatives. *BJOG* 2009; 116: 693–9.

21. Tikkanen M. Etiology, clinical manifestations and prediction of placental abruption. *Acta Obstet Gynecol Scand* 2010; 89: 732–40.

22. Dwyer BK, Beloglovkin V, Ytan L, et al. Prenatal diagnosis of placental accreta: sonography and magnetic resonance imaging? *J Ultrasound Med* 2008: 27(9): 1275–81.

23. Chou MM, Ho ES, Lee HY. Prenatal diagnosis of placenta praevia accreta by trans abdominal color Doppler ultrasound. *Ultrasound Obstet Gynecol* 2000; 15: 28–35.

24. Palacious Jarquemada JM, Bruno CH. Magnetic resonance in 300 cases of placenta accrete: surgical correlation of new findings. *Acta Obstet Gynecol Scand* 2005; 84: 716–24.

25. Royal College of Obstetricians and Gynaecologists (RCOG). Placenta praevia, placenta accrete and vasa praevia: diagnosis and management. RCOG Green-Top Guideline No 27. London: RCOG Press, January 2011.

26. Silver RM. Abnormal placentation. Clinical expert series. *Obstet & Gynecol* 2015 Sept; 126(3): 654–68.

27. Silver RM, Barbour KD. Placenta accreta spectrum. *Obstet Gynecol Clin N Am* (2015); 42: 381–402.

28. Shetty MK, Dryden DK. Morbidly adherent placenta: ultrasound assessment and supplemental role of magnetic resonance imaging. *Semin Ultrasound CT MRI*. 2015; 36: 324–31.

29. Rac MWF, Dashe JS, Wells CE, Moschos E. Ultrasound predictors of placental invasion: the placenta accrete index. *Am J Obstet Gynecol* 2015; 212: 343.e1–7.

30. Bowman ZS, Eller AG, Kennedy AM, Richards DS, Winter TC, Woodward PJ, Silver RM. Interobserver variability of sonography for prediction of placenta accrete. *J Ultrasound Med* 2014; 33: 2153–8.

31. Alfirevic Z, Tang AW, Collins S, Robson S, Jaraquemada JP. Standardised proforma for ultrasound reporting in suspected abnormally invasive placenta (AIP)– an international consensus. *Ultrasound Obstet Gynecol* 2015 Nov; 13: Doi: 10.1002/uog.15810.

32. Srisajjakul S, Prapaisilp P, Bangchokdee S. MRI of placental adhesive disorder. *Br J Radiol* 2014; 87: 20140294.

33. Magan EF, Bass JD, Chauhan SP, et al. Amniotic fluid volume in normal singleton pregnancies. *Obstet Gynecol* 1997; 90: 524.

34. Ghidini A, Schiliro M. Locatelli A. Amniotic fluid volume: when and how to take action. *Contemporary OB/Gyn* 2014; 59(6): 26–35.

35. Nwosu EC, Welch CR, Manasse P, et al. Longitudinal assessment of amniotic fluid index. *Br J Obstet Gynaecol* 1993; 100: 816–19.

36. Kollmann M, Voetsch J, Koidl C, et al. Etiology and perinatal outcome of polyhydramnios. *Ultraschall Med* 2014; 35(4): 350–6.

37. Fayyaz H, Rafi J. TORCH screening in polyhydramnios: an observational study. *J Maternal Fetal Neonatal Med* 2012; 25(7): 1069–72.

38. Nabham AF, Abdelmoula YA. Amniotic fluid index versus single deepest vertical pockets of liquor as a screening test for preventing adverse pregnancy outcome. *Cochrane Database Syst Rev* 2008; 16(3): CD006593.

Chapter 7

Ultrasound-guided diagnostic procedures

Kate Navaratnam and Zarko Alfirevic

Invasive prenatal tests, including chorionic villus sampling (CVS), amniocentesis and fetal blood sampling (FBS), allow examination of fetal chromosomes and provide information for the management of fetal infections and anemia. The specific test employed is usually dependent on the indication, parental wishes, and the specific timing of preceding screening tests.

With the arrival of noninvasive prenatal testing (NIPT), the landscape of screening and prenatal diagnosis is rapidly changing. A comprehensive understanding of prenatal diagnostic techniques is required for clinicians who provide counseling and offer choice to their patients. For a trainee undertaking the UK Royal College of Obstetricians and Gynaecologists (RCOG)'s Fetal Medicine Advance Training Skills Module (ATSM), the following requirements should be met. This chapter, however, provides a comprehensive overview of some of the invasive antenatal diagnostic tests.

(1) Understand methods of prenatal diagnosis including indications, techniques, complications and the role of fetal blood sampling.
(2) Be clinically competent at amniocentesis and have a sound knowledge of the principles and techniques of first-trimester chorionic villus biopsy.
(3) Be aware of their own clinical and professional limitations, and be comfortable with seeking advice from other specialists or professional groups.
(4) Understand the organization of prenatal screening and diagnostic services at a local and regional level.

Which test and when

Amniocentesis remains the most frequently performed ultrasound-guided diagnostic procedure in the UK,

although CVS is increasingly common following widespread introduction of the combined first-trimester Down's syndrome screening. Amniocentesis is carried out to obtain amniotic fluid for karyotyping from 15+0 weeks onwards[2]. Early amniocentesis prior to 14 completed weeks is not advisable due to a 1.7% additional risk of fetal loss when compared with amniocentesis after 15+0 weeks, and an increased risk of talipes[2]. Before the amniotic membrane is fused with the chorion, tenting of the amnion and difficulty perforating this membrane may occasionally be encountered.

CVS is usually performed between 11+0 and 13+6 weeks of gestation and involves obtaining a sample of placental villi. It can be performed using either a transabdominal or a transcervical approach. In some cases, CVS will be warranted in the 15th week, when the placenta is easily accessible and the couple do not wish to wait for amniocentesis.

There were reports of oromandibular limb hypoplasia associated with CVS prior to 10 weeks. Due to an inadequacy of subsequent evidence to refute or support this concern, it is recommended that CVS is not performed prior to 11+0 weeks[3]. Early CVS is more technically challenging due to the smaller uterus and placenta.

FBS is carried out to obtain fetal blood from the umbilical vein using a transabdominal approach. It is possible to perform the procedure from the late second trimester, and becomes less technically challenging with advancing gestation and maturity of fetal tissues.

Vesicocentesis (transabdominal aspiration of urine from the fetal bladder) and fetal urine analysis was previously considered as an indicator of the risk of postnatal renal damage secondary to fetal lower urinary tract obstruction (LUTO). This technique is no longer

Fetal Medicine, ed. Bidyut Kumar and Zarko Alfirevic. Published by Cambridge University Press. © Cambridge University Press 2016.

Table 27.1 Investigations possible from different ultrasound-guided diagnostic procedures

	Chorionic villus sampling	Amniocentesis	Fetal blood sampling
Fetal karyotype	✓	✓	✓
Fetal microarray (DNA test)	✓	✓	✓
Fetal virology	✗	✓	✓
Fetal hemoglobin	✗	✗	✓

advocated as it has low diagnostic accuracy and is not helpful in assessing for in-utero treatment[4]. See also Table 27.1.

Indications for ultrasound-guided diagnostic procedures

- High-risk Down's syndrome screening result (after combined test, second-trimester serum screening, NIPT).
- Previous history of pregnancy affected by aneuploidy or genetic disease.
- Parental translocation, or family history of genetic disease.
- Structural anomalies or markers for fetal aneuploidy identified at the dating scan or fetal anomaly screening.
- Fetal urinary tract obstruction.
- Suspected fetal viral infection, evidence of recent maternal infection on virology testing and fetal ultrasound markers.
- Evidence of fetal hemolytic anaemia, maternal sensitization with elevated fetal middle cerebral artery peak systolic velocity, fetal hydrops.

Aneuploidy screening and diagnostic tests

Currently, Down's syndrome screening may be performed in both the first and second trimesters with a national cut-off for high risk of 1:150[5]. Women undergoing first-trimester combined screening should obtain a result within the timeframe for CVS. Where second trimester serum screening is undertaken, the timing of results will mean that amniocentesis is the procedure of choice.

Many women opt for screening tests in pregnancy for an assurance of normality. Prior to embarking on any aneuploidy screening, couples should be counseled to ensure they understand the role of screening and diagnostic tests. The discussion should be individualized and explore what they hope to obtain from screening, and what they personally would consider to be an unacceptably high-risk result. It is sensible to encourage couples to consider how they would approach a high-risk result, and if diagnostic testing and termination of an affected pregnancy may be acceptable to them. If such testing or termination of pregnancy is not acceptable to the couple on religious, moral or personal grounds, then the psychological impact of a high-risk result for the remainder of the pregnancy needs to be discussed.

Counseling and consent

Consent for invasive procedures should be written. Ideally, standardized forms based on the Department of Health Consent Form 3 should be used. Specific consent advice is available from the RCOG for amniocentesis[2]. Information provided for other invasive procedures should follow a similar structure. Information should be presented in lay language with an opportunity to ask questions, and be supported by a local patient information leaflet. Provision for translation of discussion and documentation should be made for women who do not speak English, and individualized support provided for those with other special needs.

The discussion should cover the intended benefits of the procedure in ascertaining fetal karyotype and defining the presence of fetal infection or anemia as necessary. Discussion of procedure-related risks should encompass serious and frequently occurring risks[6]. The consequences of not performing the procedure, and possible alternatives, should be made clear during pretest counseling[6].

A clear record should be kept of the information provided, which should include the method of communicating results, usual reporting times and reasons to seek medical advice after the procedure[5]. Storage and disposal of samples should be discussed[6].

Associated risks

Procedure-related miscarriage. A rate of 1% above the background rate for gestational age for amniocentesis, 1–2% for CVS and 1.4% for FBS are most commonly quoted[2]. In 2007, a systematic review reported pooled pregnancy loss rates within 14 days of genetic amniocentesis of 0.6% and 0.9% for losses prior to 24 weeks, and 1.9% in total[7]. For CVS, the corresponding figures were 0.7%, 1.3 and 2% with greater heterogeneity[7]. Controls were not matched for gestational age and it was concluded that the lack of adequate controls tends to underestimate the true added risk of prenatal invasive procedures. Therefore, local procedure-related pregnancy loss rates below 1% should be quoted only if supported by robust data[2]. For procedures performed after 24 weeks, discussion of the risk of preterm birth would replace discussion of fetal loss.

Fetal bradycardia or asystole. This complication is associated with FBS and is usually transient, but prolonged bradycardia can necessitate emergency delivery by cesarean section.

Chorioamnionitis. Severe sepsis, including maternal death, has been reported but the risk is likely to be less than 1/1,000 procedures[2].

Maternal bowel injury. This complication is also rare and minimized by tracking the needle from insertion to removal with continuous ultrasound guidance.

Fetal injury. This complication is rare and described only in case reports. Parents should be reassured the risk is further minimized by the standard use of continuous ultrasound guidance.

Amniotic fluid leakage. This may be temporary or prolonged, and with the added risk of *preterm delivery*.

Failure to obtain an adequate sample. An experienced operator is likely to be successful in obtaining an adequate sample at the first attempt in 94% of CVS and amniocentesis procedures[2].

Bloodstaining of amniotic fluid. An experienced operator is likely to obtain blood stained samples in <1% of amnioceteses using continuous ultrasound guidance[2]. Prior to the standard use of continuous ultrasound guidance, bloodstaining occurred much more frequently[9].

Rapid test failure (polymerase chain reaction (PCR)). This occurs in 2.2% of cases due to bloodstaining or insufficient complement of fetal cells.

Failure of cell culture in the laboratory. This occurs in 1% of CVS and 0.5% of amniocentesis samples. This is more likely with bloodstaining of the sample.

Maternal cell contamination (MCC). This affects 1–2% of amniocentesis samples, and is more frequent with CVS samples. Further information can be offered with MCC analysis in the laboratory.

Frequently occurring risks

Mild discomfort at the needle insertion site. This is estimated to be equivalent to the experience of venepuncture for amniocentesis and transabdominal CVS with local anesthetic.

Hematoma formation. Some bleeding can occur from the FBS site, or hematoma formation. This is usually self-limiting, and hematoma resolution can be seen during ultrasound surveillance.

Techniques

Chorionic villus sampling

CVS may be conducted transabdominally or transcervically, the former being standard practice in most UK centers. Both procedures should be conducted under continuous ultrasound guidance by the operator. There is little evidence of advantage for either technique, and the choice largely depends on operator experience and access to the placenta. For either technique, the placenta should be accessible without traversing the amnion and entering the gestation sac.

Ninety-eight percent of specialist centers in the UK use local anesthetic for transabdominal CVS[8]; 10 mL 1% lidocaine is progressively infiltrated through the skin and anterior abdominal wall to the level of the uterus, with ultrasound guidance as appropriate.

It is beneficial to prime the CVS needle and syringe with a small volume of transport medium to ease aspiration of chorionic villi and preserve the architecture of the villi in the sample. In the single needle technique, an 18G needle is inserted via the same path as the local anesthetic, and introduced through the myometrium into the placenta. Chorionic villi can then be aspirated using suction, usually with a 20 mL syringe. The needle and syringe are then removed and chorionic villi

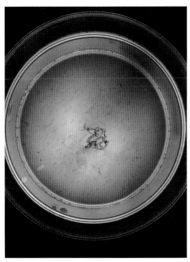

Figure 27.1 Photograph of placental fronds demonstrating an adequate sample volume and quality for analysis.

expelled into a container with transport medium. Adequacy of the sample must be checked using microscopy prior to completing the procedure – a 5–10 mg sample is sufficient for conventional cytogenetic analysis and up to 15 mg is required for molecular genetics (Figure 27.1). The double needle technique uses a 20G needle inside an 18G needle – the needle is introduced into the placenta in the same manner and the 20G needle used to aspirate the sample. The advantage of this technique is that the 18G outer needle serves as a guide, and if the sample is found to be inadequate, a second entry can be avoided. The needle should be carefully removed under continuous ultrasound control.

For transcervical CVS, the cervix is visualized with a Cuscoe's speculum. The cervix is cannulated under continuous ultrasound guidance. Techniques for obtaining the sample depend on operator experience, but there is some evidence to suggest an advantage of small biopsy forceps over aspiration cannulae.

Amniocentesis

Local anesthetic was shown to have no effect on pain scores for amniocentesis, and is used by just 4% of specialist centers in the UK[8]. Where possible, the needle path is transamniotic and the placenta is avoided. However, if transplacental passage of the needle provides the only safe access to an adequate pool of liquor, there is no evidence of increased procedure-related complications[2]. The placental cord insertion should be avoided. A 20–22G needle should be inserted under

continuous ultrasound control. The stylet of the needle can be removed when the tip is clearly into the amniotic sac, and aspiration attempted. Occasionally the needle will be visible in the sac with ultrasound but aspiration is not possible as the needle is obstructed by amniotic membrane. When this occurs the needle can be advanced slightly or rotated to free the tip. A 15–20 mL sample is generally adequate for analysis and should be transported in a plastic container. When sufficient volume has been aspirated, the stylet of the needle is reinserted and the needle removed with continuous ultrasound guidance. The color of the sample and presence of any bloodstaining should be recorded.

Fetal blood sampling

Local anaesthetic is advisable for this procedure. In some cases, particularly where FBS is combined with transfusion, fetal paralysis usually using vecuronium will need to be considered. A 20G needle is inserted at a preselected site to approach the target using continuous ultrasound control. When approaching cord vessels, the needle should be placed in light contact with the intended portion of cord, and then advanced swiftly into the target vessel. This assists with piercing the Wharton's Jelly and avoids glancing the needle off the target (Figure 27.2). The intrahepatic portion of the umbilical vein can be approached through the fetal liver or along the entry of the umbilical cord. After entering the vessel, the stylet of the needle can be removed and a 1-mL syringe aspirated to confirm intravascular placement. A 1–2 mL sample of fetal blood will be adequate for hemoglobin, fetal virology or karyotype. Blood should be aspirated into a lithium heparin tube (EDTA is used for microarray). A rapid estimate for fetal hemoglobin can be obtained with a point-of-care test, and confirmed with a full blood count (Figure 27.2).

After removing an adequate volume, the stylet of the needle is replaced and the needle removed under ultrasound guidance. It is normal to see a small amount of turbulence in the amniotic fluid surrounding the insertion site or a small echogenic area as fetal blood seals the puncture.

Performing the procedure

Preparation

The tray for invasive prenatal tests should be set-up in a uniform way for each procedure, and asepsis of the tray maintained throughout (Figures 27.3 and 27.4).

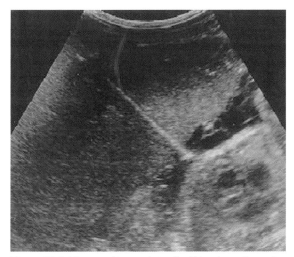

Figure 27.2 Ultrasound image during fetal blood sampling – the full length of the needle is visible.

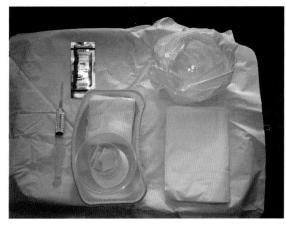

Figure 27.3 Standard tray for ultrasound-guided diagnostic procedures.

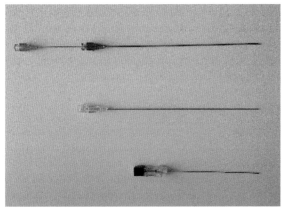

Figure 27.4 Needles for chorionic villus sampling (green/purple), fetal blood sampling (yellow) and amniocentesis (black).

When preparing for FBS, possible actions in case of persistent fetal bradycardia should be discussed with the couple. When the fetus is considered viable, arrangements should be made with the delivery suite for the possibility of a category 1 cesarean section before beginning the procedure.

A trained chaperone who can assist in supporting the patient and receiving the sample should be available. The patient should be offered the choice to be accompanied by her partner or other support person during the procedure, who can be seated at her side clear of the intended aseptic field.

The ultrasound probe should be enclosed in a sterile bag, and a separate sterile gel should be available. Use a two-dimensional ultrasound probe and select a setting for invasive procedures with a wide-angled field to assist tracking of the needle. The abdominal skin should be cleansed using disposable chlorhexidine wipes, and sterile disposable drapes applied.

Prior to commencing the procedure, an assessment should be made of the most suitable approach to the target. For amniocentesis, this will include avoiding transplacental passage of the needle where possible. The patient should be positioned supine; it may also be helpful to tilt the patient to access the target with the needle, in which case the patient should be stabilized and made comfortable by adjusting the bed or using pillows or a wedge. Contrary to common belief, a full bladder is rarely needed for invasive procedures. More often than not it is simply a hindrance that makes women more uncomfortable. For transcervical CVS, a full bladder is required, a full bladder is also required in some cases with a retroverted uterus for transabdominal CVS. FBS is possible but more technically demanding prior to 20 weeks' gestation due to smaller targets and more friable tissues. When selecting the intended targets, fixed, stable areas, such as the placental cord insertion or intrahepatic portion of the umbilical vein, are more favorable, whereas free cord loops are more inclined to move and tear. A contingency plan should be made for preferred and approachable targets in each case.

When preparing and carrying out transabdominal procedures, the two-dimensional transabdominal probe should be utilized at 90° to the floor and the uterus viewed in transverse section. The needle should be introduced in-line with the probe, and the probe slightly adjusted to keep the full length of the needle in view throughout. For all procedures, lateral movement of the needle should be avoided.

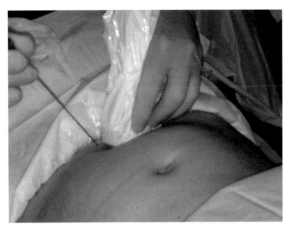

Figure 27.5 Correct alignment of two-dimensional ultrasound probe and needle.

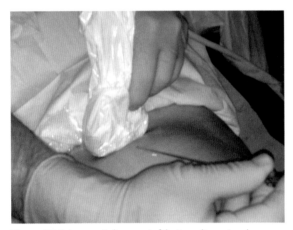

Figure 27.6 Incorrect alignment of the two-dimensional ultrasound probe and needle.

For any procedure, a more experienced operator should be consulted if two attempts at uterine insertion have failed to produce an adequate sample for analysis[2]. Where difficulties can be anticipated (obesity, multiple pregnancy, poor access to placental cord insertion), these should be prepared for in setting up the procedure, including considering support from a second experienced operator (Figures 27.5 and 27.6).

Postprocedure management

At completion of the procedure, the fetal heartbeat should be demonstrated to the woman. The needle insertion site should be cleaned and covered with a small sterile dressing, and anti-D arranged for Rhesus (Rh) negative women (250 units IM <20 weeks' gestation, 500 units >20 weeks), according to RCOG

guidance[9]. Time should be allowed to ask questions following the procedure. The procedure should be documented in a standardized format stating indication, type of procedure, needle gauge, entries, complications and provision of anti-D where applicable.

Women should be advised to expect mild discomfort at the needle insertion site and mild period-type abdominal discomfort, during the first 24–48 h for which paracetamol should be sufficient. They should be advised to avoid strenuous activity for 48 h, and activities involving bending, stretching or lifting. Many women will prefer to be at home during this time. It should be explained that this is for her comfort, but does not prevent procedure-related pregnancy loss occurring.

If more severe abdominal pain occurs, vaginal loss or bleeding, or the woman feels systemically unwell, she should seek advice from the hospital.

A rapid karyotype from quantitative fluorescent PCR (QF-PCR) result is usually available within 4 working days, microarray within 10–14 days and full culture within 21 days. The method for communicating results should also be discussed and agreed.

More complex procedures

Third trimester

Amniocentesis in the third trimester is carried out for a number of indications, most commonly, for late karyotyping and detection of suspected fetal infection in prelabor preterm rupture of the membranes (PPROM). Much of the literature on the risks of late amniocentesis predates the use of continuous ultrasound guidance. More recent series report more than one attempt in over 5% of samplings and bloodstained fluid in 5–10% of cases, and accordingly there is a suggestion that culture failure rates are increased[10]. When amniocentesis is carried out in the presence of PPROM, failure rates are higher. Serious complications, including the need for emergency delivery, are rare.

Multiple pregnancy

A high level of ultrasound expertise is essential for operators undertaking ultrasound-guided diagnostic procedures in twins and higher multiples because uterine contents have to be meticulously "mapped." This is essential to ensure that separate samples are taken for each fetus. Fetal labeling is greatly assisted by the presence of obvious fetal abnormality or discordant gender.

To minimize the risk of chromosomal abnormality being assigned to the wrong twin, invasive procedures in multiple pregnancy should only be performed by a specialist who is able to proceed to selective termination of pregnancy[2]. It is very unlikely that a specialist would be prepared to carry out a selective termination of pregnancy relying on information provided by a referring doctor, particularly in the absence of clearly identifiable ultrasound appearances. Most clinicians will use two separate puncture sites when performing amniocentesis or CVS in multiple pregnancies, although there is some experience with single-entry techniques. The procedure-related miscarriage rate is likely to be higher than in singleton pregnancies, and is estimated at 1/56 (1.8%)[11].

The role of CVS in dichorionic placentas remains controversial because of a relatively high risk of cross-contamination of chorionic tissue, which may lead to false-positive or false-negative results. This risk may be minimized if two separate needles are used. Such procedures should be performed only after detailed counseling.

Infectious diseases

In most centers, women are not routinely screened for methicillin-resistant *Staphylococcus aureus* (MRSA) carriage at booking or prior to invasive prenatal tests. If, however, women are known to be colonized with MRSA and invasive prenatal testing is indicated, the advice of the Infection Control Team should be sought. It is advisable to delay investigations by approximately 1 week, until eradication therapy is complete.

Bloodborne viruses may constitute both a risk of vertical transmission, and a potential infection control risk for operators. The risk of hepatitis B transmission is very low. Maternal viral load is the most important risk indicator, and risk increases significantly with viral loads of 7 million copies/mL or greater[12]. There is no evidence for increased hepatitis C transmission secondary to invasive prenatal testing.

Studies recommend avoiding invasive prenatal testing in human immunodeficiency virus (HIV)-positive women, but most predate the use of highly active antiretroviral therapy (HAART). Evidence suggests testing earlier in pregnancy is safe provided that antiretroviral therapy is being used and the maternal viral load is low[13]. Specialists need to be aware and inform women that the majority of evidence is based on amniocentesis, and that data on CVS are very limited.

Whenever possible, procedures should be delayed until treatment has optimized the maternal viral load[1]. Where the results of screening for maternal infection are not yet known or the woman has declined such testing, then informed consent should include discussion of the risks of vertical transmission of infection. For women in high-risk groups where no HIV test result is available, it is advisable to delay the invasive test and perform a rapid HIV test[2]. If the results indicate maternal infection, then the risk of transmission should be discussed and consideration given to starting antiretroviral therapy to reduce the viral load prior to the procedure.

Achieving and maintaining technical competence

Operators carrying out invasive prenatal tests should be trained to the competencies expected of subspecialty training in maternal and fetal medicine, such as the UK RCOG's Fetal Medicine ATSM or an international equivalent[2].

It is advised that clinical skills models, assessment of interaction with patients and supervised procedures should be an integral part of training[2]. Invasive procedures are practical skills and trainees will achieve competence at different rates. Once competency is achieved, it is proposed that skills should be maintained by carrying out at least 30 ultrasound-guided invasive procedures per annum. For revalidation purposes, operators should carry out a continuous audit of frequencies of multiple insertions, failures, "bloody" taps and postprocedure losses.

Very experienced operators, performing more than 100 procedures annually, may have higher success rates and lower procedure-related losses[14]. Expert opinion suggests that an operator's competence should be reviewed where loss rates appear high and an audit should certainly occur where they exceed 4/100 consecutive amniocenteses or 8/100 CVS[2]. A register of invasive diagnostic procedures should be kept to facilitate an annual audit, and results made accessible to patients (see below)[2].

RCOG auditable standards

- Rate of pregnancy loss at any gestation after a procedure.
- Rate of pregnancy loss <24+0 weeks after a procedure.

- Rate of pregnancy loss within 14 days of procedure.
- Local cytogenetic laboratory culture failure rates for amniocentesis and CVS.
- Proportion of procedures requiring more than one needle insertion.
- Proportion of procedures with failure to obtain an adequate sample.
- Complication rates (bloody tap, amniotic fluid leakage).
- Rate of anti-D prophylaxis for women who are RhD-negative undergoing amniocentesis or CVS.

Summary

Trainees undertaking advanced training in fetal medicine need to develop a sound understanding of ultrasound-guided diagnostic procedures, and the organization of prenatal screening and diagnostic services. With advancing technology, the options available to women continue to evolve, and clinicians must have the initiative to follow developments and adapt to new processes relevant to their patients. An organized reflective approach and mentorship are beneficial when acquiring new practical skills. Trainees are encouraged to keep a logbook of ultrasound-guided procedures they complete and learn from their experiences. All operators, new and experienced should prioritise patient safety. They should be mindful of their individual limitations, monitor individual complication rates and provide support for each other where concerns are anticipated or occur.

References

1. Royal College of Obstetricians and Gynaecologists (RCOG). Advanced Training Skills Module – Fetal Medicine, 2010. http://www.rcog.org.uk/files/rcog-corp/ED-ATSM-Fetal-Med.pdf (accessed January 30, 2014).

2. Royal College of Obstetricians and Gynaecologists (RCOG). Amniocentesis. Green-Top Guideline No. 8. London: RCOG Press, 2005.

3. Firth HV, Boyd PA, Chamberlain P, et al. Severe limb abnormalities after chorionic villus sampling at 56–66 days' gestation. *Lancet* 1991; 337: 762–3.

4. Morris RK, Quinlan-Jones E, Kilby MD, et al. Systematic review of accuracy of fetal urine analysis to predict poor postnatal renal function in cases of congenital urinary tract obstruction. *Prenat Diagn* 2007; 27: 900–11.

5. National Health Service Fetal Anomaly Screening Programme. Cut-off changes to Down's Syndrome screening, 2008. http://fetalanomaly.screening.nhs.uk/programmestatements#fileid11755 (accessed January 30, 2014).

6. Royal College of Obstetricians and Gynaecologists (RCOG). *Amniocentesis.* Consent Advice 6. London: RCOG, 2006.

7. Mujezinovic F, Alfirevic Z. Procedure-related complications of amniocentesis and chorionic villus sampling: a systematic review. *Obstet Gynecol* 2007; 110(30): 687–94.

8. Carlin AJ, Alfirevic Z. Techniques for chorionic villus sampling and amniocentesis: a survey of practice in specialist UK centres. *Prenat Diagn* 2008; 28: 914–19.

9. Royal College of Obstetricians and Gynaecologists (RCOG). Use of anti-D immunoglobulin for Rh prophylaxis. RCOG Green Top Guideline No. 22. London: RCOG Press, 2002.

10. Gordon MC, Narula K, O'Shaughnessy R, et al. Complications of third-trimester amniocentesis using continuous ultrasound guidance. *Obstet Gynecol* 2002; 99: 255–9.

11. Cahill AG, Macones GA, Stamilio DM, et al. Pregnancy loss rate after mid-trimester amniocentesis in twin pregnancies. *Am J Obstet Gynecol* 2009; 200: 257.

12. Yi W, Pan CQ, Hao J, et al. Risk of vertical transmission of hepatitis B after amniocentesis in HBs antigen-positive mothers. *J Hepatol* 2014 60(3): 523–9.

13. Maiques V, Garcia-Tejedor A, Perales A, et al. HIV detection in amniotic fluid samples. Amniocentesis can be performed in HIV pregnant women? *Eur J Obstet Gynecol Reprod Biol* 2003; 108: 137–41.

14. Blessed WB, Lacoste H, Welch RA. Obstetrician-gynecologists performing genetic amniocentesis may be misleading themselves and their patients. *Am J Obstet Gynecol* 2001; 1784: 1340–2.

Chapter

28

Fetal therapy

R. Katie Morris and Mark D. Kilby

Fetal therapy may be considered when it is of immediate benefit to the fetus, to potentially cure or ameliorate disease progression, or when prenatal therapy may reduce postnatal complications and facilitate therapy in the newborn period. Animal models have provided clinicians with an understanding of disease etiology and pathogenesis of underlying conditions that may be potentially treated in utero. However, in many cases, our understanding of this process is sadly incomplete. Cohort studies and more recently randomized controlled trials with systematic reviews and meta-analysis of their results have moved fetal therapy into the evidence-based era.

Rapid developments in fetal imaging technologies (improved two-dimensional ultrasound resolution, three-dimensional ultrasound imaging (with surface rending and internal volume acquisition) and fetal magnetic resonance imaging (MRI)), advances in therapeutic techniques (ultrasound-guided needle therapy, microendoscopy) combined with improved management of complications of fetal therapy (preventing preterm labor, amniorrhexis and neonatal care) have led to a dramatic increase in the efficacy of fetal therapies. There are still many challenges.

Medical therapy

Fetal drug therapy

The "drug" is delivered to the mother and relies upon transplacental passage. This has disadvantages of pharmacodynamic and kinetic effects both in the mother and fetus. Fetal drug therapy falls into three categories: preventative for fetal malformations (e.g., folic acid), prophylactic use to reduce or prevent neonatal complications (e.g., corticosteroids for fetal lung maturity, antibiotics or retrovirals) and drugs to treat specific fetal conditions. The latter therapies are discussed in detail in the relevant chapters, e.g. anti-arrhythmics in fetal supraventricular tachycardia (Chapter 3.3), prostaglandin synthetase inhibitors in polyhydramnios (Chapter 8.2) and immunoglobulins in alloimmune thrombocytopenia (Chapter 4.2).

Ultrasound-guided needle therapy

Fetal transfusions

The advent of ultrasound in the early 1980s allowed intrauterine transfusion to move from the percutaneous intraperitoneal fetal transfusion employed by Liley (using fluroscopic screening in the 1960s) to direct intravascular transfusions of a fetal vessel[1]. The indication for fetal transfusion is to provide therapy in the form of donor-"packed" (high hematocrit) red cells to treat fetal anemia, platelets (concentrates) for alloimmune thromobocytopenia or direct drug therapy, e.g., for incessant fetal arrhythmias. The most common indication is fetal anemia secondary to red cell alloimmunization (commonly Rhesus (Rh) disease secondary to anti-D or Kell antibodies), but also to treat parvovirus B19 infection, severe fetomaternal hemorrhage or relatively rare causes secondary to placental chorioangiomas or homozygous alpha-thalassemias (rare in Europe). The management of these conditions, the clinical decision to perform such therapy and timing of the transfusion are discussed in Chapters 15, 16 and 27.

The procedure of intrauterine transfusion is the same, regardless of the indication, but in conditions of thrombocytopenia, cord puncture is often avoided if possible. This requires a subspecialist with training and experience in performing such therapy and maternal preparation (including counseling and consent). Maternal sedation may be offered, along with prophylactic antibiotic cover and corticosteroids. It is performed as an outpatient procedure using an aseptic, minimal touch technique with continuous ultrasound guidance. A 20G needle is used either freehand or with a needle guide to puncture the chosen vessel. A sample of fetal blood is taken and analysed immediately for fetal hemoglobin (and hematocrit) estimation. The volume of blood to be transfused is then calculated using nomograms (using fetal hematocrit, donor hematocrit and estimated fetoplacental volume). The donor hematocrit should be relatively high (≥75%) to reduce the volume infused. The aim is to transfuse to a fetal hematocrit of 40–45% using maternal crossmatched, O Rh-negative, cytomegalovirus (CMV)-negative, leucodepleted, irradiated blood. The timing of repeat transfusion is individualized based on the history and severity of the anemia. Studies have estimated that the post-transfusion decline in hematocrit is 1–2% per day[2,3]. Some therapists use serial middle cerebral artery Doppler peak systolic velocity (MCA-PSV) to time fetal transfusions.

Intravascular transfusion (placental cord root or intrahepatic vein determined by access; Figure 28.1) has advantages over intraperitoneal transfusions in that a sample of fetal blood can be obtained to confirm fetal blood group and hematocrit and hemoglobin, thus aiding diagnosis[4,5]. It allows calculation of the amount to be transfused and post-transfusion measurement to be collected allowing assessment of transfusion interval. Treatment via this route is more effective when the fetus is hydropic and avoids trauma to fetal intraperitoneal organs.

Intraperitoenal transfusions rely on absorption of the red cells into the fetal circulation via the subdiaphragmatic lymphatics and thoracic duct. The presence of ascites reduces the efficacy of this process, significantly reducing absorption and increasing mortality. The main advantage of the intraperitoneal route is that it can be performed at earlier gestations (in very high-risk situations)(<18 weeks) or when access to the fetal vasculature is hampered by fetal lie. The needle is inserted through the anterior abdominal wall, below the umbilical vein but above the fetal bladder. Correct placement of the needle intraperitoneally can be confirmed by aspirating ascetic fluid in the hydropic fetus or via observing an infusion of saline into the cavity.

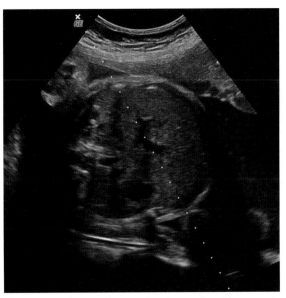

Figure 28.1 Ultrasound picture showing needle guide centered on intrahepatic vein.
Reproduced from Kilby MD et al. (eds) *Fetal Therapy.* Cambridge UK: Cambridge University Press 2012, with permission.

Complications include the risks of an invasive procedure during pregnancy and a perinatal mortality rate of 1.6–2%[6,7] due to the specific complications of umbilical cord hematoma resulting in arterial (sometimes transient) vasospasm, fetal bradycardia or fetal exsanguination from needle puncture site, leading to fetal compromise and resultant emergency premature delivery (particularly in fetal alloimmune thrombocytopenia). There is a risk of fetomaternal hemorrhage with the resultant risk of increasing maternal antibody levels or even the development of new red cell antibodies.

Outcomes for pregnancies managed with intrauterine transfusions are good with an overall survival rate of 84%, higher survival is seen in pregnancies that are nonhydropic compared to hydropic (94% versus 74%)[7]. The study with the longest follow-up is the LOTUS study from Leiden in the Netherlands[8]. A total of 291 children who underwent intrauterine transfusion for hemolytic disease of the fetus were evaluated at a median age of 8.2 (range, 2–17) years. Cerebral palsy was detected in six (2.1%) children, severe developmental delay in nine (3.1%) children, and bilateral deafness in three (1.0%) children. The overall incidence of neurodevelopmental impairment was 4.8% (14/291). In a multivariate regression analysis including only preoperative risk factors, severe hydrops was independently associated with neurodevelopmental impairment (odds ratio (OR), 11.2; 95% confidence interval (CI), 1.7–92.7)[8].

Needle aspiration for drainage of fluid from body cavities

Under ultrasound guidance any fluid-filled cavity can be aspirated. This may be performed for two reasons: either to sample the fluid for diagnostic purposes (e.g., fetal urine in lower urinary tract obstruction) or to reduce the amount of fluid within an anatomic space to prevent dilatation or compression of the associated organ (e.g., pleural effusions) until delivery can occur. Performing this procedure for the latter indication should be carefully considered as it is likely that the fluid will re-accumulate and that multiple procedures will be required. In this instance, shunting of the cavity may also be considered. In some cases, drainage of a cavity may be required prior to delivery to either facilitate vaginal delivery, e.g., abdominal cysts (enlarging the abdominal circumference with risk of dystocia) or to facilitate neonatal resuscitation and management, e.g., pleural effusions to facilitate ventilation. Palliative procedures may also be performed to facilitate vaginal delivery, e.g., drainage of a hydrocephalus, which can be performed percutaneously prior to labor or vaginally intrapartum.

Ultrasound-guided shunt insertion

Thoracic

The procedure for thoracoamniotic shunting is the same as that for vesicoamniotic shunting (VAS) as are the complications. The "pigtail" catheter is inserted into the lower pleural cavity, posterior to the midaxillary line. The main indication for shunting is an effusion, likely to be an isolated chylothorax with no chromosomal anomalies, which rapidly accumulates after thoracocentesis. The rationale for treatment is to (a) reduce the risk of pulmonary hypoplasia and (b) reduce the risks of cardiovascular compromise (and the development of hydrops fetalis). A systematic review of pulmonary drainage (shunt, surgery or drainage), including 16 observational studies and 608 fetuses, concluded that pulmonary drainage did not improve perinatal survival in cystic lung lesions (mainly congenital cystic adenomatoid malformations and pulmonary sequestrations) compared with no drainage overall. However, there was a marked

improvement with this therapy in a subgroup of fetuses with fetal hydrops fetalis (but not in the subgroup uncomplicated by fetal hydrops fetalis)[9]. Only two of the included studies looked at treatment for primary hydrothoraces and there was no significant improvement in survival with treatment; sub-group analysis according to the presence of hydrops fetalis was not possible in this group[9].

Urinary tract

Fetal VAS is the most common antenatal intervention for lower urinary tract obstruction (LUTO) and was first reported by Golbus et al in 1982[10]. The procedure is performed under ultrasound guidance with prophylactic antibiotics and maternal sedation if required. Amnioinfusion may also be required prior to shunt insertion if there is anhydramnios or severe oligohydramnios. The shunt is inserted via a trochar percutaneously and consists of a pigtail catheter (either Harrison or Rocket), with one end in the fetal bladder and the other draining into the amniotic cavity, thus bypassing the obstruction.

Data relating to the efficacy of VAS in the management of LUTO from cohort studies has been summarized in a systematic review that concluded that VAS compared to no treatment improved perinatal survival (OR 3.86; 95% CI 2.00–7.45) but that this effect was more significant in a group with poor prognosis on fetal urinalysis (OR 13.85; 95% CI, 1.25–153.05) (Figure 28.2). However, when subgroup analysis was performed to look at the effects on survival with normal renal function, there was a suggestion that VAS had an adverse effect (OR 0.50; 95% CI 0.13–1.90)[11] (Figure 28.3). Due to the biases in cohort data highlighted in the systematic appraisal of the evidence, there was a need for an randomized controlled trial (RCT) of VAS versus conservative management with long-term follow-up into childhood. The percutaneous vesicoamniotic shunting versus conservative management for fetal lower urinary tract obstruction (PLUTO) trial was a multicenter RCT with the objectives to determine if intrauterine VAS for fetal bladder outflow obstruction, compared with conservative care, improved prenatal and perinatal mortality and renal function for survivors[12]. Unfortunately, due to poor recruitment and the high numbers of parents that opted for termination of pregnancy (TOP) (46.9%), the PLUTO trial closed early to randomization in December 2010 with 31 babies in the randomized arm, 46 registered and 68

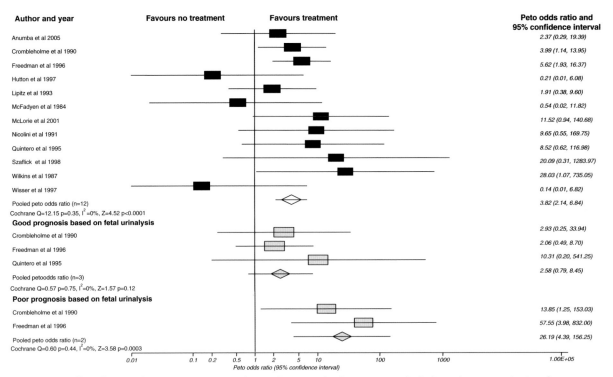

Figure 28.2 Effect of antenatal intervention on perinatal survival compared with no treatment (including voluntary termination of pregnancies) stratified by predicted prognosis.

Reproduced from Morris et al. *BJOG* 2010; 117: 1350–7, with kind permission.

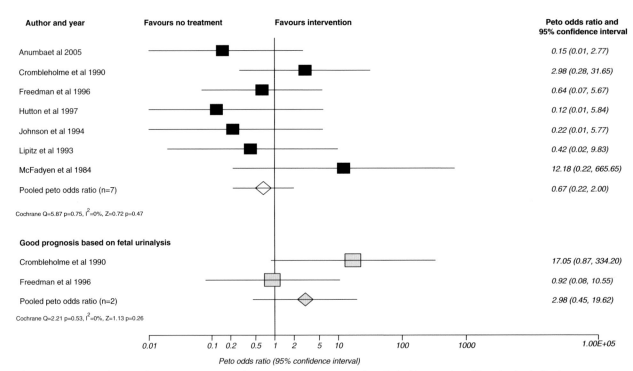

Figure 28.3 Effect of antenatal intervention compared to no treatment on postnatal survival with normal renal function (excluding intrauterine deaths and voluntary termination of pregnancy) stratified according to predicted prognosis.

Reproduced from Morris et al. *BJOG* 2010; 117: 1350–7, with kind permission.

Outcome	Randomised to VAS n = 52	Randomised to conservative management n = 48
Pregnancy loss (termination or miscarriage)	13	9
Live birth	39	39
Alive at 28 days	26	13
Alive at 1 year	23	10
Alive at 2 years	23	10
Normal renal function at 2 years	7	0

Figure 28.4 Outcomes for babies within the PLUTO trial (extrapolated to 100 babies). VAS, vesicoamniotic shunting.

pregnancies that had had a TOP. Of those randomized to VAS, 8/16 (50%) survived to 28 days compared with 4/15 (27%) of those randomized to conservative management (relative risk (RR), 1.88; 95% CI, 0.71–4.96; P = 0.27). All 12 newborn deaths were as a result of pulmonary hypoplasia in the early neonatal period. One baby in each arm of treatment subsequently died prior to 1 year of life due to renal failure. RR estimates for survival at 1 and 2 years were similar to those seen at 28 days. The conclusion was that survival appeared higher in those fetuses receiving VAS, but uncertainty in the direction and magnitude of the effect remained. Overall long-term prognosis for all babies regardless of treatment received was poor, with only two babies surviving to 2 years of age with no renal impairment (Figure 28.4).

Cohort studies have reported outcomes for survivors past 5 years of age following VAS and shown that while these children have normal quality of life scores and normal cognitive ability, a significant proportion have difficulty voiding or incontinence and recurrent urinary tract infections. Up to a third will require dialysis and/or transplantation[13].

Thus, counseling of parents faced with this diagnosis for their baby must include a multidisciplinary approach involving fetal medicine specialists, neonatologists and pediatric urologists/nephrologists, recognizing that the prenatal counseling is complex and stressful for parents. Qualitative research has shown that parents often consider TOP as the long-term outcomes are morbid with significant consequences for the family unit[14].

Fetoscopy

Diagnostic and therapeutic cystoscopy

The limitations of VAS in terms of patient selection, diagnosis of underlying pathology and inability to correct the blockage, led to the development of fetal cystoscopy by Quintero et al. in 1995[15]. The proposed advantages of this technique are that it can be used for

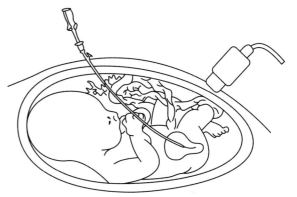

Figure 28.5 Technique for fetal cystoscopy.
Reproduced from Kilby MD et al. (eds) *Fetal Therapy*. Cambridge UK: Cambridge University Press 2012, with permission.

diagnosis of underlying pathology as well as treatment in LUTO. The most common technique is percutaneous anterograde fetal cystoscopy under maternal anesthesia (regional or local) with fetal anesthesia (fentanyl and pancuronium) under direct ultrasound guidance (Figure 28.5). A fetal urine sample can be obtained and then the bladder neck is inspected. If posterior urethral valves are identified, options for treatment and perforation of the valves are hydroablation, guide wire or laser fulguration. The finding of a nonmembrane like structure at the bladder neck suggests urethral atresia. A systematic review of the literature has assessed the effectiveness of fetal cystoscopy for diagnostic accuracy and effectiveness and demonstrated a high sensitivity (100%) and specificity (85.7%) for the correct diagnosis of LUTO[16]. However, comparing VAS to fetal cystoscopy, there appeared to be no significant improvement in perinatal survival OR 1.49 (95% CI, 0.13–16.97)(Figure 28.6). Further investigation in the form of a RCT is required to compare VAS to fetal cystoscopy[16] with long-term follow-up of babies to allow confirmation of diagnosis postnatally and long-term outcomes, such as renal function and bladder function, to be assessed. Complications of fetal cystoscopy are similar for any fetoscopic technique, with no reports

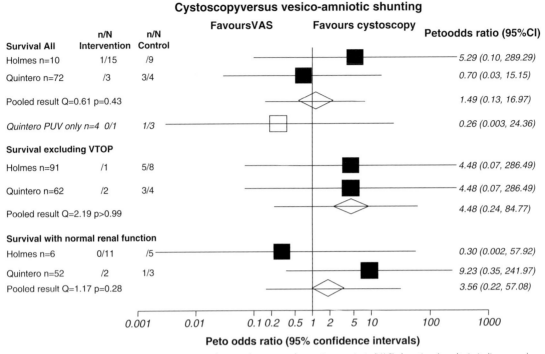

Figure 28.6 Effect of fetal cystoscopy on perinatal survival compared to vesicoamniotic (VAS) shunting (results in italics are sub-groups). VTOP, voluntary termination of pregnancy; PUV, posterior urethral valves.

Reproduced from Morris et al. *BJOG* 2010; 117: 1350–7, with kind permission.

of fetal bladder damage secondary to treatment in the small number of cases reported.

The treatment of severe twin-to-twin transfusion syndrome: fetoscopic laser coagulation

Twin-to-twin transfusion syndrome (TTTS) is a condition of monochorionic (MC) pregnancies associated with a hemodynamic imbalance between twin fetal circulations. Untreated, the condition carries a mortality rate of 80–90%. The pathology and natural history of TTTS has been detailed in Chapter 7.1.

Historically, there were three main treatment options: selective feticide, serial amnioreduction and amniotic septostomy. Serial amnioreduction was the initial mainstay of treatment as it was easy to perform and helped improve maternal symptoms secondary to distension, and reduced the risk of preterm labor. Although an improvement in Doppler studies has been reported with the use of this treatment[17], due to an uncertain mechanism, it has variable survival rates from 37–60%[17,18], with 17–33% of survivors developing neurologic damage. In the 1990s, septostomy

was introduced[19], again with the advantage of being a simple treatment, its mechanism being to equalize the pressure difference between the two sacs. Outcomes include survival rates of up to 83%[20] but long-term morbidity data is lacking. Both amnioreduction and septosotomy have the risk of rupture of membranes, intrauterine infection, placental abruption, miscarriage and preterm labor, and the latter iatrogenically converts the pregnancy to a monoamniotic one with the risk of twin and cord entanglement.

Fetoscopic laser coagulation (FLC) of placental vessels was introduced in the 1990s[21] and has been proven to be effective via RCT compared with amnioreduction[22]. It is the only treatment to address the underlying pathology by ablating the intertwin anastomoses along the chorionic plate.

A Cochrane review reported for treatment of TTTS with FLC: overall death, RR 0.87 (95% CI, 0.55–1.38); death of at least one infant per pregnancy, RR 0.91 (95% CI 0.75–1.09) and death of both infants, RR 0.67 (95% CI 0.27–2.10) when compared with amnioreduction. More babies were alive without any neurologic abnormality at the age of 6 years in the laser group than in the amnioreduction groups (RR 1.57; 95% CI 1.05–2.34

adjusted for clustering, one trial). A recent publication summarizing the outcomes for seven fetal medicine teams, with over 100 patients for each team, reported survival rates of 73–90.5% of at least one twin[23].

The treatment of stage 1 TTTS remains controversial. It can be managed with close observation, particularly if the cervical length is (reducing the risk of preterm delivery) and the condition remains stable[24]. Others recommend consideration of invasive treatment even at an early stage[22,25,26]. A cost-effective analysis, which looked at no treatment, amnioreduction and FLC, found the dominant strategy to be FLC using quality-adjusted life years (QUALYs – unit of assessment for clinical effectiveness as utilized by the National Institute for Health and Care Excellence) as an outcome measure. Amniodrainage did perform better than no treatment alone but was not as effective or cost-effective as FLC. This further supports the rationale for FLC being the first-line treatment for TTTS[25,27].

FLC is performed between 16 and 26 weeks. The technique involves either a regional or local anesthetic and a 3-mm trocar is inserted under ultrasound guidance into the recipient sac. Ideally, the trocar is inserted at right angles to the donor's longitudinal axis to allow the operator to visualize the intertwin membrane and anastomoses. The trocar is used to introduce a fetoscope and laser fibre (using either a Nd:Yag or diode laser at 40–60 Watts) and anastomoses are coagulated under direct vision (Figure 28.7). In some cases, amnioinfusion is used to facilitate the procedure, with drainage at the end to a normal maximum pool depth. Techniques for identifying and selecting vessels to be coagulated involve: the selective sequential technique (SLCPV), avoiding the AA and VV anastomoses; the nonselective technique, coagulating all vessels crossing the membrane to ensure none are missed; and the "Solomon" technique. The latter involves completing an initial selective coagulation and then coagulating a dividing line across the vascular equator. A recent RCT comparing SLCPV to the Solomon technique reported a reduction in postoperative fetal morbidity in severe TTTS. There was a reduction in twin anemia polycythemia sequence (TAPS) (3% versus 16% for the standard treatment; OR 0.16, 95% CI 0.05–0.49) and less recurrence of TTTS (1% versus 7%; OR 0.21, 95% CI 0.04–0.98). Perinatal mortality and severe neonatal morbidity did not differ significantly between the two groups[28]. Tocolysis and prophylactic antibiotics are usually employed.

Early referral to a tertiary center is important for assessment, and when FLC is being considered, centers

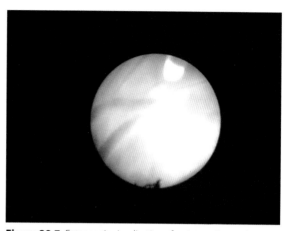

Figure 28.7 Fetoscopic visualization of an intertwin arteriovenous anastomosis. The vein is "cherry red" in color and the artery is "blue in hue." The laser fiber tip (500 μm at 1 o'clock in the image) can be visualized along with a "white patch" between the artery and vein produced by coagulation at 40W.

need to demonstrate a high throughput of cases. Morris et al. demonstrated the significance of a learning curve, not only for the center but for the individual, and the effects of experience on outcome[23]. Maternal complications of this technique range from pain due to amniotic fluid leak into the peritoneal cavity, chorioamniontis, ruptured membranes and bleeding to severe complications of placental abruption and pulmonary embolus. Maternal complications are likely to be under-reported with rates of 5.4% overall and 1.8% for severe complications as stated above[29]. Fetal complications can occur in the first 6 days (early), including single and double intrauterine death and TAPS. Late complications include recurrent or reversed TTTS, late TAPS, intrauterine death (with risks to the surviving twin if single twin demise). Recurrent TTTS and TAPS are due to residual anastomoses or revascularization of ablated anastomoses and are found in up to 33% of placentas following FLC with SLCPV[30]. As discussed earlier, the Solomon technique confers a reduction in these late complications[28]. There is a high risk of preterm labor, with 30.5% of cases delivering before 32 weeks[31]. Thus, even after successful therapy it should be recognized that the pregnancy remains high risk and many centers advocate delivery between 32 and 3 weeks.

Vascular occlusion in MC twins

Indications for selective reduction in MC twins include twin-reversed arterial perfusion (TRAP), severe intrauterine growth restriction, twins discordant for structural or chromosomal anomalies or severe TTTS, where laser therapy is not the preferred option. Historically, treatment involved open cord occlusion following hysterotomy or endoscopic placement of a cord clip. Again, due to significant maternal morbidity, management soon developed into minimally invasive techniques of two main types: cord occlusion and intrafetal ablation.

The best documented cord-occlusive technique is bipolar thermocoagulation, which is performed under ultrasound guidance with the percutaneous passage of a trochar. The umbilical cord is grasped close to the placental insertion and coagulation performed until color Doppler demonstrates no flow. Perinatal survival rates are reported up to 80%, with lower survival rates at earlier gestations (41%)[32,33]. As the use and availability of fetoscopic techniques has increased, laser coagulation of the cord or placental anastomoses has been introduced. This technique is associated with higher survival rates of 77–100%[34,35]. Cord occlusion techniques are limited by the diameter of the cord and cord edema, the former increasing with gestational age, and thus are most appropriate for earlier gestations (16–24 weeks). The rate of prelabor preterm rupture of the membranes also increases after 24 weeks. After 26 weeks, cord ligation must be employed due to the increased size of the umbilical cord and is associated with varying success rates.

Techniques for intrafetal ablation include monopolar thermocoagulation, interstitial laser and radiofrequency ablation. Intrafetal ablation is the preferred technique for MC twins complicated by TRAP sequence as it has been shown by systematic review to be technically easier (lower technical failure rates), have fewer postoperative complications (lower preterm delivery and membrane rupture prior to 32 weeks), and is more effective with longer treatment to delivery interval and higher treatment success (defined as survival of "pump" twin after 32 weeks) [35]. Intervention can be performed as early as 12 weeks but the majority of centers perform the procedure after 16 weeks (Figure 28.8). Success rates overall are reported as 85%[36].

The reduction of pulmonary hypoplasia in congenital diaphragmatic hernia: fetoscopic endoluminal tracheal occlusion

An understanding of the role of the lungs in amniotic fluid homeostasis and the importance of prenatal

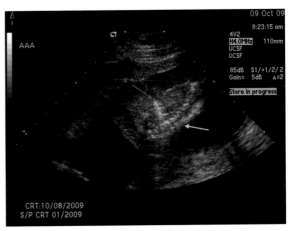

Figure 28.8 Ultrasound image taken during radiofrequency ablation.
Reproduced from Kilby MD et al. (eds) *Fetal Therapy*. Cambridge UK: Cambridge University Press 2012, with permission.

airway pressure in lung development from animal studies, has again paved the way for surgical interventions in congenital diaphragmatic hernia. Fetoscopic endoluminal tracheal occlusion (FETO) has been demonstrated to trigger lung growth in animal models[37]. Following occlusion, the accumulated lung fluid creates a positive pressure, and it is leveled by fetal breathing movement. The cyclic nature of the pressure change and tissue stretching is essential for lung tissue growth and differentiation[38]. Currently, the balloon occlusion method is preferred as it allows for tracheal growth and can be performed percutaneously via endoscopic placement. The balloon can accommodate for an increase in tracheal diameter as the fetus grows and does not cause tracheal damage[39], although laryngomalacia has been described. Traditionally, occlusion reversal was achieved by removing the balloon at the time of cesarean delivery using ex-utero intrapartum treatment (EXIT) strategy. However, animal data suggested that in-utero reversal of occlusion could lead to morphologically better lung maturation[40]. It provided the rationale for reversing the occlusion at 34 weeks' gestation in utero, either by ultrasound-guided puncture or fetoscopy, with the added advantages of allowing vaginal delivery and delivery away from the FETO center, and this has been shown to improve survival[41]. Associated complications are those of an invasive prenatal procedure (preterm premature rupture of the membranes and preterm delivery up to 25%).

In the first series of cases, the procedures were carried out between 26–28 weeks gestation and the effects were dependent on pre-existing lung size in the severe category, but reported survival rates were around 50% until discharge[41]. Later series have reported similar results, as has a recent RCT from Brazil reporting a RR for survival of 10.5 (95% CI, 1.5–74.7; P < 0.01) with FETO[42]. Several similar trials are ongoing; they are essential before widespread availability of this form of experimental fetal therapy.

Open fetal surgery

The decision to undertake fetal surgery requires extensive parental counseling followed by multidisciplinary preparation. The over-riding concern is maternal safety. Screening needs to be performed to ensure appropriate patient selection, e.g., exclusion of other structural and chromosomal anomalies and fetal MRI to assess the lesion. Steps must be taken to reduce the risk of preterm labor, e.g., earlier gestation, appropriate use of antibiotics and tocolysis. General anesthesia is preferred as it allows anesthesia for the fetus as well as the mother, and provides uterine relaxation. Further fetal anesthesia is provided by intramuscular narcotic and neuromuscular blockade prior to fetal incision. Postoperatively, tocolysis is maintained for a period. Delivery will be by elective cesarean section. Risks to the fetus are mainly those from prematurity if preterm labor occurs. For the mother, the risks are of the surgery and include chorioamnionitis, pulmonary edema, placental abruption and extrusion of the fetus through hysterotomy. In the longer term, the mother has an increased risk of scar dehiscence or rupture due to the classical uterine incision.

Myelomeningocele

Animal studies suggest a double-hit pathogenesis in neural tube defect in that the failed development of the neural tube is combined with neurologic damage with the prolonged exposure of the neurologic tissue to the intrauterine environment resulting in permanent neurologic deficit. Animal experiments of prenatal surgery support this hypothesis demonstrating that prenatal coverage preserved neurologic function and improved hindbrain herniation[43,44]. Early studies in humans demonstrated ascent in hindbrain structures on fetal MRI following surgery[45] and a decreased need for shunting postnatally in the short term[46]. The effect on lower limb function[47] and cognitive function was harder to assess[48]. These early studies were associated with high rates of perinatal

mortality (6%)[47] due to extreme prematurity and the long-term effects of a classical cesarean section for the mother[49].

In 2003, the Management of Myelomeningocele (MOMS) trial opened to recruitment. Eligible patients were singleton pregnancies between 18–25 weeks with myelomeningocele (level T1–S1 with hindbrain herniation, normal karyotype, and no other structural differences). The primary end-point was a. The trial was closed after the recruitment of 183 patients (planned 200). The composite of fetal death and the need for a shunt at 1 year occurred in 68% of the infants in the prenatal surgery group and in 98% of those in the postnatal surgery group (RR, 0.70; 97.7% CI, 0.58–0.84; P <0.001). Actual rates of shunt placement were 40% in the prenatal surgery group and 82% in the postnatal surgery group (RR, 0.48; 97.7% CI, 0.36–0.64; P <0.001). Prenatal surgery also resulted in improvement in the composite score for mental development and motor function at 30 months (P = 0.007) and in improvement in several secondary outcomes, including hindbrain herniation by 12 months and ambulation by 30 months. For morbidity there was an association with prenatal surgery and an increased risk of preterm delivery (13% before 30 weeks) and uterine dehiscence at delivery (1/3)[50].

It is imperative that the babies of the MOMS trial are followed-up long term to ensure that these medium-term benefits continue, and so that the parents and the fetal medicine community can fully assess how important the benefits conferred by prenatal surgery are when taking into account maternal and fetal risks.

Summary

Fetal therapy is a dynamic area. Advances in technology, animal studies, feasability studies and now RCTs have brought fetal therapy into the evidence-based era. This must be embraced by the fetal medicne community whilst not forgetting the ethical dilemmas of the fetus as a patient and the emotional distress that this causes for families.

References

1. Liley AW. Liquor amnil analysis in the management of the pregnancy complicated by resus sensitization. *Am J Obstet Gynecol* 1961; 82: 1359–70.

2. MacGregor SN, Socol M, Pielet BW, et al. Prediction of haematocrit decline after intravascular transfusion. *AJOG* 1989; 161: 1491–3.

3. Jones HM, Linch D, Nicolaides K, et al. Survival of transfused adult cells in the fetus. *Fetal Ther* 1986; 1: 193–5.

4. Somerset DA, Moore A, Whittle MJ, et al. An audit of outcome in intravascular transfusions using the intrahepatic portion of the fetal umbilical vein compared to cordocentesis. *Fetal Diagn Ther* 2006; 21: 272–6.

5. Nicolini U, Nicolaidis P, Fisk NM, et al. Fetal blood sampling from the intrahepatic vein: analysis of safety and clinical experience with 214 procedures. *Obstet Gynecol* 1990; 76: 47–53.

6. Van Kamp IL, Klumper F, Opekes D, et al. Complications of intrauterine intravascular transfusion for fetal anemia due to maternal red cell alloimmunisation. *AJOG* 2005; 192: 171–7.

7. Schumacher B, Moise KJ Jr. Fetal transfusion for red blood cell alloimmunisation in pregnancy. *Obstet Gynecol* 1996; 88: 137–50.

8. Lindenburg IT, Smits-Wintjens V, van Klink JM, et al., on behalf of the LOTUS study group. Long-term neurodevelopmental outcome after intrauterine transfusion for hemolytic disease of the fetus/newborn: the LOTUS study. *AJOG* 2012; 206: e1–8.

9. Knox EM, Kilby MD, Martin WL, et al. In-utero pulmonary drainage in the management of primary hydrothorax and congenital cystic lung lesion: a systematic review. *Ultrasound Obstet Gynaecol* 2006; 28: 726–34.

10. Golbus MS, Harrison M, Filly RA, et al. In utero treatment of urinary tract obstruction. *American J Obstet Gynecol* 1982; 142: 383–8.

11. Morris RK, Main G, Khan KS, et al. Systematic review of the effectiveness of antenatal intervention for the treatment of congenital lower urinary tract obstruction. *BJOG* 2010; 117: 382–90.

12. Morris RK Malin GL, Quinlan-Jones E, et al. Percutaneous vesicoamniotic shunting versus conservative management for fetal lower urinary tract obstruction (PLUTO): a randomised trial. *Lancet* 2013; 382: 1496–506.

13. Biard J-M, Johnson MP, Carr MC, et al. Long-term outcomes in children treated by prenatal vesicoamniotic shunting for lower urinary tract obstruction. *Obstet Gynecol* 2005; 106(3): 503–8.

14. Denny E, Quinlan-Jones E, Bibila S, et al. The experience of pregnant women with a diagnosis of fetal lower urinary tract obstruction (LUTO). *Midwifery* 2014; 30(6): 636–42.

15. Quintero RA, Johnson M, Romero R, et al. In-utero percutaneous cystoscopy in the management of fetal lower obstructive uropathy. *Lancet* 1995; 346: 537–40.

16. Malin G, Tonks AM, Morris RK, Gardosi J, Kilby MD. Congenital lower urinary tract obstruction: a population-based epidemiological study. *BJOG*, 2012 Nov; 119(12): 1455–64.

17. Urig M, Clewell W, Elliot P. Twin-twin transfusion sydrome. *AJOG* 1990; 163: 1522–6.

18. Saunders N, Snijders R, Nicholaides K. Theraputic amniocentesis in twin-twin transfusion syndrome appearing in the second trimester of pregnancy. *AJOG* 1991; 166: 820–4.

19. Saade G, Olson G, Belfort M. Amniotomy: a new approach to the 'stuck twin' syndrome. *AJOG* 1995; 172: 429.

20. Saade G, Belfort M, Berry D, et al. Amniotic septostomy for the treatment of twin oligohydramnios-polyhydramnios sequence. *Fetal Diagn Ther* 1998; 13: 86–93.

21. De Lia JE, Cruikshank DP, Keye WR Jr. Fetoscopic neodymium: Yag laser occlusion of placental vessels insevere twin-twin transfusion syndrome. *Obstet Gynecol* 1990; 75: 1046–53.

22. Senat MV, Deprest J, Boulvain M, et al. Endoscopic laser surgery versus serial amnioreduction for severe twin-to-twin transfusion syndrome. *NEJM* 2004; 315: 136–44.

23. Morris RK, Selman TJ, Harbidge A, et al. Fetoscopic laser coagulation for severe twin to twin transfusion syndrome: factors influencing perinatal outcome, learning curve of the procedure and lessons for new centres. *BJOG* 2010; 117: 1350–7.

24. Quintero RA. Twin-twin tansfusion syndrome. *Clin Perinatol* 2003; 30: 591–600.

25. Roberts D, Neilson JP, Kilby MD, et al. Interventions for the treatment of twin-twin transfusion syndrome. *Cochrane Database Syst Rev* 2014; 1: CD002073.

26. Ville Y. Twin-twin transfusion syndrome: time to forget the Quintero staging system? *Ultrasound Obstet Gynaecol* 2007; 30: 924–7.

27. Odibo A, Caughey A, Grobman W, et al. Selective laser photocoagulation versus serial amniodrainage for the treatment of twin-twin tansfusion syndrome: a cost effectiveness analysis. *J Perinatol* 2009; 29: 543–7.

28. Slaghekke F, Lopriore E, Lewi L, et al. Fetoscopic laser coagulation of the vascular equator versus selective coagulation for twin-to-twin transfusion syndrome: an open-label randomised controlled trial. *Lancet* 2014; 383(9935): 2144–51.

29. Merz W, Tchatcheva K, Gembruch U, et al. Maternal complications of fetoscopic laser photocoagulation (FLP) for treatment of twin-twin transfusion syndrome (TTTS). *J Perinatal Med* 2010; 38: 439–43.

30. Lewi L, Jani J, Cannie M et al. Intertwin anastomoses in monochorionic placentas after fetoscopic laser coagulation for twin-to-twin transfusion syndrome: is there more than meets the eye? *AJOG* 2006; 194: 790–5.

31. Yamamoto M, Murr E, Robyr R, et al. Incidence and Impact of perioperative complications in 175 fetoscopy guided laser coagulation of chorionic plate anastomoses in fetofetal transfusion syndrome before 26 weeks gestation. *AJOG* 2005; 193: 1110–6.

32. Deprest JA, Audibert F, Van Schoubroeck D, et al. Bipolar coagulation of the umbilical cord in complicated monochroionic twin pregnancy. *AJOG* 2000; 182: 340–5.

33. Robyr R, Yamamoto M, Y Ville. Selective feticide in complicated monochrorionic twin pregnancies using ultrasound-guided bipolar coagulation. *BJOG* 2005; 112(10): 1344–8.

34. Hecher K, Lewl L, Gratacos E, et al. Twin reversed arterial perfusion: fetoscopic laser coagulation of placental anastomoses or the umbilical cord. *Ultrasound Obstet Gynaecol* 2006; 28: 688–91.

35. Tan TY, Sepulveda W. Acardiac twin: a systematic review of minimally invasive treatment modalities. *Ultrasound Obstet Gynaecol* 2003; 22: 409–19.

36. Cabassa P, Fichera A, Prefumo F, et al. The use of radiofrequency in the treatment of twin reversed arterial perfusion sequence: a case series and review of the literature. *Eur J Obstet Gynaecol Reprod Biol* 2013; 166: 127–32.

37. Suda K, Bigras J, Bohn D, et al. Echocardiographic predictors of outcome in newborns with congenital diaphragmatic hernia. *Pediatrics* 2000; 105(5): 1106–9.

38. Jani J, Cannie M, Peralta C, et al. Lung volumes in fetuses with congenital diaphragmatic hernia: comparison of 3D US and MR imaging assessments. *Radiology* 2007; 244: 575–82.

39. Deprest J, Evrard V, Van Ballaer P, et al. Tracheoscopic endoluminal plugging using an inflatable device in the fetal lamb model. *Eur J Obstet Gynaecol Reprod Biol* 1998; 81: 165–9.

40. Flageole H, Evrard V, Piedboeuf B, et al. The plug-unplug sequence: an important step to acheive type II pneumocyte maturation in the fetal lamb model. *J Pediatr Surg* 1998; 33: 299–303.

41. Deprest J, Nicolaides K, Done E, et al. Technical aspects of fetal endoscopic tracheal occlusion for congenital diaphragmatic hernia. *J Pediatr Surg* 2011; 46: 22–32.

42. Ruano R, Yoshisaki CT, da Silva MM, et al. A randomized controlled trial of fetal endoscopic tracheal occlusion versus postnatal management of severe isolated congenital diaphragmatic hernia. *Ultrasound Obstet Gynecology* 2012; 39: 20–7.

43. Bouchard S, Davey M, Rintoul NE, et al. Correction of hindbrain herniation and anatomy of the vermis following in utero repair of myelomeningocele in sheep. *J Pediatr Surg* 2003; 38: 451–8.

44. Meuli M, Meuli-Simmen C, Hutchins GM, et al. In utero surgery rescues neurological function at birth in sheep with spina bifida. *Nat Med* 1995; 1: 342–7.

45. Sutton L, Adzick N, Bilaniuk L et al. Improvement in hindbrian herniation demonstrated by serial fetal magnetic resonance imaging following fetal surgery for myelomeningocele. *JAMA* 1999; 282: 1826–31.

46. Bruner J, Tulipan N, Paschall R, et al. Fetal surgery for myelomeningocele and the incidence of shunt dependant hydrocephalus. *JAMA* 1999; 282: 1819–25.

47. Johnson MP, Sutton L, Rintoul N, et al. Fetal myelomeningocele repair: short-term clinical outcomes. *AJOG* 2003; 189: 482–7.

48. Johnson MP, Gerdes M, Rintoul N, et al. Maternal-fetal surgery for myelomeningocele: neurodevelopment outcomes at 2 years of age. *AJOG* 2006; 194: 1145–8.

49. Wilson R, Lemerand K, Johnson M et al. Reproductive outcomes in subsequent pregnancies after a pregnancy complicated by open maternal-fetal surgery (1996–2007). *AJOG* 2010; 203: 209e1–6.

50. Adzick NS, Thom EA, Spong CY, et al. A randomized trial of prenatal versus postnatal repair of myelomeningocele. *NEJM* 2011; 364: 993–1004.

Chapter

29

The perinatal postmortem examination

Neil J. Sebire

The perinatal autopsy is an integral part of a specialist fetal medicine service and current UK guidelines recommend that the option of an autopsy, performed by specialist pediatric/perinatal pathologists, should be offered for all perinatal deaths, including miscarriages, stillbirths, terminations of pregnancy following diagnosis of fetal abnormality, and neonatal deaths[1].

Details provided in this chapter are based on UK practice and are generic as far as possible, but due to medicolegal requirements, specific details may vary by country or region.

Functions of perinatal autopsy

Autopsy findings provide data for different functions ranging from information relevant to the parents, which may influence further management, through to providing data for clinical governance and service development. The main functions are discussed below.

Determination of cause of death or major diagnosis

In the majority of adult and pediatric settings, the primary role of the autopsy is to determine the likely underlying cause of death or to determine undiscovered pathology in cases where pregnancy was untimely terminated. However, it should be recognized that in a large proportion (up to 75%) of clinically unexpected stillbirths, the precise cause of death will remain unexplained even after postmortem examination, highlighting the need for further research in this area[2]. It is important to recognize that fully confirmatory findings are also of benefit. Confirmation of the underlying cause of death or abnormality is reassuring to clinicians and parents, and may assist some parents in their grieving process.

Management of future pregnancies and siblings

As outlined above, in around 10–20% of cases, additional information from autopsy will have a direct effect on the recurrence risk and counseling of future pregnancies. For example, detection of additional malformations may lead to a specific underlying syndromic diagnosis or the identification of a hereditary disorder, and as such will modify genetic counseling and/or management of future pregnancies. The detection of such underlying genetic or metabolic disorders may also have implications for other family members. Likewise, although uncommon, placental histologic examination may reveal potentially recurrent disorders, including massive perivillous fibrin deposition and chronic histiocytic intervillositis, both of which are associated with adverse pregnancy outcome and a high risk of recurrence.

Research

In some cases, autopsy findings may provide little immediate clinical benefit for the parents, but information derived from such studies may lead to improved understanding of a variety of pathologic processes, with subsequent modification of clinical care and benefit for future patients. Previous examples include better understanding of pulmonary hypoplasia, bronchopulmonary dysplasia and hypoxic-ischemic brain injury patterns in relation to timing of insults. Autopsy data are also important when evaluating the possible effects of new treatment modalities and therapeutic interventions, including complications and side effects, new diagnostic procedures, and the pathologic features of diseases such as viral epidemics, providing data for improved health policies.

Fetal Medicine, ed. Bidyut Kumar and Zarko Alfirevic. Published by Cambridge University Press. © Cambridge University Press 2016.

Audit, quality control and teaching

Comparisons between postmortem findings and antenatal diagnoses represent an important audit function, which serves to improve diagnostic accuracy. Similarly, regular discussion at multidisciplinary team meetings regarding findings and discrepancies between clinical and postmortem findings should be encouraged to improve patient care and service provision. The postmortem examination should also play an important role in teaching medical staff, including surgeons, trainee pathologists and undergraduate medical students, to achieve the highest possible standards of care[3].

Medicolegal issues/malpractice litigation

In the UK, this function has been a relatively minor one until recently. Increasingly, the perinatal pathologist is requested to perform an autopsy investigation on behalf of HM Coroner in cases in which there is risk of litigation relating to an intrapartum or neonatal death. In these circumstances, there may be issues relating to timing of events, such as hypoxic-ischemic injury, meconium passage or iatrogenic injury. If possible litigation or negligence is suspected, the case should be referred to HM Coroner (see below).

Contribution of the perinatal autopsy to clinical care

In both adult and perinatal practice, with reduced exposure of doctors in training to autopsy, there is a perception that with improvements in medical care the relevance of autopsy is declining, but published data would suggest otherwise. A systematic review reported substantial discrepancies between clinical diagnoses and autopsy findings in many cases[4]. "Major errors" (previously unrecognized diagnosis of the cause of death) were reported in around a quarter of cases, with 10% "class I errors," defined as previously unknown conditions that may have affected patient outcome had they been diagnosed in life. A further meta-analysis demonstrated 15–40% discrepancy for major diagnoses and 30–60% discrepancy for cause of death in adults, with 45–75% of autopsies demonstrating at least one additional finding[5]. Similar data are available for perinatal autopsies, specifically, with a review of 27 studies reporting that perinatal autopsy resulted in a change in diagnosis or additional findings, which might have influenced management or counseling in

22–76% of cases[6]; in this study 35% of antenatal ultrasound diagnoses were modified by additional autopsy findings. If only studies reported in the last decade are included, significant additional information required to change the underlying diagnosis or counseling has been reduced to around 10%. This still represents a significant proportion, with a detection rate far above the majority of investigations performed in routine critical practice. See Table 29.1.

However, it should be noted that in these studies, results are derived from the final autopsy reports. The process of postmortem examination involves several procedures and the data presented do not allow information to be derived regarding which investigation provided additional information. A change in perspective from considering postmortem examination as one investigation to a more targeted investigation after death, using an algorithmic approach, would allow optimal resource use to target those in whom the various components of the autopsy are likely to be most contributory. Furthermore, in some clinical circumstances, whilst a postmortem investigation may provide information that may be useful for the purposes listed above, such as governance and quality assurance, in these settings the underlying diagnosis and counseling of parents is unchanged.

Factors influencing the value of the perinatal autopsy

Several factors influence the usefulness of autopsy, including the type of antenatal care, accuracy and availability of antenatal sonography and level of clinical expertise, which may all affect the likelihood of identifying additional findings. Autopsies performed by specialist perinatal/pediatric pathologists in tertiary centers are significantly more likely to provide useful additional information compared to those performed by general pathologists. In addition, in highly complex cases, pathologists with specific expertise in, for example, complex congenital cardiac disease or neuropathology, may be required for optimal interpretation.

Various technical variables may limit the pathologist's ability to identify abnormalities. The most important of which are the effects of secondary changes following fetal death, either in utero (maceration) or during the delivery to postmortem interval. For example, 10–20% of antenatally detected brain abnormalities cannot be confirmed at autopsy due to the degree of maceration and/or postmortem autolysis[7].

Table 29.1 Results of recent series reporting the frequency of finding additional clinical information derived from perinatal autopsies (2004–2014)

Study	Group	N	Additional findings (any)	Additional findings that changed diagnosis
Akgun 2014	PND renal	62	17/62	11/62
Godbole 2014	PND	141	65/141	35/141
Grapsa 2012	PND cystic hygroma	18	5/18[a]	—
Vimercati 2012	PND	144	73/144	24/144
Giordano 2011	PND renal	14	13/14	7/14
Hakverg 2012	PND	274	43/274[a]	—
Hauerberg 2012	PND	52	23/52	5/52
Hickey 2012	NND	164	85/164	29/164
Costa 2011	NICU	53	35/53	13/53
Ramalho 2010	PND aneuploid	57	15/57	0/57
Phadke 2010	PND	91	23/91[a]	—
Antonsson 2008	PND	112	57/112	17/112
Dickinson 2007	PND euploid	562	205/562	85/562
Papp 2007	PND aneuploid	305	195/305	0/305
Akgun 2007	PND	107	25/107[a]	—
Szigeti 2007	PND trisomy 21	184	63/184	0/184
Szigeti 2007	PND trisomy 18	70	39/70	0/70
Ramalho 2006	PND	76	30/76	9/76
Sankar 2006	PND	138	—	25/138
Ceylaner 2006	PND NTD	37	8/37[a]	—
Elder 2005	HIE NND	16	10/16[a]	—
van Dooren 2004	CDH	39	21/39[a]	—
Killeen 2004	SB NND	213	38/213	24/213
Newton 2004	Pediatric	61	29/61	12/61
Piercecchi-Marti 2004	PND	352	176/352[a]	—
Overall	**ALL**	**3,342**	**1,293/3,342 (39%)**	**296/2,408 (12%)**

[a] Not possible to determine 'type' of additional finding.
PND, prenatally diagnosed; NICU, neonatal intensive care unit; NTD, neural tube defects; NND, neonatal death; HIE, hypoxic ischemic encephalopathy; CDH, congenital diaphragmatic hernia.

It is therefore important that if an autopsy is to be performed, the body is refrigerated and the procedure performed as soon as possible after death. Some findings may also remain undetected if the autopsy is limited either to a specific body region or to specific techniques only, depending on the clinical circumstances. The number and type of ancillary investigations performed, for example, microbiological investigations or genetic testing, will also affect yield.

From a practical perspective, rapid turnaround times and high-quality postmortem reports, which include a comprehensive, inclusive and directed clinicopathologic correlation, improve the usefulness of perinatal autopsy for contributing to patient management.

Indications of particular value and of limited value

Based on available data and empirical practice, the potential value of postmortem examination to contribute to future patient management is dependent upon the clinical circumstances. For example, in termination of pregnancy (TOP) for prenatally diagnosed chromosomal abnormalities, whilst autopsy may provide confirmation and allow detection of subtle features that may contribute to detailed understanding, the underlying diagnosis, and hence patient management, is unlikely to be altered. In contrast, for a patient undergoing termination for a prenatally diagnosed abnormality, which may have a wide range of underlying etiologies such as central nervous system malformations and cystic renal disease, postmortem investigation is highly likely to provide a specific diagnosis that cannot be achieved by other means. Other examples include prenatally diagnosed skeletal dysplasias in whom the specific type of dysplasia, relevant for management of future pregnancies and prenatal testing, is often not determined until after autopsy examination.

It is impossible to provide a definitive list of indications representing "high" or "low" autopsy yields, since the individual circumstances, clinical questions and availability of specialist antenatal investigations and perinatal pathologists will vary between centers. Nevertheless, it is suggested that this process is performed locally in order to maximize use of resources and to ensure that expectations of both parents and clinicians are realistic and evidence based.

Classification systems of perinatal deaths and their issues

For the purposes of epidemiologic studies and research, a range of classification systems have been used in order to categorize the type of perinatal death and/or the underlying pathophysiologic mechanism involved. No universally accepted classification system exists. Those in use range from simple systems with only a few generic categories (e.g., the Wigglesworth[8]) to more recent and complex systems, which attempt to take account of not only autopsy findings but also any potentially relevant conditions from the clinical history or other investigations, (e.g., ReCoDe[9]). By using different classification systems, it is possible to use the same underlying datasets but significantly alter the proportion of cases in a specific category, such as "unexplained." However, the clinical and epidemiologic usefulness of each system largely depends on the purpose for which the data will be used. It is therefore important to be aware of which system was used in order that erroneous conclusions are not drawn when comparing data classified in different ways. A review of the features and relative merits of various classifications systems is available.

Prevalence of perinatal autopsy and reasons for consent refusal

Despite the potential benefits noted, perinatal postmortem rates have decreased over recent years. The perinatal autopsy rate (including late fetal losses, stillbirths, and neonatal and postneonatal deaths) reduced from 48% of potential cases in 2000 to 39% in 2003, continuing to fall in recent years, with marked regional variation across the UK. Recent data reveal a plateau for the proportion of neonatal deaths referred for consented postmortem examination, with 22% in 2003 and 21% in 2007[2]. In most cases, autopsy is offered by the clinical team, but consent is not provided by the parents. First, whilst parents' opinions regarding autopsy have been influenced by the organ retention issues at some hospitals in the UK[10], the main reasons for refusal of standard autopsy are fear that the child will be mutilated/disfigured by the procedure, and feelings that ultimately the parents may not have the answers to their questions about the cause of fetal death[11]. Cultural and religious considerations also play a role as most major religions do not explicitly prohibit the autopsy, particularly if there is a perceived benefit to public health. It is of note that in a study of women's reactions, 30% who refused autopsy subsequently regretted the decision, possibly since questions remained unanswered[12]. Secondly, clinicians find discussing the option of postmortem examination with bereaved parents difficult and distressing. This is further influenced by the complex and often lengthy consent forms now required. In conjunction with reduced exposure to autopsy, younger clinicians regard the autopsy less useful compared to senior colleagues[13]. Finally, perceptions may be influenced by the attitudes of pathologists, delays in issuing final postmortem reports, lack of clinicopathologic correlation and paucity of appropriate multidisciplinary team meetings, contributing to the notion that the autopsy is of limited value in the immediate and subsequent management of the patient and/or parents.

Types of perinatal autopsy: consented versus coronial

The vast majority of perinatal postmortem examinations require consent by one or both parents since the immediate cause of death will be known and appropriate certification can be completed. Occasionally, intrapartum and neonatal deaths may be referred to HM

Coroner, who may decide to instruct a pathologist to perform a postmortem examination on their behalf; in these circumstances, parental consent is not required and the Coroner's decision overrides that of the parents. Cases that should be referred to the Coroner include deaths of of initially liveborn infants in which:

- cause is unknown, death is sudden and unexpected
- occurred during an operation or before recovery from the effects of an anesthetic
- may have been caused by violence or neglect
- may have been due to an accident
- may have been in any other way unnatural or there are suspicious circumstances
- may be related to substandard care or malpractice (the indication most applicable to obstetric and neonatal deaths).

In general, stillbirths do not fall under the Coroner's jurisdiction since no death certificate is issued, but HM Coroner may decide to investigate in some circumstances. Once the Coroner has completed the investigation, tissue samples then fall under the Human Tissue Act and should be handled according to parents' wishes. If there is a potential issue of litigation due to neglect/malpractice by hospital staff, the case should always be discussed with HM Coroner, as a coronial autopsy may be performed and an inquest held, which results in the detailed circumstances of the case being reviewed but without assigning blame.

Consent requirements for autopsy

Following issues associated with organ retention in UK, the Human Tissue Act 2004 came into force in 2006[14], overseen by the Human Tissue Authority (www.hta.gov.uk), which publishes Codes of Practice and licenced organizations. The Act covers almost any activity related to human tissue, including postmortem examination, and requires consent for the removal, storage and use of human tissue. The Act applies to all stillbirths and neonatal deaths, but it is recommended that consent be obtained for the examination of all fetal tissue and for its use for scheduled purposes, regardless of gestational age.

Giving of consent must be a positive action following the provision of appropriate information and adequate understanding. The absence of refusal is not adequate consent. Consent must be given voluntarily by an appropriately informed person who has the capacity to agree, which in the setting of perinatal postmortem examinations will usually be one or both parents. For

stillbirths and neonatal deaths, it is recommended that, if possible, consent is obtained from the mother and, where appropriate, both parents are involved. Under the Act, consent from one parent is sufficient. However, if there is disagreement between the parents, it is recommended that this be sensitively discussed before proceeding. It is important that the consent process is not viewed as the single act of signing the consent form, but rather a process in which parents can discuss the issues, ask questions and make an informed choice.

It is usually the treating clinician's responsibility to seek consent, who should be sufficiently senior and well informed, with an adequate knowledge of the postmortem procedure. It is recommended that consenting clinicians are trained in the management of bereavement and should have witnessed a postmortem examination. As valid consent can only be given if appropriate communication has taken place, information leaflets and consent forms should be available in the main local community languages for patients whose first language is not English, and interpreters should be used.

Practical aspects of the postmortem examination

External and macroscopic examination

The request for postmortem examination should be seen as a request for a clinical consultation by a specialist colleague, and hence requires the provision of both appropriate clinical information and documentation of the particular question to be addressed. If there is uncertainty, it is always useful to discuss the case with the pathologist. Once the clinical details have been reviewed and the case discussed, the consent status is verified, the body identified, and an external examination is performed. According to the particulars of the consent, local police, and specific indications, postmortem imaging may also be performed at this stage.

The infant is weighed, measurements are taken for assessment of fetal biometry, and external features such as the degree of maceration are assessed (including skin discoloration, blistering and skin slippage), allowing the pathologist to make an approximate estimate of the duration of intrauterine retention following fetal death. Note that such estimates are not precise and may be affected by many factors, including duration of the interval between delivery and postmortem examination, gestational age, storage conditions, delays during transportation from local to specialist hospitals, the presence of infection and maternal pyrexia. It is important to emphasize that significant tissue changes begin to occur following death and delivery, and that the likelihood of adequate detailed postmortem examination reduces with increasing time for which the body is not refrigerated after delivery. Furthermore, this process of autolysis appears to occur even more quickly in cases following feticide using potassium chloride, and therefore in such cases, particularly for those with cardiac or brain abnormalities, the body should be refrigerated as soon as possible and with the minimum delay between delivery and postmortem examination.

Particular emphasis is placed on identifying external anomalies or dysmorphic features. Routine photographs are usually taken as part of the medical record, with more detailed photographs to document specific abnormalities (Figure 29.1). External examination is followed by a detailed macroscopic investigation of the body, usually via a midline incision through the anterior thorax and abdomen. A careful inspection of the internal organs is carried out, which are then removed, weighed, dissected and sampled for histologic examination. Organs are then returned to the body, which is reconstructed prior to release. Organ weight ratios may allow determination of certain pathologic processes, such as the brain:liver weight ratio (which is increased in intrauterine growth restriction), and the lung:body weight ratio, which is reduced in pulmonary hypoplasia[15]. If the head is to be examined, the scalp is incised, the skull and the brain removed for formalin fixation, which may take several weeks for complex brain anomalies.

Histologic examination

Small tissue samples of major organs are examined under the microscope for cases in which the consent status allows this, since it is recognised that many conditions will only be apparent on histologic examination, despite an organ appearing as normal macroscopically. Tissue samples are processed into small paraffin wax blocks and tissue sections on glass slides, 3–5 microns in thickness, are stained for detailed characterization of the underlying disease process as required.

Ancillary investigations

Radiology

Whilst in some circumstances it had been standard practice to perform whole-body X-ray examinations, the

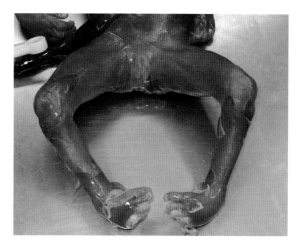

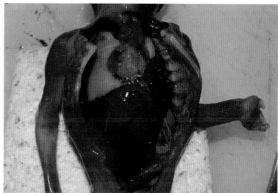

Figure 29.1 (a, b) Macroscopic photographs from perinatal autopsies demonstrating effects of maceration, such as skin slippage and bilateral talipes equinovarus (top) and congenital left-sided diaphragmatic hernia (bottom).

diagnostic yield from this approach in the era of routine antenatal ultrasound screening is very low. However, if there are structural abnormalities, in particular skeletal abnormalities, detailed whole-body radiography is mandatory, and often provides the specific underlying diagnosis. Other imaging modalities that are now becoming more common include postmortem computed tomography (CT) and MRI, but these remain outside of routine clinical practice in most areas (Figure 29.2).

Other

A wide range of other ancillary investigations may be performed according to clinical indications, including microbiologic and virologic analyses, metabolic studies (blood and bile spots for acylcarnitine profiling by tandem mass spectrometry or enzyme assays using cultured fibroblasts) and cytogenetic and DNA analysis for genetic disease.

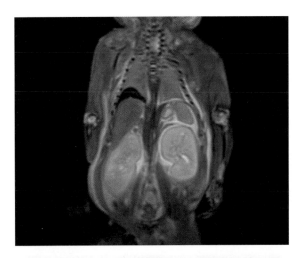

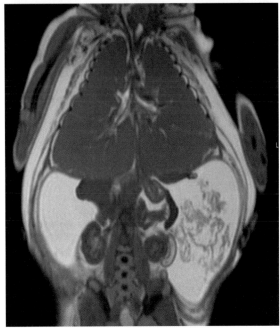

Figure 29.2 (a, b) Postmortem magnetic resonance images demonstrating enlarged hyperechogenic kidneys in a fetus with infantile polycystic kidney disease (top) and enlarged lungs with diaphragmatic eversion and massive ascites in a fetus with congenital high airway obstruction syndrome (CHAOS; bottom).

Retention of organs

Occasionally, it may be required to retain an organ temporarily for fixation and further examination. In the vast majority of cases, this will be known before the autopsy is conducted based on the clinical circumstances. Retention involves removal of the organ from the body and fixing in formalin, which hardens the tissues by crosslinking proteins, enabling more detailed

macroscopic examination and high-quality histologic sections. Such temporary retention is usually only required for the brain, which is very friable and soft, and prone to disintegrate on handling, thus limiting the extent of the examination. Formalin fixation is also recommended for detailed examination of the heart in cases with suspected complex structural cardiac malformations. It should be noted that even if an organ is temporarily retained for formalin fixation and further examination, it is usually not retained indefinitely but is reunited with the body prior to release, although this may delay funeral arrangements. Should parents wish, retained organs can be returned at a later stage, usually via their designated undertakers, for subsequent burial or cremation or parents can request the hospital to dispose of the tissue in a lawful way. It is important that parents be informed that in certain cases, particularly terminations of pregnancy or deaths with suspected brain abnormality, fixation of the brain is likely to be required for adequate examination.

Disposal of retained tissue samples, including blocks and slides

The blocks and slides taken as part of the postmortem examination are usually kept as part of the medical record in order that they can be reviewed in the future as these tissue samples may also be valuable for medical education, audit, quality control and research. Parents have the option to consent to the use of tissue for research, which may help other families in the future, and surveys of bereaved parents have shown that the majority of parents are keen to participate in research[16].

Alternatively, parents can request that all samples are disposed of, either by the hospital or parents can make their own arrangements, usually via their designated undertaker. If parents choose either of these options, it is important that they understand that subsequent review and further diagnosis will not be possible. Note that any tissue samples taken during a coronial autopsy are under the authority of the HM Coroner and remain so until their investigation has ceased.

The limited/partial postmortem examination

Parents have the option to choose a limited or partial postmortem examination, which can take several forms: limited to external examination, with or without postmortem imaging but usually including placental examination, or restricted to a particular body region (such as the chest, abdomen or head) or specific organ (e.g., heart only). The information obtained by a limited postmortem examination may in certain circumstances provide sufficient information for definitive diagnosis and appropriate genetic counseling for future pregnancies, but due to potential limitations it is suggested that all cases of limited examination are discussed with pathologists prior to examination.

Limitations of postmortem examination

Despite the potential benefits, as outlined above, it is important that parents do not have unrealistic expectations. The examination may not answer their questions, and in a significant number of cases may not establish a cause of death, particularly for clinically unsuspected third trimester stillbirths. Conversely, as outlined above, although the postmortem examination may find "nothing new," this too may be clinically helpful, providing reassurance to both clinicians and parents that nothing important had been overlooked during life.

The postmortem report

It is recommended that a final autopsy report, incorporating histologic findings and results of further investigations, is provided within 6 weeks (RCPath[17]). The report should both document the salient macroscopic and microscopic findings and results of ancillary investigations, and also contain a concise and appropriate clinicopathologic correlation and summary. Parents are entitled to a copy of the report, but it is recommended that the contents be discussed with them by their clinician prior to receipt, preferably in person, as some parents may find the technical language used in such reports insensitive or distressing.

Placental examination

Histopathologic examination of the placenta represents a subject in itself with detailed textbooks available for further reference regarding specific findings[18]. In this context, it should be recognized that examination of the placenta represents an important and intrinsic component of the perinatal autopsy. In some circumstances, for example, spontaneous miscarriage of an apparently normally formed fetus in the second trimester or an intrauterine death associated

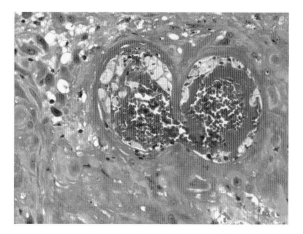

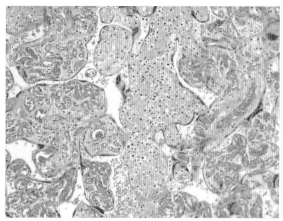

Figure 29.3 (a, b) Photomicrographs of histologic sections from perinatal autopsy cases demonstrating uteroplacental vascular disease with atherosis in a placental decidual section from a fetus with fetal growth restriction (top), and placenta showing villitis of unknown etiology (VUE; bottom).

with pre-eclampsia, placental examination is likely to provide the most significant information of the entire autopsy process. In other circumstances, for example TOP for a fetus with an underlying structural cardiac abnormality, placental examination is likely to be noncontributory. For these reasons, it is difficult to determine the relative importance and contribution of placental examination since the majority of studies report on cases with a mixture of indications. However, one study specifically reporting on autopsy investigation in stillbirths reported that cases that also underwent placental examination were significantly less likely to remain unexplained, and in around half of all cases the findings of placenta investigation were included in the classification of the stillbirth[19]. Placental examination may reveal potentially recurrent disorders,

Table 29.2 Summary of major features of selected pathologic entities that may be reported based on histologic placental examination

Pathological entity	Key features	Presumed mechanism/ cause	Recurrence
Massive perivillous fibrin deposition	Widespread fibrin surrounding villi and within the intervillous space	Haemodynamic or immune	10–50%
Chronic histiocytic intervillositis	Accumulation of histiocytes in the intervillous space	Immune	70%
Villitis of unknown etiology	Infiltration of villi by lymphocytes	Immune	10–40%
Ascending genital tract infection	Neutrophilic infiltration of fetal membranes and/or placenta	Infection	1–3-fold increase rate
Fetal thrombotic vasculopathy	Occlusive thrombi in fetoplacental vasculature	Thrombotic	Not known
Uteroplacental vascular disease	Vasculopathy affecting maternoplacental vessels with haemodynamic effects	Vasculopathic/immune	20–30%
Distal villous immaturity	Poor formation of normal terminal villi	Developmental	Not known

such as massive perivillous fibrin deposition, chronic intervillositis or villitis of unknown etiology, and may confirm the presence of chorioamnionitis and funisitis, viral pathogens or fetal thrombotic vasculopathy, some of which may have implications for future siblings or pregnancies (Table 29.2). Moreover, targeted specialist investigations can be performed, such as vascular injection studies in complicated monochorionic twin placentas(Figure 29.3).

A caveat should be noted in that many of the macroscopic and microscopic placental findings associated with an underlying pathophysiologic process related to the cause of death can also be identified in clinically uncomplicated placentas. Therefore, simply the identification of a placental lesion does not necessarily imply that this was the cause of death, and such findings should be interpreted in conjunction with other features and the clinical history. Such remains even more marked in relation to the umbilical cord in terms of its length, coiling pattern or other parameters, and it should be recognized that in many circumstances definitive comment regarding the significance of such lesions is impossible.

Future directions

Postmortem imaging and the minimally invasive autopsy

Two of the important issues that contribute to why parents do not agree to postmortem examination are the dislike of large incisions (fear of "disfigurement"), and concerns regarding organ retention. In view of this,

there has been recent interest in developing alternative methods of determining or confirming diagnoses after death. Small reports have suggested that postmortem MRI may be useful, either as an adjunct or alternative for those cases in which parents do not consent to standard autopsy. A large study funded by the UK Department of Health has been completed, blindly investigating the accuracy of postmortem MRI (with noninvasive ancillary investigations) compared with traditional open autopsy examination, and reported concordance rates for fetuses and infants of around 95% for major diagnosis or cause of death[20].

Postmortem MRI, with or without postmortem CT scanning, can provide high-quality images of both bony and soft-tissue elements, and with acquisition protocols optimized for the specific postmortem setting, excellent tissue resolution is achievable. With the development of high-field 9.4T magnetic resonance scanners, even higher spatial resolutions will be possible. Postmortem MRI allows detection of the vast majority of structural abnormalities, being particularly good for central nervous system defects. However, since a significant proportion of causes of death and other significant pathologies at autopsy can only be detected following direct inspection of organs and the use of ancillary investigations, such as histologic sampling or microbiologic investigations, postmortem imaging alone cannot replace traditional autopsies.

Nevertheless, postmortem imaging is likely to significantly change future autopsy practice. First, since anatomic detail is excellent with MRI, with the added advantage that an original dataset is captured, which can be reviewed at a later date, postmortem MRI can provide significant information as an adjunctive investigation to direct the approach of future autopsies. This is particularly important in cases of fetal neuroimaging, where the brain may be autolyzed and conventional histopathology is uninformative. Furthermore, abnormalities on antenatal ultrasound imaging, particularly relating to posterior fossa abnormalities, may often not be adequately demonstrated at autopsy, and postmortem MRI may be informative. Secondly, for some parents in whom the traditional autopsy is unacceptable, any form of postmortem examination to allow additional information to be obtained will be preferable to nothing. Thirdly, accurate reconstruction of internal organs and skeletal injuries can be done by rapid prototyping of three-dimensional MRI and CT datasets, and these may be useful for demonstration and/or teaching. Finally, and perhaps most importantly, use of postmortem imaging techniques, such as MRI, in conjunction with modification of tissue sampling techniques, such as endoscopic examination, could change the way many autopsies are performed. Fetal and infant laparoscopic-assisted autopsy is now described, with the aim of potentially replacing the conventional autopsy in certain cases by preceding MRI and subsequent laparoscopic internal examination and tissue sampling. Similar clinical information may be possible to obtain compared with standard autopsy but with no large incisions, only laparoscopic port entries required[21].

This less invasive approach appears more acceptable to parents and healthcare providers, with initial studies suggesting that almost all parents who declined consent for standard autopsy agreed to noninvasive imaging-based investigation. Furthermore, healthcare professionals feel that having these additional alternatives available rather than the binary "yes" or "no" option of standard autopsy would make the process of discussing investigation after death easier with parents[22]. For these reasons, it is highly likely that postmortem imaging in some form is likely to become of increasing importance in future for the investigation following perinatal death.

Novel ancillary investigations

Ongoing advances in laboratory diagnostic techniques, particularly in genomics, transcriptomics, proteomics and metabolomics are likely to revolutionize further the approach to postmortem investigation. Whilst at present tissue samples are predominantly obtained for histologic microscopic examination, it is likely that using small amounts of tissue for a range of OMICs studies, characteristic expression profiles will be described for both underlying disease and pathophysiologic processes. This approach will allow more reliable identification of genetic diseases, pathophysiologic mechanisms of death and tissue-specific changes from limited amounts of tissue. When combined with next-generation postmortem imaging techniques for anatomical assessment, the combined approach to determination of underlying disease processes is likely to become significantly less invasive.

Summary

Despite improvements in antenatal and neonatal care, perinatal postmortem examination continues to play an important role and will do so for the foreseeable future. However, the value of perinatal autopsy may be further improved by better communication between clinicians and pathologists, the issuing of standardized, high-quality postmortem reports with appropriate clinicopathologic correlation, shorter turnaround times, regular multidisciplinary team meetings, and further development of novel postmortem techniques, such postmortem imaging and the need for less invasive sampling, which will provide parents with additional choices.

References

1. Report of Joint Working Group, Royal College of Obstetricians and Gynaecologists (RCOG), and Royal College of Pathologists. *Fetal and Perinatal Pathology*. London: RCOG, 2001.

2. Confidential Enquiry into Maternal and Child Health (CEMACH). Perinatal Mortality 2007. Dorchester UK: Dorset Press, 2009.

3. Burton JL, Underwood J. Clinical, educational, and epidemiological value of autopsy. *Lancet* 2007; 369: 1471–80.

4. Shojania KG, Burton EC, McDonald KM, et al. Changes in rates of autopsy-detected diagnostic errors over time: a systematic review. *JAMA* 2003; 289: 2849–56.

5. Roulson J, Benbow EW, Hasleton PS. Discrepancies between clinical and autopsy diagnosis and the value of postmortem histology; a meta-analysis and review. *Histopathology* 2005; 47: 551–9.

6. Gordijn SJ, Erwich JJHM, Khong TY. Value of the perinatal autopsy: critique. *Pediatr Dev Pathol* 2002; 5: 480–8.

7. Griffiths PD, Variend D, Evans M, et al. Postmortem MR imaging of the fetal and stillborn central nervous system *AJNR Am J Neuroradiol* 2003; 24(1): 22–7.

8. Wigglesworth JS, Singer DB. *Textbook of Fetal and Perinatal Pathology*, 2nd edn. Malden: Blackwell Science, 1998.

9. Gardosi J, Kady SM, McGeown P, et al. Classification of stillbirth by relevant condition at death (ReCoDe): population based cohort study. *BMJ* 2005; 331(7525): 1113–7.

10. Gordijn SJ, Erwich JJ, Khong TY. The perinatal autopsy: pertinent issues in multicultural Western Europe. *Eur J Obstet Gynecol Reprod Biol* 2007; 132: 3–7.

11. McHaffie HE. *Crucial Decisions at the Beginning of Life. Parents' experiences of treatment withdrawals from infants.* Abingdon: Radcliffe Medical Press Ltd, 2001.

12. Rahman HA, Khong TY. Survey of women's reactions to perinatal necropsy. *BMJ* 1995; 310: 870–1.

13. McDermott M. The continuing decline of autopsies in clinical trials: is there any way back? *Arch Dis Child Fetal Neonatal Ed* 2004; 89: F198–F199.

14. UK Legislation. Human Tissue Act 2004 (http://www .opsi.gov.uk/ACTS/acts2004/ukpga_2004 0030_en_1).

15. Cox P, Marton T. Pathological assessment of intrauterine growth restriction. *BestPract Res Clin Obstet Gynaecol* 2009; 23: 751–64.

16. Cohen MC, Blakey S, Donn T, et al. An audit of parents'/guardians' wishes recorded after coronial autopsies in cases of sudden unexpected death in infancy: issues raised and future directions. *MedSci Law* 2009; 49: 179–84.

17. Royal College of Pathologists (RCPATH). Service specification for paediatric and perinatal histopathology. London: RCPATH, 1995. http:// www.rcpath.org/publications-media/publications/ service-specification-for-paediatric-and-per inatal-histopathology

18. Fox H, Sebire NJ. *Pathology of the Placenta*, 3rd edn. Philadelphia: Saunders Elsevier, 2007.

19. Heazell AE, Martindale EA. Can post-mortem examination of the placenta help determine the cause of stillbirth? *J Obstet Gynaecol* 2009; 29(3): 225–8.

20. Thayyil S, Sebire NJ, Chitty LS, et al; MARIAS collaborative group. Post-mortem MRI versus conventional autopsy in fetuses and children: a prospective validation study. *Lancet* 2013; 382(9888): 223–33.

21. Sebire NJ, Weber MA, Thayyil S, et al. Minimally invasive perinatal autopsies using magnetic resonance imaging and endoscopic postmortem examination ("keyhole autopsy"): feasibility and initial experience. *J Matern Fetal Neonatal Med* 2012; 25(5): 513–8.

22. Cannie M, Votino C, Moerman P, et al. Acceptance, reliability and confidence of diagnosis of fetal and neonatal virtuopsy compared with conventional autopsy: a prospective study. *Ultrasound Obstet Gynecol* 2012; 39(6): 659–65.

Index